Drugs
in Use

Drugs
in Use

Clinical case studies for pharmacists

Third edition

Edited by

Linda J Dodds

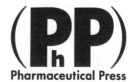

London • Chicago **Pharmaceutical Press**

Bib# 42174

Published by the Pharmaceutical Press
Publications division of the Royal Pharmaceutical Society
of Great Britain

1 Lambeth High Street, London SE1 7JN, UK
100 South Atkinson Road, Suite 206, Grayslake, IL
60030–7820, USA

© Pharmaceutical Press 2004

(**P.P**) is a trade mark of Pharmaceutical Press

First edition published 1991
Second edition published 1996
Third edition published 2004

Text design by Barker/Hilsdon, Lyme Regis, Dorset
Typeset by Photoprint Ltd, Torquay, Devon
Printed in Great Britain by TJ International, Padstow, Cornwall

ISBN 0 85369 541 5

A catalogue record for this book is available from the British
Library

For Peter, Graham and Elizabeth
and my parents Alan and Jean Birdsell

Contents

Preface

Since I first conceived this book, back in the late 1980s, the scope of clinical pharmacy practice has expanded dramatically. Back then, cutting edge pharmaceutical practice was taking place primarily in secondary care, with pharmacists contributing to clinical decision making on ward rounds, but rarely getting involved in actually writing the prescription or independently adjusting drug dosage. Fifteen years later, massive change to the NHS in the UK has led to significant changes for the profession of pharmacy, not least a new career path for pharmacists in primary care trusts and GP practices. The clinical skills that were once used almost exclusively on hospital wards are now also used to persuade GPs to review their prescribing and to practise evidence-based medicine. Whilst under Patient Group Directions and protocols, pharmacists in community pharmacies and GP surgeries as well as hospitals are treating patients not only for minor ailments but also for chronic diseases, and will soon be able to prescribe. Pharmacists are poised to take on roles at the forefront of health service modernisation in the UK, with their skills and knowledge being used to facilitate access to care and improve patient outcomes in many disease areas through medication review and medicines management. This places new and exciting demands on individual pharmacists that must be supported by undergraduate and postgraduate education, and tailored through appropriate continuing professional development.

It can be a daunting task to translate the knowledge acquired during undergraduate and postgraduate pharmacy courses into the clinical skills required to optimise the therapy of an individual patient and identify and meet all the patient's other pharmaceutical needs. Patients rarely have a single disease with a textbook presentation and many factors can influence the choice of therapy, such as concurrent diseases and treatments, previous medical and drug history, changes in clinical opinion on drug use etc. Without an appreciation of these factors it can be difficult to understand the reason for a therapy decision, to respond appropriately to questions regarding the choice of agent from a selection of similar products, or even to know when it is appropriate to offer drug-related information. If it is not clear why a particular product has been prescribed it is also more difficult to monitor its usage appropriately and to counsel the patient.

One way of acquiring the extra knowledge and skills needed to contribute effectively to the care of individual patients is to work with, and to learn from, experienced clinical pharmacists. Unfortunately, such role models are not accessible to all. This book was therefore conceived as a method of helping pharmacists to 'bridge the gap' between the acquisition of theoretical knowledge about drugs and its practical application to individual patients.

Pharmacists with considerable experience of the clinical use of drugs were asked to share their expertise by contributing a case study in an area of special interest to them. The topics chosen for inclusion in the book are ones which are either commonly encountered, associated with particular difficulties in dosage individualisation, or in which major advances in therapeutics have occurred in recent years. This third edition has been expanded to include a number of new disease areas, including dementia, osteoporosis, Type 1 diabetes and stroke. Many of the chapters featured in previous editions have had a major revision to reflect new evidence around optimal care, thus reinforcing the importance of the need for all health care practitioners to keep abreast of medical advances and changes in practice. Two new chapters also reflect the emerging importance of the need for a holistic approach to medicines management, and for a heightened awareness of the possibility of medication errors at each point in the drug use process. The chapters have been written by practitioners in primary and secondary care, illustrating the importance of clinical skills and knowledge in all patient settings.

I should like to take this opportunity to thank all the pharmacists who have contributed material for the third edition of *Drugs in Use*. Preparing case studies requires an enormous amount of time and effort and everyone involved has given unstintingly of both. Once again the authors have had to adhere to a tight schedule that was set in order to ensure the shortest possible time between the preparation of material and its publication. The reward for all this is largely the hope that the book will be of use to pharmacists who are committed to improving their clinical skills.

Linda J Dodds
June 2003

About the editor

Linda Dodds is a pharmaceutical adviser, formerly for East Kent Health Authority but now based in Ashford Primary Care Trust (PCT) where she heads a multidisciplinary clinical governance team and leads (for nine Kent and Medway PCTs) on interface and specialist drug issues. She is currently involved in the development of the curriculum for the new Medway School of Pharmacy and, from April 2004, will have a joint post between the School and the NHS.

For most of her career Linda has worked as a hospital pharmacist (most recently as Principal Pharmacist Clinical Services and Training at Kent and Canterbury Hospital). She has also contributed as an author and editor to a variety of clinical pharmacy publications, and worked as a community pharmacist. She was external examiner for the MSc in Clinical Pharmacy at the University of Otago, Dunedin, New Zealand in 1992 and 1996.

Throughout her career Linda has undertaken and published pharmacy practice research on a variety of topics. Most recently she has been involved in projects to develop Clinical Governance in Community Pharmacy and medication error reporting in primary care.

Contributors

Christopher Acomb BSc, MPharm, MRPharmS, MCPP
Clinical Pharmacy Manager, Leeds Teaching Hospital NHS Trust, Leeds, UK

Caroline A Ashley BPharm, MSc, MRPharmS
Principal Specialist Pharmacist (Renal Unit), Royal Free Hampstead NHS Trust, London, UK

Helen Bates BSc, DipClinPharm, MRPharmS
Senior Pharmacist, Burton Hospitals NHS Trust, Burton-on-Trent, Staffordshire, UK

Ruth Bednall BPharm, MSc, MRPharmS
Principal Pharmacist, General Medicine, Guy's & St Thomas' Hospital NHS Trust, London, UK

Peter Bramley BSc, MSc, MRPharmS
Chief Pharmacist, William Harvey Hospital, Ashford, Kent, UK

Susan Brammer BSc, MSc, MRPharmS
Lead Clinical Pharmacist, William Harvey Hospital, Ashford, Kent, UK

David Bryant BSc, DipClinPharm, MRPharmS
Clinical Pharmacy Team Leader, Leeds Teaching Hospitals NHS Trust, Leeds, UK

Judith A Cantrill BSc, MSc, FRPharmS
Professor of Medicines (Usage, Evaluation & Policy), School of Pharmacy & Pharmaceutical Sciences, University of Manchester, UK

Gillian F Cavell BPharm, MRPharmS
Associate Pharmacy Director, Clinical Services, King's College Hospital NHS Trust, London, UK

Anne Cole BSc, MSc, MRPharmS, NEBSSdip
Clinical Appraisal Pharmacist, Southampton University Hospitals NHS Trust, Southampton, UK

Aileen D Currie BSc(Hons), MRPharmS
Senior Pharmacist (Renal Services), Queen Margaret Hospital, Dumfermline, Fife, UK

Elizabeth Davies BSc, MRPharmS
Principal Pharmacist HIV/GUM, Chelsea & Westminster Hospital, London, UK

Stan Dobrzanski BPharm, PhD, MRPharmS
Clinical Services Manager, Bradford Hospitals NHS Trust, Bradford, UK

Linda J Dodds BPharm, MSc, MRPharmS
Specialist Pharmaceutical Advisor, Ashford PCT, Ashford, Kent, UK

Stuart Gill-Banham BSc, DipPsychPharm, MRPharmS, MCMHP
Senior Pharmacist (Mental Health), William Harvey Hospital, Ashford, Kent, UK

Colin Hardman MPharm, MRPharmS
Senior Pharmacist, United Lincolnshire Hospitals NHS Trust, Lincoln County Hospital, Lincoln, UK

Robert C A Hirst BPharm, MRPharmS
Neurosciences Care Group Pharmacist, King's College Hospital NHS TRust, London, UK

Robert Horne BSc, MSc, MRPharmS
Professor of Psychology in Health Care and Director, Centre for Health Care Research, University of Brighton, Brighton, UK

Stephen A Hudson MPharm, MRPharmS
Professor of Pharmaceutical Care, Department of Pharmaceutical Sciences, University of Strathclyde, Glasgow, UK

Alison Issott BPharm, MRPharmS
Senior Prescribing Advisor, East Kent Coastal PCT, Ramsgate, Kent, UK

Amanda Kemp BPharm, MRPharmS, DipClinPharm
Clinical Pharmacist Gastroenterology Directorate, Nottingham City Hospital NHS Trust, UK

Kym Lowder BPharm, MSc, MRPharmS
Pharmaceutical and Medicines Management Adviser, Shepway Primary Care Trust, Folkestone, Kent, UK

Jonathan Mason BSc, MSc, MPhil, DIC, MRPharmS, ACCP
Head of Prescribing and Pharmacy, City and Hackney PCT, London, UK

John McAnaw BSc, PhD, MRPharmS
*Research Fellow in Clinical Pharmacy, Department of Pharmaceutical Sciences,
University of Strathclyde, Glasgow, UK*

Duncan McRobbie MSc(ClinPharm), MRPharmS
*Principal Clinical Pharmacist, Guy's & St Thomas' Hospital NHS Trust, CHD
Advisor, London Specialist Pharmacy Services, London, UK*

Sharron Millen BPharm, DipClinPharm, MRPharmS
*Surgery Directorate Pharmacist, Clinical Governance and Risk Manager,
Southampton University Hospitals NHS TRust, Southampton, UK*

Charles Morecroft BSc(Pharm), BSc(Psychology), MSc, FRPharmS
University of Manchester, Manchester, UK

Sue Parkinson BPharm, DipClinPharm, MRPharmS
*Practice Support Pharmacist, Leeds North East PCT. Formerly, Lead
Rheumatology Pharmacist, Leeds Teaching Hospitals NHS Trust, Leeds, UK*

Carol Paton BSc, DipClinPharm, MRPharmS, MCMHP
Chief Pharmacist, Oxleas NHS Trust, Bexley, Kent, UK

Kate Richardson BPharm, ClinDip, MRPharmS
*Senior Renal Directorate Pharmacist, Barts and London NHS Trust, London,
UK*

Sandra Ross BSc, MSc, MRPharmS
Prescribing Adviser, Erewash Primary Care Trust, Ilkeston, Derbyshire, UK

Railton Scott BSc, MSc, MRPharmS, RMN
*Principal Clinical Pharmacist, South London and Maudsley NHS Trust, and
Clinical Trainer/Tutor, Brighton and Sussex University Hospitals NHS Trust,
Brighton, UK*

Sarah Stoll BSc, MSc, MRPharmS
Senior Liver Pharmacist, King's College Hospital NHS Trust, London, UK

Maxwell Summerhayes BPharm, PhD, MRPharmS
Scientific Advisor, Roche Products, Welwyn Garden City, Herts, UK

Denise Taylor DipPharm(NZ), MSc, MRPharmS, MCPP
Senior Teaching Fellow (Clinical Pharmacy), Department of Pharmacy and Pharmacology, University of Bath, Bath, UK

Derek Taylor MSc, MRPharmS, MCPP
Pharmacy Manager, Broadgreen Hospital, Royal Liverpool and Broadgreen University Hospitals NHS Trust, Liverpool, UK

Peter A Taylor BPharm, MPharm, MRPharmS
Director of Pharmacy, Airedale NHS Trust, Keighley, UK

Helen Thorp BSc, DipClinPharm, MRPharmS
Clinical Pharmacy Team Leader, Leeds Teaching Hospitals NHS Trust, Leeds, UK

Stephen Tomlin BPharm, MRPharmS, AFNPP
Principal Paediatric Pharmacist, Guy's & St Thomas' Hospital NHS Trust, London, UK

Mary P Tully MSc, PhD, MRPharmS, MPSNI
Clinical Lecturer, School of Pharmacy and Pharmaceutical Sciences, University of Manchester, Manchester, UK

Helen Williams BPharm, DipPharmPrac, MRPharmS
Pharmacy Team Leader, Cardiac Services, King's College Hospital, London, UK

Jayne Wood BSc, MPhil, MRPharmS, MCPP
Associate Director (Diagnostics and Clinical Support), Pennine Acute Hospitals NHS Trust, Fairfield General Hospital, Bury, Lancashire, UK

Notes on the use of this book

This book has been written to help demonstrate how the specialised knowledge and skills possessed by pharmacists can be applied to the care of individual patients. It is a teaching aid and should not be regarded, or used, as a pharmacology textbook.

The case studies and questions have been kept separate from the answers in order to encourage readers to formulate their own answers before reading the author's. A short reading list can be found at the end of each case study. This should help to supplement the information supplied in the answers.

The background information provided on each patient has been kept to the level that should be easily accessible to the pharmacist, either by consulting the medical notes, or through discussions with the patient's physician. Although many of the patients in this book are presented as hospital in-patients, the problems suffered by most of them, and the consequent need for pharmacist input, could as easily occur if they were living in the community and receiving care from their GP.

The questions interspersing the case presentation aim to reflect those frequently asked by other health care professionals, plus those that should be considered by a pharmacist when the prescription is seen. In some cases questions have also been inserted to help ensure the reader appreciates the specialist techniques used to assess patients with the problems under discussion. In order to ensure that the overall pharmaceutical care of the patient is considered, as well as specific problems, at least one question for each patient relates to the construction of a pharmaceutical care plan.

The observant reader will notice that the reference ranges for some laboratory indices vary between case studies. This reflects the normal practice of an individual laboratory setting its own reference ranges.

The answer sections illustrate how the questions should be approached and what factors should be taken into consideration when resolving them. The answers are based on clinical opinion current at the time of writing but they also represent, to some degree, the opinions of the authors themselves. It is thus highly likely that after studying the literature and also taking into account new drugs and new information which may have become available since the case studies were prepared, some readers will disagree with decisions arrived at by the authors. This is entirely appropriate in a book endeavouring to teach decision-making skills in complex areas where there is rarely an absolute right or wrong answer. Indeed, it is hoped that the questions raised in the case studies will generate discussion and argument between pharmacists, as it is through such debate that communication skills are developed. The ability to put forward and defend drug therapy decisions to medical colleagues is almost as important a skill to the pharmacist wishing to develop his or her clinical involvement as the ability to make such decisions.

Finally, as this book is intended for teaching purposes and not as a reference work, it has been indexed to disease states and approved drug names only.

Abbreviations

A11A	angiotensin 11 antagonist
ABCD	disc-shaped cholesteryl sulphate–amphotericin B complexes
ABLC	amphotericin B–phospholipid complexes
ACE	angiotensin-converting enzyme
ACEI	angiotensin-converting enzyme inhibitor
AchEI	acetylcholinesterase inhibitor
ACS	acute coronary syndrome
AD	Alzheimer's disease
ADAS-cog	Alzheimer's Disease Assessment Scale-cognitive subscale
ADH	antidiuretic hormone
ADL	activities of daily living
ADP	adenosine diphosphate
ADR	adverse drug reaction
AF	atrial fibrillation
AIDS	acquired immunodeficiency syndrome
ALD	alcoholic liver disease
ALG	antilymphocyte immunoglobulin
ALT	alanine aminotransferase
AMI	acute myocardial infarction
ANA	antinuclear antibody
ANC	absolute neutrophil count
APTT	activated partial thromboplastin time
ARCD	age-related cognitive decline
ARF	acute renal failure
ARR	absolute risk reduction
5-ASA	5-aminosalicylic acid
AST	aspartate aminotransferase
ATG	antithymocyte immunoglobulin
BCG	Bacillus Calmette-Guérin
BDP	beclometasone dipropionate
BEAM	carmustine–etoposide–cytarabine–melphalan
BHS	British Hypertension Society

BMD	bone mineral density
BMI	body mass index
BMT	bone marrow transplant
BNF	*British National Formulary*
BP	blood pressure
BTS	British Thoracic Society
CABG	coronary artery bypass grafting
CAN	chronic allograft neuropathy
CAPD	continuous ambulatory peritoneal dialysis
CAST	Chinese Acute Stroke Trial
CCB	calcium-channel blocker
CCF	congestive cardiac failure
CF	cystic fibrosis
CHD	coronary heart disease
CHOP	cyclophosphamide–doxorubicin–vincristine–prednisolone
CK	creatine kinase
CK-MB	creatine kinase isoenzyme specific for myocardium
CK-MB%	CK-MB expressed as a percentage of total CK
CMV	cytomegalovirus
CNS	central nervous system
COMT	catechol-O-methyltransferase
COPD	chronic obstructive pulmonary disease
COX	cyclooxygenase
CPMS	Clozapine Patient Monitoring Service
CPN	Community Psychiatric Nurse
CrCl	creatinine clearance
CRP	C-reactive protein
CSF	cerebrospinal fluid
CSM	Committee on Safety of Medicines
CT	computed tomography
CVD	cardiovascular disease
CVP	central venous pressure
DBP	diastolic blood pressure
DHEA	dehydroepiandrosterone
DLBCL	diffuse large B-cell non-Hodgkin's lymphoma
DMARD	disease-modifying antirheumatic drug
DOT	directly observed therapy
DSM	Diagnostic and Statistical Manual of Mental Disorders
DVT	deep-vein thrombosis
DXA	dual x-ray absorptiometry
EC	enteric-coated

ECG	electrocardiograph/electrocardiogram
ECT	electroconvulsive therapy
EMS	eosinophilia myalgia syndrome
EPSE	extrapyramidal side-effect
ESR	erythrocyte sedimentation rate
FBC	full blood count
FEV	forced expiratory volume
FFP	fresh frozen plasma
FP	fluticasone propionate
FVC	forced vital capacity
G-CSF	granulocyte colony-stimulating factor
GABA	gamma-aminobutyric acid
GFR	glomerular filtration rate
GM-CSF	granulocyte-macrophage colony-stimulating factor
GP	general practitioner
GTN	glyceryl trinitrate
HAART	highly active antiretroviral therapy
HAMD	Hamilton Depression (scale)
Hb	haemoglobin
HbA_{1c}	glycated haemoglobin
HCA	Health Care Assistant
HDL	high-density lipoprotein
HIV	human immunodeficiency virus
HMG-CoA	hydroxymethylglutaryl coenzyme A
HOPE	Heart Outcomes Prevention Study
HPLC	high-performance liquid chromatography
HR	heart rate
HRT	hormone replacement therapy
HSA	human serum albumin
5-HT	5-hydroxytryptamine
IBW	ideal body weight
IHD	ischaemic heart disease
IL	interleukin
INR	international normalised ratio
IPD	idiopathic Parkinson's disease
IPPV	intermittent positive pressure ventilation
iPTH	intact parathyroid hormone
IST	International Stroke Trial
JME	juvenile myoclonic epilepsy
LABA	long-acting $beta_2$–agonist
LD	loading dose
LDL	low-density lipoprotein

LFT	liver function test
MAC	*Mycobacterium avium* complex
MAG3	^{99m}Tc mercapto acetyl triglycene
MAOI	monoamine-oxidase inhibitor
MAP	mean arterial pressure
MCH	mean cell haemoglobin
MCI	mild cognitive impairment
MCV	mean cell volume
MD	maintenance dose
MDI	metered-dose inhaler
MDS	monitored-dose system
MI	myocardial infarction
MMF	mycophenolate mofetil
MMSE	Mini Mental State Examination
MSA	multiple system atrophy
NHL	non-Hodgkin's lymphoma
NICE	National Institute for Clinical Excellence
NIV	non-invasive ventilation
NMDA	*N*-methyl-D-aspartate
NNRTI	non-nucleoside reverse transcriptase inhibitor
NNT	numbers needed to treat
NPSA	National Patient Safety Agency
NSAID	non-steroidal anti-inflammatory drugs
NSTEMI	non-ST-elevated myocardial infarction
NRTI	nucleoside reverse transcriptase inhibitor
NSF	National Service Framework
NYHA	New York Heart Association
OBRA	Omnibus Budget Reconciliation Act
OGD	oesophago-gastro-duodenoscopy
OTC	over-the-counter
PBPC	peripheral blood progenitor cell
PBPCT	peripheral blood progenitor cell transplantation
PCA	patient-controlled analgesia
PCI	percutaneous coronary intervention
PCP	*Pneumocystis carinii* pneumonia
PCT	Primary Care Trust
PCV	Primary Care Visitor
PE	pulmonary embolism
PEEP	peak end expiratory pressure
PEFR	peak expiratory flow rate
PMR	polymyalgia rheumatica
POD	patient's own drugs

PPD	purified protein derivative
PPI	proton pump inhibitor
PSP	progressive supranuclear palsy
PTCA	percutaneous transluminal coronary angioplasty
PTH	parathyroid hormone
PUD	peptic ulcer disease
PV	plasma viscosity
RA	rheumatoid arthritis
RBC	red blood cell
R-CHOP	rituximab–cyclophosphamide–doxorubicin–vincristine–prednisolone
RRT	renal replacement therapy
RT	rapid tranquillisation
rt-PA	alteplase or recombinant tissue-type plasminogen activator
SBP	systolic blood pressure/spontaneous bacterial peritonitis
SD	standard deviation
SERM	selective oestrogen receptor modulator
SIMV	synchronised intermittent mandatory ventilation
SSRI	selective serotonin reuptake inhibitor
STEMI	ST-elevated myocardial infarction
SV	stroke volume
TB	tuberculosis
TCA	tricyclic antidepressant
TIA	transient ischaemic attack
TIPS	transjugular intrahepatic porto-systemic shunt
TNF	tumour necrosis factor
TPN	total parenteral nutrition
UA	unstable angina
WBC	white blood cell

Myocardial infarction

Helen Williams

Day 1 Mr BY, a 52-year-old sales representative, presented to casualty via ambulance following the onset of chest pain approximately two hours earlier while he was replacing some guttering on his house. He had tried several doses of sublingual glyceryl trinitrate (GTN), but his pain had not resolved. He had become increasingly breathless and clammy, with a tight crushing pain across his chest and left shoulder. His past medical history was documented as 'angina'. He was noted to be obese (estimated body weight above 100 kg). His drug history on admission was recorded as nifedipine and isosorbide mononitrate (doses were not stated). On examination his blood pressure was found to be 150/110 mmHg with a heart rate of 112 beats per minute.

Q1 What routine tests should be carried out to confirm a diagnosis of acute myocardial infarction (AMI)?

Mr BY was initially prescribed one dose of each of the following drugs:

- Diamorphine 2.5 mg intravenously
- Metoclopramide 10 mg intravenously
- Aspirin 300 mg orally

Q2 What actions of diamorphine are particularly useful in the acute phase of an AMI?

Q3 Why is metoclopramide necessary? What alternative anti-emetics could be considered?

Q4 Why should intramuscular injections generally be avoided in patients suffering with AMI?

Q5 What is the rationale for aspirin administration during an AMI?

Q6 What other therapies should be considered at this stage?

The electrocardiogram (ECG) showed 2–3 mm ST elevation in leads V2–V4 with some evidence of ischaemia in the lateral leads indicating that Mr BY had suffered an anterior MI.

Laboratory results were as follows:

- Qualitative troponin (bedside) negative
- Creatine kinase (CK) result not yet available
- Sodium 138 mmol/L (reference range 135–145)
- Potassium 3.8 mmol/L (3.5–5.0)
- Creatinine 104 mmol/L (45–120)
- Urea 6 mmol/L (3.3–6.7)

- Glucose 18 mmol/L (3–7.8 fasting)
- Haemoglobin 14.2 g (14–18)
- Red blood cells (RBC) 6.4×10^{12}/L (4.5–6.5)
- White blood cells (WBC) 6.1×10^9/L (4–11)
- Platelets 167×10^9/L (150–400)

Following analysis of the ECG a decision was taken to thrombolyse him. In accordance with local protocol a bolus dose of tenecteplase 50 mg was administered. Intravenous heparin and a sliding-scale insulin infusion were also initiated.

Q7   What is the rationale for thrombolysis in the management of AMI?
Q8   When should thrombolysis be administered to gain maximal benefit?
Q9   What are the contra-indications to thrombolysis?
Q10 What pharmaceutical issues should be considered when choosing a thrombolytic?
Q11 What monitoring should be undertaken for patients prescribed and administered thrombolytic therapy?
Q12 What alternative strategies could be employed when thrombolysis is contra-indicated?
Q13 Is intravenous heparin indicated for Mr BY?
Q14 What other therapies might be considered at this stage?

Mr BY was successfully thrombolysed and transferred to the Coronary Care Unit for further care. On arrival he was found still to be breathless, although his chest pain had resolved. A repeat ECG at 90 minutes post-thrombolysis showed resolution of the ST segments indicating successful thrombolysis. He had coarse crackles at the left base of the lung and a chest x-ray showed some pulmonary oedema. His blood gases showed reduced oxygen saturations on room air, so oxygen therapy was continued. Intravenous furosemide was prescribed at a dose of 80 mg over 20 minutes.

- BP 105/65 mmHg

- HR 103 beats per minute

He was prescribed:

- Diamorphine 2.5 mg–5 mg intravenously when required
- Metoclopramide 10 mg three times daily orally or intravenously, as required
- GTN 400 micrograms sublingually when required

- Humidified oxygen at 4 L/min
- Human Actrapid insulin 50 units in 500 mL to run over 24 hours according to a sliding-scale regimen
- Aspirin 75 mg orally daily

Day 2   Following three intravenous doses of furosemide, Mr BY's symptoms had settled with no further episodes of chest pain and improved oxygen saturations. A repeat chest x-ray showed a good response to diuretic therapy with resolution of pulmonary oedema. On the ward round a cardiac echo was requested by the registrar, alongside repeat blood tests.

- BP 94/63 mmHg

- HR 88 beats per minute

His biochemistry results were:

- Sodium 143 mmol/L (135–145)
- Potassium 3.1 mmol/L (3.5–5.0)
- Glucose 4.8 mmol/L (3–7.8)
- Urea 5 mmol/L (3.3–6.7)
- Creatinine 110 micromol/L (45–120)

- Haemoglobin 13.2 g/dL (14–18)
- RBC 5.2×10^{12}/L (4.5–6.5)
- WBC 6.0×10^9/L (4–11)
- Platelets 172×10^9/L (150–400)

From admission bloods:

- Total cholesterol 5.6 mmol/L (<5.0)

- Triglycerides 4.2 mmol/L (<1.8)

Q15 Outline a pharmaceutical care plan for Mr BY.
Q16 Why are his potassium levels a cause for concern? What other electrolytes should be monitored closely?
Q17 Comment on the drugs Mr BY was taking prior to admission.

Day 2 (p.m.)   Mr BY continued to respond well to treatment and was beginning to mobilise. He was haemodynamically stable (blood pressure 92/50 mmHg; heart rate 72 beats per minute). The echo report highlighted marked hypokinesia of the anteroseptal region of the left ventricle and an ejection fraction of 35–40% indicating compromised ventricular function. Mr BY was started on ramipril 1.25 mg initially then 2.5 mg twice daily thereafter, plus pravastatin 20 mg at night.

Q18 What is the rationale for angiotensin-converting enzyme inhibitors (ACEI) post-MI? How should ACEI therapy be initiated?

Q19 Should beta-blocker therapy be considered at this stage?

Q20 What advice would you give about the initiation of a beta-blocker in Mr BY?

Q21 Comment on Mr BY's cholesterol level.

Q22 How should Mr BY's cholesterol be addressed?

Q23 How should Mr BY's blood sugar levels be controlled over the longer-term?

Day 5   Mr BY had made good progress over the past three days although he was complaining of a dry cough.

- BP 92/56 mmHg
- HR 58 beats per minute
- Sodium 141 mmol/L (135–145)
- Potassium 4.2 mmol/L (3.5–5.0)

- Glucose 5.1 mmol/L (3–7.8)
- Urea 5.3 mmol/L (3.3–6.7)
- Creatinine 121 micromol/L (45–120)

He was stabilised on the following regimen for discharge:

- Aspirin tablet 75 mg orally daily
- Ramipril 2.5 mg orally twice daily
- Carvedilol 3.125 mg orally twice daily
- Pravastatin 40 mg orally at night

- Human Actrapid insulin 8 units subcutaneously three times daily
- Human Insulatard 10 units subcutaneously at night
- GTN spray 400 micrograms sublingually as required

Q24 What lifestyle issues should be discussed with Mr BY?

Q25 What issues should be highlighted during discharge counselling for this patient?

What routine tests should be carried out to confirm a diagnosis of AMI?

A1 **A 12-lead ECG should be performed and a blood sample should be taken for measurement of troponin and/or creatine kinase (CK) levels.**

A 12-lead ECG is the key diagnostic tool used to distinguish ST-elevated MI (STEMI – classic MI) from other acute coronary syndromes (including non-ST-elevated MI and unstable angina). Key ECG features of STEMI include ST elevation of more than 1 mm in two adjacent limb leads or more than 2 mm in two adjacent chest leads or the presence of new left bundle branch block.

Cardiac enzyme measurements are used to determine the presence or absence of myocardial necrosis. CK and CK isoenzyme specific for myocardium (CK-MB) have been used routinely in the diagnosis of AMI. Other cardiac markers include myoglobin and lactic dehydrogenase. All of these markers have limitations in clinical practice. For example, CK only becomes raised a number of hours after the onset of MI and as a result the usefulness of the test in the early phase of treatment to guide thrombolytic therapy is limited. In addition, CK and CK-MB levels only increase after significant degrees of infarct damage have occurred, and therefore cannot detect smaller areas of ischaemic damage. In view of the limitations of standard biochemical markers of cardiac damage, new diagnostic tests with greater sensitivity and specificity have been sought. Troponins are cardiac contractile proteins which, if raised, indicate thrombotic activity and recent myocardial damage. Troponin levels become raised within three to 12 hours after the onset of pain, even after minor damage to the cardiac muscle, and are more sensitive and specific for myocardial damage than CK or CK-MB. As troponin levels only become raised a few hours after the onset of chest pain, their utility in the acute treatment phase is limited. Serial negative tests are required over a 12- to 24-hour period after pain onset to exclude myocardial damage and allow safe discharge from hospital in patients complaining of chest pain.

Any increase in the levels of these biochemical markers indicates some degree of myocardial damage, but only in the presence of characteristic ECG changes can the diagnosis of STEMI be confirmed. In this case Mr BY presented early after the onset of symptoms and the cardiac enzymes may not yet have become raised. This emphasises the importance of the ECG in making an accurate and timely diagnosis to maximise the benefits of treatment. Repeat troponin or CK levels may be measured to confirm the working diagnosis of AMI and assess the extent of myocardial damage.

> What actions of diamorphine are particularly useful in the acute phase of an AMI?

A2 **Diamorphine has analgesic, anxiolytic and vasodilating effects.**

All of these effects are beneficial in AMI. Analgesia is required to provide immediate relief from chest pain, while vasodilatation improves blood supply to the myocardium and may contribute to the anti-ischaemic effects. As the symptoms of MI frequently cause patients to panic and further exacerbate the situation, the anxiolytic effect of diamorphine can calm the patient rapidly and facilitate the administration of further therapy. These effects are not unique to diamorphine and other opiates may be considered, although pethidine is generally avoided due to its short duration of action and propensity to increase blood pressure.

> Why is metoclopramide necessary? What alternative anti-emetics could be considered?

A3 **During the acute phase of MI, the majority of patients suffer from significant nausea and vomiting which may be further exacerbated by administration of an intravenous opiate. Metoclopramide is a suitable agent for use in this setting as it can be administered intravenously for a rapid onset of action.**

Intravenous cyclizine 50 mg up to three times daily would be a suitable alternative, although occasionally this agent may cause a significant reduction in blood pressure and, in the presence of heart failure, may reduce cardiac output.

> Why should intramuscular injections generally be avoided in patients suffering with AMI?

A4 **CK levels can be increased by intramuscular injections, which may confuse the diagnosis of AMI. In addition, the administration of drugs by the intravenous route allows a rapid and predictable onset of action.**

A number of non-cardiac problems including cardiac resuscitation, intramuscular injection, diabetes mellitus, skeletal muscle damage and alcoholism can increase CK levels, which can limit its usefulness in diagnosing MI. Similarly, troponin release is not entirely specific to myocardial ischaemia. For example, levels should be interpreted cautiously in the presence of chronic renal failure. Care should be taken when interpreting biochemical markers to exclude other reasons for raised CK levels.

What is the rationale for aspirin administration during an AMI?

A5   **In the acute phase, the administration of aspirin has been shown to reduce mortality at five weeks by approximately 23%.**

ISIS-2 demonstrated that the administration of aspirin reduces mortality and morbidity associated with AMI. A dose of 300 mg should be administered immediately, regardless of prior aspirin use. Patients should be advised to chew the tablet before swallowing to aid early absorption. Aspirin therapy has also been shown to reduce the rates of reocclusion and reinfarction. A meta-analysis of antithrombotic interventions in high-risk patients has concluded that, when used chronically, aspirin reduces the risk of MI by approximately 25%. Aspirin should therefore be continued indefinitely post-MI at a dose of 75–150 mg daily.

What other therapies should be considered at this stage?

A6   **At this stage the diagnosis is unclear. A number of potential drug therapies should therefore be under consideration.**

Heparin, glycoprotein IIb/IIIa receptor antagonists or thrombolysis with or without intravenous beta-blockers may be indicated pending test results. Patients with ongoing pain or evidence of left ventricular dysfunction may benefit from intravenous GTN. Oxygen should be administered early to improve myocardial oxygen supply and limit the extent of ischaemia.

What is the rationale for thrombolysis in the management of AMI?

A7   **Thrombolytic therapy has been shown to reduce five-week mortality in patients suffering AMI by 18%, with benefits being maintained for up to 10 years.**

The majority of MIs are caused by obstruction of blood flow in one or more coronary arteries through the formation of a blood clot. Thrombolytic therapy is targeted at breaking down the occluding thrombus through the process of fibrinolysis. Myocardial tissue does not die immediately and early reperfusion following clot dissolution may salvage areas of heart muscle where blood flow has been compromised. As a result, thrombolytic therapy may limit infarct size, preserve left ventricular function and reduce deaths. A number of clinical trials have confirmed the benefits of thrombolysis in patients with acute STEMI, most notably ISIS-2, GISSI and GUSTO. ISIS-2 demonstrated a 25% reduction in 35-day mortality through the administration of streptokinase alone in AMI, and highlighted the benefits of combining aspirin and thrombolytic therapy, when a 42% mortality reduction was seen.

When should thrombolysis be administered to gain maximal benefit?

A8 **Thrombolytic therapy should be administered as early as possible after symptom onset to gain the maximum benefit from treatment.**

The UK National Service Framework (NSF) for Coronary Heart Disease 'door-to-needle' target for the administration of thrombolytics is currently 30 minutes. Early treatment has been shown to improve survival from AMI. One study investigating the use of pre-hospital thrombolysis demonstrated a mortality of 1.2% in patients treated within 70 minutes of symptom onset, compared to 8.7% in the remainder who received therapy at 70 minutes or later. It has been calculated that for every hour earlier thrombolytic therapy is administered, an additional 1.6 lives per 1000 patients treated could be saved. Thrombolytic therapy offers significant benefits when administered up to 12 hours after symptom onset, although greater benefits are seen within the first six hours. At 12 hours and beyond, patients derive little benefit from the administration of thrombolytic therapy and other strategies should be considered.

What are the contra-indications to thrombolysis?

A9 **Contra-indications to thrombolytic therapy can be divided into those that are absolute (i.e. therapy must not be administered) and those that are relative (i.e. the benefits and risks of therapy must be considered for the individual patient requiring treatment).**

The absolute contra-indications to thrombolytic therapy are previous haemorrhagic stroke, any cerebrovascular event within the previous year, active internal bleeding and suspected aortic dissection. Relative contra-indications include uncontrolled hypertension (systolic blood pressure greater than 180 mmHg), anticoagulant therapy or bleeding disorder, recent trauma or major surgery (within the previous four weeks), prolonged cardiopulmonary resuscitation and pregnancy. The decision to administer thrombolytic therapy to a patient with relative contraindications should be made following careful consideration of the risks and potential benefits on an individual patient basis.

What pharmaceutical issues should be considered when choosing a thrombolytic?

A10 **A number of issues should be considered, including comparative efficacy, dose, method of administration and adverse effects.**

A number of thrombolytic agents are licensed for the treatment of AMI, all of which are effective, but can be distinguished from one another in terms of their pharmacokinetic and pharmacodynamic profiles. The most commonly used across the UK are currently streptokinase and alteplase. Streptokinase is supported by strong clinical trial data demonstrating mortality and morbidity benefits up to 10 years after administration, and is the cheapest thrombolytic agent available. However, it does have disadvantages, particularly the potential for allergic reactions and the development of neutralising antibodies within a few days that make re-administration inappropriate. Alteplase is also supported by strong clinical trial data, particularly when administered in a 'front-loaded' regimen. Earlier vessel patency rates have been demonstrated in clinical trials, but an increased incidence of intracranial haemorrhage has also been noted. Unfortunately, the early reperfusion achieved with alteplase has not been shown to improve survival significantly in comparison to streptokinase. Alteplase is not subject to the allergies and antibodies responses that limit the usefulness of streptokinase, but it is significantly more expensive. Both of these drugs are administered by infusion, and alteplase is given by a complex 'front-loaded' regimen, in which 65% of the total dose is given during the first 30 minutes of the 90-minute infusion.

The ideal thrombolytic would be effective, easy to administer (ideally by bolus dosing), have a low rate of complications and be at least as effective as the current gold standards. Recently, reteplase (a double-bolus agent) and tenecteplase (a single-bolus agent) have been licensed. These agents are marginally more expensive than alteplase with equivalent outcome data, but are much easier to administer. Many centres are now moving over to these therapies in an attempt to improve door-to-needle times in order to reach NSF targets, although there remains concern over the potential for these agents to precipitate intracranial bleeds, particularly in elderly patients.

What monitoring should be undertaken for patients prescribed and administered thrombolytic therapy?

A11 **Patients should be monitored closely throughout thrombolytic therapy as they are at risk of haemodynamic instability, reperfusion arrhythmias or other complications. The clinical efficacy of the thrombolysis should be assessed at 90 minutes with a repeat 12-lead ECG.**

Standard observations should be undertaken including monitoring of blood pressure (hypotension can occur), heart rate and rhythm. A repeat 12-lead ECG at 90 minutes post-thrombolysis should confirm resolution of the ST segment, thus indicating successful thrombolysis.

Complications of thrombolytic therapy include haemorrhagic stroke, occurring in approximately 1.2% of patients overall, but higher frequencies have been noted in hypertensive patients and the elderly. Other adverse effects include allergy (particularly to streptokinase), other haemorrhage [patients should be monitored for signs of bleeding such as haematuria, epistaxis (nose bleeds) and haematemesis (coffee-ground vomit)] and systemic emboli. A full blood count should be checked prior to and after treatment to ensure there is no significant drop in haemo-globin, which may indicate haemorrhage. Patients are at risk of bleeding for up to four days following the administration of thrombolytic therapy.

What alternative strategies could be employed when thrombolysis is contra-indicated?

A12 **The most effective strategy for managing AMI is primary angioplasty (direct angioplasty to the affected coronary artery, which may be combined with intracoronary stent placement). This has been shown to be superior to thrombolytic therapy in the majority of comparative studies.**

In patients presenting late (48 hours or more after the acute event), myocardial damage is likely to be irreversible. Standard therapies such as heparin, aspirin and intravenous GTN may be considered if there is ongoing pain, with referral for early angiography. The early use of intravenous beta-blockers (with or without thrombolytic therapy) is recommended in most AMI guidelines, primarily to reduce the occurrence of ischaemia-related tachyarrhythmias.

Is intravenous heparin indicated in this patient?

A13 **Yes. Intravenous heparin should be administered at the same time as tenecteplase (TNK-tPA) and be continued for a minimum period of 48 hours. The use of concomitant heparin therapy during thrombolysis is agent dependent.**

Heparin is indicated for use in combination with alteplase, reteplase and tenecteplase. The adjunctive use of heparin therapy is necessary to protect against reocclusion. By comparison, streptokinase should not be co-prescribed with heparin due to an increased risk of cerebral bleeds and a greater need for transfusions. Intravenous heparin doses should be weight-adjusted to reduce bleeding complications and should be initiated with a bolus dose followed by a continuous infusion. Careful monitoring of the activated partial thromboplastin time (APTT/APTTr) should be undertaken, particularly at initiation and after any dosage changes. In general, the aim is to achieve an APTT/APTTr twice that of the control. Alternatively, a low-molecular-weight heparin may be considered, although these remain unlicensed in combination with thrombolytic agents. Data from the ASSENT-3 study has demonstrated that a combination of enoxaparin and tenecteplase is both safe and effective in AMI.

What other therapies might be considered at this stage?

A14 **In view of Mr BY's raised blood glucose on admission, an intensive insulin regimen should be initiated to ensure tight control of his blood sugars in order to improve survival.**

Evidence from the DIGAMI study, first published in 1997, has established the importance of aggressive blood sugar management in AMI. Sliding-scale insulin therapy is recommended for the first 24 hours in all patients with a raised blood sugar (above 11 mmol/L) on admission, or any history of diet- or tablet-controlled diabetes mellitus. DIGAMI reported an absolute reduction in mortality of 11% at one year when an aggressive insulin/glucose/potassium infusion was prescribed for the first 24 hours, followed by a minimum of three months subcutaneous insulin therapy. The majority of this benefit was established in younger patients, who had no previous diagnosis of diabetes. No outcome data exist to support the use of diet or oral medication to control blood glucose in post-MI patients.

Outline a pharmaceutical care plan for Mr BY.

A15   The pharmaceutical care plan for Mr BY should include the following:

(a)   Ensure evidence-based strategies are introduced in a timely manner.
(b)   Ensure all drugs are initiated at an appropriate dose and that dose titration is undertaken.
(c)   Monitor for efficacy and adverse effects, notify relevant staff and advise on alternatives if necessary.
(d)   Ensure nursing staff are administering intravenous therapy correctly.
(e)   Ensure secondary prevention strategies are initiated.
(f)   Ensure adequate lifestyle advice has been given and that the patient is being followed-up by the appropriate specialist teams.
(g)   Ensure appropriate information on aims of therapy, dose titrations post-discharge, duration of treatment and monitoring are provided to the GP.
(h)   Counsel Mr BY on his discharge medication, including the rationale for therapy, appropriate monitoring, possible side-effects and how to deal with them, and how therapies should be continued in future.
(i)   Reinforce patient counselling with written patient information on drug therapy and through provision of appropriate aids, such as a medication record card.

Why are his potassium levels a cause for concern? What other electrolytes should be monitored closely?

A16   A reduction in serum potassium may predispose the patient to post-infarction arrhythmias. Serum magnesium and calcium should also be monitored, and corrected if necessary to further protect against arrhythmias. Serum sodium, creatinine and urea should be monitored throughout his diuretic therapy.

A significant fall in serum potassium might be expected in this patient secondary to excess catecholamine release in response to the pain and anxiety caused by his AMI. In addition, the intensive insulin/glucose infusion prescribed and the use of repeated bolus doses of a loop diuretic will further reduce his serum potassium levels.

Oral potassium supplements could be started at this point, unless there are signs of impending arrhythmias such as frequent ventricular ectopic beats or runs of ventricular tachycardia. In this situation, intravenous supplementation may be more appropriate.

Comment on the drugs Mr BY was taking prior to admission.

A17 **Mr BY's drug therapy on admission of nifedipine and isosorbide mononitrate should be reviewed.**

The SPRINT-2 study indicated that nifedipine may increase early mortality post-MI and is not associated with a reduction in cardiac events in the long-term. Therefore his nifedipine therapy should be discontinued. While isosorbide mononitrate is an effective anti-anginal agent, it has not been shown to improve outcomes in patients with coronary heart disease and more suitable alternatives with secondary prevention benefits should be considered first. Mr BY has a number of co-morbidities (hypertension, angina and raised blood glucose) which should all be considered when making decisions on drug therapy. His drug regimen on discharge should be designed to optimise cardiovascular outcomes in the long-term.

What is the rationale for angiotensin-converting enzyme inhibitors (ACEIs) post-MI? How should ACEI therapy be initiated?

A18 **A number of studies have demonstrated the benefits of ACEIs post-MI (SAVE, AIRE, GISSI-3, ISIS-4 and TRACE), with an overall reduction in 30-day mortality of 7%.**

ACEIs should be initiated in all patients post-MI (in the absence of contra-indications). The greatest benefits from therapy are seen in high-risk patients, such as those with a reduced left ventricular ejection fraction or overt clinical signs of heart failure (as in the case of Mr BY), diabetes, anterior infarcts or tachycardia. The longer-term benefits with respect to reduced morbidity and mortality in patients with cardiovascular disease were established in the HOPE study (which included post-MI patients) and, specifically in post-MI, in the AIREX study (an extension of the AIRE study).

Following publication of the GISSI-3 and ISIS-4 studies, early initiation of therapy (within 24 hours) is recommended. Where there is concern over haemodynamic instability (systolic blood pressure below 90 mmHg), ACEI initiation may be temporarily delayed, but this should be reviewed on a daily basis. ACEIs should be initiated at low doses to avoid the problem of first-dose hypotension and dose-titration should then be undertaken to achieve the optimal doses used in clinical trials. Persistent hypotension may limit the extent to which dose titration can be undertaken during the acute hospital admission. Mr BY's blood pressure and heart rate should be monitored closely throughout the initiation phase. His renal function should be checked prior to and within 48 hours of initiating ACEI therapy post-MI and should be rechecked within a few days of each dose increment. Renal dysfunction (except bilateral renal artery stenosis) is not a contra-indication to ACEI therapy. It is recommended that ACEI therapy be continued indefinitely in the absence of any clear reason to stop therapy.

Should beta-blocker therapy be considered at this stage?

A19 **Beta-blocker therapy has been shown to reduce mortality and morbidity post-MI, and should therefore be considered for Mr BY. Consideration should be made of his concurrent heart failure and reduced left ventricular ejection fraction, which may make early initiation of beta-blocker therapy inappropriate, and will also influence the choice of agent and dose regimen chosen.**

Early intravenous beta-blocker therapy is recommended in the majority of guidelines to reduce the risk of post-infarct arrhythmias. Acute intravenous therapy would have been inappropriate in the case of Mr BY due to his clinical signs of heart failure in the early phases of his illness. Long-term oral beta-blocker therapy has been studied post-MI in a number of clinical trials and an overall 20% reduction in mortality has been established through meta-analysis. The majority of benefit is attributed to a reduction in sudden cardiac death.

In this case there are additional considerations. Mr BY has clinically evident left ventricular dysfunction, an indication for beta-blocker therapy in its own right, and there is evidence that beta-blockers can be initiated safely and effectively in patients with left ventricular dysfunction post-MI. The recently published CAPRICORN study, in which patients were randomised to carvedilol or placebo at three to 21 days post-MI, demonstrated a 23% reduction in mortality over approximately one year. Beta-blocker therapy should therefore be considered for initiation over the next few days providing that Mr BY remains clinically stable, particularly with respect to his symptoms of heart failure.

The use of both ACEI and beta-blocker therapy post-MI is recommended by the NSF. It might be considered that ACEI therapy should be optimised before the addition of a beta-blocker; however, it should be remembered that while there are established benefits of ACEI dose titration, these are primarily morbidity benefits (reduced hospitalisations seen in the ATLAS study). In contrast, ACEIs and beta-blockers have both been shown to reduce mortality independently. Early initiation of agents from the two different drug classes may therefore be justified, but dose titration of each should be continued over the next few weeks to reach the maximal tolerated doses. For Mr BY, the key limitation of combined ACEI and beta-blocker therapy in the early phases will be his persistent low blood pressure following his acute event.

What advice would you give about the initiation of a beta-blocker?

A20 **The beta-blocker therapy should be introduced cautiously, starting at low dose, and with careful monitoring of heart rate, blood pressure, blood gases and symptoms of heart failure. The dose should be titrated to the maximum tolerated by doubling at two-weekly intervals, unless cardiac symptoms prohibit this. Mr BY's symptoms may be exacerbated during the titration phase. If this happens additional diuretic therapy may be required or the interval between dose titrations may need to be extended. Occasionally, a step down in beta-blocker dose may be required. Close follow-up should be arranged prior to discharge to ensure ongoing monitoring and dose titration.**

Comment on MR BY's cholesterol level.

A21 **Mr BY has a raised cholesterol level which indicates an increased risk of coronary heart disease. Lipid-lowering therapy should be initiated, as reducing serum cholesterol has been shown to reduce the risk of death, reinfarction or other cardiovascular events in this patient group.**

Cholesterol levels should be measured within 24 hours of symptom onset in patients with AMI, as after 24 hours cholesterol levels have been shown to fall and remain low for approximately three months. As the cholesterol level was taken on admission in this case, it is unreasonable to expect a fasting sample and therefore only the measured total cholesterol levels can be considered reliable. The NSF recommends treatment of all patients with total cholesterol above 5.0 mmol/L and/or low-density lipoprotein (LDL) above 3.0 mmol/L, with a target of 80–90% of patients receiving treatment at discharge, although more aggressive therapy may be warranted in view of data from the Heart Protection Study (see Answer 22).

How should Mr BY's cholesterol level be managed?

A22 **Mr BY should be given dietary advice in combination with the initiation of a statin.**

Patients should be encouraged to reduce their total fat intake and, in particular, their intake of saturated fat, and to increase their intake of vegetable and fibre. A number of booklets on healthy eating for patients with coronary heart disease are available, e.g. *Cut the Saturated Fat from Your Diet* from the British Heart Foundation. Most patients find it difficult to achieve large reductions in total cholesterol using diet alone, with average reductions in the order of 5%.

Statins reduce total cholesterol by an average of 25–35%, with greater reductions in LDL, the cholesterol subtype which correlates most closely with cardiovascular risk. Reducing cholesterol with statins has been shown to reduce the risk of death, reinfarction or other cardiovascular events in this patient group. Since the publication of the Heart Protection Study, which recruited patients with a total cholesterol above 3.5 mmol/L, many clinicians feel that statin therapy is justified at much lower levels and some believe statins should be initiated in all patients post-MI regardless of the admission cholesterol levels (although clinical guidelines at the time of writing do not yet reflect this view). The majority of clinical trial data on statins post-MI have initiated therapy three to four months after the acute event, following a dietary trial. However, for practical reasons, most clinicians now initiate therapy during the acute phase, and there is evidence emerging to indicate that this approach is safe and may further improve outcomes. Statin therapy should be started at a clinically effective dose, e.g. pravastatin 40 mg daily which has been shown to be safe and effective in trials. Mr BY's cholesterol level should be rechecked in three months and therapy should be reviewed if the levels remain high. Liver function tests should be performed annually during statin therapy (more frequently in the first year).

How should Mr BY's blood sugar levels be controlled over the longer-term?

A23 **A subcutaneous insulin regimen should be initiated on cessation of his sliding-scale intravenous insulin.**

The preferred insulin regimen for Mr BY is the combination of a long-acting (basal) insulin with short-acting soluble insulin at meal times to mimic physiologic insulin patterns. Patient assessment, careful selection of insulin dose and administration device, and the provision of adequate patient education and support is essential to ensure successful management of blood sugar levels. All patients should be referred to a diabetic clinic to ensure appropriate follow-up. In the DIGAMI study, insulin therapy was maintained for a minimum of three months post-infarction, but the optimal duration of insulin therapy has not been clearly established. Long-term control of blood sugar is important post-MI to reduce the risk of cardiac and non-cardiac complications of diabetes.

What lifestyle issues should be discussed with Mr BY?

A24 **Lifestyle advice should include the importance of diet, exercise and weight loss. Stopping smoking, modifying his diet and increasing exercise are all effective in reducing his risk of further coronary events. Mr BY should be encouraged to participate in a cardiac rehabilitation programme, where these issues will be addressed in greater depth.**

Within one year of smoking cessation, the risk of cardiac events is halved and after two to three years it has returned to that of a non-smoker. Interventions to improve smoker quit rates include counselling, use of nicotine replacement therapies and prescription of amfebutamone (bupropion). The issue of smoking cessation should be discussed with Mr BY. He should be strongly encouraged to stop smoking at this point and appropriate smoking cessation aids should be offered.

Diets low in saturated fats and supplemented with polyunsaturated fatty acids (usually from fish oils) have been shown to improve survival in patients with coronary heart disease. Adoption of a healthy balanced diet, low in saturated fats and high in vegetable and fibre, should be encouraged for Mr BY. A reduction in calorie intake is appropriate in view of Mr BY's obesity and a reduced saturated fat intake will contribute to his cholesterol lowering. Weight loss will also improve his sensitivity to insulin and may reduce the need for long-term insulin therapy.

Exercise is also important and has been shown to reduce cardiac mortality. Mr BY should be given advice on increasing his physical exercise safely and should be encouraged to attend a cardiac rehabilitation programme where he can begin to do this under supervision. Such a programme will support Mr BY in making the lifestyle changes necessary to reduce his cardiovascular risk.

What issues should be highlighted during discharge counselling for this patient?

A25 **Key areas for counselling include an explanation of the indication for and aim of each medicine, instruction on how each medicine should be taken, information on appropriate follow-up, long-term monitoring and dealing with potential adverse effects. The benefits of long-term cardiovascular risk reduction should be emphasised to encourage adherence to prescribed medication.**

It is essential to convey the importance of long-term drug treatment in patients with coronary heart disease. If the difference between risk reduction and symptom management is not clearly explained, patients may fail to adhere to therapy, particularly if they are asymptomatic. Mr BY should be advised that some of his drug doses may need to be increased over the next few weeks to achieve the optimal dose. Follow-up by a diabetic clinic and a heart failure clinic will be necessary to ensure appropriate long-term management.

All of these points should be reinforced with written information and, ideally, an individual patient's medication record card as an aide-mémoire. Additional information for patients, in the form of booklets such as *Medicines for the Heart*, is available from the British Heart Foundation. Mr BY should again be encouraged to attend a cardiac rehabilitation programme, which has been shown to improve outcome post-MI.

Further reading

ACE-Inhibitor Myocardial Infarction Collaborative Group. Indications for ACE-Inhibitors in the early treatment of acute myocardial infarction: systematic overview of individual data from 100 000 patients in randomised trials. *Circulation* 1998; **97**: 2202–2212.

Acute Infarction Ramipril (AIRE) Study Investigators. Effect of ramipril on mortality and morbidity of survivors of acute myocardial infarction with clinical evidence of heart failure. *Lancet* 1993; **342**: 821–828.

AIRE Extension (AIREX) Study. Follow-up study of patients randomly allocated ramipril or placebo for heart failure after acute myocardial infarction. *Lancet* 1997; **349**: 1493–1497.

American College of Cardiology/American Heart Association Guidelines for the Management of Patients with Acute Myocardial Infarction, 1999. Available at: www.americanheart.org/presenter.jhtml?identifier = 2865

Anon. Lifestyle measures to reduce cardiovascular risk. *MeReC Brief* 2002; **19**.

Antithrombotic Trialists' Collaboration. Collaborative meta-analysis of randomised trials of antiplatelet therapy for prevention of death, myocardial infarction, and stroke in high risk patients. *Br Med J* 2002; **324**: 71–86.

Assessment of the Safety and Efficacy of a New Thrombolytic (ASSENT-2) Investigators. Single-bolus tenecteplase compared with front-loaded alteplase in acute myocardial infarction. The ASSENT-2 randomised double-blind trial. *Lancet* 1999; **354**: 716–722.

Assessment of the Safety and Efficacy of a New Thrombolytic Regimen (ASSENT-3) Investigators. Efficacy and safety of tenecteplase in combination with enoxaparin, abciximab, or unfractionated heparin. The ASSENT-3 randomised trial in acute myocardial infarction. *Lancet* 2001; **358**: 605–613.

Dargie HJ (for the CAPRICORN Investigators). Effect of carvedilol on outcome after myocardial infarction in patients with left-ventricular dysfunction; the CAPRICORN randomised trial. *Lancet* 2001; **357**: 1385–1390.

Department of Health. *National Service Framework for Coronary Heart Disease.* Department of Health, London, 2000.

Erhardt L, Herlitz J, Bossaert L *et al*. Task Force on the Management of Chest Pain. *Eur Heart J* 2002; **23**: 1153–1176.

Fibrinolytic Therapy Trialists' (FTT) Collaborative Group. Indications for fibrinolytic therapy in suspected acute myocardial infarction: collaborative overview of early mortality and major morbidity results from all randomised trials of more than 1000 patients. *Lancet* 1994; **343**: 311–322.

Fourth International Study of Infarction Survival Collaborative Group (ISIS-4). A randomised factorial trial assessing early oral captopril, oral mononitrate and intravenous magnesium sulphate in 58 050 patients with suspected acute myocardial infarction. *Lancet* 1995; **345**: 669–685.

Freemantle N, Cleland J, Young P *et al*. Beta-blockade after myocardial infarction. Systematic review and meta-regression analysis. *Br Med J* 1999; **318**: 1730–1737.

Goldbourt U, Behar S, Reicher-Reiss H *et al*. Early administration of nifedipine in suspected acute myocardial infarction (SPRINT-2). *Arch Intern Med* 1993; **153**: 345–353.

Gruppo Italiano per lo Studio della Streptochinasi nell'Infarto Miocardico. Effectiveness of intravenous thrombolytic treatment in acute myocardial infarction. *Lancet* 1986; i: 397–402.

Gruppo Italiano per lo Studio della Sopravvivienza nell'Infarto Miocardico. GISSI-2: a factorial randomised trial of alteplase versus streptokinase and heparin versus no heparin among 12 490 patients with acute myocardial infarction. *Lancet* 1990; **336**: 65–71.

Gruppo Italiano per lo Studio Dell Sopravvivienza nell'Infarto Miocardico. GISSI-3: the effects of lisinopril and transdermal glyceryl trinitrate singly and together on 6-week mortality and ventricular function after acute myocardial infarction. *Lancet* 1994; **343**: 1115–1122.

GUSTO Investigators. An international randomized trial comparing four thrombolytic strategies for acute myocardial infarction. *N Engl J Med* 1993; **329**: 673–682.

Heart Outcomes Prevention Evaluation Study Investigators. Effects of an angiotensin-converting-enzyme inhibitor, ramipril on cardiovascular events in high-risk patients. *N Engl J Med* 2000; **342**: 145–153.

Heart Protection Study Collaborative Group. MRC/*BHF* heart protection study of cholesterol lowering with simvastatin in 20 536 individuals: a randomised placebo-controlled trial. *Lancet* 2002; **360**: 7–22.

International Study Group. In-hospital mortality and clinical course of 20 891 patients with suspected acute myocardial infarction between alteplase and streptokinase with or without heparin. *Lancet* 1990; **336**: 71–75.

ISIS-1 (First International Study of Infarct Survival) Collaborative Group. Randomised trial of intravenous atenolol among 16 027 cases of suspected acute myocardial infarction: ISIS-1. *Lancet* 1986; ii: 57–66.

ISIS-2 (Second International Study of Infarct Survival) Collaborative Group. Randomised trial of intravenous streptokinase, oral aspirin, both or neither among 17 187 cases of suspected acute myocardial infarction: ISIS-2. *Lancet* 1988; ii: 349–360.

ISIS-3 (Third International Study of Infarct Survival) Collaborative Group. ISIS-3: a randomised comparison of streptokinase vs tissue plasminogen activator vs anistreplase and of aspirin plus heparin vs aspirin alone among 41 299 cases of suspected acute myocardial infarction. *Lancet* 1992; **339**: 753–770.

Kober L, Torp-Pedersen C, Clarsen JE *et al.* Trandolapril Cardiac Evaluation (TRACE). *N Engl J Med* 1995; **333**: 1670–1676.

LaRosa JC, He J, Vupputuri S. Effect of statins on risk of coronary disease: a meta-analysis of randomized controlled trials. *J Am Med Assoc* 1999; **282**: 2340–2346.

LATE Study Group. Late assessment of thrombolytic efficacy (LATE) study with alteplase 6–24 hours after onset of acute myocardial infarction. *Lancet* 1993; **342**: 759–766.

Malmberg K, Norhammer A, Wedel H *et al.* Glycometabolic state at admission: important risk marker in conventionally treated patients with diabetes mellitus and acute myocardial infarction: long-term results from the Diabetes and Insulin-Glucose Infusion in Acute Myocardial Infarction (DIGAMI) study. *Circulation* 1999; **99**: 2626–232.

Moon J, Kalra P, Coats A. DANAMI-2: is primary angioplasty superior to thrombosis in acute MI when the patient has to be transferred to an invasive centre? *Int J Cardiol* 2002; **85**: 199–201.

National Institute for Clinical Excellence. *Inherited Clinical Guideline – Prophylaxis for Patients Who Have Experienced a Myocardial Infarction.* NICE, London, 2001. Available at: www.nice.org.uk/docref.asp?d = 16479

National Institute for Clinical Excellence. *Technology Appraisal Guidance No 52. Guidance on the Use of Drugs for Early Thrombolysis in the Treatment of Acute Myocardial Infarction.* NICE, London, 2002. Available at: www.nice.org.uk/pdf/52_Thrombolysis_fullguidance.pdf

Packer M, Poole Wilson PA, Armstrong PW *et al.* Assessment of Treatment with Lisinopril and Survival (ATLAS). *Circulation* 1999; **100**: 2312–2318.

Pfeffer MA, Braunwald E, Moyé LA *et al.* (on behalf of the SAVE investigators). Effect of captopril on mortality and morbidity in patients with left ventricular dysfunction after myocardial infarction: results of the Survival and Ventricular Enlargement Trial. *N Engl J Med* 1992; **327**: 669–677.

Ridker PM, Hebert PR, Fuster V *et al.* Are both aspirin and heparin justified as adjuncts to thrombolytic therapy for acute myocardial infarction. *Lancet* 1993; **341**: 1574–1577.

Sacks FM, Pfeffer MA, Moye LA *et al.* The effect of pravastatin on coronary events after myocardial infarction in patients with average cholesterol levels. *Am J Cardiol* 1991; **68**: 1436–1446.

Scandinavian Simvastatin Survival Study Group. Randomised trial of cholesterol lowering in 4444 patients with coronary heart disease: the Scandinavian Simvastatin Survival Study. *Lancet* 1994; **344**: 1383–1389.

Second Joint Task Force of the European Society of Cardiology, European Atherosclerosis Society and European Society of Hypertension. Prevention of coronary heart disease in clinical practice. Recommendations. *Eur Heart J* 1998; **19**: 1434–1503.

Swedberg K, Held P, Kjekshus J *et al.* (on behalf of the CONSENSUS II Study Group). Effects of the early administration of enalapril on mortality in patients with acute myocardial infarction. Results of the Co-operative New Scandinavian Enalapril Study II (CONSENSUS II). *N Engl J Med* 1992; **327**: 678–684.

Task Force for the Diagnosis and Treatment of Chronic Heart Failure, European Society of Cardiology. Guidelines for the diagnosis and treatment of chronic heart failure. *Eur Heart J* 2001; **22**: 1527–1560.

Weaver WD, Cerqueria M, Hallstrom AP *et al.* Pre-hospital vs hospital initiated thrombolytic therapy: the myocardial infarction triage and intervention trial. *J Am Med Assoc* 1993; **270**: 1211–1216.

Wood DA, Durrington P, Poulter N *et al.* (on behalf of the Societies). Joint British recommendations on prevention of coronary heart disease in clinical practice. *Heart* 1998; **80**(suppl. 2): S1–S29.

Yusuf S, Peto R, Lewis J, Collins R et al. Beta blockade during and after myocardial infarction: an overview of the randomised trials. *Prog Cardiovasc Dis* 1985; **27**: 335–371.

2

Ischaemic heart disease

Duncan McRobbie

Case study and questions

Day 1 Mr CW, a 62-year-old businessman, presented to A & E complaining of central chest pain which was only partly relieved by the glyceryl trinitrate (GTN) spray he carried with him. On examination he was tachycardic, with a blood pressure of 156/90 mmHg.

He had a previous medical history of angina. His attacks had become more frequent over the last few weeks, but this was the first one that had not been completely relieved by his GTN spray. He was also a diet-controlled Type 2 diabetic and his random blood sugar was 11 mmol/L and his glycated haemoglobin (HbA$_{1c}$) was 7.2% at admission.

He also had a history of hypercholesterolaemia with his last recorded fasting cholesterol being 7.2 mmol/L. He had never been hospitalised for his heart condition.

His father had died of a heart attack at age 68. His mother and his sister were still living. He was married with three adult sons, none of whom had any cardiac complaints. He smoked 30 cigarettes a day and his job required him to entertain regularly, resulting in him drinking 20–30 units of alcohol a week. He weighed 95 kg with a body mass index (BMI) of 31.

His regular medicine consisted of:

- Aspirin 75 mg enteric-coated tablet, one daily
- Ranitidine 150 mg orally twice a day
- Nicorandil 10 mg orally twice a day
- Isosorbide mononitrate sustained-release 60 mg orally every morning
- Atenolol 100 mg orally daily
- Simvastatin 20 mg orally at night
- GTN spray sublingually when required

Q1 Discuss Mr CW's risk factors for coronary heart disease.

Q2 What are the aims of treatment in angina?

Q3   Comment on the appropriateness of each of Mr CW's medicines on admission. Would you recommend any changes?

Q4   What other medications could have been added to this therapy regimen?

After initial assessment he was referred to the cardiology team who documented that he had no obvious symptoms of jaundice, anaemia, cyanosis, clubbing or oedema. His abdominal and respiratory examinations revealed nothing of note. His 12-lead electrocardiogram (ECG) showed transient ST segment changes (above 0.05 mV) that developed during symptomatic episodes, but resolved when asymptomatic. No Q waves were observed. His urea and electrolytes were within the normal reference ranges, and his full blood count revealed nothing remarkable. His creatine kinase isoenzyme specific for myocardium (CK-MB) fraction was less than 4%. A troponin-T test was planned for 12 hours after the initial onset of his chest pain.

Q5   What is the reason for performing a CK-MB fraction and troponin T test?

An acute myocardial infarction (AMI) was excluded and the cardiologist's impression was that he was suffering from unstable angina (UA).

Q6   What is UA and what are the implications for Mr CW?

Q7   Identify pharmaceutical care needs for this patient during the acute phase of his hospitalisation.

Mr CW was admitted to the coronary care unit for medical management. He was prescribed:

- Aspirin 150 mg orally once daily
- Clopidogrel 300 mg orally for one dose, then 75 mg orally daily
- Enoxaparin 95 mg twice a day subcutaneously
- Eptifibatide 17 mg immediately by intravenous bolus, then 11.4 mg/h by intravenous infusion
- GTN intravenous infusion 50 mg in 50 mL at a rate of 1–5 mg/h titrated to response
- Actrapid insulin intravenous sliding scale to keep blood sugars between 4 and 8 mmol/L
- Atenolol 100 mg orally daily
- Simvastatin 40 mg orally at night

His pain settled on the medication regimen.

Q8   Comment on the rationale for the combination of antiplatelet therapy prescribed.

Q9   What risks are associated with the use of combination antiplatelet therapy?

Q10   How should Mr CW be monitored?

Q11   How should Mr CW's GTN infusion be 'titrated to response'?

After 12 hours of treatment his troponin-T result was positive. He was consented for angiography/angioplasty with or without coronary artery stent insertion or coronary artery bypass grafting (CABG) for the following morning.

Q12   What is meant by interventional cardiology?

Day 2   The angiogram revealed 90% occlusion of the left anterior descending coronary artery. An angioplasty was performed and a coronary artery stent was successfully inserted.

His medication immediately after the procedure was:

- Aspirin 150 mg orally daily
- Clopidogrel 75 mg orally daily
- Eptifibatide 11.4 mg/h by intravenous infusion
- Actrapid insulin sliding-scale to keep blood sugars between 4 and 8 mmol/L
- Atenolol 100 mg orally daily
- Simvastatin 40 mg orally at night
- GTN spray two puffs sublingually when required

Q13   What is the place of drug-eluting stents. Would one have benefited Mr CW?

Q14   Was it appropriate to discontinue his enoxaparin?

Q15   Why has his nicorandil and isosorbide mononitrate therapy not been restarted?

Mr CW's femoral sheaths were removed 12 hours after the procedure and the eptifibatide was discontinued.

Day 3   Mr CW's CK-MB was not elevated on the day following the procedure, indicating that no further myocardial damage had occurred during the procedure. Ramipril 2.5 mg orally once daily was initiated. Mr CW remained pain-free and his discharge was planned for the following day, with a referral to the cardiac rehabilitation team and a cardiology out-patient appointment made for six weeks later. His blood pressure and renal function remained stable. Metformin 850 mg orally twice a day was initiated.

Q16   Why was metformin initiated?

Day 4   Mr CW remained pain-free. His blood pressure remained stable at 150/85 mmHg.

His discharge medication was:

- Aspirin 150 mg orally daily for one month, then 75 mg daily
- Clopidogrel 75 mg orally daily
- Atenolol 100 mg orally daily
- Ramipril 2.5 mg orally daily
- Metformin 850 mg orally twice a day
- Simvastatin 40 mg orally at night
- GTN spray two sprays sublingually when required

Q17   How long should Mr CW remain on his antiplatelet therapy?

Q18   What information should be communicated to the GP?

Q19   What points would you wish to discuss with Mr CW prior to discharge?

Q20   Should Mr CW be offered nicotine replacement therapy?

Discuss Mr CW's risk factors for coronary heart disease.

A1 **Mr CW presents with many factors which increase his risk of coronary heart disease (CHD). Fixed factors include: his age, being male, having a previous history of ischaemic heart disease (IHD) and a family history of IHD. Modifiable factors include: hypertension, diabetes, hypercholesterolaemia, cigarette smoking and obesity.**

People who have multiple risk factors for heart disease are typically three to five times more likely to die, suffer a heart attack or other major cardiovascular event than people without such conditions or risk factors. People who have already had a heart attack, have angina or who have undergone coronary revascularisation are at particularly high risk. Identifying and treating those at greatest risk is one of the highest priorities of the National Services Framework for Coronary Heart Disease.

Various tools are available that allow clinicians to calculate quickly and easily an individual's cardiovascular risk (e.g. Joint British Societies Coronary Risk Prediction Chart, Sheffield Risk Table). These allow for calculation of risk status in patients without a confirmed diagnosis of ischaemic heart disease; however, as Mr CW has already been diagnosed and treatment initiated, his risk cannot now be calculated using these tools.

As well as having pre-existing CHD, Mr CW has a number of modifiable risk factors for CHD.

(a) Hypertension. Hypertension is defined as systolic blood pressure (SBP) of ≥ 140 mmHg, diastolic blood pressure (DBP) of ≥ 85 mmHg or the use of antihypertensive drugs. The Framingham Heart Study demonstrated that hypertensive patients have an excess risk of CHD, stroke, peripheral artery disease and heart failure compared with patients with normal blood pressure. Hypertensive individuals with one or more major CHD risk factors make up the bulk of the hypertensive population and more aggressive blood pressure targets are set for these people. As Mr CW has diabetes, the British Hypertension Society recommends a target blood pressure of 140/80 mmHg or lower.

(b) Diabetes. The mortality rates from coronary heart disease are up to five times higher for people with diabetes, while the risk of stroke is up to three times higher. Mr CW has both elevated random blood sugars and an elevated HbA_{1c}.

(c) Smoking. The risk of cardiovascular disease (CVD) is two to four times higher in heavy smokers (those who smoke at least 20 cigarettes per day) than in those who do not smoke. Other reports estimate the age-adjusted risk for smokers of more than 25 cigarettes per day is five to 21 times that of non-smokers.

(d) High cholesterol levels. Studies have repeatedly demonstrated the benefit of reducing cholesterol, especially low-density lipoprotein (LDL) cholesterol, in patients with CHD. Earlier studies focused on patients with 'elevated' cholesterol, but the recently published Heart Protection Study demonstrated that all patients with coronary risk factors will benefit from reduction of their serum cholesterol level.

(e) Obesity. Obese patients are at an increased risk for developing many medical problems, including insulin resistance and Type 2 diabetes, hypertension, dyslipidaemia, CVD, stroke and sleep apnoea. Excess body weight is also associated with substantial increases in mortality from all causes, in particular, CVD. A study in US nurses estimated this increase in risk to be two- to three-fold that of lean persons. Mr CW has a BMI of 31 which makes him 'obese' according to the World Health Organization classification.

What are the aims of treatment in angina?

A2 **The National Service Framework for Coronary Heart Disease states that the aims of treatment for stable angina are:**

(a) **To relieve symptoms.**
(b) **To prolong life and minimise cardiac risk.**

Treatment to relieve symptoms should include the use of sublingual nitrates for immediate symptom control plus beta-blockers and/or nitrates and/or calcium antagonists for long-term symptom control.

In order to minimise his cardiovascular risk, Mr CW should receive advice and treatment about how to adjust his modifiable risk factors.

(a) Stop smoking.
(b) Increase physical activity.
(c) Decrease alcohol consumption.
(d) Manage his diabetes.
(e) Advice and treatment to maintain his blood pressure below 140/80 mmHg.

(f)   Continue low-dose aspirin therapy to reduce the chance of future cardiac events.

(g)   Continue statin therapy, plus dietary advice to lower serum cholesterol concentrations to less than 5 mmol/L (LDL cholesterol to below 3 mmol/L) or by 20–25% (whichever is greater).

(h)   Education about the symptoms of heart attack and, should they develop, instruction to seek help rapidly by calling '999'.

Comment on the appropriateness of each of Mr CW's medicines on admission. Would you recommend any changes?

A3   **The choice of agents is appropriate. Aspirin and statin therapy reduce the risk of further cardiovascular events. Nitrates and nicorandil therapy decrease the frequency and severity of his anginal symptoms, while beta-blockers are the mainstay of anti-anginal therapy as they reduce both symptoms and risks. However, a number of adjustments to his current therapy should be considered.**

(a)   Aspirin.

People at increased risk of heart disease, including men older than 40 years of age, post-menopausal women and younger persons with heart disease risk factors (smoking, diabetes or hypertension) will benefit from low-dose (75–150 mg/day) aspirin. Regular aspirin use in these groups was linked to a 28% reduction in cardiac events.

For 1000 patients with a 5% risk of cardiac events in the next five years, aspirin would prevent six to 20 myocardial infarctions (MIs). At the same time, aspirin would cause zero to two haemorrhagic strokes and two to four major gastrointestinal bleeding episodes. If the five-year risk was 1%, only one to four infarctions would be prevented, but just as many bleeding events would occur.

In an extensive review of the literature, the Antiplatelet Trialists Collaboration demonstrated an absolute risk reduction of 2% per year in patients with established coronary artery disease.

As Mr CW is known to have coronary artery disease he would benefit from remaining on his aspirin, however, there is no evidence that enteric-coated aspirin products reduce gastrointestinal bleeding episodes, so a switch to dispersible aspirin should be considered and he should be encouraged to take the dose after a meal.

(b) Ranitidine.

Gastrointestinal bleeding and dyspepsia are more frequent with aspirin than with placebo. However, the absolute risk of these occurring is small and patients should not be automatically initiated on acid-suppression medication. In addition, the combination of enteric-coated preparations, which are specifically designed to dissolve in the higher pH of the duodenum, with an H_2-antagonist which reduces acid secretion in the stomach, is not logical.

If Mr CW has a previous history of gastrointestinal bleeding or dyspepsia, a low dose of a proton pump inhibitor (e.g. lansoprazole 15 mg daily) has been shown to be superior to H_2-antagonists at reducing the risk of gastrointestinal bleeding in patients on aspirin. If he has no previous history, acid suppression is probably not required.

(c) Statins.

Numerous trials have demonstrated the benefit of statins with respect to lowering serum cholesterol. Primary prevention studies, including WOSCOPS and the Heart Protection Study have consistently demonstrated the benefit of lowering total and LDL cholesterol. Substantially more benefit is gained in patients with established CHD. Current recommendations are to reduce total cholesterol to less than 5 mmol/L or by 20–25%, whichever will result in the lower serum cholesterol value. Mr CW's cholesterol is considerably above 5 mmol/L and, provided he is compliant with his current therapy, his dose should be increased to 40 mg simvastatin.

(d) Beta-blockers.

Various studies have demonstrated the beneficial effect of beta-blockers in angina and they are now considered first-line therapy. Beta-blockers achieve a decrease in myocardial oxygen demand by blocking beta-adrenergic receptors, thereby decreasing heart rate and the force of left ventricular contraction. Beta-blockers are particularly useful in exertional angina. Patients treated optimally should have a resting heart rate of around 60 beats per minute.

The Atenolol Silent Ischaemia Study showed a trend for atenolol to be superior to placebo in reducing anginal attacks and cardiac complications. The results demonstrated that seven patients need to be treated to prevent one primary end-point (death, resuscitation from ventricular tachycardia, non-fatal MI, UA or worsening angina, or revascularisation), but 55 needed to be treated to prevent one death.

Beta-blockers should be used with caution in patients with diabetes as the production of insulin is under adrenergic system control and thus their concomitant use may worsen glucose control. Beta-blockers can also mask the symptoms of hypoglycaemia and patients in whom the combination is considered of value should be warned of this; however most clinicians now believe that the benefits of taking beta-blockers, even in diabetics, outweigh the risks and they are frequently prescribed.

Mr CW's pulse should be monitored to ensure his dose is appropriately titrated, and his concordance with the medication assured.

(e) Nitrates.

Decreased myocardial oxygen consumption can be achieved by decreasing the vasomotor tone of the blood vessels. Various vasoactive substances, most notably endothelium-derived relaxing factor and nitric oxide, have been identified. Nitrates, which release nitric oxide when metabolised, have an established role in the treatment and prevention of angina.

The problem of tolerance with nitrates (where increased doses are required to achieve the same effect) means that short-acting preparations need to have their timings staggered to achieve an eight-hour nitrate-free period every day; however, this can be overcome with the use of a modified-release preparation. Whilst modified-release nitrate formulations provide a nitrate-free period, they also confer a treatment-free period, usually just before waking. This is of concern as it is the period of greatest risk for an acute coronary event. For this reason nitrates are not optimal first-line monotherapy. In addition, trials have so far not established any mortality gain from the use of oral nitrate preparations, although their role in providing symptom relief is well established.

GTN spray is an important diagnostic tool in establishing the severity of anginal pain. Its rapid onset of action results in relief of anginal pain, while failure to relieve this pain through the use of repeated (up to six) sprays indicates progression of stable angina to a more acute condition (UA or MI). The spray formulation has largely replaced sublingual GTN tablets as it does not oxidise on contact with air and therefore retains effectiveness for up to three years.

Mr CW should be regularly questioned as to his usage of GTN spray and its effectiveness.

(f) Nicorandil.

Nicorandil combines the properties of an organic nitrate with a potassium channel activator. It causes dilation of coronary arteries and arterioles and decreases systemic vasculature resistance. In small studies monotherapy appears to be as effective as other anti-anginal medication. The recently published IONA trial demonstrated a positive effect on mortality, and may raise nicorandil above nitrates in the anti-anginal prescribing hierarchy. Mr CW is on a small dose of nicorandil and this could be increased if anginal symptoms are not being controlled.

What other medications may have been added to this therapy regimen?

A4   **Calcium-channel blockers (CCBs) are effective at reducing anginal symptoms and angiotensin-converting enzyme inhibitors (ACEIs) have an emerging role in reducing the development of coronary events in patients with ischaemic heart disease.**

(a)   CCBs.

While short-acting CCBs have been implicated in the exacerbation of angina due to the phenomenon of 'coronary steal', longer-acting preparations of dihydropyridines, e.g. amlodipine and nifedipine LA, have demonstrated symptom-relieving potential similar to beta-blockers.

CCBs with myocardial rate control as well as vasodilatory properties (e.g. diltiazem) and those with predominantly rate-controlling effects (e.g. verapamil) have also been shown to improve symptom control, reduce the frequency of anginal attacks and increase exercise tolerance. They should be avoided in patients with compromised left ventricular function and conduction abnormalities. They should also be used with caution in patients already receiving beta-blockers, as bradycardia and heart block have been reported with this combination.

(b)   ACEIs.

While they are well-established treatments for heart failure, the vasoactive properties of ACEIs are still to be fully understood.

The Heart Outcomes Prevention Study (HOPE) provided compelling evidence that ramipril will reduce cardiovascular death, non-fatal MI, stroke, heart failure and the need for revascularisation in patients with angina, but without heart failure. The HOPE investigators randomised over 9500 patients with ischaemic heart disease to receive either ramipril (titrated to 10 mg a day) or placebo as well as conventional anti-anginal therapy. At the end of four years the ramipril group had a 3% absolute risk reduction of MI, stroke or cardiovascular death compared to the placebo group. A significant number of patients achieved, and were maintained, on the 10 mg dose and the drop-out rate in both groups was the same. There was a small decrease in blood pressure in the ramipril group (136/76 mmHg compared to 139/77 mmHg) which may have contributed to some, but not all, of the effect.

Further evidence for the benefit of ACEIs with respect to reducing cerebrovascular events has been provided by the PROGRESS study.

What is the reason for performing a CK-MB fraction and troponin-T test?

A5 **CK-MB and troponin T are tests used to identify whether myocardial damage has occurred. The tests are used to help differentiate between different types of myocardial chest pain.**

The term acute coronary syndrome (ACS) covers a group of conditions with a common theme of myocardial ischaemia. There is considerable emphasis placed on accurate diagnosis of these conditions, as their drug management differs considerably. Traditionally, four factors contribute to the diagnosis of ACS: history, examination, electrocardiogram and cardiac markers. The ideal cardiac marker should be present in the myocardial tissue only, released into the systemic circulation in a direct proportion to the amount of myocardial injury, then remain in the circulation long enough to provide a therapeutic window, and be assessed by a cheap, easy to perform and readily available assay. Currently no such marker exists.

CK is a muscle-bound protein released into the systemic circulation after muscle damage. CK-MB is still an acceptable diagnostic test. Rapid, cheap and accurate assays are available; however, it loses specificity in the setting of skeletal muscle injury or surgery. It has low sensitivity during the early (first six hours after the onset of symptom) and late (over 36 hours after onset of symptoms) phases. In combination with a positive history and sustained ECG changes, a CK-MB of greater than 4% indicates that a MI has occurred.

Cardiac troponins are more sensitive and specific markers of myocardial necrosis. Their ability to detect minor myocardial damage enhances their prognostic value beyond CK-MB levels. Troponin T is a protein which binds strongly to tropomycin on the filaments of myocardial tissue, and it is released into the blood system when the myocardium is damaged. 'Troponin-positive' patients with normal CK-MB values at presentation have an increased risk of death and cardiac complications compared to those who are 'troponin-negative'. There is also an excellent linear correlation between increasing troponin levels and worsening outcome. Troponin T and I are the preferred markers as the isoform C shows significant similarity with smooth and skeletal muscle.

Troponin T has low sensitivity in the early stages of symptoms and tests should be carried out eight to 12 hours after the onset of chest pain. Its long half-life (up to two weeks) means that it has limited ability to detect reinfarction.

The combination of the patient's history (previous diagnosis of, and worsening of angina, plus chest pain at rest), transient ECG changes, normal CK-MB with a raised troponin T, led the cardiologist to a diagnosis of UA.

What is UA and what are the implications for Mr CW?

A6 **UA can be defined as new onset angina at rest or prior existing angina which is increasing in severity, duration or frequency. Unstable angina results from the rupture of atheromatous plaques in the coronary vasculature, which initiates the formation of platelet plugs. This is a dynamic process with endogenous antiplatelet factors in competition with platelet-activating factors. Without aggressive management a significant number of patients will develop a thrombus which may completely occlude a coronary blood vessel, resulting in an MI.**

The conditions grouped as acute coronary syndrome (ACS) often present with similar symptoms of chest pain which is not, or only partially relieved, by GTN. These conditions include AMI, UA and non-ST-elevated MI (NSTEMI). AMI with persistent ST segment elevation on the ECG usually develops Q waves indicating transmural infarction (see Chapter 1). UA and NSTEMI present without persistent ST segment elevation and are managed differently, although a similar early diagnostic and therapeutic approach is employed.

Unstable angina is defined as angina that occurs at rest or with minimal exertion, or new (within one month) onset of severe angina or worsening of previously stable angina. Modern approaches consider NSTEMI (or non-Q wave MI) to be a more severe state of the same clinical syndrome.

There are about 115 000 new patients diagnosed each year with UA or NSTEMI in England and Wales. Despite the use of standard therapy the rate of adverse outcomes (such as death, non-fatal MI or refractory angina requiring revascularisation) remains at 5–7% at seven days and about

15–30% at 30 days; 5–14% of patient with UA die within the first year of diagnosis.

Patients presenting with UA can be classified into three categories depending on their risk of death or developing an AMI. High-risk patients (those with ST segment changes during chest pain, chest pain within 48 hours, troponin T-positive patients and those presenting already on intensive anti-anginal therapy) can be effectively managed with aggressive medical and interventional therapy. This results in lower event rates (development of AMI) and costs. Mr CW is classified as a high-risk patient and would be suitable for interventional therapy.

> Identify Mr CW's pharmaceutical care needs during the acute phase of his hospitalisation.

A7 **The pharmaceutical care needs of Mr CW can be viewed in the context of his key therapeutic aims which are to:**

(a)   Reduce his chance of death or MI.
(b)   Control his symptoms of chest pain.
(c)   Reduce his long-term cardiovascular risk.

Each of these three priorities should be evaluated in order to ensure that:

(a)   Mr CW is prescribed all necessary drug therapies at an optimal dose.
(b)   The drug therapy is safe.
(c)   The drug therapy is effective.
(d)   He can comply with the drug therapy.

> Comment on the rationale for the combination of antiplatelet therapy prescribed.

A8 **Aspirin, clopidogrel and low-molecular-weight heparins each inhibit different platelet activation pathways. This combination has been shown to be superior to the use of individual antiplatelet agents in reducing the risk of AMI in UA. Eptifibatide inhibits the binding of fibrinogen to receptors on platelets and prevents platelet adhesion. This drug is especially beneficial in patients with UA who are going to undergo percutaneous coronary intervention.**

Ischaemia develops as a result of decreased myocardial perfusion caused by platelet aggregation following the disruption of an atherosclerotic plaque. After vessel wall injury platelets initially adhere to the site of the injury with von Willebrand factor acting as a binding ligand. This process initiates a cascade of platelet activation which is stimulated via numerous mechanisms of which collagen, thrombin, thromboxane A_2, serotonin, and adenosine diphosphate (ADP) are the most significant. These stimulants cause a change in platelet conformation and the activation of glycoprotein IIb/IIIa receptors on the surface of the platelet. Platelet aggregation (platelet plugging) results from the binding of these receptors with fibrinogen and the eventual development of a thrombus which may partially or completely occlude the coronary artery. The development of these platelet plugs is a dynamic process, with endogenous antiplatelet factors attempting to effect clot dissolution. Pharmaceutical intervention is aimed at reducing platelet activation and aggregation.

The combination of aspirin (150 mg) and enoxaparin (1 mg/kg twice a day) is now recognised to be superior to aspirin and unfractionated heparin (5000 units stat then 30 000 units/24 hours with the aim of keeping the activated partial thromboplastin time (APTT) 1.5–2.5 times that of the control). The combination of these agents has a pharmacological logic, as they act on different platelet activation pathways, and their use results in a decrease in incidence of MI and death. The addition of the ADP inhibitor clopidogrel (300 mg initially, then 75 mg daily), confers significant additional benefit to the combination of thromboxane A_2 inhibitor and antithrombin agent, especially in the acute phase.

While decreasing platelet activation via these mechanisms is important, over 90 other factors that activate platelets have been identified and the prevention of platelet aggregation via inhibition of the glycoprotein IIb/IIIa receptor has attracted particular attention in recent years. The glycoprotein IIb/IIIa receptor inhibitors eptifibatide or tirofiban should be considered, especially as Mr CW has a raised troponin level. There is a financial implication to using these products, as well as an increased risk of bleeding; however, these drugs have demonstrated a significant reduction in death and MI in high risk patients, with the maximum benefit seen in high risk patients who go on to percutaneous transluminal coronary angioplasty (PTCA), as PTCA disrupts atheromatous plaques and initiates the platelet activation cascade.

The use of glycoprotein IIb/IIIa inhibitors is now recommended by the National Institute for Clinical Excellence as an adjunct to percutaneous coronary intervention (PCI) for all patients with diabetes undergoing elective PCI and for those patients undergoing complex procedures.

The chosen drug should be initiated before the start of the procedure and continued for 12 hours after the end of the procedure.

The results of trials involving thrombolytic therapy, either alone or in combination with a glycoprotein IIb/IIIa receptor antagonist in UA, have so far not shown any benefit, but have resulted in a significant increase in the risk of bleeding complications.

What are the risks associated with the use of combination antiplatelet therapy?

A9 **The main risks associated with combination antiplatelet therapy are an increase in bleeding events and an increase in thrombocytopenia.**

The combination of antiplatelet agents has the benefit of reducing platelet adherence, but the risk of increased bleeding. Bleeding events are usually defined as fatal, major bleeds or minor bleeds. The definition of the latter two are not necessarily consistent between trials, making interpretation of data difficult.

Using aspirin alone is not without risk. While there is no increase in the number of fatal bleeds that occur, there is a 2% absolute increase in major and minor bleeds.

Adding heparin (either unfractionated or low-molecular-weight) increases the absolute risk of major and minor bleeds to about 7%. Again, no increase in fatal bleeds has been noted.

Better awareness of the bleeding risks associated with the combination of glycoprotein IIb/IIIa inhibitors and heparin has resulted in a dramatic decrease in reported bleeding rates. A meta-analysis of glycoprotein IIb/IIIa trials indicated the risk of major bleeds to be 1.4% on heparin alone and 2.5% on a glycoprotein IIb/IIIa inhibitor plus heparin. Minor bleeds were not reported and there was no increase in intracranial haemorrhage.

The ESPRIT study pre-treated patients undergoing stent procedures with aspirin and clopidogrel (or ticlopidine, another thienopyridine), dose-adjusted heparin and either placebo or eptifibatide. The bleeding rate for both major and minor bleeds increased in the eptifibatide group (1 versus 0.4% and 2.8 versus 1.7% respectively).

The CURE study demonstrated a significant increase in overall bleeding from 5 to 8.5% in patients taking clopidogrel and aspirin compared to those taking aspirin only (minor bleeding: 5.1 versus 2.4%; major bleeding: 3.7 versus 2.7%).

Although traditionally, laboratory testing has been used to titrate the dose of unfractionated heparin there is no routine assay for monitoring either low-molecular-weight heparin or glycoprotein IIb/IIIa receptor antagonist therapy. One advantage of low-molecular-weight heparin is that its antifactor Xa activity is predictable, obviating the need to monitor anticoagulant activity in the majority of cases.

Unfractionated heparin, low-molecular-weight heparin and the glycoprotein IIb/IIIa receptor inhibitors have all been associated with thrombocytopenia. Thrombocytopenia can be defined as a fall in platelet count to below 100 000 cells/microlitre, but again this definition is not consistent across all trials.

ESSENCE compared enoxaparin and dose-adjusted heparin in UA and reported a thrombocytopenia rate (defined as a drop in platelet count of over 50% from baseline) of 2.5% in the enoxaparin group and 3.7% in the unfractionated heparin group.

Abciximab, the first glycoprotein IIb/IIIa inhibitor marketed, appears to be the one most prone to cause thrombocytopenia. A review of three abciximab studies demonstrates a significant increase in thrombocytopenia from 2.03 to 3.73%. All patients also received unfractionated heparin. Only two patients in the ESPRIT study developed thrombocytopenia. Both were in the eptifibatide arm.

There was no increase in the incidence of thrombocytopenia between the clopidogrel and placebo arm in the CURE study.

How should Mr CW be monitored?

A10   **Mr CW should be monitored for symptoms of ischaemic chest pain and for side-effects of medicines.**

Monitoring for ischaemic chest pain should include ECG monitoring and evaluation of his cardiac markers (CK-MB) after the angioplasty, to ensure no periprocedural ischaemic event occurred.

Antiplatelet agents should be monitored for signs of bleeding and thrombocytopenia. Dyspepsia should also be monitored and a proton pump inhibitor may be required. Mr CW's blood sugars should be controlled to 4–8 mmol/L, and his pulse and blood pressure should be monitored to ensure the effectiveness of the beta-blocker. His renal function should be monitored every few days to ensure there is no decrease in creatinine clearance after the initiation of the ACEI.

Measuring cholesterol levels after an acute event does not provide accurate results, but he should be monitored for other side-effects of statins, e.g. myalgia. Liver function tests should be compared to baseline 12 weeks after initiation of a statin or after changing the dose (as in Mr CW's case).

How should Mr CW's GTN infusion be 'titrated to response'?

A11 **Intravenous nitrates reduce myocardial oxygen demand by reducing the workload of the heart. Traditionally, intravenous nitrates are made up to a strength of 1 mg/mL by diluting 50 mg GTN in 50 mL of normal saline and running the infusion into a peripheral venous line via a syringe driver. The drug should be initiated at a dose of 5 micrograms/kg/min and the dose increased until the patient is pain-free or until headaches become intolerable or hypotension (systolic blood pressure less than 100 mmHg) necessitates dose reduction.**

Discuss the implications of interventional cardiology.

A12 **Interventional cardiology encompasses various invasive procedures which aim to improve myocardial blood delivery, either by opening up the blood vessels or replacing them. PCIs open stenosed coronary vessels and are less invasive than coronary bypass surgery, where the coronary vessels are replaced.**

A percutaneous (through the skin) transluminal (through the lumen of the blood vessels) coronary (into the heart) angioplasty (surgery or repair of the blood vessels) (PTCA) was first carried out on a conscious patient by Andeas Gruentzig in Zurich in 1977. Now over 2 million people a year undergo this procedure. The procedure is less invasive than coronary artery bypass graft (CABG) surgery, although the overall effectiveness and cost-effectiveness are not established.

PTCA involves the passing of a catheter via the femoral artery and aorta into the coronary vasculature under radio-contrast guidance. Inflation of a balloon at the end of the catheter in the area of the atheromatous plaques opens the lumen of the artery.

For patients undergoing PTCA there is a risk of death, MI and long-term restenosis. This is reduced by insertion of a coronary artery stent. Over the last 10 years the proportion of patients undergoing PCTA in which a stent is implanted has increased markedly. In 2000 the British Society of International Cardiology reported that stents were used in 83% of all PTCA procedures.

After stent insertion there is a short-term risk of thrombus formation until the endothelial lining of the blood vessel has been re-established. Traditional anticoagulation with warfarin required patients to be heparinised and therefore hospitalised, until a therapeutic international normalised ratio was achieved. This was replaced by the combination of the ADP receptor antagonist ticlopidine and aspirin, which while effective had a high incidence of neutropenia. The combination of the newer antiplatelet agent clopidogrel (300 mg initiated pre-procedure and 75 mg daily thereafter) and aspirin (325 mg daily) has been shown to be safer and equally as effective, and to decrease the length of hospital stay. The clopidogrel should be continued for four weeks and the aspirin, at a lower dose, indefinitely.

What is the place of drug-eluting stents. Would one have benefited Mr CW?

A13   **Diabetic patients face a greater risk of complications and events following coronary intervention and there is some evidence that drug-eluting stents may be more effective at reducing the risk of restenosis in this population.**

Restenosis occurs after PCI due to hyperplasia of the new intimal lining of the blood vessels. Restenosis rates following PTCA were originally as high as 40%; however, stent implantation reduced restenosis to less than 30% and intracoronary brachytherapy (irradiation of the blood vessel) to less than 10%. Drug-eluting stents appear to reduce restenosis rates to 0–5%.

Drug-eluting stents are balloon expandable stents which have been impregnated with a variety of agents to prevent restenosis. Immunosuppressants (e.g. sirolimus – RAVEL and SIRIUS studies) and antineoplastic agents (e.g. paclitaxel – TAXUS-I and ELUTES studies) have both so far shown dramatic reductions in restenosis rates at one year.

Trials are currently ongoing or planned with migration inhibitors such as batimastat and halofunginone and with enhanced healing agents including vascular endothelial growth factor, 17-beta-estradiol and hydroxymethylglutaryl coenzyme A (HMG-CoA) reductase inhibitors.

The cost-effectiveness of drug-eluting stents remains unresolved. In the UK a bare metal stent is considerably cheaper than the current commercially available drug-eluting stent; however, the overall need for repeat treatments due to restenosis currently occurs in approximately 15–20% of all patients (source British Cardiovascular Intervention Society; www.bcis.org.uk). National Guidance on this issue is expected.

Was it appropriate to discontinue his enoxaparin?

A14   **Yes. It is important to discontinue heparin at the end of the procedure and at least four hours before the femoral sheaths are removed to prevent haematomas and oozing at the incision site.**

In trials comparing low-molecular-weight heparin with unfractionated heparin, where patients went on to revascularisation (ESSENCE and TIMI 11B), the low-molecular-weight heparin was discontinued pre-procedure and substituted with unfractionated heparin. The unfractionated heparin was discontinued at the end of the procedure. A recent consensus document reviewed the available literature and suggested that low-molecular-weight heparin can be used as a safe alternative to unfractionated heparin, in combination with a glycoprotein IIb/IIIa receptor inhibitor.

Why has his nicorandil and isosorbide mononitrate therapy not been restarted?

A15 **PCI procedures result in less anginal pain and this opportunity should be taken to reduce Mr CW's tablet load.**

Discontinuation of anti-anginal drugs, particularly those for symptom relief, would be beneficial at this time. These drugs can be re-initiated should symptoms recur; however, drugs prescribed to reduce his long-term cardiovascular risk should be continued.

Why was metformin initiated?

A16 **To provide better control of his diabetes.**

Cardiovascular disease remains the major cause of morbidity and mortality in the diabetic population who continue to have a three- to five-fold greater risk of developing CVD than do non-diabetic persons. Prospective data have linked elevated HbA_{1c} with increased CV morbidity and mortality, and in both the Diabetes Control and Complications Trial and the United Kingdom Prospective Diabetes Study reduction in HbA_{1c} resulted in a decreased incidence of CVD.

Metformin can be used as monotherapy as an adjunct to diet. It has approximately equal effect on fasting blood glucose and HbA_{1c} as sulphonylureas, but should be considered first-line in obese patients like Mr CW as body weight is significantly lower after long-term metformin, compared with sulphonylurea treatment. A suphonylurea can be added to the metformin therapy if appropriate blood sugars are not achieved.

How long should Mr CW remain on his oral antiplatelet therapy?

A17 **In order to prevent intrastent thrombus formation, the combination of aspirin and clopidogrel should be continued for a month. Aspirin should be continued indefinitely. The decision to continue clopidogrel would depend on whether Mr CW experienced further angina.**

Clopidogrel (with aspirin) has replaced ticlopidine (with aspirin) as an effective strategy to decrease intracoronary thrombus after stent insertion. Early trial work suggested that 28 days of this combination was sufficient to reduce events in both planned and unplanned cases (e.g. UA).

   PCI-CURE demonstrated that patients pre-treated with clopidogrel and aspirin had a better 30 day outcome than patients who received aspirin only pre-PCI. The follow-up results (eight months after PCI) were less impressive. In the absence of any clear data, many cardiologists base the length of clopidogrel course on the severity of the patient's anginal condition.

What information should be communicated to the GP?

A18 **Apart from the traditional information provided (drug name, dose and frequency), GPs find guidance on duration of treatment, monitoring, new patient allergies and any changes in therapy particularly important.**

The summary information for Mr CW would comprise:

(a)   Drugs started

   (i)   Clopidogrel 75 mg for one month only after stent insertion. A full blood count should be performed in one week (if not done in hospital) to check for thrombocytopenia.
   (ii) Ramipril 2.5 mg initiated. Increase the dose by 2.5 mg intervals until target dose of 10 mg daily is achieved or side-effects occur (drop in blood pressure, decreased renal function or intolerable cough). Continue treatment long-term.
   (iii) Metformin initiated to control blood sugars. Review renal function annually and stop if renal function decreases. Review blood sugars regularly and add other oral hypoglycaemic agents as required.

(b) Dose changed

　(i) Aspirin EC changed to 75 mg dispersible form as no benefit from use of enteric-coated form. Continue long-term. Review for dyspepsia.

　(ii) Simvastatin. Dose increased to 40 mg daily. Cholesterol levels should be checked in six weeks together with liver function tests. Continue therapy long-term.

(c) Drugs stopped

　(i) Ranitidine, as no clear indication for use.

　(ii) Nicorandil. Successful PTCA should reduce chest pain. Re-initiate only if chest pain reoccurs.

　(iii) Isosorbide mononitrate, as nicorandil.

(d) As before

　(i) Atenolol and GTN spray.

What points would you wish to discuss with Mr CW prior to discharge?

A19 **Patient adherence to their medication regimens is associated with how satisfied they are with the quality of information they have received about their medicines and not necessarily the quantity of the information they receive. It is therefore important to establish Mr CW's need for information and to provide this as far as possible.**

Patient beliefs about medicines are influenced by many factors. These can largely be divided into beliefs about the importance of the medicine and concerns about the medicine's harmful effects. In order to assure the patient's concordance with medication regimens it is necessary to address each individual patient's beliefs and concerns.

One approach to counselling Mr CW may be to divide the medication prescribed into those used to reduce risk of heart attacks and death, and those for symptom control. Key points to be discussed will relate to side-effects and what to do if they occur, the need to continue medication until told otherwise and to ensure he does not run out of medication.

In relation to each prescribed medicine, specific information might include:

(a) Aspirin long-term is used to reduce the chance of a heart attack by reducing the formation of clots in the blood system, in particular the blood vessels that feed the heart muscle. The dose should be taken after food (not on an empty stomach), as aspirin can cause indigestion. If indigestion is a problem, this should be reported to the patient's GP who may prescribe a drug to counter this effect.

(b)   Clopidogrel is used to enhance the effect of aspirin while the stent settles. It only needs to be taken for one month and can then be discontinued. If a blood test has not been done in hospital (to check platelets), this should be done after a week. The patient's GP can do this.

(c)   Simvastatin. There are primarily two types of fats that circulate in the blood: low-density lipoproteins (LDLs), which cling to the blood vessel wall, resulting in narrowing of blood vessels, and high-density lipoproteins (HDLs) which do not narrow blood vessels. The target for cholesterol lowering is to reduce the total amount of cholesterol in the blood, but also to shift the balance of fats by decreasing LDL and increasing HDL. Cholesterol lowering drugs work best in conjunction with a low fat diet. It is therefore important to reduce intake of animal fats, including cheese and dairy products which contain the LDLs. Fish and olive oil contain the good HDLs. Antioxidants are thought to be beneficial, and are found in fresh fruit and salads. These are normally obtained as part of a fully balanced diet and there is little evidence that taking any additional vitamin supplements makes any difference (vitamin E or betacarotene). The target for total cholesterol should be a level less than 5 mmol/L. The GP should do a blood test in six weeks' time to see how much cholesterol reduction has occurred, and to check for side-effects of the medicine. It may be necessary to increase the dose if the target has not been achieved. Appointments to take blood should be booked with the surgery. Blood should normally be taken in the morning and ideally the patient should not have eaten before the blood is drawn. Simvaststin works best if taken at night; however, sleep disturbances can occur. Any muscle aches and pains should be reported immediately to the patient's GP.

(d)   Atenolol. Chest pain (angina) occurs when the heart muscle requires more oxygen than the blood vessels can deliver (because they are narrowed with cholesterol). Often angina occurs when the heart beats faster or harder than normal. Atenolol (a beta-blocker) reduces the workload of the heart, thereby reducing the heart's need for oxygen. This therefore reduces angina. Atenolol will reduce the heart rate increase that normally occurs during exercise or emotion. Patients often feel tired when first starting on atenolol, although will usually adjust to this. Other common side-effects include cold hands and cold feet and impotence in men. Any of these should be discussed with the patient's GP who may initially try other medicines from the same class of medicines. Patients with angina usually need to take a beta-blocker for a protracted period of time.

(e) Ramipril has been shown to decrease further damage to the heart. The ideal dose is 10 mg daily and the GP will try to increase the dose to this target; however, not all patients can tolerate this dose. Ramipril (as well as atenolol) can decrease blood pressure. This has positive effects, provided the blood pressure does not decrease too much. The GP will monitor this. Ramipril can sometimes cause cough which may occur at night. If this becomes bothersome, this should be reported to the GP, who may change the medicine. Ramipril may also be required long-term.

(f) GTN spray is used when symptoms of chest pain occur. Simply resting (sitting down and taking deep breaths) may sometimes alleviate chest pain, however if this has not occurred after 5 minutes, the spray should be used. Two puffs should be sprayed onto the tongue or the inside of the cheek. Symptoms of flushing or headache mean that the drug is working and will go away relatively quickly. If the chest pain is not relieved after five minutes then another two sprays should be used. Should this be unsuccessful, then urgent medical attention should be sought (usually by going to casualty or dialling '999'), as a clot may be forming in the arteries that feed the heart. It is important to carry the spray at all times and it is often easier to have two or three sprays (one at work, in the car, etc.). If the patient notices that they need to use the spray more frequently they should tell their GP who may adjust their regular medicines.

Should Mr CW be offered nicotine replacement therapy?

A20 **Yes. Any and every opportunity should be taken to encourage Mr CW to stop smoking.**

High-quality research has demonstrated that there are simple treatments and important lifestyle changes that can reduce cardiovascular risk substantially, and that can slow and perhaps even reverse progression of established coronary disease. When used appropriately, these interventions can be more cost-effective than many other treatments currently provided by the NHS.

Within a matter of months after smoking cessation, CHD risk begins to decline. Within two to three years of smoking cessation, the risk decreases to approximately the level found in people who have never smoked, regardless of the amount smoked, duration of the habit and the age at cessation.

A meta-analysis of structured cessation programmes has indicated that nicotine replacement therapy nearly doubles smokers' chances of successfully stopping smoking (18 versus 11%). Mr CW should be offered advice on stopping smoking and encouraged to attend specialist smokers' clinics to further improve his chances of quitting.

Further reading

Antiplatelet Trialists' Collaboration. Collaborative overview of randomised trials of antiplatelet therapy I: prevention of death, myocardial infarction and stroke by prolonged antiplatelet therapy in various categories of patients. *Br Med J* 1994; **308**: 81–106.

Boersma E, Harrington RA, Moliterno DJ et al. Platelet glycoprotein IIb/IIIa inhibitors in acute coronary syndromes: a meta-analysis of all major randomised clinical trials. *Lancet* 2002; **359**: 189–198.

Braunwald E, Antman EM, Beasley JN *et al*. ACC/AHA guideline update for the management of patients with unstable angina and non-ST-segment elevation myocardial infarction: a report of the American College of Cardiology/American Heart Association Task Force on Practice Guidelines (Committee on the Management of Patients with Unstable Angina). *Circulation* 2002; **106**: 1893–1900.

CURE. Effects of clopidogrel in addition to aspirin in patients with acute coronary syndromes without ST segment elevation. *N Eng J Med* 2001; **345**: 494–502.

De Lorgeril M, Salen P, Martin J-L *et al*. Mediterranean diet, traditional risk factors, and the rate of cardiovascular complications after myocardial infarction. Final report of the Lyon Diet Heart Study. *Circulation* 1999; **99**: 779–785.

Department of Health. *National Service Framework for Coronary Heart Disease*. Department of Health, London, 2001.

Department of Health. *National Service Framework for Diabetes*. Department of Health, London, 2001.

Duggan C, Feldman R, Hough J et al. Reducing adverse prescribing discrepancies following hospital discharge. *Int J Pharm Pract* 1998; **6**: 77–82.

Heart Protection Study Collaborative Group. MRC/BHF Heart Protection Study of cholesterol lowering with simvastatin in 20,536 high risk individuals: a randomised placebo-controlled trial. *Lancet* 2002; **360**: 7–22.

Heart Outcomes Prevention Evaluation Study Investigators. Effects of an angiotensin-converting-enzyme inhibitor, ramipril on cardiovascular events in high-risk patients. *N Engl J Med* 2000; **342**: 145–153.

Johansen K. Efficacy of metformin in the treatment of NIDDM: meta-analysis. *Diabetes Care* 1999; **22**: 33–37.

Kereiakes DJ, Montalescot G, Antman EM *et al*. Low-molecular-weight heparin therapy for non-ST-elevation acute coronary syndromes and during percutaneous coronary intervention: an expert consensus. *Am Heart J* 2002; **144**: 615–624.

Munday A, Kelly B, Forrester JWE *et al*. Do general practitioners and community pharmacists want information on the reasons for drug therapy changes implemented by secondary care? *Br J Gen Pract* 1997; **47**: 563–566.

National Institute for Clinical Excellence. *Guidance on Glycoprotein IIb/IIIa Inhibitors for Acute Coronary Syndromes*. NICE, London, 2002.

Pi-Sunyer FX. Medical hazards of obesity. *Ann Intern Med* 1993; **119**: 655–660.

Raw M, McNeill A, West R. Smoking cessation guidelines for health professionals. A guide to effective smoking cessation interventions for the health care system. *Thorax* 1998; **53**[suppl. 5(1)]: S1–38.

Working Group for the Study of Transdermal Nicotine in Patients with Coronary Artery Disease. Nicotine replacement therapy for patients with coronary artery disease. *Arch Intern Med* 1994; **154**: 989–995.

3

Hypertension

Charles Morecroft and Mary P Tully

Day 1 Mr CT, a 71-year-old man, was admitted to hospital after a fall due to a blackout while shopping. He had been unable to get up as his right arm and leg were numb, so a passer-by had called an ambulance. When he arrived at A & E the numbness was improving; however, the x-ray showed a hairline fracture of the pelvis, and he was admitted for observation and pain relief.

His previous medical history was unremarkable, he was taking no medication and he had never experienced a similar blackout before. He was overweight (90 kg), smoked 20–25 cigarettes per day and drank over 21 units of alcohol a week. On examination, he had a blood pressure of 170/110 mmHg and a pulse rate of 75 beats per minute. There was severe bruising to his lower back and left arm, caused by the fall. Further observations of his blood pressure confirmed that Mr CT was hypertensive. Talking with Mr CT established that both his father and his grandfather died from a heart condition.

His serum biochemistry and haematology results were:

- Sodium 138 mmol/L (reference range 135–145)
- Potassium 4.1 mmol/L (3.5–4.5)
- Creatinine 95 micromol/L (60–120)
- Urea 6.7 mmol/L (2.5–7.5)
- Haemoglobin 15.2 g/dL (12–18)
- Serum total cholesterol 6.5 mmol/L
- Blood glucose 5.5 mmol/L

Q1 Should an elderly gentleman such as Mr CT be treated for hypertension?

Q2 What is the recommended first-line treatment for Mr CT's hypertension?

Q3 What other therapy(ies) would you recommend?

Q4 Outline a pharmaceutical care plan for Mr CT.

Day 2 Mr CT's numbness disappeared completely within 24 hours and aspirin 75 mg daily was started in order to help prevent further transient ischaemic attacks. The medical staff also prescribed paracetamol 1 g up to four times a day when required for his pain and bendroflumethiazide 2.5 mg in the morning. They requested twice-daily blood pressure monitoring.

Q5 How quickly can a response to his antihypertensive therapy be expected and what level of blood pressure should be aimed for?

Day 4 During the night Mr CT complained to the house officer on call that he was still in a lot of pain and that the paracetamol was not helping. The house officer prescribed diclofenac 50 mg to be taken when required, up to three times a day with or after food.

Q6 Was this appropriate treatment for Mr CT?

Day 6 Mr CT was feeling much better, he had stopped smoking and the bruising was beginning to disappear. He was discharged from hospital on bendroflumethiazide 2.5 mg in the morning, aspirin 75 mg in the morning, simvastatin 10 mg at night and paracetamol 1 g four times a day plus codeine 30 mg up to four times a day when required for pain. He was advised to make an appointment with his GP to ensure his care continues uninterrupted.

Q7 What are Mr CT's risk factors for cerebro/cardiovascular events, other than hypertension?
Q8 What general advice should he be given?

Month 4 Mr CT attended his routine out-patient appointment. His blood pressure was slightly reduced, but was still high at 165/100 mmHg. He was prescribed atenolol 50 mg in the morning, in addition to the bendroflumethiazide.

Q9 Was this additional medication appropriate for the further treatment of his hypertension?
Q10 How should treatment with diuretics and beta-blockers be monitored?

Month 7   Mr CT made an appointment to see his GP because he was constantly feeling 'under the weather', and he could never get his hands and feet to warm up. He complained that at this time of the year he was often cold, but that he had 'never had a winter like it'. He also complained that he was getting a lot of pain in his legs when he was walking. On examination, Mr CT was found to have a blood pressure of 140/95 mmHg and a pulse of 48 beats per minute. His hands were cold to touch. He had lost some weight and was now 83 kg. Investigation for signs of a urinary tract infection proved negative.

Q11   Could Mr CT's symptoms be related to his medication?

The GP discontinued the atenolol permanently and the bendroflumethiazide temporarily for two days, and started Mr CT on captopril 6.25 mg twice daily. He took a sample of blood and asked Mr CT to come back in two days for another blood test and to make an appointment to see him again in one week.

Q12   What is the rationale for using angiotensin-converting enzyme inhibitors (ACEIs) in hypertension?
Q13   How should ACEI treatment be started in an elderly person such as Mr CT?
Q14   How should treatment with ACEIs be monitored?
Q15   What advice should be given to Mr CT about his treatment?

Mr CT returned to his GP after one week and his blood pressure was recorded as 160/95 mmHg. He said that he had felt a little dizzy for the first day, but that he felt fine now. The biochemistry results for the pre-treatment blood test were:

- Sodium 135 mmol/L (135–145)
- Potassium 3.6 mmol/L (3.5–4.5)
- Creatinine 125 micromol/L (60–120)

- Urea 9.7 mmol/L (2.5–7.5)

and for the post-treatment sample:

- Sodium 137 mmol/L (135–145)
- Potassium 3.9 mmol/L (3.5–4.5)
- Creatinine 210 micromol/L (60–120)

- Urea 11.6 mmol/L (2.5–7.5)

Q16 Why has Mr CT's renal function deteriorated so quickly?

Q17 What options are there for the further treatment of Mr CT's hypertension?

Month 12 Mr CT returned to the out-patient clinic and his blood pressure was noted to be stabilised at 145/85 mmHg on bendroflumethiazide 2.5 mg in the morning and modified-release nifedipine 40 mg twice daily.

Should an elderly gentleman, such as Mr CT, be treated for
hypertension?

A1   **Yes. There is good evidence that treating hypertension in
elderly people is highly effective at preventing cerebro/
cardiovascular events.**

For many years, the perceived risk of adverse drug reactions (ADRs) from
antihypertensive drugs, together with the lack of knowledge about benefits, was such that many elderly people did not receive treatment. Recent
outcome trials (e.g. STOP-hypertension, SHEP, Treatment of Hypertension
in the Elderly) have indicated a clear benefit of lowering blood pressure up
to the age of 80 years. For those patients over the age of 80, the ongoing
Hypertension in the Very Elderly Trial will provide some guidance. The
trial evidence to date indicates a potential 33% reduction in stroke
mortality, 26% reduction in coronary mortality and a 22% decrease in
cardiovascular mortality between the treatment and control groups. Antihypertensive treatment is thus indicated and beneficial for people aged 60
and above, when their systolic blood pressure is greater than 160 mmHg
even if their diastolic remains within normal limits. Hypertension is one
of several risk factors for cerebro/cardiovascular events, and the British
Hypertension Society (BHS) and the National Service Framework (NSF) for
Coronary Heart Disease now recommend consideration of these risk factors and their possible treatment. For patients over 80 years of age, the
decision to treat will depend on their general level of health and concomitant disease(s). For example, the short-term risks of treating a frail
lady of 81, who suffers from postural hypotension, poor mobility and
frequent falls due to severe Parkinson's disease, might outweigh any
potential benefits she might gain in the long-term.

Mr CT has no concomitant diseases and, with a history of transient
ischaemic attack (TIA), should potentially receive considerable benefit
from the treatment of his hypertension and a reduction of his other risk
factors.

What is the recommended first-line treatment for Mr CT's
hypertension?

A2   **A low dose of a thiazide diuretic.**

BHS guidelines recommend the use of a stepped programme for the
treatment of hypertension: the first step is either a thiazide diuretic or a

beta-blocker. Work carried out by the Medical Research Council has shown that diuretics are more effective in treating hypertension in elderly patients; however, treatment must be tailored to the individual patient and any concomitant diseases they may have.

The action of thiazide diuretics in hypertension is due to a decrease in extracellular fluid volume and a possible vasodilator effect. The mechanism of action of beta-blockers is not clear, but their blockade of $beta_1$ receptors may be important. They reduce cardiac output, alter baroreceptor reflex sensitivity and reduce plasma renin secretion.

Diuretics are cautioned or contra-indicated in the presence of gout, diabetes mellitus and prostatic hypertrophy. They should also be used with caution in patients who have reduced mobility, as urgency to micturate may lead to incontinence and resultant dependence. Beta-blockers are cautioned or contra-indicated in the presence of peripheral vascular disease, asthma, heart failure and diabetes mellitus.

Mr CT has no conditions that would prohibit the use of either class of drug. As diuretics are still considered drugs of first choice in elderly patients, a dose of bendroflumethiazide 2.5 mg daily, or an equivalent dose of another agent, is recommended. Doses greater than this do not have any additional benefit in terms of blood pressure reduction and increase the risk of electrolyte disturbances. Doses as low as 1.25 mg have also been shown to be effective in some cases. Once daily administration of bendroflumethiazide increases the potential for compliance with treatment. With these low doses, there is no need for the concomitant prescription of potassium-sparing diuretics or potassium unless there is evidence of hypokalaemia.

What other therapy(ies) would you recommend to be prescribed?

A3 **Other recommended therapies for Mr CT would include those to reduce the risk of further TIAs as well as adequate pain relief.**

Despite the benefits of antihypertensive medication, population studies have demonstrated that hypertensive patients continue to have a substantially higher risk of coronary heart disease and stroke than non-hypertensive individuals, even after several years of treatment.

As Mr CT has both hypertension and a history of TIA, the BHS guidelines recommend that both aspirin 75 mg and a statin (HMG CoA reductase inhibitor) are prescribed as secondary prevention. The use of a statin has been shown to reduce the risk of further coronary events.

If Mr CT had not had a history of TIA, the use of a statin and aspirin could have been considered in the context of primary prevention. The decision to prescribe statins for well-controlled hypertensive patients, as primary prevention is based upon the patient's serum cholesterol level (5 mmol/L or above) and their 10–year coronary heart risk calculation (30% or less; estimated by using the Joint British Society cardiovascular risk charts). The HOT trial suggests that for well-controlled hypertensive patients over 50 years, prescribing aspirin 75 mg daily can reduce cardiovascular events by 15% and myocardial infarction by 36%. However, the risk of non-cerebral bleeding does increase and this would have to be balanced against the benefits of coronary heart disease for individual patients. Had Mr CT had no further risk factors (not the case), then prescribing aspirin 75 mg daily could potentially increase morbidity and mortality because the risk of bleeds would outweigh any potential cardiovascular benefits.

Adequate pain relief may be obtained by prescribing paracetamol 1 g up to four times a day plus the addition of codeine phosphate 15–30 mg up to four times a day when required. Using separate formulations, rather than a co-codamol 30/500 preparation, will ensure that pain relief is adequate, whilst the side-effects associated with codeine use such as constipation will be kept to a minimum.

Outline a pharmaceutical care plan for Mr CT.

A4   The pharmaceutical care plan should identify and address each of Mr CT's problems. It should indicate what monitoring is necessary to ensure the desired therapeutic outcomes are reached.

(a) Problems
   (i)   Cause of fall, i.e. TIA.
   (ii) Pain due to bruising and hairline fracture.
   (iii) Hypertension.
   (iv) Patient's possible anxiety and lack of confidence.

(b) Plan

   (i)   Prescribe aspirin and reduce his risk factors for TIA (hypertension, smoking, obesity).
   (ii) Ensure adequate pain relief is provided with paracetamol with or without codeine.

(iii)   Prescribe appropriate antihypertensive therapy and reduce his risk factors for hypertension (smoking, obesity, high salt intake).
(iv)   Prescribe HMG CoA reductase inhibitor (statin).
 (v)   Ensure he has an adequate understanding of his medication regimen, in order to maximize his compliance.
(vi)   Discuss with the patient ways to reduce his risk factors for cerebro/cardiovascular events.

(c)   Monitoring: all therapy should be monitored for efficacy and side-effects

 (i)   Aspirin. Check for ADRs.
(ii)   Pain relief. Enquire about efficacy of pain relief and add codeine if necessary. Mention to the patient the possibility that constipation may occur as increasing quantities of codeine are taken.
(iii)   Antihypertensive therapy. Monitor blood pressure, sodium, potassium, urea and creatinine levels.
(iv)   Cholesterol lowering. Regular monitoring of total cholesterol, high-density lipoprotein and triglyceride levels.

How quickly can a response to his antihypertensive therapy be expected and what level of blood pressure should be aimed for?

A5   **Low-dose diuretics can take several weeks to reach maximum efficacy. An optimal target blood pressure for Mr CT is a systolic pressure of less than 140 mmHg and a diastolic of less than 85 mmHg.**

Thiazide diuretics have been shown to take as long as 12 weeks to reach maximal effect and, except in severe hypertension, treatment should be unaltered for a minimum of four weeks, to ensure an adequate therapeutic trial of the chosen drug. A common problem associated with the management of hypertension is changing the dose or treatment too quickly. It is also prudent not to lower blood pressure aggressively in an elderly patient, as a real risk of falls due to hypotension exists. Ideally, if an elderly patient has a history of falls, blood pressure measurements should be taken while the patient is both standing and sitting to check for a postural drop.

The HOT study has produced clearer guidance regarding the target blood pressure to be achieved and given reassurance that reducing diastolic blood pressure to below 80 mmHg does not increase cardiovascular risk. Current guidelines recommend an optimal blood pressure to aim for (i.e. a minimum recommended goal) and a higher blood pressure target for those patients who fail to attain the optimal level. For Mr CT, the BHS recommends an optimal blood pressure target of below 140/85 mmHg, with a blood pressure of at least below 150/90 mmHg being reached. It is important that both systolic and diastolic blood pressures reach the target pressures. (Note that other national guidelines vary in the levels of blood pressure recommended.)

Was this appropriate treatment for Mr CT?

A6 **No, this treatment was not appropriate.**

Surveys of the incidence and prevalence of ADRs in the elderly population show that gastrointestinal symptoms and bleeding due to non-steroidal anti-inflammatory drugs (NSAIDs) are common. In particular, NSAIDs can mask the pain of the peptic ulcer disease until severe bleeding or haematemesis occurs. Renal dysfunction can also be precipitated, because of a reduction of prostaglandin-mediated renal blood flow. In addition, NSAIDs can antagonize the antihypertensive action of diuretics by inhibiting diuretic-induced sodium and water excretion. This effect is most pronounced with indometacin, but all NSAIDs have this potential. Fortunately, it is usually only clinically significant with long-term NSAID treatment. If treatment lasts less than one week, it is unlikely to have a major impact on blood pressure levels.

As outlined in the pharmaceutical care plan, Mr CT should be given a short course of an adequate dose of codeine, e.g. 15–30 mg, to be taken up to four times a day with regular paracetamol. The pharmacist should monitor for efficacy and ADRs, particularly constipation, nausea and confusion.

What are Mr CT's risk factors for cerebro/cardiovascular events, other than hypertension?

A7 **(a) Family history of heart conditions.**

   (b) Ethnicity.

   (c) History of TIA.

   (d) Smoking.

   (e) Drinking.

(f)   **Being overweight.**

(g)   **High cholesterol levels.**

Consideration of all these factors, along with his age and blood pressure levels (prior to treatment) probably place him at high risk of further cerebro/cardiovascular events.

British South Asians and Blacks appear to have a higher prevalence of hypertension than White Europeans. The efficacy of antihypertensive medication also varies with ethnicity, e.g. beta-blockers, ACEIs and angiotensin II receptor antagonists can be less effective in Blacks. When calculating the estimated coronary heart disease risk for patients from ethnic minorities it is possible that the value given will be an underestimation.

What general advice should he be given?

A8   Mr CT should be given advice on adherence, alteration of diet, weight reduction, increased exercise, and the benefits that would be derived from stopping smoking and reducing his alcohol consumption.

(a)   Adherence. Contrary to received wisdom, elderly people are not less likely to be compliant with drug treatment than are younger patients. However, they are more likely to be taking complex medication regimens, have difficulty with dexterity or vision, or have cognitive dysfunction, all known to decrease compliance in patients of all ages. When Mr CT was admitted to hospital he was on no treatment. The ward pharmacist should ensure that Mr CT understands how to take his medication regimen and should check that he can, for example, open child-resistant tops and read the container labels. The pharmacist should ensure that the patient is given advice and information on why he is taking this medication regimen, and what may happen if he does not. Any advice given should be endorsed with leaflets and a selection of suitable website addresses, if appropriate.

(b)   A low-sodium diet. The BHS guidelines recommend the adoption of dietary change for all patients, regardless of whether or not they are receiving active pharmacological treatment. There is some evidence that sodium restriction will result in a small reduction in systolic blood pressure (an average decrease of 8 mmHg). While an aggressive reduction is difficult, a high sodium intake can negate the effectiveness of diuretics, so Mr CT should receive advice about using salt substitutes, not using salt in cooking and reducing his intake of high sodium foods. Increasing the amount of potassium in the diet can also forestall any possible ADRs due to diuretics, and is in itself hypotensive. This can easily be achieved by using salt substitutes such as Lo-salt and increasing the amount of fruit, particularly bananas, in his diet.

(c)   Weight reduction. There is an association between overweight and hypertension for patients of all ages, although it is reduced in elderly patients. A decrease in weight usually brings about a corresponding, albeit small, reduction in blood pressure. However, compliance to weight-reducing diets is a problem and they are not easily maintained. The usual aim is to change specific areas, particularly the amount of fat consumed. While Mr CT is overweight he is not obese, so anti-obesity drugs will be of little benefit. He should be encouraged to take responsibility for his weight reduction and referred to a dietitian for advice on a low-fat diet.

(d)   Regular exercise, particularly walking or swimming (30–45 minutes), can bring about a modest reduction in blood pressure. The exercise has to be maintained, as any benefit is lost 14 days after the exercise ceases. As Mr CT experienced a fall due to a TIA, he may be anxious about increasing his activity due to loss of confidence following his fall. In addition, any anxiety may also lead to an increase in his blood pressure. Counselling may be offered to help him deal with these issues.

(e)   Smoking cessation. The Medical Research Council study highlighted the association between smoking and cardiovascular mortality in elderly people. Mr CT should be given advice about smoking cessation programmes and support groups. However, note that nicotine replacement patches and chewing gum are contra-indicated in patients with a recent history of cerebrovascular accidents, including TIAs, so these cannot be recommended. Although amfebutamone (bupropion) is not contra-indicated, it may cause an increase in blood pressure and its use is therefore cautioned.

(f)   Some groups of over-the-counter (OTC) medications may cause problems for antihypertensive patients and all patients should be advised to consult their community pharmacist before purchasing any OTC medications. For example, antacids can reduce the adsorption of ACEIs and oral sympathomimetic decongestants can cause an increase in blood pressure. Mr CT should also be advised to be cautious of medication, both prescribed and OTC which have a high sodium content, e.g. Gaviscon or medications presented in an effervescent formulation.

Was this additional medication appropriate for the further treatment of his hypertension?

A9   Yes, this was appropriate treatment.

Diuretic and beta-blocker combination therapy is a logical progression for Mr CT. Diuretic therapy in the treatment of hypertension has a relatively flat dose–response curve. Therefore, increasing the dose of Mr CT's bendroflumethiazide will only result in an increased incidence of ADRs for minimal reduction of his blood pressure. However, before beta-blocker treatment is started it is important to check that he does not have undiagnosed heart failure, as this is a common sequelae to hypertension in this age group. If heart failure is present, the use of an ACEI, in addition to a diuretic, would be more appropriate.

The addition of a second antihypertensive from another pharmaco-logical group is based on complementary action to, or countering the reflex action of, the first drug. In clinical practice, it is usual to choose either an ACEI or Beta-blocker plus either a Calcium-channel blocker or Diuretic (the ABCD rule), although in Mr CT's case, another option would have been to treat with a single drug from the AB antihypertensives before combination therapy was started.

Current research indicates that patients whose blood pressure re-sponds poorly to a drug that stimulates the renin system may respond better to one that inhibits the system. For example, AB antihypertensives block the renin system, whereas CD antihypertensives stimulate it. Treat-ment using this rule begins with monotherapy chosen from an AB or CD antihypertensive. If the target blood pressure is not reached, then Step 2 would involve changing over to an antihypertensive chosen from the other pair. For example, treatment initiated using a diuretic which failed to reduce blood pressure would be stopped and replaced with either an ACEI or beta-blocker. If the target blood pressure was still not attained, then step three would involve the addition of a second antihypertensive from the initial pair (A or B plus C or D).

Using this stepwise approach helps achieve one of the aims of hypertension therapy, which is to obtain maximum control of the blood pressure with minimum therapy, thus reducing possible side-effects and increasing the degree of compliance.

The pharmacist should ensure that Mr CT received further counsel-ling about his medication, due to the increasing complexity of his drug regimen. The pharmacist should also take the opportunity to enquire how he has been able to reduce his other risk factors. Once the correct dose of each respective agent has been established, there may be a case for using a combined preparation, if one exists, to simplify his regimen.

How should treatment with diuretics and beta-blockers be monitored?

A10   In addition to the obvious monitoring for efficacy, bendroflumethiazide and atenolol should be monitored according to their respective ADR profiles.

Thiazide diuretics can cause hypokalaemia, hyperuricaemia and impaired glucose tolerance. However, only potassium levels are usually monitored routinely, unless there is a reason to suspect that other levels might be affected. Potassium levels might be expected to drop by up to 0.6 mmol/L with the maximum decrease occurring during the first three months of treatment. Potassium supplements should only be given if the potassium level goes below 3.5 mmol/L or if there is concomitant treatment with digoxin: the majority of patients will not require them. Of particular concern in elderly patients is hypovolaemia and syncope (faints), and Mr CT should be specifically asked whether he has experienced dizzy spells and falls.

Unlike diuretics, beta-blockers do not require biochemical monitoring. A 25% drop in heart rate is evidence of effective beta-blockade, but heart rate should be monitored for signs of more significant bradycardia. A watchful eye should be kept for the signs and symptoms of bronchospasm and heart failure. Atenolol is a water-soluble beta-blocker; the lipid-soluble agents, such as propranolol, can cause sleep disturbance and nightmares.

Could Mr CT's symptoms be related to his medication?

A11   Yes. Fatigue, bradycardia and peripheral vasoconstriction are side-effects of beta-blockers.

The action of beta-blockers on cardiac output causes a decrease in peripheral blood flow. As a result, susceptible patients may suffer from cold extremities or Raynaud's phenomenon. Intermittent claudication, with pain on walking, due to decreased blood supply to the lower leg muscles, may be worsened. Although beta-blockers with intrinsic sympathomimetic activity such as celiprolol do not have this effect, it is more usual to change to a different drug group if a patient suffers significantly from such side-effects.

Urinary tract infections in elderly people do not always cause classic symptoms of polyuria and dysuria, but may present with chills and general malaise. Therefore, Mr CT's GP correctly excluded this as a cause of his current symptoms.

What is the rationale for using ACEIs in hypertension?

A12   **ACEIs act by a number of mechanisms to reduce blood pressure.**

The renin–angiotensin–aldosterone system plays a central role in hypertension, producing the potent vasoconstrictor angiotensin II and releasing aldosterone. ACEIs competitively block the enzyme responsible for the conversion of angiotensin I to the active angiotensin II. They promote sodium excretion, both by reducing aldosterone levels and by causing renal vasodilation. They reduce the breakdown of the vasodilatory bradykinins and inhibit local formation of angiotensin II in the tissues. In elderly patients, low renin levels are common, but ACEIs still seem effective in reducing blood pressure. They can also be helpful for patients with claudication because of their vasodilatory effects.

The HOPE study concluded that ramipril should be given to patients who are at high risk of stroke. The study found that ramipril reduced the incidence of stroke even though only a modest reduction in blood pressure was noted. Fewer patients in the ramipril group had a fatal stroke and functional impairment was less. It is unclear whether this is a specific drug effect or a class effect of ACEI or simply the effect of lowering blood pressure.

Research into hypertension therapy is concentrating on the role of the renin–angiotensin–aldosterone system. Losartan is a newer antihypertensive which is a specific blocker of angiotensin II receptors. The LIFE study indicated that losartan was more beneficial than atenolol for those high-risk patients with left ventricular hypertrophy, but its use in other groups of patients has not yet been established.

How should ACEI treatment be started in an elderly person such as Mr CT?

A13   **Treatment should be started at a low dose to prevent hypotension.**

The first dose of most ACEI can cause a sudden and profound drop in blood pressure, particularly in individuals who are treated with concomitant diuretics. A low dose should be administered initially, with the first dose preferably at night before lying down. If diuretics have been used, as in Mr CT's case, they should be discontinued for a few days prior to treatment with ACEIs to reduce the drop in blood pressure. Elderly people do not tolerate sudden drops in blood pressure as well as do younger patients. This is due to the decreased sensitivity of the baroreceptors, which monitor blood pressure. As a result they are at greater risk of falls and their sequelae. Although the ACEI perindopril is promoted as lacking this 'first-dose' hypotensive effect, captopril still remains the agent of choice as a test dose because of its fast onset of action. In maintenance therapy, however, it must be given twice daily, so another agent, such as lisinopril or ramipril, may be preferable.

How should treatment with ACEIs be monitored?

A14   **ACEIs are associated with few serious side-effects. Renal dysfunction may occur, so monitoring of renal function tests (urea and creatinine) is required.**

The deterioration in renal function can be dramatic and serum urea and creatinine must be checked prior to treatment and shortly after starting an ACEI. Potassium levels may increase, because of the inhibition of aldosterone, and should be monitored. For this reason ACEIs should not be co-prescribed with potassium-sparing diuretics. Haematological abnormalities are rare, but neutropenia due to captopril is more common in patients with renal dysfunction. A dry, irritating cough occurs in up to 15% of patients and should be actively enquired about. It is thought to be mediated by an increase in bradykinin levels.

What advice should be given to Mr CT about his treatment?

A15   **Mr CT should be given advice about the potential side-effects associated with captopril and further counselling about complying with his drug regimen.**

Mr CT should be asked to take the first dose of captopril at bedtime and told that he should be careful about rising too quickly from a lying position. He has already been told not to take his bendroflumethiazide for the next two days and the pharmacist should make sure that this is clearly understood. Mr CT should be warned about the possibility of a cough, which should not cause him undue concern, but he should tell his doctor if it occurs. Previously he was told to increase his potassium intake and to use Lo-salt, but this recommendation now needs to be revised, as it may result in hyperkalaemia. As with any patient with an increasingly complex drug regimen, tactful enquiries should be made as to how well he manages to take his treatment as prescribed. He should receive further advice on how to take his medication. Counselling about drug treatment should be ongoing: a single session is unlikely to have a lasting impact.

Why has Mr CT's renal function deteriorated so quickly?

A16   **ACEIs may cause abrupt renal dysfunction, especially in the presence of renal artery stenosis.**

Renal artery stenosis, or narrowing, produces a decreased glomerular filtration pressure. Angiotensin II constricts the efferent glomerular arteriole and helps to increase the pressure gradient across the glomerulus. This necessary effect is antagonised by ACEIs and renal hypoperfusion results. Although there was no previous evidence that Mr CT had renal stenosis, the risk of silent renal artery stenosis is increased if peripheral vascular disease is present. Mr CT's GP correctly acted with caution in doing renal function tests at baseline and again soon after starting ACEI treatment.

What options are there for the further treatment of Mr CT's hypertension?

A17   **Further treatment could include calcium-channel blockers, alpha-blockers or methyldopa or combinations of these agents.**

There are three classes of calcium-channel blockers: dihydropyridine derivatives (e.g. nifedipine, amlodipine, nicardipine), benzothiazine derivatives (e.g. diltiazem) and papaverine derivatives (e.g. verapamil). They are quite similar in their efficacy as antihypertensive agents. They act on different sites to slow calcium influx into vascular smooth muscle cells, causing vasodilation and reduced blood pressure. They have varying degrees of negative inotropic effects, with verapamil having the greatest effect and nicardipine the least. They are, therefore, cautioned or contra-indicated in the presence of heart failure. The Syst-Eur study has shown that dihydropyridine calcium-channel blockers are a suitable alternative for elderly patients when thiazides are ineffective, contra-indicated or not tolerated. These would therefore be a suitable alternative for Mr CT, as they have a minimum of cardiac adverse effects and the vasodilatory effects will help his peripheral vascular disease.

Alpha$_1$-blocking agents, such as prazosin, doxazosin and terazosin, act as vasodilators upon both arterioles and veins. They have the advantages of not decreasing cardiac output, and of having a positive effect on cholesterol and triglyceride levels. Also, they would not exacerbate the peripheral vascular disease suffered by Mr CT. However, there is a risk of first-dose and postural hypotension, particularly with prazosin. The newer agents can be prescribed as single daily doses. If Mr CT proves unable to tolerate a calcium-channel blocker, or if calcium-channel blocker therapy proved to be ineffective, one of these agents would be the logical next step.

Other possibilities include methyldopa, hydralazine and minoxidil. Methyldopa has been shown to decrease mortality due to stroke in elderly patients, but has central nervous system side-effects including sedation. This limits its usefulness in elderly patients. Hydralazine and minoxidil are direct-acting vasodilators, but their adverse effects limit their use to situations where other agents have been shown to be ineffective. Clonidine, guanethidine and reserpine are used only in the last resort, in combination with other agents, due to their side-effect profiles.

Further reading

Bosch J, Yusuf S, Pogue J *et al*. Use of ramipril in preventing stroke: double blind randomised trial. *Br Med J* 2002; **324**: 699–702.

Dahlof B, Devereux RB, Kjeldsen SE *et al*. Cardiovascular morbidity and mortality in the Losartan Intervention For Endpoint reduction in hypertension study (LIFE): a randomised trial against atenolol. *Lancet* 2002; **359**: 995–1005.

Dahlof B, Lindholm LH, Hanson L *et al*. Morbidity and mortality in the Swedish trial in old patients with hypertension (STOP-Hypertension). *Lancet* 1991; **338**: 1281–1285.

Dickerson JE, Hingorani AD, Ashby MJ *et al*. Optimisation of anti-hypertensive treatment by crossover rotation of four major classes. *Lancet* 1999; **253**: 2008–2013.

Duggan J. Benefits of treating hypertension in the elderly: should age affect treatment decisions? *Drugs and Ageing* 2001; **18**: 631–618.

Hansson L. How far should we lower blood pressure in the elderly? *Cardiovasc Drugs Therapy* 2001; **15**: 275–279.

Hansson L, Zanchetti A, Carruthers SG *et al*. Effects of intensive blood-pressure lowering and low-dose aspirin in patients with hypertension: principal results of the Hypertension Optimal Treatment (HOT) ran-domised trial. *Lancet* 1990; **335**: 827–838.

Heart Outcomes Prevention Evaluation Study Investigators. Effects of an angiotensin-converting-enzyme inhibitor, ramipril on cardiovascular events in high-risk patients. *N Engl J Med* 2000; **342**: 145–153.

Kaplan NM. Ethnic aspects of hypertension. *Lancet* 1994; **344**: 450–452.

Kinirons M, Jackson S. Hypertension in the elderly. *Practitioner* 1997; **241**: 686–690.

Lever AF, Ramsey LE. Treatment of hypertension in the elderly. *J Hypertens* 1995; **13**: 571–579.

Medical Research Council Working Party. MRC trial of treatment of hyper-tension in older adults: principal results. *Br Med J* 1992; **304**: 505–412.

National High Blood Pressure Education Program Working Group Report on Hypertension in the Elderly. *Hypertension* 1994; **23**: 275–285.

Mulrow CD, Cornell JA, Herrera CR *et al.* Hypertension in the elderly. Implications and generalizability of randomized trials. *J Am Med Assoc* 1994; **272**: 1932–1938.

O'Donnell CJ, Kannel WB. Epidemiological appraisal of hypertension as a coronary risk factor in the elderly. *Am J Geriat Cardiol* 2002; **11**: 86–92.

Raynor DK. Patient compliance: the pharmacist's role. *Int J Pharm Pract* 1992; **1**: 126–135.

Ramsay L, Williams B, Johnston G *et al.* Guidelines for the management of hypertension: report of the third working party of the British Hypertension Society. *J Hum Hypertens* 1999; **13**: 569–592.

SHEP Co-operative Research Group. Prevention of stroke by anti-hypertensive drug treatment in older persons with isolated systolic hypertension. *J Am Med Assoc* 1991; **265**: 3255–3264.

Staessen JA, Fargard R, Thijis L *et al.* For the Systolic Hypertension-Europe (Syst-Eur) Trial Investigators. Morbidity and mortality in the placebo-controlled European Trial on Isolated Hypertension in the Elderly. *Lancet* 1997; **360**: 757–764.

West R, McNeill A, Raw A. Smoking cessation guidelines for health care professionals: an update. *Thorax* 2000, **55**: 987–999.

Wood DA, Durrington P, Poulter N *et al.* (on behalf of the Societies). Joint British recommendations on prevention of coronary heart disease in clinical practice. *Heart* 1998; **80**(suppl. 2): S1–S29.

Useful addresses

National Service Framework for Older People and the National Service Framework for Coronary Heart Disease can be found on the Department of Health website www.doh.gov.uk/nsf/. Examples of patients' experiences of hypertension and links to other patient-related medical sites can be found on the DIPex website: www.dipex.org

Leaflets

BHS information service
www.hyp.ac.uk/bhsinfo
www.hyp.ac.ul/bhs

Smoking cessation
wwww.givingupsmoking.co.uk

General information for patients
www.hbpf.org.uk
www.medlinfo.co.uk
www.healthnet.org.uk

4

Cardiac failure

Stephen A Hudson and John McAnaw

Day 1 Mrs HMc, a 71-year-old lady weighing 53 kg who had been treated for chronic heart failure for three years, was referred to hospital by her GP with a suspected exacerbation. She had been well until three months earlier, when she had started complaining of increasing tiredness, some difficulty sleeping, and shortness of breath on walking and also at night. Mrs HMc also reported periods of discomfort in the chest, which she described as 'palpitations' rather than tightness or pain. Mrs HMc also has a history of atrial fibrillation and hypertension.

Medication on admission:

- Bendroflumethiazide 2.5 mg daily
- Furosemide 40 mg daily
- Enalapril 10 mg daily
- Digoxin 125 micrograms daily
- Warfarin 3 mg daily
- Co-codamol 8/500 tablets, two when required

On examination she was pale and her temperature was 37.3°C, pulse 130 beats per minute and irregular, and her blood pressure (lying) was 155/89 mmHg. Her jugular venous pulse was elevated 3 cm, and pitting oedema was present in both feet and ankles. The apex of the beat was difficult to locate, and crepitations were present in the right and left lung fields. There was slight enlargement of the liver beyond the costal margin, but no tenderness. The results of plasma biochemistry and haematology investigations on admission were:

- Sodium 137 mmol/L (reference range 135–145)
- Potassium 3.7 mmol/L (3.5–5.0)
- Urea 12.4 mmol/L (2.6–6.6)
- Creatinine 140 micromol/L (80–120)
- Haemoglobin 10.1 g/dL (12–16)

- Mean cell volume 71 femtolitres (77–91)
- Mean cell haemoglobin concentration 0.30 g/dL (0.32–0.36)

- Digoxin 1.0 microgram/L (0.8–2)

An electrocardiogram (ECG) demonstrated rapid atrial fibrillation (AF) without ischaemic changes or signs of infarction. An echocardiogram confirmed left ventricular systolic dysfunction with an ejection fraction of 35%.

A diagnosis was made of cardiac failure, complicated by the presence of atrial fibrillation and anaemia associated with iron-deficiency.

Q1 How can atrial fibrillation and anaemia exacerbate cardiac failure in a patient such as Mrs HMc?
Q2 What symptoms of cardiac failure does Mrs HMc exhibit?
Q3 What are the immediate therapeutic aims for Mrs HMc?
Q4 What evidence-based treatments should be considered for Mrs HMc, and why?
Q5 Can a knowledge of digoxin pharmacokinetics guide digoxin dose optimisation? What dose would you recommend for Mrs HMc?

Day 5 Mrs HMc was discharged home with a New York Heart Association (NYHA) functional assessment of II/III and on the following medication:

- Digoxin 187.5 micrograms once daily
- Furosemide 40 mg each morning
- Enalapril 10 mg twice daily

- Ferrous sulphate 200 mg three times daily after food
- Warfarin 3 mg daily
- Bisoprolol 1.25 mg daily

A two-week follow-up appointment was arranged.

Q6 Outline your pharmaceutical care plan for Mrs HMc.

Day 20 Mrs HMc was seen in the out-patient heart failure clinic. She still seemed to be symptomatic at home and had some difficulty in climbing stairs. Oedema was still present in both ankles and her pulse was 108 beats per minute.

Q7 Which medical conditions and drug treatments are known to exacerbate cardiac failure?
Q8 What is the likely explanation for Mrs HMc's persisting cardiac failure?

Mrs HMc's digoxin dose was increased to 250 micrograms daily, and her diuretic requirements were increased to furosemide 40 mg each morning and 20 mg at lunchtime. She was asked to return to clinic in two weeks.

Day 35 Mrs HMc was visited at home by her GP after a week-long deterioration in her condition. She felt unwell, tired but restless and nauseated. She had been unsociable and had not been out of the house for three days. She was readmitted to hospital with suspected digoxin toxicity.

Q9 What symptoms might lead you to suspect digoxin toxicity?

Q10 What is the role of plasma digoxin assay and when should blood samples be drawn?

Q11 What clinical factors predispose patients to digoxin toxicity, and why do you think Mrs HMc might be demonstrating these symptoms?

On examination in hospital Mrs HMc's pulse was found to be 52 beats per minute and regular. She was still nauseated, withdrawn and a little confused. An ECG demonstrated sinus rhythm with no abnormalities. Blood was sampled for urea, electrolytes, international normalised ratio (INR) and plasma digoxin. Her plasma potassium was 3.7 mmol/L (3.5–5.0) and her plasma digoxin concentration was 2.7 micrograms/L (1.0–2.0).

Q12 What are the cardiac effects of digoxin toxicity?

Q13 Apart from stopping the drug, how can digoxin toxicity be managed?

Due to Mrs HMc demonstrating signs and symptoms of digoxin toxicity at the plasma digoxin concentration required to control her AF, digoxin was discontinued and amiodarone commenced. She improved mentally within 24 hours and became mobile over the following two days. She was discharged after five days on the following therapy:

- Furosemide 40 mg each morning, and 20 mg at lunchtime
- Enalapril 10 mg twice daily
- Amiodarone 200 mg three times a day
- Ferrous sulphate 200 mg three times daily after food
- Warfarin 3 mg daily
- Bisoprolol 5 mg daily

Q14 What issues would you add to or change in the pharmaceutical care plan originally developed for Mrs HMc and described in Answer 6?

Day 70 Mrs HMc was complaining of increasing shortness of breath and further ankle swelling.

Q15 What treatment options might you consider next to manage Mrs HMc's cardiac failure?

How can atrial fibrillation and anaemia exacerbate cardiac failure in a patient such as Mrs HMc?

A1 **The heart fails when its output falls short of the perfusion needs of the tissues. This may present as 'low-output' or 'high-output' failure. Mrs HMc's persistent arrhythmia could be contributing to low-output failure, or her iron-deficiency anaemia to high-output failure.**

'Low-output' failure can occur when the heart pump is compromised by ventricular damage (e.g. ischaemia or infarction), persistent arrhythmia, valve disorder or outflow obstruction which results in a reduction in the rate of oxygen and nutrient delivery to the tissues.

In AF, the contractions of the atria are disorganised and frequent electrical impulses (more than 600 per minute) pass down the conducting fibres. The ventricles cannot contract at this rate, owing to the refractoriness of the conducting system (the atrio-ventricular node). Instead they contract irregularly, at a rate usually between 100 and 200 beats per minute. Cardiac output is reduced as a result of reduced ventricular filling arising from the loss of normal atrial contraction and the short diastole (caused by the high ventricular rate).

The poor control of Mrs HMc's AF is thus likely to be exacerbating her cardiac failure. This may be reversed by an improvement in the control of her AF.

'High-output' failure can occur in the presence of iron-deficiency anaemia, where the capacity for the blood to transport oxygen to the tissues is reduced due to the low haemoglobin content of the red cells. In response to severe depletion of oxygen the heart can increase cardiac output in an effort to increase the blood supply to the tissues and therefore compensate for the reduced rate of oxygen delivery. The resulting increased demands placed on the heart can exacerbate symptoms of cardiac failure in a patient such as Mrs HMc.

What symptoms of cardiac failure does Mrs HMc exhibit?

A2 **Dyspnoea, oedema and raised jugular venous pulse, pallor, and tiredness.**

In a patient with stable heart failure, presenting symptoms are often described using the NYHA classification of functional status outlined overleaf. This system allows the grading of heart failure symptoms

NYHA classification of functional status of the patient with heart failure	
I	No symptoms with ordinary physical activity (such as walking or climbing stairs)
II	Slight limitation with dyspnoea on moderate to severe exertion (climbing stairs or walking uphill)
III	Marked limitation of activity: less than ordinary activity causes dyspnoea (restricting walking distance and limiting climbing to one flight of stairs)
IV	Severe disability, dyspnoea at rest (unable to carry on physical activity without discomfort)

experienced by the patient by severity, and is frequently used to describe populations of heart failure patients studied in clinical trials.

Dyspnoea occurs on exertion and on lying down (orthopnoea). Orthopnoea may progress to attacks of gasping at night, termed paroxysmal nocturnal dyspnoea, which are relieved by sitting or standing up. These symptoms arise from a reduced output from the left ventricle, which in turn results in an impaired blood supply to the tissues and organs where the function of muscle, kidney and nervous systems are particularly affected. Mrs HMc could be described as NYHA Stage II/III.

In cardiac failure, retention of sodium and fluid leads to oedema collecting in the lungs, ankles, wrists and abdomen. When the patient is lying down, oedema is redistributed, and in the lungs this produces cough or breathlessness.

Congestion of blood in the lungs produces increased pulmonary capillary pressure which leads to pulmonary oedema and shortness of breath. Due to the reduced compliance of the congested lungs, more effort is required to expand them. Failure of the right ventricle leads to congestion and oedema in the peripheral tissues. Venous congestion may be demonstrated in the reclining patient by visible elevation of the jugular venous pulse in the neck.

Muscle fatigue resulting from the decreased blood supply further diminishes tolerance to exercise. Symptoms are often insidious in onset, especially in the elderly, as patients may adjust their lifestyle to accommodate a loss of tolerance to exercise. Other symptoms resulting from a reduced blood supply to the tissues of the brain, kidneys, liver and gut are confusion, renal failure, enlargement of the liver (hepatomegaly) and abdominal distension, anorexia, nausea, and abdominal pain. The patient's complexion may be pale, and the hands cold and sweaty, due to stimulation of the sympathetic nervous system in response to reduced cardiac output.

What are the immediate therapeutic aims for Mrs HMc?

A3   (a)   **Treat her AF to control the ventricular rate.**

Digoxin is recommended for use in patients with heart failure and concurrent atrial fibrillation. It is often highly effective; however, plasma drug concentrations at the upper end of the therapeutic range of 0.8–2 micrograms/L are normally required. Digoxin causes an increase in myocardial intracellular ionic calcium secondary to the inhibition of sodium extrusion from the myocardial cell. The positive inotropic effect secures the contractile force of the myocardium; however, this effect of digoxin may not be maintained during long-term administration. Concentrations of digoxin above 1.5 micrograms/L usually result in a reduction in electrical discharge from the sino-atrial node, together with a slowing of conduction and increasing refractoriness of the atrioventricular node. It is digoxin's effects on the atrio-ventricular node that are relevant to the management of AF and the subsequent control of ventricular rate.

   (b)   **Investigate and treat her suspected iron-deficiency anaemia.**

A dietary and drug history is required, together with any history of blood loss from the body (e.g. gastrointestinal, post-menopausal, urinary). Laboratory tests should include serum iron, total iron-binding capacity and serum ferritin levels, to confirm or refute true iron-deficiency. Treatment would most likely involve the use of ferrous sulphate tablets 200 mg three times daily. A course of oral iron treatment may last up to six months. This is to ensure that body iron stores are replenished, which necessitates treatment continuing beyond the restoration of haemoglobin concentration to within normal limits.

   (c)   **Control her oedema and symptoms of cardiac failure.**

Diuretic therapy is normally prescribed for the control of sodium and water retention, although Mrs HMc's oedema may reduce once her AF and the associated cardiac failure are successfully controlled.

   There are two main classes of diuretic available for the treatment of cardiac failure: thiazides and loop diuretics. Thiazides are not usually used as sole diuretic therapy, being reserved for cases of very mild cardiac failure where renal function is not compromised. Most patients with symptoms of cardiac failure require a more potent loop diuretic, usually bumetanide or furosemide. Torasemide is a newer loop diuretic but seems to offer little advantage over the previous two drugs in this class, although there is little experience with its use in practice.

Loop diuretics produce a more vigorous diuresis than thiazides, and thus carry a greater risk of causing hypovolaemia in the short-term. A too rapid and profound diuresis can exacerbate cardiac failure by reducing the circulating blood volume and can also increase the patient's uraemia (pre-renal azotemia). In practice, furosemide 40 mg is considered equipotent to bumetanide 1 mg. Clinical trials indicate that 5–10 mg torasemide is equivalent to furosemide 40 mg. Thiazides, on the other hand, produce a less profound diuresis, but pose the greater long-term risk of hypokalaemia and hyponatraemia, particularly in elderly patients. The thiazides have a longer duration of action (average 12–24 hours) than the loop diuretics (average four to six hours), but have a low ceiling effect. Bendroflumethiazide produces a maximum effect at 5 mg: any further increase in dose provides no added benefit, but increases the chance of adverse effects such as hyperglycaemia and hyperuricaemia.

Thiazide diuretics also lose effectiveness when renal function is markedly impaired, particularly when the patient's creatinine clearance is below 25 mL/min. For these reasons, thiazide use in cardiac failure is usually reserved as an add-on to a loop diuretic in order to produce a synergistic effect. Metolazone in particular is reserved for synergistic use with a loop diuretic and can produce profound diuresis with potentially dramatic effects on electrolyte balance.

Mrs HMc is exhibiting signs and symptoms of acute congestive cardiac failure (CCF) whilst being prescribed furosemide 40 mg, therefore an increase in dose is warranted during her hospital stay to control these symptoms. Due to this increase in her diuretic dose, Mrs HMc's potassium level must be monitored closely, as hypokalaemia increases the risk of digoxin toxicity. If required, potassium-sparing diuretics or adequate potassium supplements (e.g. 40–80 mmol/day) should be co-prescribed. Combination diuretic plus potassium products such as Burinex K (bumetanide 0.5 mg plus potassium 7.7 mmol) are not suitable as their potassium content is too low.

(d)   Ensure effective antithrombotic prophylaxis.

AF predisposes to stroke, particularly in patients with rheumatic heart disease, congestive heart failure, arterial hypertension, diabetes mellitus or uncontrolled thyrotoxicosis. Recent randomised controlled trials have investigated the use of warfarin and aspirin for the prevention of first stroke (primary prevention) or further stroke (secondary prevention) in patients with AF. These trials have shown that anticoagulation reduces the risk of thromboembolic stroke by two-thirds in men and women with persistent or paroxysmal non-rheumatic AF. Anticoagulation mainly has a role in primary prevention of stroke, with some benefit also shown in the prevention of a further stroke for those with a history of stroke. Warfarin should therefore be a therapeutic option for those patients over 65 years of age with non-valvular AF and at least one other risk factor for stroke. In the case of Mrs HMc, three risk factors are present: age over 65, history of hypertension and presence of heart failure. Therefore warfarin is the best treatment option for her. However, the benefits and risks of warfarin therapy should be considered very carefully in those patients over 75 years old. Only where warfarin is refused by the patient or contra-indicated should the use of aspirin 75–300 mg be considered. Although aspirin is considered to be a safer option, and a simpler and cheaper alternative to warfarin in the prevention of stroke in patients with AF over the age of 75, it is less effective than warfarin. In patients with AF under 65 years with no risk factors for stroke such as diabetes mellitus or hypertension, the benefits of anticoagulant therapy are marginal (less than 2% reduction of risk).

(e)   Control her blood pressure.

Control of underlying hypertension is important in order to reduce her risk of haemorrhagic stroke and other cardiovascular problems such as coronary heart disease, myocardial infarction and organ damage. The optimum blood pressure to be achieved in Mrs HMc is < 140/85 mmHg, therefore her current blood pressure of 155/89 mmHg demonstrates poor blood pressure control. Mrs HMc is currently prescribed two anti-hypertensive agents (bendroflumethiazide 2.5 mg daily, and enalapril 10 mg daily) but there is scope to reduce her blood pressure by further optimising the dose of angiotensin-converting enzyme inhibitor (ACEI).

What evidence-based treatments should be considered for Mrs HMc, and why?

A4   **In recent years a number of studies have demonstrated benefits in morbidity and mortality for patients with chronic heart failure due to left ventricular systolic dysfunction. The resulting evidence base for treatment supports the use of ACEIs, beta-blockers, low-dose spironolactone, angiotensin II antagonists (AIIA) and hydralazine/nitrate combinations. Although digoxin has been shown to improve morbidity and reduce the number of hospital admissions in patients with heart failure, its effect on mortality is still controversial.**

(a)   ACEIs. Large studies (CONSENSUS II, SOLVD-T, SOLVD-P and V-HeFT II), have shown that ACEIs, in combination with diuretics (with or without digoxin), can improve symptoms and prolong life in all grades of heart failure, as well as improve exercise tolerance. In those patients who have suffered a myocardial infarction, similar improvements in outcomes have also been demonstrated (SAVE, AIREX and TRACE). ACEIs are thus regarded as a 'cornerstone' in the management of heart failure. Progression of heart failure from mild to severe is reduced, as is hospitalisation, and survival is improved in all grades of heart failure. Some conditions, such as renovascular stenosis, aortic stenosis or outflow tract obstruction, are relative contra-indications to ACEIs; however, ACEIs tend to be well tolerated by most patients.

ACEI act upon the renin–angiotensin–aldosterone system, and produce vasodilation by blocking the sequence of events leading to the production of the circulating vasoconstrictor angiotensin II and subsequent effects mediated by aldosterone. Through impairment of aldosterone formation, ACEIs also benefit heart failure by reducing sodium and water retention, thereby reducing venous congestion. The reduction in venous congestion contributes to an improved cardiac output which in turn improves renal perfusion leading to a reduction in oedema. ACEIs are therefore able to interrupt the cycle of secondary physiological events that occur in response to cardiac failure.

The major problems with all ACEIs are first-dose hypotension (worsened by an upright posture), skin rashes and renal toxicity signified by proteinuria. First-dose hypotension is particularly marked in patients who have recently received high doses of diuretics. The sensitivity of blood pressure to the introduction of an ACEI results from the high circulating angiotensin levels which maintain the blood pressure in circumstances of reduced blood volume secondary to diuresis. To minimize acute hypotension, high diuretic doses should thus be curtailed, if possible for a few days prior to starting treatment with the ACEI, and a small first dose of the drug should be administered at bedtime. In patients at risk of hypotension, captopril is most commonly used. Even though captopril has the disadvantage of a faster onset of effect, it has the advantage of a shorter duration of action in the event of an exaggerated response. Other patients at particular risk of this first-dose effect include patients who have activation of the renin–angiotensin system and secondary hyperaldosteronism (such as patients with liver disease).

After the initiation of an ACEI, the dose is titrated towards that used in clinical trials associated with improvements in morbidity and mortality, e.g. enalapril 10–20 mg twice daily. Where a target dose is not achievable in a patient due to poor tolerance, the maximum tolerable dose is an acceptable alternative. As ACEIs can have a pronounced effect on blood pressure, it is important that dose titration towards a target dose is accompanied by blood pressure measurements after each increase in dose.

The ACEIs are all prodrugs apart from captopril and lisinopril. The use of prodrugs means that there may be patient variability in response, affected by the bioavailability and the varying ability of patients to convert the prodrug into the active form. All ACEIs licensed, at the time of writing, for CCF are predominantly eliminated by the kidney and require dosage adjustment in renal failure (creatinine clearance less than 60 mL/min). ACEIs can also impair renal function, although this is most likely to occur in a patient with pre-existing renal impairment or renal artery stenosis. This effect can occur with any member of the class and therefore renal function should be carefully monitored when initiating therapy and after any subsequent increase in dose.

The risk of hyperkalaemia precludes the use of potassium supplements or potassium-sparing diuretics with ACEIs, unless potassium levels are carefully monitored.

Unwanted immunological effects on the skin and proteinuria occur more often with captopril than with the other agents and are thought to be due to its sulphydryl group. However, these are rare side-effects in the usual therapeutic dose range, unless the patient has a connective tissue disorder such as rheumatoid arthritis. Alteration or loss of taste, cough and mouth ulcers are also recognised side-effects of ACEIs, but are not specific to any one agent.

(b)   Beta-blockers. Beta-blockers were previously considered to be contra-indicated in patients with heart failure, however recent clinical trials involving carvedilol, bisoprolol and metoprolol SR (US Carvedilol, CIBIS II, MERIT-HF and COPERNICUS) have shown that they have a beneficial effect on morbidity and mortality in all grades of heart failure as an adjunct to ACEIs and diuretic therapy. In the UK at the time of writing only carvedilol and bisoprolol are licensed for the treatment of patients with chronic heart failure.

Beta-blockers counteract the chronic sympathetic over-activity that occurs when the heart fails to maintain sufficient cardiac output. They inhibit arterial constriction and the direct effects of noradrenaline (norepinephrine) and circulating catecholamines on the heart. These effects reduce the demands placed on the heart, thereby lessening the structural and physiological changes that occur with chronic heart failure. Clinical trial evidence has shown that initiation at a low dose and careful upward titration of dose is necessary to institute beta-blocker therapy safely. Titration is usually carried out over a period of weeks or months, during which time patients are likely to suffer from an initial worsening of symptoms at each dose increment. The goal is to titrate the dose towards the doses used in clinical trials that led to morbidity and mortality benefits, e.g. bisoprolol 5–10 mg daily. However, it is accepted that not all patients will be able to tolerate such doses and therefore the maximum tolerated dose would be an acceptable alternative.

Close monitoring is needed during the initiation and titration of beta-blocker therapy in order to identify excessive bradycardia or marked deterioration of symptoms. The occurrence of these symptoms may limit the use of beta-blocker therapy in certain patients. Other limiting side-effects related to beta-blocker therapy may include fatigue and loss of libido.

(c)   AIIAs. AIIA therapy should only be considered where a patient is truly intolerant of an ACEI, as clinical trials have not shown AIIAs to be superior to ACEIs (ELITE I and ELITE II).

AIIAs can reduce sodium and water retention by preventing the release of aldosterone (reduction in venous congestion), and angiotensin II-mediated arterial vasoconstriction (reduction in afterload). As with the ACEIs, these effects combine to improve cardiac output and renal perfusion, thus leading to an improvement in symptoms and a reduction in oedema.

ACEIs remain the agent of choice in the treatment of heart failure, therefore AIIAs are mainly used where there is true intolerance to an ACEIs or where side-effects are extremely troublesome for the patient, such as a persisting dry cough. As with the use of ACEIs, monitoring of renal function and plasma potassium concentration is important on initiation of therapy or after any increase in dose. This is of particular importance in more elderly patients or those who have a compromised renal function.

(d)   Hydralazine/nitrate combination. Directly acting agents such as hydralazine and organic nitrates exert a selective action on arteries and veins respectively. Although less effective than the ACEI in reducing mortality, the combination of hydralazine in doses of 300 mg/day with isosorbide dinitrate at a dose of 160 mg/day has been associated with significant improvement in morbidity and mortality (VHeFT and VHeFT II).

The nitrate component leads to vasodilation on the venous side, which reduces the rate of return of blood to the heart and the tendency of the ventricles to overfill. This in turn results in a reduction in pulmonary congestion and a reduction in symptoms. In order to achieve a balanced effect on the heart, nitrates are mostly used in combination with an arterial vasodilator such as hydralazine, which reduces the arterial pressure against which the heart must work. The net effect is an improvement in cardiac output and a reduction in symptoms.

This combination of hydralazine plus nitrate can be used as an alternative to an ACEI where patients show ACEI intolerance (ACE-induced renal dysfunction or intractable cough) or a contraindication to ACEI use (bilateral renal artery stenosis, aortic stenosis, hypersensitivity). In practice, it is more common to see isosorbide mononitrate being used in conjunction with hydralazine instead of isosorbide dinitrate. This is due to the fact that the isosorbide 5-mononitrate metabolite derived from isosorbide dinitrate is responsible for producing venodilation. To reduce the risk of nitrate tolerance developing, it is important that an asymmetric dosing regimen is used to ensure a nitrate-free period.

There is a need to monitor the compliance of patients prescribed an asymmetric dosing regimen, and to monitor for side-effects such as postural hypotension, headache or dizziness. As there is a risk of hydralazine-induced systemic lupus erythematosus, it is also important to monitor patients for the appearance of a rash on the face (shaped like a butterfly) or neck.

(e) Digoxin. Digoxin has been shown to have a neutral effect on mortality, but is associated with a reduction in hospital re-admission rate and an improvement in symptoms of patients who remain symptomatic despite adequate doses of an ACEI and diuretics (DIG). Digoxin is recommended for use in NYHA III–IV heart failure as an adjunct to ACEI and diuretic therapy. Other studies have shown that when digoxin is discontinued in patients in sinus rhythm, there is a worsening of symptoms (RADIANCE and PROVED), therefore only a trial of digoxin discontinuation can demonstrate whether a patient in sinus rhythm is continuing to benefit from the drug.

As discussed earlier, digoxin increases the force of contraction of the heart through direct stimulation of the heart muscle, thereby improving cardiac output. It also improves cardiac output in patients with atrial fibrillation through suppression of the atrioventricular node and control of ventricular rate. There is also some evidence to show that digoxin is linked to a decrease in sympathetic nerve activity as well as increased vagal stimulation. Both of these actions may be involved in the beneficial effects seen with digoxin.

Although the use of digoxin is associated with the treatment of atrial fibrillation, its use for patients with heart failure in sinus rhythm can lead to improved symptom control with much lower doses than those used to treat atrial fibrillation. There are no target plasma drug concentrations for the use of digoxin in sinus rhythm, therefore the dose is titrated against the symptoms. Due to the long half-life associated with digoxin and the fact that it has a narrow therapeutic range, initiation of treatment involves the calculation of a suitable loading dose and subsequent maintenance dose to give to the patient. This will ensure that the plasma drug concentration is within the accepted range. Although drugs like digoxin with a low therapeutic index require close patient monitoring for signs and symptoms of toxicity or lack of effect, routine plasma drug concentration monitoring is not recommended. Therapeutic drug monitoring is usually reserved for the confirmation or exclusion of toxicity, assessment of compliance or confirmation of the plasma drug concentration following an increase in dose. Thus, most of the monitoring of digoxin therapy involves clinical assessment to identify poor control of symptoms, or to detect potential toxicity evidenced by symptoms such as nausea, vomiting, depressed appetite, visual disturbances or diarrhoea.

(f)   Spironolactone. Spironolactone has been proven to decrease mortality significantly in patients with NYHA III–IV grades of heart failure at a dosage of 25 mg daily in patients who are already receiving standard therapy including ACEIs, diuretics and digoxin (RALES).

Spironolactone is an aldosterone antagonist, and therefore prevents aldosterone-mediated sodium and water retention, sympathetic activation and parasympathetic inhibition, all of which have a detrimental effect on the failing heart. Spironolactone also helps provide a more complete blockade of the renin–angiotensin–aldosterone system, which is activated in the presence of heart failure.

Spironolactone should now be considered as a standard addition to therapy for patients with a functional assessment of NYHA III–IV where there are persisting symptoms despite adequate treatment with an ACEI and diuretic. Although this agent is potassium-sparing, the low dose has been shown to have a minimal effect on plasma potassium concentrations when used in combination with an ACEI (potassium-conserving).

Although the use of spironolactone at a dose of 25 mg daily has been shown to be safe in conjunction with an ACEI it is still important that plasma potassium is carefully monitored and practitioners must be vigilant for any signs and symptoms of hyperkalaemia developing.

In summary, the place of the agents discussed can be expressed in an algorithm where the use/addition of therapeutic agents is linked to NYHA functional assessment as follows:

Grade of heart failure symptoms	Drug therapy indicated
No symptoms (NYHA I)	**ACEI** If contra-indicated or poorly tolerated, consider **AIIA** or either **digoxin** or **hydralazine + isosorbide dinitrate**
Symptoms (NYHA II)	Addition of diuretic (usually loop diuretic). Where appropriate, consider **carvedilol** or **bisoprolol** (both licensed for use in heart failure in the UK)
Symptoms (NYHA III or IV)	Where appropriate, consider further addition of **carvedilol** or **bisoprolol** **spironolactone** **digoxin** **metolazone** **hydralazine + isosorbide dinitrate**

It is important to point out that although most of the above combinations have been shown to improve symptoms, the Val-HeFT III trial highlighted that the combination of an ACEI, an AIIA plus a beta-blocker led to an increase in mortality and therefore this combination should be avoided.

Can a knowledge of digoxin pharmacokinetics guide digoxin dose optimisation? What dose would you recommend for Mrs HMc?

A5 **Yes. Digoxin pharmacokinetics are relevant to the selection of a dosage regimen both when the drug is being initiated or when it is adjusted, as in Mrs HMc's case. Mrs HMc should**

**have her dose increased to 187.5 micrograms daily. In order
to achieve steady-state plasma levels rapidly, she should first
receive a loading dose of 500 micrograms (given as
250 micrograms twice daily for one day only).**

Therapeutic plasma concentrations of digoxin (1–2 micrograms/L) will
not be achieved until concentrations in the body compartments are
equilibrated. Digoxin is slowly absorbed and bioavailability is incomplete. Digoxin is only 25% bound to plasma proteins and the drug
distributes slowly into a large apparent volume of distribution (approximately 7 L/kg body weight). Thus, to ensure a rapid onset of the drug's
therapeutic effects when therapy is initiated, most patients are given a
loading dose of digoxin. As 99% of digoxin in the body is tissue-bound,
primarily to skeletal and cardiac muscle and minimally within body fat, a
suitable oral loading dose can be calculated from the patient's lean body
weight on the basis of 12–15 micrograms/kg. As Mrs HMc is a thin
woman, her actual body weight should have been used to calculate the
dose, so a suitable loading dose at the initiation of digoxin therapy would
have been approximately 795 micrograms orally, that is 750 micrograms
given as three doses of 250 micrograms at six-hourly intervals to reduce
side-effects of nausea and vomiting.

If Mrs HMc had been in urgent need of digitalisation at the time of
digoxin initiation, e.g. if she had been suffering from acute dyspnoea as a
result of her cardiac failure, intravenous digoxin therapy might have been
more appropriate to control her tachycardia. An intravenous dosage
regimen must, however, take into account the increased bioavailability of
the drug by this route: the dose should be 70% of that calculated for oral
administration and the total dose should, whenever possible, be divided
into aliquots, with an interval of one to two hours between injections to
allow proper clinical evaluation. However, digitalisation in hospital often
requires only the use of oral digoxin administered at suitable intervals
over six to 24 hours.

If a loading dose is not given to the patient on initiation of therapy,
then the maximum clinical effect of a maintenance dose (MD) would
only be seen after the serum digoxin level is at steady state (i.e. when
digoxin excretion equals daily digoxin intake), which is usually after four
or five half-lives. In Mrs HMc's case, this would have been 17–21 days.

When calculating an appropriate MD of digoxin for Mrs HMc,
several factors need to be considered. The first is her renal function. The
half-life of digoxin is normally 36–40 hours. Since the drug is excreted
approximately 70% unchanged in the urine, any impairment of renal
function will extend the half-life and must therefore be taken into

account. Mrs HMc's plasma creatinine level can be used to estimate her creatinine clearance (CrCl). When the equation of Cockcroft and Gault is used, it can be calculated that Mrs HMc has a CrCl of 27 mL/min, which indicates that caution must be taken in choosing an MD. The extension of digoxin half-life can be calculated from:

$$\text{Extension in half-life} = \frac{1}{(1 - Fe) + (Rf \times Fe)}$$

where Fe = fraction of drug excreted unchanged in urine (for digoxin, 0.7) and Rf = fraction of normal renal function (patient's CrCl/100, for Mrs HMc = 0.27).

For Mrs HMc, the calculated extension in half-life is 2, i.e. her predicted digoxin half-life is double that of a person with normal renal function. Thus, as a guide, her renal impairment should be compensated for by a 50% reduction in MD.

The choice of MD can also be guided by estimating the proportion of the loading dose that will be excreted each day, and which must therefore be replaced, using the formula:

% loading dose excreted each day = (14% + patient's CrCl/5)

For Mrs HMc, this gives a figure of 19% of the loading dose being excreted each day. If the loading dose were 750 micrograms, then the MD should be 142 micrograms.

A third method of calculating an appropriate MD is to use population values from reference texts. To do this the patient's renal function, expressed as CrCl, is first estimated using the Cockcroft and Gault equation. The estimated CrCl can then be used to predict the digoxin clearance for the patient. If the patient is more than 15% overweight their ideal body weight rather than their true body weight should be used in these calculations.

Digoxin clearance (ml/min/kg) = 0.88 CrCl (ml/min/kg) + 0.33

where 0.88 is a coefficient which allows for a degree of heart failure (if no heart failure then coefficient = 1). It is then necessary to convert digoxin clearance in mL/min/kg into L/h for the next stage:

$$\text{Average steady-state level of digoxin } (C_{ss}) = \frac{F \times S \times D}{Cl \times \tau}$$

where F = bioavailability (0.6 for tablets), S = salt factor = 1, D = dose (in micrograms), Cl = digoxin clearance (in L/h) and τ = dosing interval (in hours). If it is necessary to convert the plasma concentration from micrograms/L to nanomol/L, then the C_{ss} value must be multiplied by 1.28.

Using this method, doses of 125, 187.5 and 250 micrograms would predict levels of approximately 1.3, 1.9 and 2.5 micrograms/L, respectively, for Mrs HMc. This method can also be used in reverse after a plasma concentration has been measured, in order to calculate a patient's true digoxin clearance. This individualised clearance estimate can then be used when calculating the effects of altering dosages; however, as linear kinetics apply and plasma concentrations vary in proportion to dose, if the dosing interval remains constant, such calculations are often unnecessary. This approach to dosage individualisation only applies if the dosage history is accurate, the sample is taken at the correct time, and the patient's medical condition is stable.

However, these dosing recommendations can only be a guide to Mrs HMc's requirements, as interindividual variations in clinical response limit the usefulness of pharmacokinetic methods. In particular, doses needed to control AF may produce plasma concentrations that would be judged excessive (e.g. 2.5–3.5 micrograms/L) compared with the usually quoted reference range of 1–2 micrograms/L that is relevant to cardiac failure in general. Although in Mrs HMc the MD needs to be reduced because of her renal function, her dose requirement may increase as her renal function improves following the control of her cardiac failure.

Mrs HMc is already on digoxin and her plasma digoxin concentration estimate indicates a need to increase the dose. The required interim loading dose (LD) to increase her plasma digoxin from the present 1.0 micrograms/L to a new target of, say, 1.8 micrograms/L (an increase of 0.8 micrograms/L) can be estimated as:

LD = Target increase (microgram/L) × vol. of distribution of digoxin (L)

Using 7 L/kg as digoxin volume of distribution and knowing Mrs HMc's body weight to be 52 kg:

LD = 0.8 × 7 × 52 = 291 micrograms

This is equivalent to 291/0.6 or 485 micrograms after oral bioavailability (0.6) has been taken into account.

In summary, an MD of 187.5 micrograms/day would be more appropriate for Mrs HMc as it is estimated this will produce a plasma digoxin concentration of approximately 1.9 micrograms/L. The new steady state will take several days to achieve if the MD is merely increased from 125 to 187.5 micrograms, but the required serum concentration can be achieved within 24 hours by giving an oral loading dose of approximately 500 micrograms (prescribed as 250 micrograms twice daily).

Outline your pharmaceutical care plan for Mrs HMc.

A6 **The main points to be considered for her pharmaceutical care plan are as follows:**

(a) Atrial fibrillation
   (i) Ensure appropriate drug therapy is prescribed to control her AF.
   (ii) Ensure an appropriate digoxin maintenance regimen is prescribed.
   (iii) Monitor urea and electrolyte levels regularly, particularly plasma creatinine and potassium.
   (iv) Counsel the patient and advise other health care professionals on the signs and symptoms of digoxin toxicity.

(b) Iron deficiency anaemia
   (i) Ensure an appropriate form and dose of oral iron supplement is prescribed.
   (ii) Counsel the patient on the potential side-effects of oral iron therapy.
   (iii) Monitor relevant haematological markers, e.g. haemoglobin, mean cell haemoglobin concentration.

(c) Cardiac failure
   (i) Ensure appropriate diuretic therapy is prescribed.
   (ii) Monitor the patient for improvement in signs and symptoms of CCF, e.g. decreased shortness of breath, decreased peripheral oedema, etc.
   (iii) Monitor for side-effects/adverse events associated with increased ACEI dosage.
   (iv) Monitor daily weight as a measure of fluid loss or retention to assess the appropriateness of diuretic therapy.
   (v) Monitor patient tolerance of bisoprolol therapy during titration towards target dose.
   (vi) Monitor all prescribed and over-the-counter medication use to ensure that medications known to exacerbate cardiac failure are avoided whenever possible or caution exercised where such a medication is deemed appropriate, e.g. a non-steroidal anti-inflammatory drug (NSAID), corticosteroids, antidepressants, antihistamines.

(d) Antithrombotic therapy
   (i) Ensure future changes to concomitant therapy account for interactions with warfarin.

(ii)   Counsel the patient on the purpose and potential side-effects of warfarin therapy.

(iii) Monitor the patient's INR routinely.

(e)   Control of blood pressure
   (i)   Ensure that control of blood pressure improves in response to changes in Mrs HMc's therapeutic plan.
   (ii) Monitor blood pressure routinely.

Which medical conditions and drug treatments are known to exacerbate cardiac failure?

A7   **Medical conditions include iron-deficiency anaemia, thyrotoxicosis, mitral valve disease and atrial fibrillation. A large number of drug treatments may exacerbate cardiac failure through a variety of mechanisms.**

Drug treatments that can exacerbate cardiac failure include:

(a)   NSAIDs, corticosteroids, carbenoxolone, liquorice, lithium and products containing high sodium levels (effervescent formulations, some antacid preparations) can all cause sodium and/or water retention.

(b)   Tricyclic antidepressants may depress heart function and they may also predispose the patient to cardiac arrhythmias.

(c)   Beta-blockers in high doses produce negative inotropic and chronotropic effects.

(d)   Class I and class III anti-arrhythmic agents (except amiodarone) cause negative inotropic effects and may lead to arrhythmias.

(e)   Calcium-channel blockers (diltiazem, verapamil, first-generation dihydropyridines) all produce negative inotropic and neuroendocrine effects.

(f)   Antihistamines, erythromycin and antifungal agents prolong the QT interval and may lead to arrhythmias.

What is the likely explanation for Mrs HMc's persisting cardiac failure?

A8   **Mrs HMc's pulse rate suggests continuing poor control of her AF.**

Loss of control of cardiac failure and AF may accompany digoxin toxicity, and this possibility needs to be excluded by inquiring about other symptoms of digoxin toxicity. Alternatively, Mrs HMc may be poorly compliant with the current digoxin regimen and this might explain the lack of control.

In her case, compliance was assured and toxicity ruled out, therefore the dose of digoxin prescribed was judged to be still suboptimal for control of AF.

What symptoms might lead you to suspect digoxin toxicity?

A9 **The loss of control of her cardiac failure, her nausea, fatigue and her complaint of restlessness.**

Digoxin toxicity may easily go unrecognised, but is commonly signalled by gastrointestinal and/or central nervous system symptoms. These symptoms may be vague and insidious in onset, such as fatigue, apathy or restlessness, insomnia, confusion, abdominal discomfort or change in bowel habits (especially diarrhoea). More overt signs are anorexia, nausea, vomiting, lethargy and psychosis. Visual disturbances (blurring, haloed or yellow vision, red–green colour blindness) are well documented, but are not often among the first symptoms volunteered by the patient.

What is the role of plasma digoxin assay and when should blood samples be drawn?

A10 **Although digoxin has a low therapeutic index, there is little evidence to support the routine assessment of the plasma digoxin concentration in patients prescribed this medication. Overuse of the digoxin plasma assay is both common and wasteful, and plasma drug concentration measurement should be reserved for the initiation of treatment, confirmation or exclusion of digoxin toxicity, or to confirm patient compliance with the drug. If an assay is appropriate, blood should be sampled for digoxin between six and 24 hours after a dose is administered.**

The slow distribution of the drug confers two-compartment pharmacokinetic characteristics. The equilibration between drug in the plasma and that in the myocardium (and other tissues) continues for up to six hours after a dose. Up to six hours after a dose, the plasma digoxin concentration reflects drug distribution and is unrelated to the amount of digoxin in the tissues, and therefore its effect on the myocardium. In addition, assay results cannot be interpreted if the sampling times are unrecorded or inappropriate.

What clinical factors predispose patients to digoxin toxicity, and why do you think Mrs HMc has experienced symptoms of toxicity?

A11 **Hypokalaemia, hypomagnesaemia, hypercalcaemia, alkalosis, hypoxia and hypothyroidism can all predispose to digoxin toxicity; however, the development of digoxin toxicity in Mrs HMc probably occurred as a result of the high plasma digoxin concentration that appears necessary to control her AF.**

Hypokalaemia, hypercalcaemia and hypomagnesaemia all lead to an increase in responsiveness of tissues to digoxin's cardiac effects and to toxic symptoms in general. The most common contributor to digoxin toxicity is hypokalaemia and plasma digoxin concentrations can only be interpreted in conjunction with a plasma potassium measurement.

Alkalosis and hypoxia also potentiate digoxin toxicity, whereas hypothyroidism increases responsiveness to digoxin and elevates plasma concentrations by decreasing the drug's clearance and apparent volume of distribution.

What are the cardiac effects of digoxin toxicity?

A12 **Arrhythmias and loss of control of cardiac failure.**

Digoxin increases the automaticity and slows conduction in all cardiac cells. Cardiotoxicity may occur without other warning symptoms and the cells of the atrio-ventricular and sino-atrial nodes are particularly affected. Common arrhythmias include atrio-ventricular block with supraventricular tachycardias, junctional or escape rhythms, ventricular ectopic beats and ventricular tachycardia. Sinus bradycardia and sino-atrial arrest may occur. Loss of control of cardiac failure may also be a feature of digoxin toxicity.

Apart from stopping the drug, how can digoxin toxicity be managed?

A13 **By correcting any underlying factors contributing to digoxin toxicity and, if clinically necessary, by using resins or digoxin-specific antibody fragments to increase digoxin elimination.**

If present, hypokalaemia should be corrected, unless the presence of atrio-ventricular block contra-indicates potassium use. When heart block persists, lidocaine and similar anti-arrhythmic agents (such as propranolol and phenytoin) are recommended, and cardiac pacing is indicated.

Attempts to reduce digoxin concentrations by dialysis are ineffective, as 99% of drug in the body is tissue bound and not in the plasma. The use of oral resins such as colestyramine and colestipol (bile acid chelating agents which also bind digoxin) can increase elimination by interrupting enterohepatic circulation of the drug; however, severe toxicity requires the use of the digoxin-specific antibody fragment preparation Digibind by the intravenous route.

Digoxin has a much higher affinity for the digoxin-specific antibody fragment than for its receptor (Na,K-dependent ATPase) and hence is attracted away from its receptors in the heart tissue. The inactive complex that is formed is readily excreted by the kidney. The dosage of digoxin-specific antibody fragment depends on the amount of digoxin to be neutralised. There are various methods available for the calculation of digoxin-specific antibody fragment required, depending upon how the toxicity occurred, the age of the patient and whether or not a measured plasma digoxin concentration is available.

The digoxin level in Mrs HMc's case probably does not warrant the use of digoxin-specific antibody fragment. However, if she showed life-threatening signs of cardiac toxicity after digoxin withdrawal and the correction of any electrolyte imbalances, then digoxin-specific antibody fragment would be an option. Under those circumstances, the formula below should be used to calculate the amount of Digibind required (rounding up to the nearest number of whole vials):

$$\text{Dose (no. of vials)} = \frac{\text{serum digoxin conc. (µg/L)} \times \text{weight (kg)}}{100}$$

For Mrs HMc:

$$\text{Dose} = \frac{3.4 \times 53}{100} = 2 \text{ vials}$$

The contents of each vial would need to be dissolved in sterile Water for Injections by gentle mixing. This solution may then be diluted further to any convenient volume with sterile saline suitable for infusion. The final solution should be infused over a 30-minute period through a 0.22-micrometre membrane filter to remove any incompletely dissolved aggregates of Digibind.

Under circumstances in which cardiac arrest is imminent, then Digibind can be given as a bolus intravenous injection. ECG and electrolyte monitoring are required for at least 24 hours following Digibind administration.

What issues would you add to or change in the pharmaceutical care plan originally developed for Mrs HMc, and described in Answer 6?

A14 **Pharmaceutical care activity related to the treatment of iron deficiency anaemia, the treatment of cardiac failure, the provision of thromboprophylaxis and the control of blood pressure would remain unchanged, but the plans related to the management of her AF must be changed. In addition, the interaction of amiodarone and warfarin, which is due to inhibition of warfarin metabolism, leads to an increased anticoagulant effect, and would prompt more frequent monitoring of the INR and adjustment of her warfarin dose during the amiodarone titration period.**

In considering which agent to prescribe as a replacement for digoxin, rate-limiting calcium-channel blockers (verapamil, diltiazem, nifedipine) and class I anti-arrhythmic agents were best avoided, due to the fact that they would aggravate Mrs HMc's heart failure. Increasing the dose of beta-blocker might have been attempted as long as Mrs HMc was able to tolerate the higher dose, as this group of agents can still aggravate heart failure symptoms although proven to be beneficial with regard to mor-bidity and mortality. The prescription of amiodarone was thus the most appropriate choice of alternative anti-arrhythmic agent.

The care plan changes around the management of her AF include removal of issues related to the prescription and use of digoxin, with the following additions relating to the introduction of amiodarone.

(a)   Ensure reduction in the daily dose of amiodarone occurs over an acceptable time period to an appropriate maintenance dose.
(b)   Ensure that appropriate control of AF is achieved with amiodarone.
(c)   Monitor thyroid function six-monthly.
(d)   Monitor liver function.
(e)   Counsel the patient and advise other health care professionals on the signs and symptoms of adverse effects of amiodarone therapy.

Amiodarone acts by increasing the refractory period of conducting tissues in the heart. The dose of amiodarone on initiation of therapy is usually 200 mg three times daily, reducing by 200 mg each week until a main-tenance dose of 200 mg daily is achieved (or the lowest dose required to control the arrhythmia). Amiodarone has an unusual pharmacokinetic profile with high protein binding, a very high volume of distribution due to extensive deposition in tissues and also a long half-life (one to two months). Amiodarone can cause hypo- or hyperthyroidism and so baseline and then regular thyroid function tests are essential. It can also produce corneal microdeposits in the eye; vision is usually unaffected although some patients might be dazzled by car headlights at night, therefore this should be discussed with those still intending to drive. Phototoxic skin reactions can also occur and sunscreen protection is often required. Hepatotoxocity is also a risk for patients taking amiodarone, and where signs or symptoms develop therapy must be stopped immediately.

> What treatment options might you consider next to manage Mrs HMc's cardiac failure?

A15 **Optimise her diuretic therapy, consider the reintroduction of digoxin or start treatment with spironolactone.**

Where symptoms of sodium and water retention continue, there is further scope to increase the dose of furosemide being prescribed. In cases where oedema is resistant, the addition of metolazone is often necessary. However, any increase in diuretic therapy will require careful monitoring of Mrs HMc's renal function, and plasma concentrations of potassium and other electrolytes.

Digoxin has been shown to have a neutral effect on survival but to improve symptoms of cardiac failure and reduce the rate of rehospitalisation. The doses required are much less than those needed to control AF, therefore Mrs HMc might still benefit from a reintroduction of this agent. Care must be taken if this option is taken, as the plasma concentration of digoxin is increased by amiodarone, and therefore the clinical and laboratory monitoring for signs and symptoms of digoxin toxicity discussed earlier must be reintroduced.

Although spironolactone is a potassium-sparing diuretic, it can usually be safely prescribed alongside an ACEI at a dose of 25 mg daily without causing hyperkalaemia in patients with NYHA III-IV. When co-prescribed, a more complete block of the renin–angiotensin–aldosterone system is achieved, thus accounting for the additional morbidity and mortality benefits observed in clinical trials. However, there have been cases where hyperkalaemia has developed so monitoring of renal function and plasma electrolytes is mandatory for patients prescribed this combination therapy.

Further reading

Berry C, McMurray J. CHF: a GP guide to management. *Practitioner* 2002; **246**: 669–672, 675–681.

CIBIS-II Investigators and Committees. The Cardiac Insufficiency Bisoprolol Study II (CIBIS-II): a randomised trial. *Lancet* 1999; **353**: 9–13.

Cohn J, Archibald DG, Ziesche S *et al*. Effect of vasodilator therapy on mortality in chronic congestive heart failure. Results of a Veterans Administration Cooperative Study. *N Engl J Med* 1986; **314**: 1547–1552.

Cohn J, Johnson G, Ziesche S *et al*. A comparison of enalapril with hydralazine-isosorbide dinitrate in the treatment of chronic congestive heart failure. *N Engl J Med* 1991; **325**: 303–310.

Cohn JN, Tognoni G. A randomized trial of the angiotensin-receptor blocker valsartan in chronic heart failure. *N Engl J Med* 2001; **345**: 1667–1675.

Hall AS, Murray GD, Ball SG. Follow-up study of patients randomly allocated ramipril or placebo for heart failure after acute myocardial infarction: AIRE Extension (AIREX) Study. Acute Infarction Ramipril Efficacy. *Lancet* 1997; **349**: 1493–1497.

Hermann DD. Beta-adrenergic blockade 2002: a pharmacologic odyssey in chronic heart failure. *Congest Heart Fail* 2002; **8**: 262–269, 283.

Kober L, Torp-Pederson C, Carlsen JE *et al*. A clinical trial of the angiotensin-converting-enzyme inhibitor trandolapril in patients with left ventricular dysfunction after myocardial infarction. Trandolapril Cardiac Evaluation (TRACE) Study Group. *N Engl J Med* 1995; **333**: 1670–1676.

MERIT-HF Study Group, Effect of metoprolol CR/XL in chronic heart failure: Metoprolol CR/XL Randomised Intervention Trial in Congestive Heart Failure (MERIT-HF). *Lancet* 1999; **353**: 2001–2007.

Packer M, Coats AS, Fowler, MB *et al*. Effect of carvedilol on survival in severe chronic heart failure. *N Engl J Med* 2001; **344**: 1651–1658.

Packer M, Gheorgiade M, Young JB *et al*. Withdrawal of digoxin from patients with chronic heart failure treated with angiotensin-converting-enzyme inhibitors. RADIANCE Study. *N Engl J Med* 1993; **329**: 1–7.

Packer M, Bristow MR, Cohn JN *et al*. The effect of carvedilol on morbidity and mortality in patients with chronic heart failure. US Carvedilol Heart Failure Study Group. *N Engl J Med* 1996; **334**: 1349–1355.

Peterson RC, Dunlap ME. Angiotensin II receptor blockers in the treatment of heart failure. *Congest Heart Fail* 2002; **8**: 246–50, 256.

Pfeffer M, Braunwald E, Moye LA *et al*. Effect of captopril on mortality and morbidity in patients with left ventricular dysfunction after myocardial infarction. Results of the survival and ventricular enlargement trial. The SAVE Investigators. *N Engl J Med* 1992; **327**: 669–677.

Pitt B, Zannad F, Remme WJ *et al*. The effect of spironolactone on morbidity and mortality in patients with severe heart failure. Randomized Aldactone Evaluation Study Investigators. *N Engl J Med* 1999; **341**: 709–717.

Pitt B, Poole-Wilson PA, Segal R *et al*. Effect of losartan compared with captopril on mortality in patients with symptomatic heart failure: randomised trial – the Losartan Heart Failure Survival Study ELITE II. *Lancet* 2000; **355**: 1582–1587.

Pitt B, Segal R, Martinez FA *et al*. Randomised trial of losartan versus captopril in patients over 65 with heart failure (Evaluation of Losartan in the Elderly Study, ELITE). *Lancet* 1997; **349**: 747–752.

Rocha R, Williams GH. Rationale for the use of aldosterone antagonists in congestive heart failure. *Drugs* 2002; **62**: 723–731.

Squire B. Angiotensin converting enzyme inhibition in heart failure: clinical trials and clinical practice. *Cardiovasc Drugs Ther* 2002; **16**: 67–74.

Studies of Left Ventricular Dysfunction (SOLVD) Investigators. Effect of enalapril on survival in patients with reduced left ventricular ejection fractions and congestive heart failure. *N Engl J Med* 1991; **325**: 293–302.

Studies of Left Ventricular Dysfunction (SOLVD) Investigators. Effect of enalapril on mortality and the development of heart failure in asymptomatic patients with reduced left ventricular ejection fractions. *N Engl J Med* 1992; **327**: 685–691.

Swedberg K, Held P, Kjekshus J *et al*. Effects of the early administration of enalapril on mortality in patients with acute myocardial infarction. Results of the Co-operative New Scandinavian Enalapril Survival Study II. *N Engl J Med* 1992; **327**: 678–684.

The Digitalis Investigation Group (DIG). The effect of digoxin on mortality and morbidity in patients with heart failure. *N Engl J Med* 1997; **336**: 525–533.

Uretsky B, Young JB, Shahidi FE *et al*. Randomized study assessing the effect of digoxin withdrawal in patients with mild to moderate chronic congestive heart failure: results of the PROVED trial. PROVED Investigative Group. *J Am Coll Cardiol* 1993; **22**: 955–962.

5

Acute renal failure

Kate Richardson

Day 1 Mrs NC, a 69-year-old woman, was admitted urgently at the request of her GP. His letter detailed the following history. Mrs NC had collapsed at the elderly people's home where she lived. The warden said she had been complaining of nausea and loss of appetite for two or three days (her current weight was 51 kg) and had vomited that morning. She had fallen on the previous day but had recovered quickly.

She had a long history of biventricular cardiac failure which had been controlled for some time with furosemide 80 mg in the morning, isosorbide mononitrate 20 mg twice daily and captopril 6.25 mg twice daily, although a degree of ankle oedema had recently necessitated an increase in the dose of furosemide to 120 mg in the morning. However, this increase had precipitated gout, which had been manifested by pain in the distal interphalangeal joint of both great toes. The pain had been treated with diclofenac 50 mg three times daily for the previous 21 days.

The patient herself was a poor historian. On examination she was pale and tired-looking, with sunken eyes. Her pulse was 120 beats per minute while her blood pressure was 105/70 mmHg lying and 85/60 mmHg standing. Ankle oedema was absent and there was no evidence of pulmonary oedema. Her extremities were cold and there was a marked reduction in skin turgor.

Mrs NC's serum biochemistry results were:

- Sodium 131 mmol/L (reference range 135–150)
- Potassium 5.5 mmol/L (3.5–5.0)
- Bicarbonate 17 mmol/L (22–31)
- Creatinine 312 micromol/L (60–110)
- Urea 27.2 mmol/L (3.2–6.6)
- Glucose 4.8 mmol/L (3.5–6.0)
- Mean cell volume 71 femtolitres (77–91)
- Osmolarity 306 mOsmol/kg (275–295)

A diagnosis of sodium and water depletion with consequent renal hypo-perfusion was made. An infusion of 1 L sodium chloride 0.9% every four to six hours was prescribed, and the following investigations were re-quested: full blood count; culture and sensitivity of blood and urine; 24-hour urine collection for determination of creatinine clearance; urinary sodium, urea and osmolarity; chest and abdominal x-ray.

Q1 Could Mrs NC's drug therapy have contributed to her renal problems?

Q2 What is the aim of intravenous sodium chloride 0.9% therapy?

Q3 What would you include in a pharmaceutical care plan for Mrs NC?

Q4 Which methods of assessing and monitoring Mrs NC's status would you recommend?

Day 2 The 24-hour urine collection yielded a volume of only 290 mL. Other data obtained from analysis of Mrs NC's urine included:

- Sodium 43 mmol/L
- Urea 117 mmol/L
- Creatinine 20.12 mmol/L
- Osmolarity 337 mOsmol/kg

The low urine volume obtained despite the concurrent volume expansion indicated that further measures were required to prevent the develop-ment of acute tubular necrosis. Mannitol was considered inappropriate in this patient, so furosemide 250 mg was administered by slow intravenous infusion. A further dose of 500 mg was administered after six hours, but neither dose produced an increase in urine production. A diagnosis of established acute tubular necrosis causing acute renal failure (ARF) was made. The following recommendations were proposed: daily fluid charts; daily weights; daily serum urea and electrolyte estimations; dietary restrictions (consult dietitian).

Q5 Why was mannitol therapy inappropriate for Mrs NC?

Q6 Would you have recommended the use of high-dose intravenous furosemide at this point?

Q7 Would you have used dopamine in this patient?

Q8 What dietary considerations are necessary for Mrs NC?

Day 4 Mrs NC complained of having muscle cramps at night, with the result that quinine sulphate 300 mg at night was prescribed. She also complained of diarrhoea which was described by the nursing staff as black and tarry in appearance. A full blood count revealed a normo-chromic and normocytic anaemia with a haemoglobin of 8.1 g/dL (12–16 g/dL). Ranitidine 150 mg at night was prescribed.

Serum biochemistry results revealed the following:

- Sodium 137 mmol/L (135–150)
- Potassium 7.1 mmol/L (3.5–5.0)
- Calcium 2.04 mmol/L (2.25–2.6)
- Bicarbonate 19 mmol/L (22–31)
- Phosphate 1.8 mmol/L (0.9–1.5)
- Albumin 34 g/L (33–55)
- Urea 31.7 mmol/L (3.2–6.6)
- Creatinine 567 micromol/L (60–110)
- pH 7.28 (7.36–7.44)

A 10-mL bolus dose of calcium gluconate 10% was administered intravenously, immediately followed by an intravenous injection of 10 units of soluble insulin with 50 mL of 50% glucose solution; the latter was written up for three further administrations over the next 12 hours. Therapy with Calcium Resonium 15 g orally four times daily was also initiated. A monitor was ordered to observe for cardiac toxicity; however, no ECG changes were apparent.

Q9 Would you have recommended quinine sulphate 300 mg at night to treat Mrs NC's nocturnal cramps?

Q10 What factors may have contributed to Mrs NC's low haemoglobin? Is ranitidine therapy appropriate?

Q11 Is Mrs NC's hyperkalaemia being treated appropriately? Should Mrs NC's hypocalcaemia, hyperphosphataemia and acidosis be treated at this point?

Q12 What factors should be considered when initiating drug therapy for a patient in ARF?

Day 7 Mrs NC complained of breathlessness which was increased on lying flat and examination showed her to have developed crepitations in both lung bases. She complained of nausea, and was noted to be drowsy and to have developed a flapping tremor.

Her serum biochemistry results included:

- Potassium 6.6 mmol/L (3.5–5.0)
- Bicarbonate 17 mmol/L (22–31)
- Urea 40.5 mmol/L (3.2–6.6)
- Creatinine 588 micromol/L (60–110)
- pH 7.24 (7.36–7.44)

It was decided to treat Mrs NC by haemodialysis. Once haemodialysis had been initiated it was felt that she would be a good candidate for total parenteral nutrition (TPN) and arrangements were made for a Hickmann catheter to be inserted.

Q13 What were the indications for dialysis in Mrs NC?

Q14 What forms of dialysis therapy are available, and what are their advantages and disadvantages?

Q15 What factors affect drug therapy during dialysis?

Q16 What factors would you take into account when formulating a TPN regimen for Mrs NC?

Day 12 Mrs NC developed a temperature of 39.6°C and a tachycardia of 120 beats per minute. Subjectively she complained of headache and feeling 'awful'. A full blood count revealed a neutrophil count of 10.5×10^9/L $(2.2–7.0 \times 10^9)$. A diagnosis of septicaemia was made, and blood samples were sent for culture and sensitivity. All in-dwelling catheters were removed and the following therapy was written up:

- Cefotaxime 1 g intravenously every 12 hours
- Gentamicin 80 mg intravenously every 24 hours
- Metronidazole 500 mg intravenously every eight hours

Q17 Is this therapy appropriate for Mrs NC's septicaemia?

Q18 What are the dangers associated with prescribing gentamicin for Mrs NC? How should her gentamicin therapy be monitored?

Day 14 Microbiological assays revealed the infective organism to be *Staphylococcus aureus*. Gentamicin and metronidazole therapy were discontinued and, as Mrs NC was clinically much improved, cefotaxime was continued as sole antibiotic therapy.

Day 19 Mrs NC, now free of infection, passed over 4 L of urine. It was felt that she was over the worst and that she would continue to improve.

Q19 Did Mrs NC follow the normal course of ARF? What is her prognosis?

Could Mrs NC's drug therapy have contributed to her renal problems?

A1   **Yes. Mrs NC's furosemide and/or diclofenac therapy may have contributed to her admission.**

Mrs NC demonstrates many of the traditional signs of sodium and water depletion, including tachycardia, hypotension, postural hypotension, reduced skin turgor, reduced ocular tension (the cause of the sunken eyes), collapsed peripheral veins and cold extremities. Evidence that Mrs NC had suffered some degree of renal impairment can be seen by the elevation in her serum urea and creatinine levels, together with the other biochemical abnormalities. The symptoms that Mrs NC suffers which cannot be explained by the sodium and water depletion (nausea, loss of appetite and vomiting) can be attributed to her high blood urea level (uraemia). ARF is defined as a rapid deterioration (several hours to several days) of renal function associated with the accumulation of nitrogenous waste in the body that is not due to pre-renal or post-renal factors.

One of the physiological responses to sodium and water depletion is a reduction in renal perfusion, which may in turn lead to intrinsic renal damage with a consequent acute deterioration in renal function. The condition may be caused by any significant haemorrhage, or by septicaemia, in which the vascular bed is dilated thereby reducing the circulating volume. It may also be caused by excessive sodium and water loss from the skin, urinary tract or gastrointestinal tract. Excessive loss through the skin by sweating occurs in hot climates and is rare in the UK, but it also occurs after extensive burns. Gastrointestinal losses are associated with vomiting or diarrhoea. Urinary tract losses often result from excessive diuretic therapy but may also occur with the osmotic diuresis caused by hyperglycaemia and glycosuria in a diabetic patient (for this reason a random blood glucose level was performed on Mrs NC).

Mrs NC had vomited, but seemingly only once, and at a late stage in her illness, so that it was more likely to be a symptom of her condition rather than the cause. It is considerably more likely that her plight has been brought about by the diuresis induced by her recently increased furosemide therapy.

Despite a large blood supply, the kidneys are always in a state of incipient hypoxia because of their high metabolic activity and any condition that causes the kidney to be underperfused may be associated with an acute deterioration in renal function. However, such a deterioration may also be produced by nephrotoxic agents, including drugs. Non-steroidal anti-inflammatory drugs (NSAIDs), in particular, are associated with renal damage and even a short course of an NSAID (such as diclofenac) has been associated with ARF especially in older patients. The main cause of NSAID-induced renal damage is inhibition of prostaglandin synthesis in the kidney, particularly prostaglandins E_2, D_2 and I_2 (prostacyclin). These prostaglandins are all potent vasodilators, and consequently produce an increase in blood flow to the glomerulus and the medulla. In normal circumstances they do not play a large part in the maintenance of the renal circulation; however, in patients with increased amounts of vasoconstrictor substances (such as angiotensin II) in the blood, vasodilatory prostaglandins become important in maintaining renal blood flow. The maintenance of blood pressure in a variety of clinical conditions, such as volume depletion (which Mrs NC has), biventricular cardiac failure (which she had also had) or hepatic cirrhosis with ascites, may rely on the release of vasoconstrictor substances. In these circumstances, inhibition of prostaglandin synthesis may cause unopposed renal arteriolar vasoconstriction, which again leads to renal hypoperfusion. NSAIDs thus impair the ability of the renovasculature to adapt to a fall in perfusion pressure or to an increase in vasoconstrictor balance.

Angiotensin-converting enzyme inhibitors (ACEIs) may also produce a reduction in renal function by preventing the angiotensin II-mediated vasoconstriction of the efferent glomerular arteriole, which contributes to the high-pressure gradient across the glomerulus. This problem is important only in patients with renal vascular disease, particularly those with bilateral stenoses, and is consequently rare. Its aetiology is as follows: when there is a significant degree of renal artery stenosis, renal perfusion falls. To maintain the pressure gradient across the glomerulus, efferent arteriolar resistance must rise. This is predominantly accomplished by angiotensin-induced efferent vasoconstriction. If ACEIs are administered this system is rendered inoperable and there is no longer any way of maintaining effective filtration pressure. This leads to a fall in glomerular filtration rate and ARF. In these circumstances deterioration in renal function is seen shortly after ACEI initiation. As Mrs NC has been taking her captopril therapy for a while, it is unlikely to have contributed to her current problems.

Iatrogenic factors including fluid and electrolyte imbalance and drug nephrotoxicity can be identified in over 50% of cases of hospital-acquired ARF and also play a large role in many cases of community-acquired ARF. It has been estimated that up to 20% of individuals over the age of 65 are prescribed diuretics, with a lesser number receiving NSAIDs; consequently, there is a large population of elderly patients susceptible to renal damage in the event of any insult to the kidney. ARF which requires dialysis is fortunately rare, with only 50–70 patients per million of the population affected annually, but less severe degrees of impairment may occur in up to 5% of hospital in-patients.

What is the aim of intravenous sodium chloride 0.9% therapy?

A2 **The aim of therapy is to restore her extracellular fluid volume.**

The initial therapeutic aim in the management of ARF is immediate correction of reversible causes. Support of renal perfusion, with either volume infusion or therapeutics that improve renal oxygen delivery, should be considered before any attempt to improve urinary flow. The fluid infused should mimic the nature of the fluid lost as closely as possible and should therefore be blood, colloid or saline. Patients should be observed continuously and the infusion stopped when features of volume depletion have been resolved, but before volume overload has been induced.

A diagnosis of acute deterioration of renal function due to renal underperfusion carries with it the implication that restoration of renal perfusion will reverse the renal impairment. Mrs NC is depleted of both water and sodium ions. Sodium chloride 0.9% is therefore an appropriate choice of intravenous fluid, as it replaces both water and sodium ions in a concentration approximately equal to plasma. Situations occasionally arise where a patient is hyponatraemic but not water-depleted, as a result of either sodium depletion or water retention; such a condition may be treated with an infusion containing sodium chloride in excess of its physiological concentration, e.g. sodium chloride 1.8% or higher. Similarly, should water depletion with hypernatraemia occur, isotonic solutions that are either free of, or low in, sodium are available, e.g. glucose 5%, or sodium chloride 0.18% with glucose 4%. Possibly the most common cause of ARF is the peripheral vasodilation which occurs in septic shock. In such cases it would be appropriate to infuse a colloid as well as sodium chloride as this would help restore the circulating volume. It is important to remember, however, that not all shocked patients are hypovolaemic and some, notably those in cardiogenic shock, could be adversely affected by a fluid challenge.

The effect of fluid replacement therapy on urine flow and central venous pressure should be carefully monitored. Central venous pressure provides a guide to the degree of fluid deficit and reduces the risk of pulmonary oedema resulting from over-rapid transfusion. If the kidneys do not respond to replacement treatment, the probable diagnosis is acute tubular necrosis, but it is common practice, although often not correct practice, to try other measures, such as treatment with mannitol and loop diuretics, to try to turn the condition towards recovery.

What would you include in a pharmaceutical care plan for Mrs NC?

A3 **The pharmaceutical care plan for Mrs NC should include the following:**

(a) Her drug therapy must be reviewed in order to ensure that any agents which might be contributing to her condition are discontinued.

(b) It must be ensured that the optimum drug therapy is prescribed to achieve the desired therapeutic outcome.

(c) All drug therapy should be monitored for efficacy and safety.

(d) It is essential that, when it becomes appropriate, Mrs NC is counselled about her prescribed medicines and any other factors which may affect her in the future (e.g. avoidance of over-the-counter NSAIDs).

(e) Mrs NC must be assessed to ensure she can manage her prescribed medication at discharge. Further counselling or compliance aids must be given if appropriate.

(f) Steps must be taken to ensure that prescribed therapy is continued after discharge.

Which methods of assessing and monitoring Mrs NC's status would you recommend?

A4 **(a)   Creatinine clearance (CrCl).**

Creatinine is a byproduct of normal muscle metabolism and is formed at a rate proportional to the mass of muscle. It is freely filtered by the glomerulus, with little secretion or reabsorption by the tubule. When muscle mass is stable, any change in plasma creatinine reflects a change in its clearance by filtration. Consequently, measurement of CrCl gives an estimate of the glomerular filtration rate (GFR). The ideal method of calculating CrCl is by performing an accurate collection of urine over 24 hours and taking a plasma sample midway through this period. The following equation may then be used:

$$\text{CrCl} = \frac{U \times V}{P}$$

where U = urine creatinine concentration (micromol/L), V = urine flow rate (mL/min), P = plasma creatinine concentration (micromol/L). This provides an accurate measure of GFR providing that all of the urine over the 24-hour period is collected.

Using this formula, it is possible to calculate Mrs NC's CrCl as 13 mL/min. A quicker and less cumbersome method is to measure the plasma creatinine concentration and collect those patient factors that affect the mass of muscle, i.e. age, sex and weight (preferably ideal body weight). This allows an estimation of CrCl to be made from average population data. The equation of Cockcroft and Gault is a useful way of making such an estimation:

$$\text{CrCl} = \frac{F \times (140 - \text{age}) \times \text{weight (kg)}}{\text{plasma creatinine (micromol/L)}}$$

where F = 1.04 (females) or 1.23 (males).

Assuming the normal CrCl to be 120 mL/min, this enables classification of renal impairment, as follows: mild, a GFR of 20–50 mL/min; moderate, a GFR of 10–20 mL/min; severe, a GFR of less than 10mL/min. Using the method of Cockroft and Gault, Mrs NC's CrCl can be estimated as 12 mL/min and her renal impairment could thus be classified as moderate verging on severe.

There are however limitations to using this equation and in the following situations caution needs to be exercised when interpreting the assessment:

(i)   Obesity: use ideal body weight (IBW).
(ii) Muscle wasting: CrCl will be overestimated.
(iii) Oedematous patients: use IBW.
(iv) Ascites: use IBW and consider the dilutional effect on serum creatinine.
(v)   ARF: when two serum creatinine levels measured in 24 hours differ by more than 20 micromol/L this may represent non-steady-state serum creatinine levels, therefore the degree of renal impairment may be underestimated. In such instances, urea levels may be a better guide to deteriorating renal function.

(b)   Urine analysis.

A healthy kidney that is underperfused will attempt to compensate for the condition by retaining sodium and water, a response mediated by aldosterone and antidiuretic hormone. Thus, the urine produced will be low in sodium (less than 10 mmol/L), but otherwise concentrated, with a high urea (greater than 250 mmol/L) and osmolarity (greater than 500 mOsmol/kg). However, damaged kidneys fail to reabsorb sodium adequately, which results in high urinary sodium concentrations (greater than 30 mmol/L). In addition, the urea concentration mechanisms fail, which results in reduced urinary urea (less than 150 mmol/L). Urine osmolarity also falls too close to that of plasma. It follows, therefore, that examination of the urine enables assessment of the renal state. Various indexes using these data have been produced, but their value is more theoretical than practical.

(c)   Serum urea levels.

These are commonly used to assess renal function; however, the rate of production of urea is considerably more variable than that of creatinine and it fluctuates throughout the day in response to the protein content of the diet. It may also be elevated by dehydration or an increase in protein catabolism, such as occurs in haemorrhage into the gastrointestinal tract or body tissues, severe infections, trauma (including surgery) and high-dose steroid therapy. The serum urea level is therefore an unreliable measure of renal function, but it is often used as a crude test because it does give information on the patient's general condition and state of hydration.

(d)   Fluid charts and weight.

Fluid charts are frequently used in patients with sodium and water depletion, but they are often inaccurate and should not be relied upon exclusively. Records of daily weight are more reliable but are rarely available before renal failure is diagnosed.

(e)   Central venous pressure.

This is of value in assessing circulating volume. The normal range is 10–15 cm of water.

(f)   Serum electrolyte levels.

Plasma potassium should be measured regularly because hyperkalaemia, which occurs in ARF, may be fatal.

Why was mannitol therapy inappropriate for Mrs NC?

A5 **Mannitol therapy is inappropriate because Mrs NC has cardiac failure.**

The rationale for using mannitol arises from the theory that tubular debris may contribute to the oliguria of ARF by causing mechanical obstruction and that the use of an osmotic diuretic may wash out the debris. A dose of 0.5–1.0 g/kg as a 10–20% infusion is recommended, but only after the circulating volume has been restored (this caution holds true for any diuretic therapy). However, intravenous mannitol will, before producing a diuresis, cause a considerable increase in the extracellular fluid volume by attracting water from the intracellular compartment. This expansion of the extracellular volume is potentially dangerous for patients with cardiac failure, especially if a diuresis is not produced. In addition, mannitol has no renoprotective effects and can cause significant renal impairment by triggering osmotic nephrosis. It may also increase tubular workload by increasing solute delivery.

Would you have recommended the use of high-dose intravenous furosemide at this point?

A6 **Yes, providing Mrs NC is euvolaemic before it is started.**

As well as producing substantial diureses, all loop diuretics have been shown to increase renal blood flow, probably by stimulating the release of renal prostaglandins. This haemodynamic effect can be inhibited by diclofenac and other NSAIDs. It is thought that the use of loop diuretics may thereby help salvage renal tissue, although evidence to support this hypothesis is difficult to find. It is, however, undeniable that any increase in urine volume produced will simplify the future management of Mrs NC by reducing the risk of fluid overload and hyperkalaemia. The patient must be euvolaemic before furosemide is considered, then doses of up to 1 g may be given intravenously at a rate of not more than 4 mg/min, since higher infusion rates may cause transient deafness. The addition of metolazone orally may also be considered. Metolazone, which is by itself a weak diuretic, has been shown to act synergistically with loop diuretics to produce a more effective diuresis.

Would you have used dopamine in this patient?

A7 **No.**

Dopamine has been used for many years as a renoprotective agent, but recently it has been shown there is no benefit in using low-dose dopamine infusion in patients with renal dysfunction and systemic inflammatory response syndrome. The theory behind its use is that dopamine at low doses (e.g. 1–5 micrograms/kg/min) has a vasodilator effect on the kidney. At slightly higher doses (e.g. 5–20 micrograms/kg/min) inotropic effects on the heart produce an increase in cardiac output. This dual effect increases renal perfusion. However, at even higher doses (e.g. 20 micrograms/kg/min and above) dopamine also acts on alpha-receptors causing peripheral and renal vasoconstriction, which results in impairment of renal perfusion. As with furosemide, dopamine may produce increases in urine volume even in those patients who progress to ARF. However, dopamine also has a number of potential disadvantages, even at low doses: it may increase cardiac contractility and systemic resistance, and it has been reported to cause tissue necrosis. It has also been suggested that desensitisation of renal dopaminergic receptors occurs with prolonged administration. Despite many clinical trials, dopamine has not been shown to affect the course of ARF favourably, and this, together with the disadvantages associated with its use, has led to it falling out of favour.

What dietary considerations are necessary for Mrs NC?

A8 **In a patient with ARF the aim is to provide sufficient nutrition to prevent the breakdown of body tissue, especially protein, and to enhance wound healing and resistance to infection.**

The diet should provide all the essential amino acids in a total protein intake of about 0.6 g/kg body weight/day. This should reduce the symptoms of uraemia, such as nausea, vomiting and anorexia. A higher intake of protein stimulates its use as an energy source, which results in increases in blood urea concentrations, while any further reduction in protein intake brings about endogenous protein catabolism, again causing blood urea to increase. Fat and carbohydrate should be given to maintain a high energy intake of about 2000–3000 kcal/day or more in hypercatabolic patients, as this helps prevent protein catabolism and promote anabolism. However, it should be borne in mind that any excessive amounts of carbohydrate can increase production of carbon dioxide and induce respiratory failure in these patients. Finally, to avoid the commonly encountered problem of hyperkalaemia, potassium intake should be kept as low as possible. Sodium and phosphorus intake should also be limited.

Unfortunately, as uraemia causes anorexia, nausea and vomiting, many severely ill patients are unable to tolerate a diet of any kind. In such cases TPN should be considered.

Would you have recommended quinine sulphate 300 mg at night to treat Mrs NC's nocturnal cramps?

A9 **Yes.**

Muscle cramps are common in patients with renal failure, probably as a result of electrolyte imbalances, and patients are often prescribed quinine salts in doses of 200–300 mg at night. The efficacy of this form of treatment is dubious and few comparative trials have been performed. Nonetheless, some patients insist that it does work and as it does not pose any risk to renal patients, it may be worth trying. The dose of quinine does not require alteration in renal failure.

What factors may have contributed to Mrs NC's low haemoglobin? Is ranitidine therapy appropriate?

A10 **Mrs NC's low haemoglobin may be a result of reduced erythropoietin secretion, but it is more likely to be the result of gastrointestinal bleeding, thus ranitidine therapy is appropriate.**

Erythropoietin, the hormone that stimulates production of red blood cells, is produced almost exclusively by the kidney and a normochromic normocytic anaemia due to reduced erythropoietin secretion is a very common symptom of chronic renal failure. However, the time course of ARF is often too short for this type of anaemia to become a problem and, although it may be present in a patient on the verge of chronic renal failure who has an acute crisis, this does not appear to be the case for Mrs NC.

Anaemia may also arise if there is a haemolytic element to the condition (e.g. severe septicaemia) or if a haemorrhage occurs, either as the cause of the ARF or as a result of it. While stress ulcers are not uncommon in acutely ill patients, uraemic gastrointestinal haemorrhage is a recognised consequence of ARF. It probably occurs as a result of reduced mucosal cell turnover owing to high circulating levels of uraemic toxins. Gastrointestinal haemorrhage is also a well recognised consequence of treatment with NSAIDs such as diclofenac, which Mrs NC had been taking prior to admission.

Mrs NC has passed melaena (black, tarry stools) and has been diagnosed as having had a gastrointestinal bleed. This is therefore the most likely cause of her low haemoglobin. H_2-receptor antagonists or proton pump inhibitors are effective therapy in this situation, and it is unlikely that any one would be more advantageous than another. Ranitidine was thus an appropriate choice of treatment and it was also appropriate to prescribe it at a reduced dosage, as Mrs NC's estimated GFR was less than 10 mL/min at this stage in her illness.

> Is Mrs NC's hyperkalaemia being treated appropriately? Should Mrs NC's hypocalcaemia, hyperphosphataemia and acidosis be treated at this point?

A11 **Yes. The methods used to treat Mrs NC's hyperkalaemia are appropriate. However, Mrs NC's calcium and phosphate levels and serum pH, although abnormal, are not sufficiently deranged to warrant treatment yet.**

(a)   Hyperkalaemia. Hyperkalaemia is a particular problem in ARF, not only because of reduced urinary potassium excretion, but also because of potassium release from cells. Particularly rapid rises are to be expected when there is tissue damage, as in burns, crush injuries and sepsis, although this is not the case for Mrs NC. She is, however, acidotic and this aggravates the situation by provoking potassium leakage from healthy cells. It is worth noting that ACEIs can increase potassium. However, in this case, it is much more likely to be due to the ARF as Mrs NC has been on captopril for some time.

Hyperkalaemia may be life-threatening as a result of causing cardiac arrhythmias and, if untreated, may result in asystolic cardiac arrest. Emergency treatment is necessary if the serum potassium is above 7.0 mmol/L (as in Mrs NC's case) or if there are ECG changes. Emergency treatment consists of:

(i)   10–20 mL of calcium gluconate 10% intravenously. This has a stabilizing effect on the myocardium but no effect on the serum potassium concentration.

(ii)   10 units of soluble insulin plus 50 mL of 50% glucose. The insulin stimulates potassium uptake into cells, thus removing it from the plasma. The glucose counteracts the hypoglycaemic effects of the insulin.

      (iii)   Calcium Resonium 15 g three or four times a day, orally or by enema. This ion-exchange resin binds potassium in the gastro-intestinal tract, releasing calcium in exchange. It is used to lower serum potassium over a period of hours or days, and is required because the effect of insulin and glucose therapy is only temporary. Both the oral and the rectal routes of administration have disadvantages. Administration of large doses by mouth may result in faecal impaction, which is why it is recommended that lactulose should be co-prescribed. The manufacturer recommends that the enema be retained for nine hours: retaining the enema is not usually the problem, rather the reverse. Oral therapy is not contra-indicated after a gastrointestinal bleed, so this is probably more appropriate for Mrs NC. Using a calcium-exchange resin is also appropriate as she is hypocalcaemic. She, and the nursing staff, should be counselled not to mix it with orange juice to improve the taste as this is also high in potassium.

      (iv)   200–300 mL of sodium bicarbonate 1.4% intravenously may be used in addition to insulin and glucose therapy. As well as stimulating potassium reuptake by cells, this helps to correct the acidosis of ARF. However, it is rarely used because of the fluid and electrolyte load it contains and it is particularly inappropriate for Mrs NC because of her history of cardiac failure.

(b)   Hypocalcaemia. Calcium malabsorption, probably secondary to disordered vitamin D metabolism, often occurs in ARF. However, it usually remains asymptomatic, as tetany of skeletal muscles and convulsions do not usually occur until plasma concentrations are as low as 1.6–1.7 mmol/L. Should it become necessary, oral calcium supplementation with calcium gluconate or lactate is usually adequate. Although vitamin D may be used to treat the hypocalcaemia of ARF, it rarely has to be prescribed. Effervescent calcium tablets should be avoided as they invariably contain a high sodium and potassium load. It should also be noted that correction of acidosis can lead to symptoms of hypocalcaemia developing (see (d)). Ionised calcium is important for cellular activation of the membrane potential and when acidosis is corrected ionised calcium drops, which causes symptomatic hypocalcaemia. There is a realistic and fairly often seen phenomenon in which giving sodium bicarbonate corrects acidosis but lowers ionised calcium, which may lead to fitting.

(c)   Hyperphosphataemia. Phosphate is normally excreted by the kidney. Phosphate retention and hyperphosphataemia may also occur in ARF, but usually only to a slight extent, and the condition rarely requires treatment. Should it become necessary, phosphate-binding agents may be used to retain phosphate ion in the gut. The most common agents are calcium-containing agents, e.g. Calcichew (calcium carbonate), Phosex (calcium acetate) and less commonly Titralac (calcium carbonate 420 mg plus glycine 180 mg). Aluminium hydroxide is infrequently prescribed, although it is an excellent phosphate binder. This is for two reasons: there is a slight risk that aluminium may be absorbed from the gut and deposited in bones to give a severe form of fracturing bone disease; also aluminium accumulation over long periods of time is associated with the risk of dementia. Aluminium levels can be monitored to minimise these risks. More recently, calcium-based phosphate binders have been associated with reports of calciphylaxis and calcium–phosphate complexes being deposited in the organs and blood vessels. Research is thus underway to develop non-calcium, non-aluminium-containing phosphate binders, e.g. Renagel (already licensed) and lanthanum.

(d)   Acidosis. The inability of the kidney to excrete hydrogen ions may result in a metabolic acidosis, which again is not in itself a serious problem, although it may contribute to hyperkalaemia. It may be treated orally with sodium bicarbonate 1–6 g/day in divided doses, although if elevations in plasma sodium preclude the use of sodium bicarbonate, extreme acidosis (plasma bicarbonate of less than 10 mmol/L) is best treated by dialysis.

Although Mrs NC does not currently require treatment of her electrolyte abnormalities, it is essential that she is carefully monitored for any further derangement.

What factors should be considered when initiating drug therapy for a patient in ARF?

A12   How the drug to be prescribed is absorbed, distributed, metabolised and excreted, and whether it is intrinsically nephrotoxic, are all factors that must be considered. The pharmacokinetic behaviour of many drugs may be altered in renal failure.

(a)   Absorption. Oral absorption in ARF may be reduced, owing to vomiting or diarrhoea, although this is of limited clinical significance, and to slowing of the gastrointestinal tract due to 'soggy gut' syndrome.

(b) Metabolism. The main hepatic pathways of drug metabolism appear to be unaffected in renal impairment. The kidney is also a site of metabolism in the body, but the effect of renal impairment is clinically important in only two cases:

   (i) Vitamin D. The conversion of 25-hydroxycholecalciferol to 1,25-dihydroxycholecalciferol (the active form of vitamin D) occurs in the kidney and the process is impaired in renal failure. Patients in ARF thus occasionally require vitamin D replacement therapy and this should be in the form of 1-hydroxycholecalciferol (alfacalcidol) or 1,25-dihydroxycholecalciferol (calcitriol).

   (ii) Insulin. The kidney is the major site of insulin metabolism and the insulin requirements of diabetic patients in ARF are often reduced.

(c) Distribution. Changes in distribution may be altered by fluctuations in the degree of hydration or by alterations in tissue or plasma protein binding. The presence of oedema or ascites tends to increase the volume of distribution, whereas dehydration tends to reduce it. In practice, these changes are only significant if the drug's volume of distribution is small (less than 50 L).

Plasma protein binding may be reduced, owing either to protein loss or to alterations in binding because of uraemia. For certain highly bound drugs the net result of reduced protein binding is an increase in free drug, so care must be taken when interpreting plasma concentrations of such drugs. Most analyses measure total plasma concentration, i.e. free plus bound drug. A drug level may therefore fall within the accepted concentration range, but still result in toxicity because of the increased proportion of free drug. However, this is usually only a temporary effect. Since the unbound drug is now available for elimination, its free concentration will eventually return to its original value, albeit with a lower total bound plus unbound level. As a consequence, the total drug concentration may fall below the therapeutic range although therapeutic effectiveness is maintained. It must be noted that the time required for the new equilibrium to be established is about four or five elimination half-lives of the drug and this itself may be altered in renal failure. Some drugs that show reduced plasma protein binding include diazepam, morphine, phenytoin, levothyroxine, theophylline and warfarin. Tissue binding may also be affected. For example, the displacement of digoxin from skeletal muscle binding sites by metabolic waste products results in a significant reduction of its volume of distribution in renal failure.

(d)   Excretion. Alterations in the renal clearance of drugs in renal impairment is by far the most important parameter to consider when making dosing decisions. Generally, a fall in renal drug clearance indicates a decline in the number of functioning nephrons. The GFR, of which CrCl is an approximation, can be used as an estimate of the number of functioning nephrons. Thus, a 50% reduction in GFR will suggest a 50% decline in renal clearance.

Renal impairment often necessitates drug-dosing adjustments; however, loading doses of renally excreted drugs are often necessary in renal failure because the prolonged elimination half-life leads to a prolonged time to reach steady state. The equation for loading dose is the same in renal disease as normal thus:

Loading dose (mg) = target conc. (mg/L) × vol. of distribution (L)

The volume of distribution may be altered (see above) but generally remains unchanged.

It is possible to derive other formulas for dosage adjustment in renal impairment. One of the most useful is:

$$DR_{rf} = DR_n \times [(1 - F_{eu}) + (F_{eu} \times RF)]$$

where DR_{rf} = dosing rate in renal failure, DR_n = normal dosing rate, RF = extent of renal impairment (i.e. patient's creatinine clearance in mL/min divided by the ideal creatinine clearance of 120 mL/min) and F_{eu} = fraction of drug normally excreted unchanged in the urine. For example, if RF = 0.2 and F_{eu} = 0.5, DR_{rf} will be 60% of normal.

An alteration in total daily dose can be achieved by altering either the dose itself, the dosage interval or a combination of both as appropriate. Unfortunately for this method, it is not always possible readily to obtain the fraction of drug excreted unchanged in the urine. In practice it is thus often simpler to use the guidelines to prescribing in renal impairment found in the *British National Formulary* and these are adequate for almost all cases.

(e)   Nephrotoxicity. Some drugs are known to be capable of damaging the kidney by a variety of mechanisms. The commonest forms of damage are interstitial nephritis (hypersensitivity reaction with inflammation affecting those cells lying between the nephrons) and glomerulonephritis (thought to be caused by the passive trapping of immune complexes in the glomerular tuft eliciting an inflammatory response). The list of potentially nephrotoxic drugs is a long one, but the majority cause damage by producing hypersensitivity reactions and are quite safe in most patients. Some drugs, however, are directly nephrotoxic and their effects on the kidney are consequently more predictable. Such drugs include the aminoglycosides, amphotericin, colistin, the polymyxins and ciclosporin. The use of any drug with recognised nephrotoxic potential should be avoided in any patient if at all possible. This is particularly true in patients with pre-existing renal impairment or renal failure, such as Mrs NC. Inevitably, occasions will arise when the use of potentially nephrotoxic drugs becomes necessary and on these occasions constant monitoring of renal function is essential.

In conclusion, the simplest solution to prescribing in renal failure is to choose a drug that is:

   (i) Less than 25% excreted unchanged in the urine.
  (ii) Unaffected by fluid balance changes.
 (iii) Unaffected by protein-binding changes.
  (iv) Has a wide therapeutic margin.
   (v) Not nephrotoxic.

What were the indications for dialysis in Mrs NC?

A13 **Her severe uraemic symptoms (nausea, reduced consciousness, flapping tremor) and evidence of pulmonary oedema indicate that dialysis would be of value for Mrs NC.**

Dialysis should be started in a patient with ARF when there is: hyperkalaemia of above 7 mmol/L; increasing acidosis (pH of less than 7.1 or plasma bicarbonate of less than 10 mmol/L); severe uraemic symptoms such as impaired consciousness; fluid overload with pulmonary oedema; or any combination of the above which may threaten life.

What forms of dialysis therapy are available and what are their advantages and disadvantages?

A14 **There are traditionally two types of dialysis: haemodialysis and peritoneal dialysis. Both put the patient's blood on one side of a semipermeable membrane and a dialysate solution on the other. Exchange of metabolites occurs across the membrane. In haemodialysis, blood is diverted out of the body and passed through an artificial kidney (dialyser), and returned to the patient, whereas in peritoneal dialysis the**

fluid is run in and out of the patient's abdominal cavity, and the peritoneum itself acts as the semipermeable membrane. A third option for Mrs NC is haemofiltration.

In haemodialysis, blood is taken from an arterial line, heparinised, actively pumped through a dialyser where diffusion and ultrafiltration occur, and returned to the patient via the venous line. The dialyser contains synthetic semipermeable membranes which allow the blood to come into close proximity with the dialysate. Metabolites and excess electrolytes pass from the blood to the dialysate, while by increasing the pressure of the blood, water can also be removed from the patient. Haemodialysis is performed two or three times a week and the duration of a single dialysis is usually about four hours. One disadvantage of haemodialysis is its dependence on expensive technology. The capital cost is considerable and the technique requires specially trained staff, so it is infrequently undertaken outside a renal unit. Haemodialysis also produces rapid fluid and electrolyte shifts which may be dangerous. However, it does treat renal failure much more rapidly than peritoneal dialysis and is therefore essential in hypercatabolic renal failure where urea is produced faster than peritoneal dialysis can remove it. Haemodialysis can also be used in patients who have recently undergone abdominal surgery, when peritoneal dialysis is inadvisable.

Continuous ambulatory peritoneal dialysis (CAPD) is usually performed manually by the patient at least four times a day. Pre-warmed dialysate is run into the peritoneum via an in-dwelling silastic catheter where it dwells for a variable length of time (usually four hours) before being drained out and fresh fluid run in. Peritoneal dialysis is relatively cheap and simple, does not require the facilities of a renal unit, and its use is consequently more widespread. It does, however, have the disadvantages of being uncomfortable and tiring for the patient, producing a fairly high incidence of peritonitis and also permitting protein loss, as albumin crosses the peritoneal membrane.

Both haemodialysis and CAPD can be used for acute renal replacement therapy (RRT) although currently more units use haemodialysis or a continuous RRT modality. Haemodialysis will reverse metabolic abnormalities much more quickly than CAPD.

Haemofiltration can also be used in ARF and is usually used in an intensive care setting. Haemofiltration is continuous and provides better removal of large molecular weight solutes and often better cardiovascular stability and blood pressure. It provides solute clearance by convection as solutes are dragged down a pressure gradient with water. Large volumes of filtrate are removed and need to be replaced. Haemodiafiltration combines dialysis with large volume ultrafiltration.

What factors affect drug therapy during haemodialysis?

A15 **Whether or not the drug is significantly removed by dialysis.**

Drugs that are not removed will require dose reductions in order to avoid accumulation and possible toxic effects. Alternatively, drug removal by intermittent dialysis or haemofiltration may be sufficient to require a dosage supplement to ensure adequate therapeutic efficacy.

In general, because haemodialysis, peritoneal dialysis and haemofiltration depend on filtration, the processes can be considered analogous to glomerular filtration. Thus, drug characteristics which favour clearance by the glomerulus are similar to those that favour clearance by dialysis or haemofiltration. They include low molecular weight, high water solubility, low protein binding, small volume of distribution and low metabolic clearance. With continuous haemofiltration the situation is more manageable than in intermittent processes as there are fewer oscillations in drug elimination.

Unfortunately, a number of other factors which depend on the dialysis process itself also affect clearance by dialysis. For haemodialysis, these include the duration of the dialysis procedure, the rate of blood flow to the dialyser, the surface area and porosity of the dialyser, and the composition and flow rate of dialysate. For peritoneal dialysis they include the rate of peritoneal exchange and the concentration gradient between plasma and dialysate.

Thus it is usually possible to predict whether or not a drug will be removed by dialysis, but it is very difficult to quantify the process, except by direct measurement, and this is rarely practical. It is therefore unsurprising that a single, comprehensive guide to drug dosage in dialysis is non-existent. However, limited data for specific drugs are available in the literature and many drug manufacturers have information on the dialysability of their products, some of which is included in the product data sheets. Thus, the most practical method of treating patients undergoing dialysis is to accumulate appropriate dosage guidelines for drugs which are likely to be used in patients with renal impairment and then to use those drugs only.

As drug clearance by haemofiltration is much more predictable than by dialysis, it is possible that standardised guidelines on drug elimination may become available in the future. In the meantime, a set of individual drug dosage guidelines similar to those described above is useful in practice.

What factors would you take into account when formulating a TPN regimen for Mrs NC?

A16 **Factors that should be considered when formulating a TPN regimen for Mrs NC include her fluid balance, calorie and protein requirements, electrolyte balance and requirements, and vitamin and mineral requirements.**

It must be noted that introducing large amounts of fluid during TPN may contribute to fluid overload, therefore dialysis may need to be adjusted to take this into account. Mrs NC's basic calorie requirements are similar to those of a non-dialysed patient (see Answer 8), although protein requirements may occasionally be increased with concurrent haemodialysis because of amino acid losses (increased amounts of protein may also be required with concurrent peritoneal dialysis because of plasma protein losses).

Although lipid emulsions may theoretically reduce the efficiency of dialysis their use does not have any noticeable effect. It is, however, useful to infuse the TPN solution into the blood as it is being returned to the body after haemodialysis, because this ensures that it is available to the patient before being presented to the filter.

Electrolyte-free amino acid solutions should be used as they allow the addition of the precise quantities of sodium and potassium required. As potassium is removed by dialysis, rigorous control of potassium intake becomes less important; potassium and sodium requirements can be calculated on an individual basis, depending on the patient's plasma levels. There is usually no need to try to normalise plasma calcium and phosphate as they will stabilize at acceptable levels with dialysis. If necessary, phosphate binders may be prescribed. Water-soluble vitamins are removed by dialysis, but the standard daily doses usually included in TPN fluids more than compensate for this. Magnesium and zinc supplementation may be required because tissue repair often increases requirements.

Once TPN is started, it will be necessary to monitor Mrs NC's plasma urea, creatinine and electrolytes daily, in order to make the appropriate alterations to her nutritional support and/or dialysis. Her serum glucose should also be checked at least every six hours, as patients in renal failure sometimes develop insulin resistance. Her serum pH should be checked initially to see whether the addition of amino acid solutions is causing or aggravating metabolic acidosis. It would also be worth checking her calcium, phosphate and albumin levels regularly, in case intervention becomes necessary. When practical, daily weighing gives a useful guide to fluid balance.

Is this therapy appropriate for Mrs NC's septicaemia?

A17   **No. Cefotaxime should be replaced by an agent with broader activity against Gram-positive organisms, such as a penicillin (e.g. ampicillin, amoxicillin or co-amoxiclav).**

Patients in ARF are prone to infection and septicaemia and this is a common cause of death in this population. Between 50 and 80% of all dialysis patients are carriers of *Staphylococcus aureus* and/or *Staphylococcus epidermidis*. Bladder catheters and intravenous lines should thus be used with care in order to reduce the chance of bacteria gaining access to the patient. Leucocytosis is sometimes seen in ARF and does not necessarily imply infection, but when seen in conjunction with pyrexia, as in Mrs NC, simple caution mandates aggressive treatment. Samples of blood, urine and any other material should be sent for culture before antibiotic therapy is started. Therapy should be prescribed to cover as wide a spectrum as possible until a causative organism is identified.

Aminoglycoside therapy is appropriate for Mrs NC as this class of compounds is highly active against most Gram-negative organisms as well as having useful activity against *S. aureus*: gentamicin is also inexpensive. Metronidazole is highly active against anaerobic organisms. Cefotaxime is a 'third-generation' cephalosporin with increased sensitivity against Gram-negative organisms, although this is balanced by reduced activity against some Gram-positive organisms, notably *S. aureus*. It can be useful when given in combination with an aminoglycoside, but it would be more advantageous to Mrs NC to use an agent with greater activity against Gram-positive organisms, e.g. ampicillin or one of its analogues such as amoxicillin or co-amoxiclav. All penicillins may cause renal damage, most commonly acute interstitial nephritis, but the damage is a hypersensitivity reaction and therefore unpredictable and it is not an absolute contra-indication to penicillin use.

What are the dangers associated with prescribing gentamicin for Mrs NC? How should her gentamicin therapy be monitored?

A18   **Gentamicin can cause nephrotoxicity and toxicity to the eighth cranial nerve. Regular monitoring for these side-effects, and of Mrs NC's gentamicin serum levels, is essential.**

Treatment with an aminoglycoside is justified for the reasons given in Answer 17; however, all aminoglycosides are potentially nephrotoxic, being associated with damage to the proximal tubule. Aminoglycosides can also precipitate ARF. Because of this, they should generally be avoided in renal impairment; however, their bactericidal activity against an extremely broad spectrum of Gram-negative organisms means that they are often prescribed for seriously ill patients with systemic infections. They are excreted solely by the kidney, so accumulation may lead to a vicious circle of increasing drug levels causing further renal deterioration and hence further accumulation. The risk of nephrotoxicity is increased when their use is combined with other nephrotoxic drugs, notably the loop diuretics. Mrs NC was prescribed the loop diuretic furosemide at an early stage of this admission, but her diuretic therapy has now been discontinued; however, if it is required again, the doses of aminoglycoside and loop diuretic must be staggered as much as possible.

In addition to being nephrotoxic, aminoglycosides are toxic to the eighth cranial nerve and may produce vestibular symptoms (i.e. loss of sense of balance) or adversely affect hearing. Such symptoms should thus be checked for on a regular basis.

Although aminoglycosides are often given in two to three divided doses over 24 hours, there is much evidence that administration once a day reduces the risk of toxicity while maintaining at least equivalent efficacy. Also, due to its accumulation in renal failure, gentamicin may only need to be administered every 24 hours or even less frequently. Other practical advantages include simplified dose calculation, a decrease in personnel time for drug administration and lower costs of consumables. In practice, in many renal units 'stat' doses of gentamicin, e.g. 80 mg, are given to patients with moderate to severe renal impairment. The levels are monitored, and when the level is less than 2 mg/L, the dose of 80 mg is re-administered. Alternatively, the *Renal Drug Handbook* (Bunn and Ashley) gives recommendations for once daily gentamicin dosing according to GFR.

In general, it is thought that the risk of nephrotoxicity and eighth cranial nerve toxicity is associated with peak serum concentrations persistently above 10 mg/L and, perhaps more importantly, troughs persistently above 2 mg/L, although persistently low levels do not guarantee freedom from nephrotoxicity.

Did Mrs NC follow the normal course of ARF? What is her prognosis?

A20   Yes. Mrs NC's illness followed the typical course of ARF and her survival to this stage is a good prognostic sign.

Acute tubular necrosis, the commonest form of ARF, usually occurs as a consequence of severe shock or as a result of sodium and water depletion giving rise to hypotension and generalised vasoconstriction, which in turn give rise to renal ischaemia. This was the sequence that resulted in Mrs NC's ARF. Acute tubular necrosis may also develop unattended by any circulatory disturbance, e.g. through direct damage to the renal parenchyma that can result from toxic or allergic reactions to drugs or other substances.

The course of ARF may be divided into two phases. The first is the oliguric phase, which is characterised by a urine volume of 200–400 mL in 24 hours, a volume at which the kidney is unable to concentrate the urine sufficiently to excrete the products of metabolism. This inevitably leads to uraemia and hyperkalaemia unless adequate management is provided. This oliguric phase usually lasts no longer than seven to 14 days, but it may last for up to six weeks. If the patient does not die in this period, he or she will enter the second phase which is characterised by a urine volume that rises over a few days to several litres. This, the diuretic phase, lasts for up to seven days and corresponds to the recommencement of tubular function. Patients who survive into this phase, as Mrs NC has, have a relatively good prognosis. Recovery of renal function takes place slowly over the following months, although the GFR rarely returns to its initial level. The elderly recover function more slowly and less completely.

The mortality of ARF varies according to the cause, but overall it is about 50%. Death due to uraemia and hyperkalaemia is rare now. The major causes of death are septicaemia and, to a lesser extent, gastrointestinal haemorrhage. Death is more common in patients aged over 60.

Acknowledgement

I would like to thank Alexander Harper who wrote the original chapter and gave permission for it to be used as the basis for this update.

Further reading

Albright RC. Acute renal failure: a practical update. *Mayo Clin Proc* 2001; **76**: 67–74.

Aronoff GR, ed. *Drug Prescribing in Renal Failure*. 4th edn. American College of Physicians, Philadelphia, PA, 1999.

Bunn R, Ashley C. *The Renal Drug Handbook*. Radcliffe Medical Press, Oxford, 1999.

Davison AM, Cameron JS, Grunfeld J-P *et al.*, eds. *Oxford Textbook of Clinical Nephrology*, 2nd edn. Oxford University Press, Oxford, 1997.

Dishart MK, Kellum JA. An evaluation of the pharmacological strategies for the prevention and treatment of acute renal failure. *Drugs* 2000; **59**: 79–91.

Firth J. Acute renal failure. *Medicine* 1999; **27**: 24–29.

Lamiere N, Vanholder R. New perspectives for prevention/treatment of ARF. *Curr Opin Anaesthesiol* 2000; **13**: 105–112.

Levy J, Morgan J, Brown E. *Oxford Textbook of Dialysis*. Oxford University Press, Oxford, 2001.

Warrell DA, Cox TM, Firth JD *et al.*, eds. *Oxford Textbook of Medicine*, 4th edn. Oxford University Press, Oxford, 2003.

6

Chronic renal failure managed by continuous ambulatory peritoneal dialysis

Aileen D Currie

Case study and questions

Day 1 Mr FB, a 34-year-old, insulin-dependent diabetic man with end-stage renal failure managed by continuous ambulatory peritoneal dialysis (CAPD), was admitted to the renal ward with a two-day history of abdominal pain and malaise. He had noticed that his CAPD effluent had become very cloudy over the previous 24 hours. It was his first admission to the renal unit at this hospital.

Mr FB had had insulin-dependent diabetes since childhood and had required CAPD for the last two years because of diabetic nephropathy. He continued to work as a personnel officer and had got married last year. He had recently been referred to the urology department for treatment of erectile dysfunction.

On admission, Mr FB was noted to be unwell, with a pulse rate of 68 beats per minute, a blood pressure of 180/90 mmHg and a temperature of 38.9°C. His weight was 61 kg, which was slightly above his normal dry weight. Clinical examination revealed moderate hypertension, mild ankle oedema and abdominal tenderness.

Drug therapy at the time of admission was:

- Calcium 500 mg (as carbonate) (Calcichew), chew twice a day before food
- Perindopril 2 mg orally daily
- Clonazepam 0.5 mg orally at night, when required for restless legs

- Ispaghula husk, one sachet orally twice daily when necessary
- Lactulose liquid 20 mL orally twice daily when necessary
- Co-dydramol, two tablets orally four times daily when necessary
- Insulin Human Mixtard 30 Pen-fill cartridge, 18 units subcutaneously each morning and 12 units subcutaneously each evening using the Novopen device (Novo Nordisk)

Mr FB's dialysis therapy consisted of 2 L exchanges four times daily, using the Dianeal PD4 Solo System. The three daytime exchanges were with dialysate containing 1.36% glucose ('weak' bags) and the overnight exchange was with dialysate containing 2.27% glucose ('medium' bag).

His serum biochemical and haematological results were as follows:

- Glucose 7.9 mmol/L (reference range 3.3–6.1)
- Potassium 4.2 mmol/L (3.6–5.4)
- Creatinine 566 micromol/L (50–140)
- Calcium 2.16 mmol/L (2.15–2.65)
- Phosphate 2.30 mmol/L (0.8–1.4)
- Sodium 134 mmol/L (133–144)
- Alkaline phosphatase 220 international units/L (70–300)
- Intact parathyroid hormone (iPTH) 500 nanograms/L (10–55)
- Red blood cells (RBC) 3.23×10^{12}/L (4.5–6×10^{12})
- White blood cells (WBC) 8.1×10^9/L (4–11×10^9)
- Haemoglobin (Hb) 8.8 g/dL (11.5–18)
- Haematocrit 0.258 (0.4–0.54)
- Serum ferritin 87.0 micrograms/L (25–350)

A sample of dialysate effluent was sent for microbiological screening.

Mr FB was diagnosed as having peritonitis with fluid overload and hyperglycaemia. He was noted to be hypocalcaemic, hyperphosphataemic and anaemic, and was complaining of pruritus.

Q1   Should the results of the microbiological cultures be obtained before initiating antibiotic therapy?

Q2   What treatment would you recommend for Mr FB's peritonitis and why?

Q3   Will Mr FB's dialysis and insulin regimens need adjustment during the initial course of treatment?

Q4   Why is Mr FB hypocalcaemic and hyperphosphataemic and how would you recommend he be treated? What are the alternative therapeutic options?

Q5   What alternatives to clonazepam are available to treat restless legs?

Q6   What are the reasons for pruritus in renal patients and what treatment would you recommend for Mr FB?

Mr FB was prescribed vancomycin 30 mg/kg and tobramycin 6 mg/L to be added to his first exchange, this exchange was to have a dwell time of at least six hours. Tobramycin was continued with each of his subsequent exchanges at a dose of 6 mg/L. Heparin was also prescribed to be added at a dose of 1000 units/L with each exchange.

Q7   Why is heparin being added to Mr FB's CAPD bags?

Day 2   Mr FB's condition was still not improving and his weight was increasing. He was becoming slightly breathless and his ankle oedema was still present. His dialysis regimen was still four exchanges a day. The dialysis effluent remained cloudy and his abdomen tender. It was discovered that the heparin was not being added to the bags.

   The CAPD regimen was altered to three exchanges with 2.27% (medium) and one with 1.36% (weak) solutions and the laboratory was phoned to try to expedite his culture results.

Day 3   Microbiological culture revealed infection with the Gram-negative organism *Proteus mirabalis*, which was sensitive to tobramycin and ceftazidime but not vancomycin. As a result, the tobramycin was continued with each exchange and intravenous ceftazidime was started. The vancomycin was discontinued, as the organism was not sensitive to it.

Q8   What dose of ceftazidime is required to treat Mr FB's peritonitis and can it be given intraperitoneally?

Day 4   Mr FB's condition was beginning to improve, and his bags were less cloudy and his abdominal pain was resolving. His weight was reducing and his ankle oedema improving, and he was less breathless. As this was Mr FB's first in-patient episode since transferring to the unit it was decided to review all his medication on the evening ward round.

Q9   What information and recommendations would you prepare for the review with respect to Mr FB's:
   (a)   Phosphate binder?
   (b)   Analgesia?
   (c)   Laxative regimen?
   (d)   Antihypertensive therapy?
   Indicate briefly other possible therapeutic options where appropriate.

Q10   What recommendations would you make for the treatment of Mr FB's anaemia?

Day 5   Mr FB's condition was still improving. His pulmonary and ankle oedema had resolved and his dialysis regimen was returned to his normal exchanges (three 'weak' and one 'medium' bag every 24 hours). His dialysate effluent was less cloudy and his abdomen was less tender; however, Mr FB was having a problem with drainage of his dialysate exchanges. An abdominal x-ray was taken which revealed constipation.

Therapy with recombinant human erythropoietin (epoetin beta: NeoRecormon) was commenced to treat his anaemia. Intravenous iron supplementation (iron sucrose 200 mg once weekly for five weeks) was started at the same time as epoetin to ensure adequate iron status for the epoetin to be effective. It was arranged that the course of iron therapy would be continued after discharge at the weekly nurse-led clinic.

Alfacalcidol was initiated to correct Mr FB's relative hypocalcaemia and suppress the renal bone disease indicated by his high serum alkaline phosphatase and iPTH. He was also counselled on the appropriate way to take his phosphate binders and the importance of concordance with therapy.

His dose of perindopril was increased.

Ispaghula husk therapy was discontinued and the dose of lactulose liquid changed to a regular night-time dose with senna tablets to be taken as needed.

Co-dydramol was replaced by paracetamol as analgesic therapy.

Day 11 Mr FB continued to improve. His CAPD effluent had now been clear for six days, so discharge was planned for the following day.

Day 12 His medication on discharge was:

- Calcium 500 mg (as carbonate) (Calcichew) chew one tablet three times daily before food
- Perindopril 4 mg orally daily
- Clonazepam 0.5 mg orally at night for restless legs
- Alfacalcidol 1 microgram orally three times a week
- Senna, two tablets orally at night when required
- Lactulose liquid 10 mL orally at night
- Paracetamol 500 mg, two tablets orally four times daily when necessary for pain relief
- Insulin Human Mixtard 30 Pen-fill cartridges, 18 units subcutaneously each morning and 12 units subcutaneously each evening using the Novopen device
- Epoetin beta, NeoRecormon 3000 units subcutaneously twice weekly
- Cetirizine 5 mg orally daily when required for relief from itch

An out-patient clinic appointment was made to continue his course of iron and to check that his peritoneal fluid remained clear.

Q11 What are the key elements of a pharmaceutical care plan for Mr FB at discharge?

Day 19   Mr FB returned to clinic and mentioned that he has been started on sildenafil 25 mg orally for his erectile dysfunction.

Q12 Outline the oral therapeutic options for erectile dysfunction. Which is most appropriate for Mr FB?

Should the results of the microbiological cultures be obtained before initiating antibiotic therapy?

A1 Definitely not.

Delay in treatment can lead to the infection, which is usually confined to the peritoneal cavity, becoming systemic. Infection can also damage the peritoneum, reducing its efficiency as a dialysis membrane in the long-term. Empirical antibiotic therapy should therefore be started as soon as peritonitis is clinically diagnosed.

What treatment would you recommend for Mr FB's peritonitis and why?

A2 The concomitant use of intraperitoneal vancomycin and tobramycin in accordance with the local, clinically audited protocol. Intravenous antibiotic therapy is not warranted for Mr FB as a systemic infection is unlikely.

Recurrent episodes of peritonitis can lead to damage to the peritoneum and result in CAPD treatment failure and the patient needing to commence haemodialysis.

An antibiotic regimen that is effective against all the major Gram-positive and Gram-negative pathogens, in particular *Staphylococcus* and *Pseudomonas* species and *Enterobacteriaceae*, is required. Sixty percent of all cases of peritonitis are caused by Gram-positive organisms, 20% by Gram-negative organisms, 5% are fungal and in 15% of cultures no growth is found. Evidence to date favours the intraperitoneal route of drug administration. This route enables precise therapeutic and non-toxic concentrations of the antibiotics to be delivered directly to the site of infection.

Vancomycin has excellent antimicrobial activity against Gram-positive *Staphylococcus* and *Streptococcus* species, the most common causative organisms of CAPD peritonitis, although recent recommendations have been made that vancomycin should only be used for methicillin-resistant *Staphylococcus aureus* due to the problems with emerging resistance. Tobramycin has excellent antimicrobial activity against a broad range of Gram-negative organisms and some Gram-positive organisms.

The local protocol for a patient such as Mr FB is as follows:

Day 1   Empirical therapy. Sample of dialysis effluent sent to pathology for culture and sensitivity tests. Vancomycin 30 mg/kg and tobramycin 6 mg/L to be added to 2 L dialysis fluid and instilled for a six-hour dwell time. Thereafter, tobramycin 6 mg/L in 2 L dialysis fluid to be given with each exchange. Heparin 1000 units/L should be added to each of the four daily bags.

Day 2   Tobramycin 6 mg/L intraperitoneally via each of the day's four dialysis bags. Heparin 1000 units/L also to be added to each bag.

Day 3   The results of the microbiological culture of the sample of drained dialysis fluid taken on day 1 should be known. Intraperitoneal antibiotic therapy adjusted as follows:

Gram-positive organism sensitive to vancomycin and tobramycin. Maintain on both antibiotics. If sensitive to only one, stop the prescription for the other.

Gram-negative organism. Continue on tobramycin only if sensitive. If not, give the appropriate antibiotic either orally, intraperitoneally or intravenously.

Culture negative. Maintain on tobramycin only. The use of heparin 1000 units/L in each bag should be continued if the bags are still cloudy.

Day 4   Review. If the bags are still cloudy add in another antibiotic (depending on reported sensitivities). Continue with tobramycin 6 mg/L intraperitoneally as above, if indicated.

Days 5–6   Continue with tobramycin 6 mg/L intraperitoneally as above, if indicated. If continuing therapy with vancomycin is indicated, another dose of 30 mg/kg should be given via the intraperitoneal route.

Days 7–10 Tobramycin 6 mg/L intraperitoneally should be continued as above, if indicated. If a further dose of vancomycin is required levels should be taken at day 10. Another dose should not be given until the vancomycin trough level is less than 10 mg/L.

Vancomycin has been shown to be relatively stable (less than 10% loss in potency) in CAPD fluid for at least 24–48 hours. Aminoglycosides are much less stable in the low pH of glucose-containing CAPD fluids. However, the use of bags that have had tobramycin added for 48 hours have demonstrated clinical efficacy on an ongoing basis. It is advisable to add the two antibiotics to 'weak' rather than 'strong' dialysis bags, as the latter tend to have a more acidic pH. Vancomycin and tobramycin have a stability of about eight hours when combined at these concentrations at body temperature. Heparin addition has minimal effect on antibiotic stability.

Although not relevant in Mr FB's case, if the dialysis effluent had still not been clearing after 10 days, antibiotic therapy should have been continued for a further four days. If this had still not been successful, CAPD intraperitoneal catheter removal would usually be indicated.

When given by the intraperitoneal route, both vancomycin and tobramycin are absorbed systemically, particularly through an infected and inflamed peritoneal membrane. This may lead to potentially ototoxic and nephrotoxic serum levels (the latter being relevant for patients who still have some remaining renal function), particularly after an extended course of treatment. Accumulation of vancomycin and tobramycin to potentially toxic levels does not occur in patients with end-stage renal failure after 10 days' therapy.

Netilmicin, although more expensive than tobramycin, is reported to be the least toxic of the aminoglycosides and is an alternative to tobramycin.

There are many other reported regimens for the effective treatment of CAPD peritonitis including the use of oral quinolones such as cipro-floxacin. Cephalosporins and aminoglycosides have a synergistic activity and can also be used to treat peritonitis very effectively.

In cases of fungal peritonitis, intraperitoneal fluconazole and oral flucytosine (available on a named-patient basis) are generally used although usually catheter removal is also required.

Will Mr FB's dialysis and insulin regimens need adjustment during the initial course of treatment?

A3   **Yes. Inflammation of the peritoneal membrane as a result of his peritonitis causes an increase in its permeability. Glucose absorption becomes more rapid, which results in a faster dissipation of the osmotic gradient that is essential for ultrafiltration. This will also raise his serum glucose levels.**

Peritoneal inflammation has already affected Mr FB in two ways: firstly, the loss of ultrafiltration has caused him to become fluid-overloaded and, secondly, the increased glucose absorption has caused his hyperglycae-mia. To correct fluid overload, the number of dialysis fluid exchanges should be increased and more 'medium' bags should be used. This reduces the dwell time of the dialysate in the peritoneum, thereby maintaining the osmotic gradient. Additionally, the more frequent use of the more hypertonic dialysate will remove the excess fluid from Mr FB.

To achieve serum glucose control, subcutaneous insulin should be stopped and an infusion of short-acting insulin started using a syringe pump. The insulin dose can be given in accordance with a sliding scale based on blood glucose measurements. As soon as Mr FB's peritonitis and fluid overload is controlled, he can revert to subcutaneous insulin therapy and four dialysis exchanges daily. The use of hypertonic dialysate can cause peritoneal discomfort and Mr FB should be warned about this. Another reason for 'strong' bags (3.86% glucose) being used only as a last resort is due to the fact that their long-term use damages the peritoneal membrane.

Insulin can also be administered by the intraperitoneal route which can produce more even glucose control, although for the best effect it should be administered into an empty abdomen which leads to time constraints for the patient. The other disadvantages to this route of administration is that an increased dose is required if it is added with the dialysate, because of dilution and adsorption of the insulin onto the plastic bag, plus it leads to a slightly increased incidence of peritonitis. Thus, in most units insulin therapy is administered subcutaneously.

Why is Mr FB hypocalcaemic and hyperphosphataemic and how would you recommend he be treated? What are the alternative therapeutic options?

A4 **Reduced synthesis of calcitriol (the physiologically active form of vitamin D) in the failing kidney results in reduced serum calcitriol levels and reduced calcium absorption from the gut. This, together with hyperphosphataemia and reduced bone resorption, causes hypocalcaemia. Mr FB requires alfacalcidol therapy orally in a pulsed regimen (e.g. 1 microgram at night three times weekly). Alternative therapeutic options are oral or parenteral calcitriol or parenteral alfacalcidol.**

Hypocalcaemia and a reduction in the direct suppressive action of calcitriol on the parathyroid gland results in an increased secretion of PTH. Uraemia also reduces the sensitivity of the parathyroid gland to calcium and inhibition of binding of calcitriol to receptors in the parathyroid gland also leads to raised PTH levels. As it is not possible for the failing kidney to increase synthesis of calcitriol in response to the increased serum PTH levels (which would result in a decrease in PTH levels in a patient with normal renal function), the serum PTH levels remain chronically elevated and hyperplasia of the parathyroid glands occur. The resultant secondary hyperparathyroidism is central to the development of renal osteodystrophy.

Renal osteodystrophy covers the four main types of bone disease: secondary hyperparathyroidism, osteomalacia, mixed renal osteodystrophy and adynamic bone disease. Renal osteodystrophy results in a reduction in bone mineral density, osteopenia and metastatic calcification, and is due to reduced phosphate excretion and reduced vitamin D production.

Mr FB's hypocalcaemia should be treated with oral alfacalcidol which is metabolised to calcitriol in the liver. An initial dose of 1 microgram three times a week would be appropriate. This dose can be adjusted according to his response. During therapy his serum calcium level should be monitored regularly, particularly as he is on a calcium-based phosphate binder. If Mr FB becomes hypercalcaemic, stopping the alfacalcidol should quickly result in a reduced serum calcium level. Significant hyperphosphataemia should always be corrected prior to correcting hypocalcaemia, as elevated phosphate and calcium levels can result in metastatic calcification of soft tissue.

The oral administration of calcitriol or alfacalcidol results in a rise in serum calcitriol and calcium, which suppresses PTH secretion to some extent. To suppress serum PTH to normal levels, large oral doses of calcitriol (or alfacalcidol) would have to be given and hypercalcaemia would quickly ensue. It has been shown that giving alfacalcidol at a higher dose (1–4 micrograms) as a pulsed (three times a week) regimen causes greater suppression of PTH by down regulation of PTH receptors without as big an increase in calcium levels. Hypercalcaemia is the rate-limiting step to treatment of hyperparathyroidism. Giving the dose of alfacalcidol at night has also been shown to be better as less calcium is absorbed. It is important not to over suppress PTH as this can lead to adynamic bone disease: PTH level of 1.5–3 times the normal level should be aimed for.

Parathyroidectomy is not normally required until the PTH is above 1000 nanograms/L. This is referred to as tertiary hyperparathyroidism, when the PTH remains elevated despite normal calcium and phosphate levels.

Future developments for the management of renal osteodystrophy are non-calcium vitamin D analogues that mimic calcium by acting on calcium-sensing receptors on PTH cells.

What alternatives to clonazepam are available to treat restless legs?

A5 **Restless legs is a condition which affects many dialysis patients and tolerance to treatment can be a problem so a drug holiday is sometimes required. Alternative treatments include carbamazepine or tricyclic antidepressants.**

Restless legs is characterised by the involuntary jerking of legs during sleep or rest and can be as disturbing for the patient's partner as it is for themselves.

The cause of restless legs is unknown although various hypotheses have been put forward for example iron deficiency anaemia and uraemic polyneuropathy. It can be exacerbated by phenytoin, neuroleptics and antidepressants.

First-line treatment is usually with clonazepam at a dose of 0.5 mg at night increasing gradually to 4 mg, although in practice doses above 1 mg can cause daytime drowsiness and are rarely used. Dependence may become a problem and treatment should be withdrawn gradually if a treatment-free period is required or when changing to an alternative treatment. If clonazepam does not work, carbamazepine, 100 mg at night increasing to 300 mg at night may be used. Other drugs which have been used in restless legs syndrome are chlorpromazine, levodopa, cabergoline, naloxone, clonidine, propranolol, tricyclic antidepressants, haloperidol, baclofen and even a tot of brandy.

In Mr FB's case his risk factors for restless legs would be chronic renal failure and iron deficiency anaemia. At the moment his clonazepam is working, but a drug holiday could be suggested to maintain the drug's efficacy.

What are the reasons for pruritus in renal patients and what treatment would you recommend for Mr FB?

A6 **Pruritus is common in renal failure due to uraemia, iron deficiency, hyperparathyroidism, dialysis itself, hyperphosphataemia and dry skin. Release of histamine from mast cells causes itching, and high histamine levels have been found in patients with chronic renal failure and have been linked with uraemic pruritus. First-line treatments include antihistamines and topical agents.**

Mr FB has poorly controlled phosphate levels which may be the main reason for his pruritus, so he should be counselled on the effects of high phosphate levels. In renal failure the itch can be very difficult to treat so a combination of systemic and topical agents tend to be used. The topical agents include moisturising lotions and creams containing urea or menthol. Sedative antihistamines tend to work better than the non-sedative ones and have the advantage of helping the patients sleep at night when the itch tends to be worse; however, as Mr FB worked he wanted a non-sedative alternative. The drug of choice tends to be cetirizine at a dose of 5 mg daily. It is best to avoid the antihistamines which may cause an increased risk of arrhythmias, as renal patients are prone to rapid electrolyte changes. Other drugs which can be used are naltrexone injection and thalidomide capsules.

It is also important to treat some of the other causes of Mr FB's pruritus, namely his iron deficiency and renal bone disease.

Why is heparin being added to Mr FB's CAPD bags?

A7 **Heparin is being added to each bag of CAPD fluid to help break down the fibrin that appears in the peritoneum as a result of peritonitis and which contributes to the cloudy appearance of the CAPD effluent. The breakdown of the fibrin helps prevent blockage of the CAPD catheter.**

Heparin additions should continue until the CAPD effluent becomes clear. The dose of heparin per bag varies considerably between renal units and is somewhat empirical.

In this unit the addition of 1000 units/L of heparin per bag has been found to be a simple and effective regimen. Although not the case with Mr FB, a proportion of patients always have a cloudy fibrinous CAPD effluent that is not associated with peritonitis. These patients add heparin to each of their CAPD bags routinely.

What dose of ceftazidime is required to treat Mr FB's peritonitis and can it be given intraperitoneally?

A8 **Sensitivities have shown that the organism is sensitive to ceftazidime, so a dose of 500 mg every 24 hours intravenously is appropriate. Ceftazidime can also be given intraperitoneally.**

As Mr FB is not improving he should be started on a course of intravenous ceftazidime at a dose of 500 mg every 24 hours. Cephalosporins can be very neurotoxic in renal patients and as they are renally excreted a marked dose reduction is required to prevent drug accumulation. Ceftazidime could also be given intraperitoneally at a dose of 125–250 mg/2 L.

This drug is stable in combination with tobramycin in PD fluid for 16 hours at room temperature. As a single agent in PD fluid it is stable for four days at room temperature.

> What information and recommendations would you prepare for the review, with respect to Mr FB's:
> (a) Phosphate binder?
> (b) Analgesia?
> (c) Laxative regimen?
> (d) Antihypertensive therapy?
>
> Indicate briefly other possible therapeutic options where appropriate.

A9 **(a) Phosphate binder.**

Mr FB's calcium carbonate therapy should be increased to 500 mg calcium three times daily. Mr FB's compliance with his phosphate binders should also be queried, based on his low calcium level. Following this change in therapy, his serum phosphate and calcium levels should be monitored regularly and the dose of calcium carbonate adjusted in response to changes in these concentrations. A low-calcium dialysate could be considered if hypercalcaemia proved to be a problem.

Serum phosphate levels rise in patients with renal failure once the glomerular filtration rate (GFR) is less than 30–40 mL/min, mainly due to the decreased renal excretion of phosphate. The resulting hyperphosphataemia plays a major role in the development of secondary hyperparathyroidism and, consequently, renal osteodystrophy, because excessive PTH release is stimulated by the hyperphosphataemia-induced hypocalcaemia and hypocalcitriolaemia. Management of hyperphosphataemia centres around a combination of dialysis and the binding of orally ingested phosphate in the gut to prevent its systemic absorption. A phosphate-binding agent is usually the salt of a di- or trivalent metallic ion.

Aluminium, usually as the hydroxide, used to be widely used as a phosphate binder. However, some aluminium is systemically absorbed from the binding agent and is toxic, causing encephalopathy, osteomalacia, proximal myopathy and anaemia. Aluminium salts also cause constipation, which can quickly lead to drainage problems in CAPD patients. Aluminium absorption can also be increased if patients are on ulcer healing drugs which increase the pH of the gut.

Alternatives to aluminium include calcium salts, usually the carbonate. Calcium carbonate has been used with some success in chronic haemodialysis patients. However, calcium has a relatively low phosphate-binding capacity, necessitating the use of doses up to 10 g daily.

The dose of calcium carbonate required to control serum phosphate in CAPD patients is, however, generally lower (1.2–3.78 g daily), probably due to the continuous removal of serum phosphate by this method of dialysis. However, unpredictable episodes of hypercalcaemia, due to systemic calcium absorption, are often a problem in this patient group. Both calcium carbonate and aluminium hydroxide should be taken 5–10 minutes before food to ensure an optimal phosphate-binding effect and also to reduce calcium and aluminium absorption.

Another alternative is calcium acetate (Phosex). The acetate salt of calcium has a stronger phosphate-binding effect and less calcium is absorbed compared with calcium carbonate. Calcium acetate should be taken with meals, which may also help to remind the patients to take them. It is of most use in people with calcium levels at the higher end of the range.

Sevelamer (Renagel) has the advantage of being a non-absorbed phosphate-binding poly(allylamine hydrochloride) polymer which is free of aluminium and calcium. It has a stronger affinity for phosphate than the other binders and doesn't affect calcium or aluminium levels. Renal units now often calculate the product of the calcium and phosphate levels (Ca × P) as this gives a more accurate measurement of total body calcium content compared with measuring calcium or phosphate concentrations alone. Ca × P product levels greater than 4.5 $mmol^2/L^2$ may lead to an increased incidence of vascular calcification, left ventricular hypertrophy and sudden cardiac death. (Mr FB's Ca × P product is 5 $mmol^2/L^2$). For this reason there is increasing interest in the use of non-calcium-containing phosphate binders such as sevelamer as a way of minimising calcium intake. Sevelamer should be taken with food to optimise the phosphate-binding effect and to reduce nausea. The product has a further advantage that it can reduce low-density lipoprotein cholesterol levels by 20%; however, it does have the disadvantage that between one to five 800 mg tablets must be taken with each meal and it is considerably more expensive than calcium-containing binders. At the moment it is only licensed for haemodialysis patients.

For both haemodialysis and CAPD patients, if serum phosphate is high and a significant amount of calcium is systemically absorbed from the calcium carbonate (a problem that is more likely if large doses are being used), there is a risk of metastatic calcification of soft tissue. Calcium salts are also constipating. However, an added advantage of a carbonate salt is that it helps correct the metabolic acidosis that is prevalent in patients with end-stage renal failure.

Other phosphate binders under trial include lanthanum. Results with lanthanum are encouraging although limitations may be due to the fact that it is not known what the effects of accumulation of lanthanum are.

Calcium carbonate in an increased dose thus remains the phosphate binder of choice for Mr FB.

(b)   Analgesia.

Co-dydramol therapy should be discontinued and replaced by paracetamol 500 mg, up to two tablets four times daily when necessary. If Mr FB's pain is continuous, regular therapy should be recommended.

Co-dydramol (containing paracetamol 500 mg and dihydrocodeine 10 mg), is not commonly used, as it is not the analgesic of choice in renal failure. Dihydrocodeine and its active metabolites accumulate in renal failure, enhancing side-effects such as constipation and sedation. This has probably contributed to Mr FB's feeling of lethargy and his need for laxatives. There is no conclusive evidence that co-dydramol is a significantly stronger analgesic than paracetamol alone.

If pain relief is not achieved with paracetamol, a non-steroidal anti-inflammatory drug could be considered, although such a drug may cause gastrointestinal bleeding and reduce any residual renal function Mr FB may have. A cyclooxygenase-2 inhibitor may be the drug of choice from this group, as they are reported to have little effect on renal function and fewer gastrointestinal problems at normal therapeutic doses, although in practice both side-effects can still occur.

Co-proxamol or co-codamol 8/500 could also be considered as an alternative, but sedation, constipation and respiratory depression can also occur with these compounds.

(c)   Laxative regimen.

Lactulose should be prescribed regularly. Ispaghula husk sachets should be discontinued and paracetamol should be prescribed as analgesia in place of co-dydramol. Senna should be commenced.

Constipation in CAPD patients can lead to obstruction of drainage of the dialysate from the peritoneum. Three factors are probably contributing to Mr FB's constipation:

  (i)   His calcium phosphate-binder (however, aluminium phosphate-binders also cause constipation).
 (ii)   The use of an analgesic containing dihydrocodeine, a synthetic narcotic analgesic with morphine-like action.
(iii)   Inappropriate 'when necessary' use of his prescribed laxatives.

Lactulose acts as both an osmotic and a bulking laxative. Because of its physiological mode of action it is unsuitable for use on a 'when necessary' basis and should be prescribed regularly. Lactulose can also produce a significant reduction in colonic pH, which may reduce the formation and systemic absorption of ammonium ions and other nitrogenous toxins, thus aiding the control of uraemia. It is not significantly absorbed and is unlikely to affect Mr FB's diabetic control adversely. A suitable starting dose is 10 mL once or twice daily, with adjustment according to response. The concomitant use of ispaghula husk sachets is illogical and can even lead to constipation. Senna is a stimulant laxative and can be used on a when required basis in combination with regular lactulose to maintain adequate bowel movements.

(d)   Antihypertensive therapy.

Increase Mr FB's antihypertensive therapy to perindopril 4 mg.

Hypertension in end-stage renal failure is attributed to either increased cardiac output, or increased peripheral vascular resistance, or both. Increased cardiac output reflects volume expansion secondary to sodium and water retention and/or the anaemia of chronic renal failure. Increased peripheral resistance may reflect an increase in circulating renin and angiotensin II or, possibly, decreased levels of vasodilators such as prostaglandins, bradykinin or renal medullary lipids. Hypertension is occasionally controlled by dialysis, but most patients, including Mr FB, need antihypertensive medication.

Beta-blockers have the potential to affect diabetics by increasing the frequency of hypoglycaemic attacks and delaying the rate of recovery, and by impairing carbohydrate tolerance. This risk is lessened by the use of the more cardioselective beta-blockers such as atenolol or metoprolol. Atenolol is excreted renally and therefore needs dosage adjustment in renal failure. Metoprolol is cleared hepatically and needs no dosage adjustment, although small initial doses are advised in renal failure.

Although there is no absolute contra-indication to beta-blocker therapy in Mr FB, it is not the treatment of choice. If a beta-blocker is desired, metoprolol therapy would be most appropriate. As Mr FB suffers from erectile dysfunction it would be best to avoid a beta-blocker.

An appropriate antihypertensive for Mr FB from a pharmacological viewpoint, is an angiotensin-converting enzyme inhibitor (ACEI), which causes vasodilation and reduced sodium retention by reducing the amount of circulating angiotensin II.

Formularies and drug information texts usually recommend avoidance of ACEIs or that they be used with extreme caution in renally impaired patients. They can cause a deterioration in renal function if the patient has renal artery stenosis. Consequently, renal function must be monitored regularly after treatment initiation and, if the renal function deteriorates, ACEI therapy must be stopped immediately.

The kidney is the major route of excretion of most ACEIs. To prevent accumulation and consequent hypotension and other adverse drug reactions in the renally impaired, therapy should be initiated with small doses, which should then be conservatively increased until the desired hypotensive effect is achieved. There is little to choose clinically between captopril, enalapril, lisinopril and other newer ACEIs. Captopril, with a shorter half-life, has acute activity which is useful for testing response to ACEIs prior to initiating routine therapy, because ACEIs can cause a profound 'first dose' drop in blood pressure in patients with renal failure. Perindopril, fosinopril and some of the newer ACEIs offer the potential of once-daily dosing as well as being either hepatically or dual metabolised which prevents the problem of accumulation in renal failure. When renal patients first start one of the newer ACEIs they take the first dose at night, if it is a patient on haemodialysis they would be advised to take the first dose at night on a non-dialysis day. This unit has always found ACEIs to be very effective in the management of hypertension in patients with renal failure. Furthermore, there are reports that ACEIs reduce thirst, which is potentially useful in those dialysis patients who have a tendency to fluid overload as a result of excessive drinking. A first step to control Mr FB's hypertension is thus to optimise the use of perindopril by increasing the dose to 4 mg daily.

Angiotensin II receptor antagonists can also be used in renal failure either instead of an ACEI if there have been problems with side-effects, e.g. cough, or in combination with ACEIs in patients with very resistant hypertension.

Nifedipine would also be an effective choice for Mr FB. However, headache, facial flushing and oedema are more common than usual in renally impaired patients. Longer-acting calcium antagonists, e.g. amlodipine, are associated with a lower incidence of such side-effects and would be suitable in this situation.

The vasodilators hydralazine, doxazosin and minoxidil are not contra-indicated in renal failure, but are not the antihypertensives of choice for Mr FB. Hydralazine and minoxidil should be used with a beta-blocker to reduce reflex tachycardia. Nausea can be problematic and a syndrome such as systemic lupus erythematosus can be induced when high doses of hydralazine are used long-term. Postural hypotension, drowsiness and nasal stuffiness can be problems with doxazosin, although this drug offers the advantage of a once daily dosage regimen.

The sensitivity of patients to all these drugs in end-stage renal failure is increased and, if used, therapy must be initiated with small doses.

> What recommendations would you make for the treatment of Mr FB's anaemia?

A10 **Mr FB should be treated with subcutaneous recombinant human erythropoietin (epoetin), a bioengineered form of the hormone. His iron deficiency should also be treated with intravenous iron therapy.**

Mr FB's anaemia is probably the major contributor to his continuous feeling of lethargy and fatigue. This, combined with other central nervous system and non-central nervous system-related disorders caused primarily by the hyperaemia of anaemia, results in a diminished quality of life. The anaemia of chronic renal failure is probably caused by a deficiency in the renal production of the hormone erythropoietin, which results in reduced bone marrow erythropoiesis. Other contributing factors include the inhibition of erythropoiesis by uraemic toxins, a shortening of red cell survival, uraemic bleeding, iron deficiency, aluminium toxicity and hyperparathyroidism.

Before the introduction of epoetin, red blood cell transfusions were the cornerstone of management of the anaemia of chronic renal failure, but erythroid marrow suppression, human leucocyte-associated antigen (HLA) antibody induction and iron overload made this treatment very unpopular. Iron and/or folic acid are given if the patient is found to be deficient.

The ready reconstituted epoetin beta (NeoRecormon) presented in a pre-filled syringe will help Mr FB self-administer his dose. Epoetin alfa (Eprex) used to be an alternative choice for this indication; however, reports of its use causing pure red cell aplasia led to its withdrawal from subcutaneous use. Red cell aplasia is a very rare condition that results in the failure of the production of erythroid elements (i.e. red blood cell precursors) in the bone marrow which leads to profound anaemia. This is possibly due to an immune response to the protein backbone of the molecule. The antibodies formed as a result of this immune response render the patient unresponsive to the therapeutic effects of epoetin alfa, epoetin beta and darbepoetin. It is now recommended that epoetin alfa should only be administered by the intravenous route.

For patients undergoing CAPD, an initial dose of 50 international units/kg twice weekly is administered. (Product literature says 20 international units three times a week, but in practice some units start with higher doses). This dose should be increased by 25% at monthly intervals until Mr FB's target haemoglobin level is reached. A slow rise in haemoglobin (not more than 1–2 g/dL/month) should minimize aggravation of Mr FB's hypertension and avoid other reported haemodynamically induced side-effects, such as seizures and clotting of vascular access. The hypertension sometimes seen during epoetin therapy is probably due to a reverse of the vasodilation caused by chronic anaemia. Mr FB's blood pressure should be regularly monitored and, if necessary, controlled by adjustment of his antihypertensive therapy.

Depletion of available iron is common during epoetin therapy because of the greatly increased marrow requirements. Mr FB's iron status should be regularly monitored and intravenous iron administered if his serum ferritin is below 100 micrograms/L in order to maintain an effective response to epoetin therapy. It takes 20 micrograms/L of ferritin to increase a patient's haemoglobin concentration by 1 g/dL, therefore patients on epoetin therapy require higher than normal iron stores to get an adequate response. Ferritin is not an ideal measurement of iron status as it can be increased during infective or inflammatory periods. Therefore in people with high ferritin levels it is best to also measure transferrin saturation, which should be greater than 20%, or the percentage of hypochromic red blood cells, which should be less than 10%. The percentage of hypochromic red blood cells is a measure of the number of individual red blood cells with a haemoglobin content of less then 28 g/dL. The improved appetite that accompanies epoetin therapy can also increase potassium intake, which in turn can necessitate the institution of some dietary control.

As Mr FB's ferritin is only 87 micrograms/L he should be commenced on an accelerated course of iron sucrose at the same time as his epoetin therapy is initiated. The total dose of iron which he requires can be calculated from the following equation:

Body weight (kg) × (13 – actual Hb) × 2.4 + 500 (storage iron)

He should receive this at a dose of 200 mg once weekly after his peritonitis has resolved, as intravenous iron treatment is associated with an increased risk of infection. He could receive this at a nurse led clinic. Once his iron stores are replete, he should receive a dose of 200 mg iron sucrose at each clinic visit, which he will attend every two to three months. Giving intravenous iron can reduce the dose of epoetin required to achieve the desired haemoglobin and result in cost savings. An alternative to iron sucrose is CosmoFer, the new formulation of iron dextran which can be given as a total-dose infusion and can be useful for patients who live far from the renal unit or who have very fragile veins.

The new formulation of iron dextran has a smaller molecule size and therefore fewer anaphylactic reactions occur. Iron tablets are not ideal in the dialysis population due to increased risk of gastrointestinal side-effects, poor bioavailability and interactions with phosphate binders leading to reduced efficacy of both drugs. As a result, iron tablets are rarely used.

Our target haemoglobin level is 10–12 g/dL (haematocrit 0.30–0.40). Once this target has been reached, the dose of epoetin is reduced and adjusted to maintain the haemoglobin at this desired level.

Intravenous administration of epoetin is effective but requires a higher dose than via the subcutaneous route to achieve the same rise in haemoglobin, thus reducing the cost effectiveness of this route. Epoetin has also been shown to be effective by the intraperitoneal route; however, early studies indicated that much larger doses than those used intravenously or subcutaneously were needed for effective therapy

An advancement in this area of anaemia management is darbepoetin (Aranesp). This stimulates erythropoiesis in the same way as epoetin therapy. It has a half-life three times as long as the endogenous protein and epoetin due to an extra two sugar residues on the molecule which causes a reduction in its hepatic metabolism. Due to its longer half-life, darbepoetin only has to be administered once a week or once a fortnight. The starting dose is 0.45 micrograms/kg weekly as a subcutaneous treatment or intravenous injection. In the case of Mr FB, subcutaneous treatment would be the route of choice so he could self-administer at home. The dose is increased in the same way as with epoetin therapy.

What are the key elements of a pharmaceutical care plan for Mr FB at discharge?

A11   **The key elements are to ensure that Mr FB understands the reasons for the changes in his drug regimen and can comply with his prescribed medication when at home, and that there is full communication with the Primary Care Team who will share his care after discharge. This communication should include details of his drug therapy and the monitoring required to ensure the desired therapeutic outcomes are met.**

Although Mr FB's oral drug regimen is relatively simple, it is good clinical practice to counsel him before discharge. If necessary a time-designated, compartmentalised compliance aid (such as the Dosette), could be supplied. This would allow oral solid doses to be assembled in advance. He should be informed that the calcium carbonate tablets should be chewed before swallowing and taken five to 10 minutes before meals, and that the 'sweet-tasting' lactulose liquid should now be taken regularly. He was already proficient at subcutaneous insulin dosing and monitoring his blood glucose levels, so he should not have a problem with his subcutaneous epoetin injections. Mr FB should be reminded not to take any other drugs, either purchased or prescribed, without first checking with the renal unit.

Communication with the Primary Care Team can be facilitated by a comprehensive and timely discharge letter, and issue of a medication record card. This unit issues a printed medication record card at discharge to help communicate information on medication at discharge with the Primary Care Team. Mr FB should be reminded to present the card for updating whenever he (or somebody on his behalf) visits a doctor, dentist, hospital or community pharmacist.

Our hospital operates a shared care protocol for epoetin. Patients are supplied by the hospital for the first three months and then the GP takes over the supply although the hospital continues to monitor treatment. At discharge, Mr FB's GP should be sent a discharge letter which includes his up-to-date medication record, together with information on epoetin. Mr FB should also be given a copy of the information to give to his community pharmacist.

Under this protocol Mr FB's haemoglobin will be measured by his GP or district nurse, and the results analysed in the hospital. Any necessary dosage recommendations are then forwarded to the GP.

> Outline the oral options available for erectile dysfunction. Which is most appropriate for Mr FB?

A12 **As a renal dialysis patient, Mr FB is entitled under Schedule 11 to receive oral treatment for his erectile dysfunction. Sildenafil 25 mg is an appropriate choice for him.**

Mr FB could be suffering from erectile dysfunction due to his diabetes, hypertension, chronic renal failure or his anaemia. We are already treating his anaemia and hypertension but this has not solved his problem. It is important to avoid beta-blockers and alpha-blocker therapy for his hypertension as they can cause erectile dysfunction. However, ACEIs have also been implicated.

Sildenafil inhibits phosphodiesterase type 5, causing an increase in cyclic GMP levels which results in corporal smooth muscle relaxation. This restores natural erectile function in response to sexual stimulation. It has a 56% success rate in diabetics and a 71% success rate in peritoneal dialysis patients. As Mr FB is not on any anginal medication, then he is eligible for sildenafil. He should be advised to take it on an empty stomach, 30 minutes to four hours prior to sexual intercourse. In renal failure an initial dose of 25 mg should be used and the dose slowly increased as required. Sildenafil is relatively well tolerated in renal failure.

Apomorphine (Uprima) is another oral alternative. This is a dopamine agonist used to enhance pro-erectile stimuli via a central mechanism. It is administered by the sublingual route therefore works faster than sildenafil, so can be taken 20 minutes pre-intercourse. In renal failure an initial dose of 2 mg is recommended. As there is not a much information on the efficacy of apomorphine in renal failure, Mr FB was commenced on sildenafil 25 mg.

Acknowledgements

I would like to thank Raymond Bunn for giving permission for his original chapter to be used as the basis for this revised case.

Further reading

Advisory Committee on Peritonitis Management. Peritoneal dialysis-related peritonitis – treatment recommendations – 1996 update. *Perit Dial Int* 1996; **16**: 557–573. For updates, see: www.ispd.org/guidelines/articles

Bunn R, Ashley C. *The Renal Drug Handbook*, 1st edn. Radcliffe Medical Press, Abingdon, Oxon, 1999.

Casadevall N, Nataf J, Viron B *et al.* Pure red cell aplasia and antierythropoietin antibodies in patients treated with recombinant erythropoietin. *N Engl J Med* 2002; **346**: 469–475.

Cassidy MJD. Renal Osteodystrophy. *Medicine* 1999; **27**(6): 37–40.

Currie A, O'Brien P. Renal replacement therapies. *Pharm J* 2001; **226**: 679–683.

Drüeke TB, Bárány P, Cazzola M *et al.* Management of iron deficiency in renal anaemia: guidelines for the optimal therapeutic approach in erythropoietin treated patients. *Clin Nephrol* 1997; **48**: 1–8.

Gokal R. Long-term CAPD therapy. *Br J Renal Med* 1998; **3**: 20–22.

Gokal R. Peritoneal dialysis. *Medicine* 1999; **27**(6): 47–49.

Morlidge C, Richards T. Managing chronic renal disease. *Pharm J* 2001; **226**: 655–657.

Quellhorst E. Insulin therapy during peritoneal dialysis. Pros and cons of various forms of administration. *J Am Soc Nephrol* 2002; **13**: S92–S96.

Richardson D, Bartlett C, Will EJ. Optimising erythropoietin therapy in haemodialysis patients. *Am J Kidney Dis* 2001; **38**: 109–117.

Silverberg DS, Blum M, Peer G *et al.* Intravenous ferric saccharate as an iron supplement in dialysis patients. *Nephron* 1996; **72**: 413–417.

7

Renal transplantation

Caroline A Ashley

Case study and questions

Day 1 (a.m.) Thirty-eight-year-old Mr JO was urgently admitted from home for a cadaveric renal transplant. He had a six-year history of renal impairment, having first presented to his GP with persistent headaches. He had also complained of weakness, fatigue and generally 'not feeling well', and on investigation was found to have a markedly elevated serum creatinine. He was diagnosed as having chronic renal failure. For the last five years he had been in end-stage renal failure, receiving intermittent haemodialysis three times a week, while awaiting a transplant. A donor kidney was now available.

His drug therapy on admission was:

- Calcichew (calcium carbonate 1250 mg), two tablets three times daily
- Alfacalcidol 1 microgram three times a week
- Folic acid 5 mg daily
- Ketovite, one tablet daily
- Amlodipine 10 mg twice daily
- Perindopril 4 mg daily
- Venofer 100 mg intravenously once a month.
- Erythropoietin 2000 international units subcutaneously three times a week

Mr JO was a non-smoker who rarely drank alcohol. He was married with an eight-year-old daughter and worked as a draughtsman, although he had recently been having difficulty maintaining his job due to the frequent dialysis sessions.

On examination Mr JO was reported to be pale, but generally quite well. He was mildly hypertensive (blood pressure 135/85 mmHg) and had a pulse of 70 beats per minute, but had no oedema or signs of cardiac failure. His urine output was less than 50 mL/day. Mr JO weighed 72 kg.

His serum biochemistry and haematology results were:

- Creatinine 672 micromol/L (reference range 60–120)
- Phosphate 1.66 mmol/L (0.8–1.4)
- Sodium 140 mmol/L (135–146)
- Potassium 4.0 mmol/L (3.5–5.0)
- Calcium 2.44 mmol/L (2.1–2.6)

- Urea 12.8 mmol/L (3.0–6.5)
- Haemoglobin 10.2 g/dL (13.5–18.0)
- White blood cells (WBC) 5.2 × 10^9/L (4–10 × 10^9)
- Liver function tests within normal limits

Day 1 (p.m.)   Mr JO was prepared for transplant. One hour prior to the operation he was given 180 mg ciclosporin (approximately 2.5 mg/kg) intravenously, 75 mg azathioprine (approximately 1 mg/kg) intravenously and 1.2 g co-amoxiclav intravenously. The latter was given to cover the surgery and insertion of a central line.

During the transplant, at the release of the vascular clamps, he was given 1 g methylprednisolone intravenously.

Q1   How should these injections be administered?
Q2   What are the therapeutic aims on return from theatre?
Q3   Which immunosuppressant(s) would you recommend be prescribed subsequently and why?

On return to the renal unit later that evening, Mr JO was started on:

- Ciclosporin 180 mg intravenously, to be repeated every 12 hours
- Azathioprine 75 mg intravenously, to be repeated once each day

- Methylprednisolone 16 mg intravenously, to be repeated once each day

Q4   How should ciclosporin therapy be monitored?
Q5   Which parameters should be monitored when azathioprine is prescribed?

Hourly fluid balance charts, temperature, blood pressure and respiration rate monitoring were started. Mr JO initially had a urine output of 40 mL/h. He was given Monosol (an electrolyte replacement solution containing glucose, calcium, sodium, magnesium, chloride and lactate), 1 L intravenously, plus the replacement volume to match his urine output each hour, using the central venous pressure (CVP) as a guide to fluid balance. He was also given 100 mL 20% human serum albumin. The kidney initially failed to diurese, so infusions of furosemide (10 mg/h) and low-dose dopamine (2.5 micrograms/kg/min) were set up.

Mr JO's blood pressure was noted to be 125/95 mmHg but, in order to keep the transplanted kidney well perfused, it was decided that antihypertensive therapy was not necessary. He was, however, started on ranitidine to prevent stress ulceration.

Two hours post-operatively, serum biochemistry and haematology results were:

- Sodium 139 mmol/L (135–146)
- Potassium 3.6 mmol/L (3.5–5.0)
- Urea 8.3 mmol/L (3.0–6.5)
- Creatinine 412 micromol/L (60–120)

- Haemoglobin 9.0 g/dL (13.5–18.0)
- WBC 5.8×10^9/L $(4.0–10.0 \times 10^9)$

Q6 What dosage of ranitidine is appropriate for this indication?

Day 3 Mr JO was well, apyrexial and his urine output was good (approximately 150 mL/h). The dopamine infusion was stopped and it was decided to give his remaining intravenous medications by the oral route.

Serum biochemistry and haematology results were:

- Creatinine 208 micromol/L (60–120)
- WBC 6.5×10^9/L $(4.0–10.0 \times 10^9)$

- Ciclosporin 263 nanograms/mL (target level 250–350 by HPLC of whole blood)

Q7 What oral doses of immunosuppressants would you recommend?

Nifedipine 10 mg orally when required was prescribed as an antihypertensive, to be used if Mr JO's diastolic blood pressure was greater than 100 mmHg.

Q8 Would you have recommended nifedipine as an antihypertensive for Mr JO?

Day 4 Serum biochemistry and haematology results were:

- Creatinine 215 micromol/L (60–120)

- WBC 6.1×10^9/L $(4.0–10.0 \times 10^9)$

Day 5 Mr JO became pyrexial with a temperature of 37.5°C and the kidney site was slightly tender. His blood pressure was 130/100 mmHg.

Serum biochemistry and haematology results were:

- Creatinine 270 micromol/L (60–120)

- WBC 6.4×10^9/L (4.0–10.0)

- Lymphocytes 3.2×10^9/L (1.0–3.5)
- Ciclosporin 268 nanograms/mL (250–350)

A MAG3 (^{99m}Tc mercapto acetyl triglycene) scan showed reduced perfusion of the kidney, and it was decided that Mr JO was suffering from an episode of acute rejection, which was confirmed by renal biopsy.

Q9 How should Mr JO's acute rejection episode be managed?

Day 8 Mr JO was looking better. His serum creatinine level had fallen to 143 micromol/L and the graft site was no longer tender. His ciclosporin level (trough) was 285 nanograms/mL.

Day 15 Mr JO again became pyrexial and the transplant had become tender and increased in size. There was no obvious infection.
Serum biochemistry and haematology results were:

- Creatinine 378 micromol/L (60–120)
- WBC 5.6×10^9/L (4.0–10.0×10^9)
- Lymphocytes 3.9×10^9/L (1.0–3.5 $\times 10^9$)
- Ciclosporin 282 nanograms/mL (250–350)

Renal biopsy showed severe acute rejection, and it was decided that Mr JO required further immunosuppression with anti-thymocyte immunoglobulin (ATG).

Q10 What precautions should be taken when starting ATG?
Q11 How should the dose be calculated?
Q12 How should ATG be administered?
Q13 How does ATG differ from antilymphocyte immunoglobulin (ALG)?
Q14 Should the doses of his other immunosuppressants be adjusted during ATG therapy?

Day 15 A subclavian line was inserted and a 10-day course of ATG started. The initial dose of ATG administered was 175 mg (2.5 mg/kg).

Day 16 Lymphocytes 1.09×10^9/L, dose of ATG = 175 mg.

Day 17 Lymphocytes 0.31×10^9/L, dose of ATG = 100mg.

Day 18 Lymphocytes 0.15×10^9/L, dose of ATG = 100 mg.

Day 19 Lymphocytes 0.07×10^9/L, dose of ATG omitted.

Day 20 Lymphocytes 0.14×10^9/L, dose of ATG = 100 mg.

Day 21 Lymphocytes 0.26×10^9/L, dose of ATG = 175 mg.

Day 22 Lymphocytes 0.21×10^9/L, dose of ATG = 175 mg.

Day 23 Lymphocytes 0.16×10^9/L, dose of ATG = 100 mg.

Day 24 Lymphocytes 0.20×10^9/L, dose of ATG = 175 mg.

Day 25 Mr JO was showing a marked improvement, with increased renal perfusion shown by a MAG3 scan.
His serum biochemistry and haematology results were:

- Creatinine 131 micromol/L (60–120)
- WBC 3.1×10^9/L (4.0–10.0)
- Ciclosporin 261 nanograms/mL (250–350)

Q15 What changes might be made to Mr JO's oral immunosuppressive medication at this point?

Mr JO was now well, with good renal function, so he was discharged home, to attend out-patients three times a week initially, to monitor his progress.

Q16 What pharmaceutical care plans should be made in preparation for Mr JO's discharge?

Mr JO was discharged on the following medication:

- Tacrolimus 3 mg orally twice daily
- Mycophenolate mofetil 500 mg orally three times daily
- Prednisolone 15 mg orally each morning
- Ranitidine 150 mg orally twice daily
- Amphotericin lozenges, one to be sucked four times each day
- Aspirin 75 mg once daily
- Co-trimoxazole 480 mg once daily

Q17 How long should Mr JO remain on immunosuppressants?
Q18 How long is Mr JO likely to require ranitidine and amphotericin therapy?
Q19 What points would you cover when counselling Mr JO about his medication?

Day 35   Mr JO became pyrexial again, but this time the transplant site was not tender. He had developed a dry cough, had some shortness of breath and exhibited a marked deterioration in blood oxygen saturation on exertion. He had also developed a swinging fever, and a chest x-ray showed diffuse interstitial shadowing.

His serum biochemistry and haematology results were:

- Creatinine 118 micromol/L (60–120)
- WBC 3.9×10^9/L $(4.0$–$10.0 \times 10^9)$
- Platelets 129×10^9/L (140–400)
- Tacrolimus 13.2 nanograms/mL (5–15)

Blood and mid-stream urine samples were sent to microbiology and virology for culture.

Q20 What has predisposed Mr JO to infection?
Q21 What types of infection is Mr JO susceptible to?

Mr JO was diagnosed as having a pneumonitis due to cytomegalovirus (CMV).

Q22 What treatment would you recommend?

Over the next 14 days Mr JO's temperature returned to normal and he appeared to be progressing well. His urine output was approximately 2 L/24 hours and his blood gases were improving.

At three months post-transplant, Mr JO was discharged back to the care of his GP, attending the hospital for transplant out-patient appointments every three months.

Day 122   Mr JO presented to the renal unit as an emergency. He mentioned that he had recently been treated for a chest infection with erythromycin by his GP. His urine output had fallen to 750 mL in the last 24 hours and he had become oedematous. He was prescribed intravenous furosemide 40 mg twice daily to relieve the oedema. A MAG3 scan showed deterioration of renal perfusion, but a biopsy of the transplant showed no evidence of rejection. Tacrolimus nephrotoxicity was diagnosed.

Serum biochemistry and haematology results were:

- Creatinine 380 micromol/L (60–120)
- WBC 5.3×10^9/L $(4.0$–$10.0 \times 10^9)$
- Tacrolimus level 27 nanograms/mL (5–15)

Q23 What could have caused tacrolimus toxicity?
Q24 Which drugs interact with tacrolimus?
Q25 How can tacrolimus nephrotoxicity be differentiated from rejection?

How should these injections be administered?

A1 **(a)** **Ciclosporin 180 mg in 250 mL glucose 5% over at least 60 minutes.**

Ciclosporin for injection should be diluted at least one in twenty, i.e. the minimum volume for 150 mg (3 mL) is 60 mL. It may be diluted in either 0.9% sodium chloride or glucose 5%. The manufacturer's data sheet recommends administration over two to six hours, but there is rarely sufficient time for this with cadaveric transplants. Faster infusion rates are associated with a higher incidence of nausea and vomiting. Mr JO should be observed throughout the infusion as ciclosporin injection contains polyethoxylated castor oil, which has been reported to cause anaphylactoid reactions.

(b) **Azathioprine 75 mg in 50 mL 0.9% sodium chloride or glucose/saline over 30 minutes.**

If a slow infusion is not practicable, azathioprine may be given as a slow bolus over at least one minute. Azathioprine injection is a very alkaline, irritant solution and therefore the bolus should be flushed with 50 mL 0.9% sodium chloride or glucose/saline after administration.

(c) **Co-amoxiclav 1.2 g in 100 mL sodium chloride 0.9% over 30–40 minutes.**

Again, an alternative method is by reconstitution with 20 mL Water for Injections followed by administration by slow bolus injection over three to four minutes.

(d) **Methylprednisolone 1 g in 100 mL glucose 5% infused over at least 30 minutes.**

The reconstituted solution may also be diluted with 0.9% sodium chloride or glucose/saline. It must be given slowly to minimise the cardiac arrhythmias, circulatory collapse and cardiac arrests associated with rapid infusions.

What are the therapeutic aims on return from theatre?

A2 (a) **Volume expansion using a combination of crystalloid fluids and blood/colloids. The latter are given to maintain a high CVP. Clear fluids are given to replace the urine output volume for volume. HSA (human serum albumin) or Gelofusine are usually given as the colloid.**

(b) **Maintain good renal perfusion, using dopamine (2.5 micrograms/kg/min) and/or furosemide (10–20 mg/h) if the urine output is less than 50 mL/h and ensure Mr JO is volume-replete. Mannitol has been used in the past to obtain a diuresis, but it has been shown to have an osmotic effect on renal tubules, is itself nephrotoxic and exacerbates the nephrotoxicity of ciclosporin.**

(c) **Control any post-operative hypertension. This will reduce the risk of fitting and/or renal damage.**

(d) **Treat any systemic vasoconstriction using vasodilators.**

(e) **Maintain adequate immunosuppression to prevent rejection.**

(f) **Avoid infection.**

(g) **Recheck plasma electrolytes (risk of rapidly rising potassium levels) and haemoglobin (to ensure Mr JO is not bleeding) on return from theatre.**

Which immunosuppressant(s) would you recommend be prescribed subsequently and why?

A3 **Mr JO should receive combined immunosuppressive therapy with azathioprine, corticosteroids and ciclosporin. Combining immunosuppressants provides a synergistic effect, allowing lower doses of each agent, and a lower incidence of toxicity and rejection. Most centres use 'triple therapy', employing a combination of newer and older immunosuppressive agents, e.g. (ciclosporin or tacrolimus) plus (azathioprine or mycophenolate) plus prednisolone.**

Rejection occurs when Mr JO's grafted kidney is recognised as 'foreign' and is attacked by his immune system. On recognition of the 'foreign' tissue, the lymphokine interleukin (IL)-2 causes T lymphocytes in his lymph nodes to differentiate into T helpers (lymphocytes that provide information to B lymphocytes about the antigens), T-cytotoxic cells (killer lymphocytes that cause direct damage to 'foreign' cells) and

T suppressors (which suppress B lymphocytes and prevent multiplication and antibody formation). Sensitised lymphocytes return to the graft site in large numbers, reacting with the antigenic material and releasing lymphokines ('messenger' substances), which attract macrophages to the site. These, together with T-cytotoxic cells, destroy the grafted kidney.

Immunosuppression either reduces to ineffective numbers the number of cells reacting against the transplanted organ or it inhibits their normal function.

Prophylactic regimens against rejection vary between transplant centres. The main immunosuppressants used are: ciclosporin; tacrolimus; azathioprine; prednisolone; mycophenolate mofetil (MMF); sirolimus; polyclonal antibodies such as ATG and ALG; monoclonal antibodies such as basiliximab, daclizumab and OKT$_3$.

(a)   Azathioprine. This is metabolised to 6-mercaptopurine, which disrupts purine metabolism and consequently interferes with DNA synthesis and cell proliferation, thereby reducing lymphocyte function.

(b)   Corticosteroids. These have several possible mechanisms of action, e.g. anti-inflammatory activity (which profoundly alters the effector phases of graft rejection, including macrophage function), blocking the production of IL-1 and IL-2 (lymphokines), and causing the sequestration of circulating lymphocytes and monocytes in lymphoid tissue, particularly the bone marrow.

Adverse effects are commonly encountered and include cushingoid appearance, hypertension, hyperglycaemia, weight gain, increased susceptibility to infection and personality changes. Long-term complications include skin and muscle atrophy and avascular necrosis of bone.

(c)   Ciclosporin. This appears to act primarily by blocking the production of IL-2 by T-helper cells through inhibition of their messenger RNA. Unlike azathioprine it is not myelosuppressive. Ciclosporin is used initially at oral doses of 5–10 mg/kg/day, reducing over several months to maintenance doses as low as 3 mg/kg/day without an apparent increase in graft rejection. Individual patient handling is very variable and doses must be tailored according to ciclosporin levels.

Neoral is an oral formulation of ciclosporin in a form that undergoes micro-emulsification in the presence of water. In addition, absorption of Neoral from the gastrointestinal tract is not bile-salt dependent. This results in improved absorption and a less variable bioavailability, allowing a greater control of blood levels; however, careful monitoring of blood levels is still essential. Toxic effects include nephrotoxicity and hypertension.

(d) Tacrolimus (FK506). This is a macrolide immunosuppressant that suppresses T-cell activation and T-helper cell-dependent B-cell proliferation, as well as the formation of lymphokines such as IL-2 and IL-3, and beta-interferon through similar mechanisms to ciclosporin. Oral absorption is estimated to be approximately 20% in kidney transplant patients. An initial dose of 0.1 mg/kg/day in two divided doses is generally used, again with the dose being adjusted according to blood levels.

From studies comparing ciclosporin with tacrolimus as primary immunosuppressants following renal transplantation, tacrolimus has been shown to be the more potent of the two, and is associated with a lower incidence of acute allograft rejection. Tacrolimus has been shown to cause nephrotoxicity, neurotoxicity and cardiotoxicity, although the incidence of these side-effects is much less with the lower doses now used in clinical practice.

(e) MMF is a prodrug of mycophenolic acid, and acts by inhibiting the intracellular *de novo* pathway for purine synthesis. Most cells also possess a salvage pathway, but T lymphocytes do not, thereby rendering them unable to synthesise purines, which in turn prevents successful cell replication. MMF is therefore similar to azathioprine, but is more selective in its pharmacological effect.

(f) Sirolimus is a novel immunosuppressive agent which inhibits T-cell proliferation by inhibiting cytokine-mediated signal transduction pathways. It has been used in combination with ciclosporin and prednisolone to lower the incidence of early acute rejection. However, its place in therapy will probably prove to be in the treatment of chronic rejection, or chronic allograft nephropathy.

(g) Monoclonal antibodies, e.g. basiliximab (chimeric) and daclizumab (humanised). These bind to the CD25 antigen on human T lymphocytes to prevent the T lymphocytes from expressing IL-2, thus inhibiting the activation of T-cytotoxic cells and thereby effectively hiding the graft from the recipient's immune system, resulting in a reduced incidence of acute rejection. These agents are very expensive, so some units use these agents for every transplant, whereas others reserve them just for high-risk transplants, i.e. one where the patient is highly sensitised from previous transplants or blood transfusions, or where the cross-match is not favourable.

OKT3 is a murine monoclonal antibody used only for the treatment of severe acute rejection unresponsive to other therapies. It is associated with side-effects such as rigors, high fever, abdominal pain and pulmonary oedema, and is rarely used now.

(h) Polyclonal antibodies, e.g. ATG (rabbit) and ALG (horse). These remove circulating T lymphocytes, and block their formation and proliferation in response to antigenic stimuli. They react with a wide variety of receptors on T cells. Traditionally, a 10-day course of either low-dose ATG or ALG was given as induction therapy after a 'high-risk' transplant, but their use now tends to be reserved for salvage therapy in patients whose acute vascular rejection episodes are not responding to high-dose steroids.

How should ciclosporin therapy be monitored?

A4 **By regular review of blood levels of ciclosporin, glucose and potassium, liver function tests, plasma lipid levels, and blood pressure.**

(a) Ciclosporin levels may be monitored in two ways:

   (i) Trough levels should be taken before the morning dose every two to three days until therapy is stabilised, then monthly, or two to three days after any dosing change. A diurnal variation in ciclosporin clearance occurs and therefore sampling should be at a fixed time each day. Times to achieve peak levels are variable (one to six hours after oral dosing); trough levels provide more consistent results. The risk of rejection is greatest shortly after transplant and pathophysiological changes occur rapidly. The half-life of ciclosporin has been reported to be six to 40 hours and hence two to three days is the time usually required to achieve steady-state concentrations.

   (ii) Profiling of the absorption of ciclosporin is a concept of therapeutic drug monitoring designed to further optimise the clinical efficacy of the drug but at the same time minimise adverse effects. A trough (C_0), followed by a single blood concentration measured two hours after ciclosporin administration (C_2) has been shown to be a significantly more accurate predictor of total drug exposure than trough concentrations alone. Although this would be the ideal way to monitor exposure to ciclosporin in all transplant patients, in practice it is difficult to achieve this in the out-patient clinic setting as it requires two blood samples to be taken exactly two hours apart. Hence its use is often restricted to the in-patient setting when initiating therapy.

      Whole-blood, plasma or serum samples may be used but quoted therapeutic ranges differ, depending on the sample type and the assay method. Ciclosporin in blood distributes between erythrocytes (50%), leucocytes (10%) and plasma (40%).

Several assay techniques are available: high-performance liquid chromatography (HPLC) is regarded as being the gold standard, but is laborious and costly. Radioimmunoassay gives a wide variation in results and is seldom used now. Fluorescence polarisation immunoassay is a rapid and sensitive method, but measures ciclosporin metabolites as well as the parent drug, so tends to give levels 10–16% higher than those obtained by HPLC. EMIT is an enzyme immunoassay developed to measure microamounts of drugs in human biological fluids. Since it detects only the parent drug, its results correlate well with those of HPLC and it is now the assay used in the majority of renal units to monitor whole-blood ciclosporin levels. Using a standard triple-therapy immunosuppression regimen, it is usual to aim for 12-hour trough levels of 250–350 nanograms/mL for the first two months, reducing to a target level of 150–250 nanograms/mL for the next four to six months. Thereafter, in a stable graft, levels of 100–150 nanograms/mL are acceptable. These levels do vary according to local protocol.

(b)   Liver function tests. Reversible dose-related hepatotoxicity may be seen, resulting in increases in serum bilirubin and liver enzymes.
(c)   Serum glucose levels. Hyperglycaemia may develop as a result of ciclosporin or concomitant corticosteroid therapy.
(d)   Serum potassium levels. Toxic levels of ciclosporin are often associated with hyperkalaemia.
(e)   Blood pressure monitoring. Hypertension is frequently observed and has been associated with seizures. It is not generally dose-related, but may result from the vasoconstrictive effects of the drug.
(e)   Plasma lipids levels. As ciclosporin can cause reversible increases in plasma lipids, serum cholesterol and triglycerides should be regularly monitored.

Which parameters should be monitored when azathioprine is prescribed?

A5   **Haematology and liver function.**

Full blood counts, including platelets, should be carried out at least weekly for the first two months and then less frequently. Azathioprine causes dose-related, reversible bone marrow suppression, which is usually seen early in therapy, but can develop on long-term treatment. Liver function tests should also be performed, as cholestatic and/or reversible dose-related hepatotoxicity can develop.

What dosage of ranitidine is appropriate for this indication?

A6 **Initially, ranitidine 50 mg intravenously three times daily, changing to 150 mg orally twice daily when Mr JO is able to take oral medication.**

Ranitidine is excreted via the kidneys and dosage is usually halved if the glomerular filtration rate (GFR) is less than 10 mL/min. Mr JO still has a high serum creatinine level, but it is lower than pre-transplant. Most of the equations available to estimate the creatinine clearance from the serum creatinine are inaccurate if there are acute changes in renal function. Accepting these inaccuracies, an estimated GFR for Mr JO is between 10 and 15 mL/min. Future serum creatinine results should be monitored to check renal function is continuing to improve.

What oral doses of immunosuppressants would you recommend?

A7 **Prednisolone 20 mg orally each morning, azathioprine 75 mg orally each morning, and ciclosporin 300 mg orally twice each day.**

Oral absorption of prednisolone is 'normal' in renal transplant patients. Methylprednisolone and prednisolone differ in anti-inflammatory potency: 5 mg prednisolone is equivalent to 4 mg methylprednisolone, therefore 20 mg prednisolone is equivalent to 16 mg methyl-prednisolone.

Azathioprine oral absorption is variable in renal transplant patients, but generally the same dose is given orally as intravenously.

Oral absorption of ciclosporin is relatively slow, variable and incomplete. One study of adult renal transplant patients demonstrated a mean bioavailability of 35 ± 25% in the first month post-operatively. Therefore the oral dose of ciclosporin is two to three times the intravenous dose. However, at doses greater than 300 mg twice daily, patients invariably develop high ciclosporin levels, so dosing should be based on ideal rather than actual body weight. The last measured ciclosporin level was high and therefore Mr JO should be given just less than twice the intravenous dose orally, and levels measured after two days.

Would you have recommended nifedipine as an antihypertensive for Mr JO?

A8   Yes.

Renal patients often have high renin profiles resulting in systemic vaso-constriction and hypertension. Vasoconstriction may also be catecholamine-mediated and this may also partly explain the hyper-tension associated with ciclosporin. Vasodilators are probably the most appropriate method of reducing the blood pressure acutely.

Nifedipine is a vasodilator and does not require dosage adjustment in renal failure. Amlodipine is more commonly used now, since it has a longer duration of action, and tends not to be associated with some of the undesirable effects that nifedipine can cause such as severe headache.

Recent research has indicated that oral nifedipine may cause increa-ses in GFR and renal blood flow, despite a substantial decrease in blood pressure. As vasoconstriction appears to play a role in acute as well as chronic ciclosporin-induced renal dysfunction, nifedipine may counter-act these effects on renal vasculature. However, some patients on nifedi-pine develop marked vasodilation-dependent oedema, which may cause alarm by suggesting renal impairment.

It is also worth noting that the manufacturers of ciclosporin state that concurrent administration of nifedipine has resulted in a higher incidence of gingival hyperplasia when compared with ciclosporin alone.

Intravenous antihypertensives such as glyceryl trinitrate, hydrala-zine and labetalol are usually reserved for more severe hypertension. Overzealous treatment of hypertension could compromise the function of the transplanted kidney by reducing renal perfusion.

How should Mr JO's acute rejection episode be managed?

A9   Methylprednisolone 500 mg to 1 g intravenously in 100 mL 5% glucose administered over 60 minutes once each day for three days.

Acute rejection is most commonly seen five to 10 days post-transplant. The three agents most commonly used to treat acute rejection are: methylprednisolone, monoclonal and polyclonal antibodies.

(a)   Methylprednisolone. This is the cheapest alternative and has been demonstrated to reverse 72–83% of first allograft rejections. Gen-erally, two consecutive rejection episodes may be treated with this drug. Thereafter, concern for the total corticosteroid dose given increases and other strategies need to be considered.

(b) Monoclonal (OKT3) and polyclonal (ATG/ALG) antibodies. These are very expensive and their use tends to be reserved either for third or subsequent rejection episodes, or for severe acute rejection not responsive to intravenous methylprednisolone. It should be noted that the chimeric/humanised monoclonal antibodies, basiliximab and daclizumab, are ineffective in the treatment of an established severe rejection episode.

Methylprednisolone 1 g/day for three days is the preferred option for Mr JO's first rejection episode.

What precautions should be taken when starting ATG?

A10 (a) **Give a test dose of ATG (5 mg diluted in 100 mL 0.9% sodium chloride administered via a central line over one hour). This is to check Mr JO's tolerance, as ATG has been associated with anaphylaxis, due to allergy to rabbit protein.**

(b) **Ensure intravenous adrenaline (epinephrine), hydrocortisone and chlorphenamine are available during administration of the first dose, and ready for use if required urgently.**

(c) **Administer ATG via a large vein, preferably a central line, to avoid thrombophlebitis and localised pain.**

How should the dose be calculated?

A11 **The initial dose is 2.5–5.0 mg/kg ATG (Imtix Sangstat brand) per day until the biological signs and symptoms improve. A typical course length would be five to 14 days (often 10). Each subsequent day's dosage is determined by monitoring the patient's WBC and lymphocyte counts. The aim is to maintain a WBC count of 2–4 $\times$ 10^9/L and a total lymphocyte count of 0.2–0.5 $\times$ 10^9/L. ATG dosing schedules vary with local protocol.**

Some centres administer ATG using alternate-day regimens to minimise the risk of neutropenia. If the lymphocyte count falls below 0.1 $\times$ 10^9/L, the next dose of ATG should be omitted.

Platelets should also be monitored during treatment and any thrombocytopenia below 50 000/mm^3 will require interruption of treatment.

How should ATG be administered?

A12 Each 25 mg vial should be diluted in 50 mL 0.9% sodium chloride, but in practice, on the prescriber's responsibility, a higher concentration (e.g. 1 mg/mL) may be administered, so that the sodium and fluid load is not too great for the patient. Alternatively, glucose 5% may be used as the diluent. The infusion is usually administered over 8–12 hours via a large vein. Any associated fever or shivering may be relieved by administering chlorphenamine or hydrocortisone intravenously one hour prior to the infusion.

How does ATG differ from ALG?

A13 ALG and ATG primarily differ in the animal used for their production. The name ATG is usually reserved for the substance produced in rabbits and ALG for that produced in horses.

Both are prepared by hyperimmunisation of the respective animals with human T-cell lymphocytes. The immunoglobulins produced are purified and concentrated. The choice of agent depends on the patient's ability to tolerate horse or rabbit proteins. Generally, ATG is considered to be the more potent of the two and there appears to be a higher incidence of adverse reactions to horse-derived products.

Should the doses of his other immunosuppressants be adjusted during ATG therapy?

A14 Mr JO's azathioprine therapy should be stopped while the ATG course is in progress. Both drugs are myelosuppressive and concurrent use may cause a marked leucopenia necessitating the withdrawal of the ATG. The prednisolone and ciclosporin doses should initially be unchanged; however, three days before the end of the ATG course, the prednisolone dose should be doubled, as practice has shown episodes of acute rejection may occur shortly after stopping ATG.

Immediately the ATG course finishes, the azathioprine should be restarted at a reduced dose which should be gradually increased (e.g. weekly) if the WBC count remains stable. The prednisolone therapy is then reduced over three to four days to the maintenance dose of 20 mg each morning.

The ciclosporin should remain at the current dose, provided blood level monitoring indicates that this is still appropriate.

> What changes might be made to Mr JO's oral immunosuppressive medication at this point?

A15 **Since Mr JO has now experienced two acute rejection episodes on his current immunosuppressive regimen, it might be useful to change his prescription to employ more potent agents.**

Ciclosporin and tacrolimus are considered to be alike in mode of action, but tacrolimus is the more potent of the two. In the same way, azathioprine and mycophenolate have similar pharmacological effects, but mycophenolate is thought to be more specific and more potent. Hence, it is not uncommon for a patient receiving ciclosporin, azathioprine and prednisolone who experiences several acute rejection episodes to be switched to an alternative regimen, such as tacrolimus, mycophenolate and prednisolone, with the aim of preventing further rejection episodes.

The risk of acute rejection is greatest in the first three to six months, after which some kind of adaptive process appears to occur, although a patient may experience a rejection episode any time during the life of the transplant, especially if the patient omits taking their immunosuppressive medication. Once the risk of acute rejection is less, the doses of the immunosuppressive drugs are usually reduced down to maintenance levels. This reduces the incidence and severity of side-effects without compromising graft function.

> What pharmaceutical care plans should be made in preparation for Mr JO's discharge?

A16 **The pharmaceutical care plan for Mr JO should include the following:**

(a) Ensure there is agreement as to who will be responsible for Mr JO's community care. If Mr JO's care is to be fully managed in the community it is essential that there is sufficient liaison with Mr JO's local (regular) community pharmacist to ensure continuity of medication supply, and that there is a suitable shared care protocol in place, such that his GP is aware of Mr JO's current medication, the monitoring required and of any clinically important drug interactions. Mr JO, his GP and his community pharmacist should be given information on how to obtain specialist advice, either from the renal pharmacy specialist or the hospital renal team.

(b) Mr JO should receive appropriate discharge medication counselling. This should ensure he understands the purpose of, and the directions given with, his medication. Patients should generally receive an accurate written treatment record card. The packaging of the medication should be appropriate to Mr JO's needs. It is important to check if any compliance aids are necessary.

How long should Mr JO remain on immunosuppressants?

A17 **Immunosuppressive therapy can rarely be stopped completely after transplant. Even the briefest cessation may precipitate rejection. Intensive immunosuppression is, however, usually only required for the first few weeks post-transplant or during a rejection crisis. Subsequently the graft may often be maintained on relatively small doses of immunosuppressive drugs and hence fewer adverse drug effects are experienced by the patient.**

In addition, the aim of immunosuppressive therapy nowadays is to tailor the drug regimen to the needs of the individual patient, in order to maximise efficacy, and at the same time minimise side-effects. Although acute rejection episodes are not as common, and are easily treated, even modern immunosuppressive agents appear to have little effect on chronic rejection, or as it is now known, chronic allograft nephropathy (CAN). The precise mechanism of this process is not fully understood, but there is some evidence that long-term use of some immunosuppressive drugs such as ciclosporin may contribute to the process. Long-term use of ciclosporin or tacrolimus is also known to be nephrotoxic, so there is now a move to switch patients to agents with an antiproliferative effect, such as sirolimus or mycophenolate, which theoretically will prevent the histological changes seen in CAN and so prolong the life of a transplanted kidney. There are ongoing long-term studies to investigate the effects of this change in therapy.

How long is Mr JO likely to require ranitidine and amphotericin therapy?

A18 **Ranitidine therapy is likely to continue whilst Mr JO remains on high-dose prednisolone, but will probably be reduced to a maintenance dose of 150 mg at night as his condition stabilizes. Amphotericin may be required as long as Mr JO**

receives immunosuppressive therapy. In practice, it is likely to be stopped three to six months post-transplant and restarted only if oral candidiasis recurs. Prophylactic oral amphotericin may be needed if Mr JO requires any further courses of antibiotics.

Many units also routinely prescribe aspirin 75 mg daily, plus co-trimoxazole 480 mg daily for all renal transplant patients. Co-trimoxazole is used for the first three months post-transplant as prophylaxis against *Pneumocystis carinii* pneumonia (PCP), while there is evidence that the antiplatelet effect of low-dose aspirin helps to prevent thrombosis of the transplant renal artery, thereby maintaining good perfusion of the transplant kidney.

What points would you cover when counselling Mr JO about his medication?

A19 **In addition to explaining the purpose of each drug the following information should be given:**

(a)   MMF

    (i)   Although it was initially advised to take MMF on an empty stomach, this factor is now not thought to be so important, and indeed, many patients take their MMF after food to minimise gastrointestinal adverse effects. In addition, since the most common side-effect of MMF is diarrhoea, many units have found it useful to initiate therapy at a low dose, e.g. 250 mg three times a day, and increase it over a period of a few days to the full dose of 1 g twice daily. Some patients prefer to take the full dose as 500 mg four times daily, to minimise the incidence of diarrhoeal episodes.

    (ii)   Mr JO should report any unusual bleeding or bruising as this could indicate bone marrow suppression.

(b)   Tacrolimus

    (i)   Try to maintain a consistent schedule with regard to the time of day the tacrolimus is taken. Ideally, twice-daily regimens should be taken at regular 12-hourly intervals. If possible take at least one hour before or two to three hours after meals in order to achieve maximal absorption. The capsules should be swallowed with fluid, preferably water. Grapefruit juice should be avoided since it contains the flavonoid naringenine which inhibits cytochrome P450 3A4, thus increasing blood tacrolimus levels.

    (ii)   Try to make early morning clinic appointments if tacrolimus blood levels are to be monitored. Do not take that morning's tacrolimus dose until the blood sample has been taken. This will ensure a trough serum level is measured.

(c)   Prednisolone

    (i)   Take at approximately the same time each day, preferably in the morning in order to mimic diurnal production of endogenous steroids.

    (ii)   Always carry a steroid card. It must also be ensured that Mr JO understands the written instructions on the card.

(d)   Ranitidine

    (i)   Take one dose in the morning and the second dose at night, with food if supper is eaten.

(e)   Amphotericin lozenges

    (i)   Take at regular intervals throughout the day.

    (ii)   Suck the lozenges slowly.

    (iii)   If taken near to meal times, suck after meals rather than before.

(f)   Aspirin

    (i)   Take one tablet each day, with or after food.

    (ii)   The tablet may be dispersed in water, or can be swallowed whole, whichever the patient finds easiest.

(g)   Co-trimoxazole

    (i)   Take one tablet each day until advised by the renal unit that treatment is no longer necessary.

(h)   General

    (i)   Do not discontinue any of the medication unless advised by the doctor.

    (ii)   Mr JO should be particularly advised to seek further expert advice either from the community pharmacist or the hospital specialists if over-the-counter medications are required.

    (iii)   Keep all medication out of the reach of children.

    (iv)   Report to the doctor any signs of infection including sore throats.

What has predisposed Mr JO to infection?

A20 **Corticosteroids, mycophenolate mofetil and tacrolimus all increase Mr JO's susceptibility to infection. In addition, Mr JO had recently undergone a course of ATG, which would impair his lymphocyte function and hence his resistance to infection for several months afterwards.**

What types of infection is Mr JO susceptible to?

A21 **After the first one or two months post-transplantation, patients are susceptible to most opportunistic infections.**

Mr JO could develop fungal infections (e.g. *Candida*, *Aspergillus*), protozoal infection (e.g. PCP), viral infection [e.g. cytomegalovirus (CMV), herpes] or common or uncommon bacterial infections (including reactivation of past tuberculosis). He would also contract common illnesses such as flu more easily than usual, and find it harder to recover from such infections.

CMV disease is very common in renal transplant patients, especially in the first few months. It is characterised by a swinging fever, and can manifest as pneumonitis, accompanied by breathlessness and blood oxygen desaturation, interstitial shadowing on the chest x-ray, and a reduced platelet and white blood cell count. Other organs that can be affected are the liver (causing CMV hepatitis, with raised liver enzymes), the gastrointestinal tract (causing acute diarrhoea) and the bone marrow (resulting in severe bone marrow depression).

What course of treatment would you recommend?

A22 **CMV disease may be treated with either intravenous ganciclovir or with oral valganciclovir. Foscarnet is extremely nephrotoxic and should not be used unless the patient has failed to respond to a prolonged course of ganciclovir therapy. Ganciclovir is renally excreted, so the dose will have to be adjusted according to Mr JO's renal function.**

Estimating Mr JO's creatinine clearance does not pose quite the same problems as in the immediate post-transplant period, since his serum creatinine results now appear more stable. However, the Cockcroft and Gault formula is not always accurate in transplant patients, since they have only one functioning kidney. Mr JO's estimated creatinine clearance is 76 mL/min, but a 24-hour urine collection measured his GFR as being 63 mL/min.

For patients with this level of renal function it is recommended that the appropriate dose of ganciclovir is 5 mg/kg twice a day, given intravenously in 100 mL sodium chloride 0.9% over one hour. Since treatment will last at least 14 days, insertion of a central line may be advisable. If Mr JO was well enough to be treated as an out-patient, he may be prescribed valganciclovir 900 mg twice daily orally (unlicensed indication). During treatment, Mr JO's renal function and full blood count should be closely monitored to detect signs of ganciclovir toxicity. It would also be wise to reduce temporarily, or discontinue the dose of MMF, since treatment with MMF can hinder the immune response to viruses, making it much harder to eradicate them effectively.

What could have caused tacrolimus toxicity?

A23 **Erythromycin and tacrolimus co-administration.**

Acute reversible nephrotoxicity has been associated with tacrolimus levels greater than 20 nanograms/mL, although it can occur at levels much lower than this. Mr JO's tacrolimus levels may have been increased by prior erythromycin therapy. Studies in healthy adults suggest that erythromycin can substantially reduce the plasma clearance of tacrolimus, by inhibition of the cytochrome P450 3A4 system. Patients who experience tacrolimus toxicity often exhibit a fine tremor, and are found to be hypertensive, due to vasoconstriction within the kidney. It is also worth noting that it is most unlikely that the administration of intravenous furosemide 40 mg worsened Mr JO's established tacrolimus nephrotoxicity. Only diuretic doses large enough to cause a marked hypovolaemia would be likely to have such an adverse effect.

Which drugs interact with tacrolimus?

A24 (a) **Drugs reported to increase the nephrotoxicity of tacrolimus include: aciclovir, ganciclovir, aminoglycosides, amphotericin B, co-trimoxazole, ciprofloxacin, furosemide (and other potent diuretics), cephalosporins, vancomycin, gyrase inhibitors and non-steroidal anti-inflammatory drugs.**

(b) **Drugs reported to increase tacrolimus levels, by inhibition of metabolism, include: clarithromycin,** erythromycin, ketoconazole, fluconazole, itraconazole, methylprednisolone, protease inhibitors, tamoxifen, omeprazole, danazol, diltiazem and verapamil.

(c) Drugs reported to decrease tacrolimus levels, by induction of metabolism, include: phenytoin, phenobarbital, carbamazepine, rifampicin, metamizole and isoniazid.

(d) Tacrolimus is extensively bound to plasma proteins, so there is the possibility of interactions with other drugs known to have high affinity for plasma proteins, e.g. oral anticoagulants and oral antidiabetic agents.

How can tacrolimus nephrotoxicity be differentiated from rejection?

A25 **Tacrolimus nephrotoxicity is difficult to differentiate from organ rejection.**

Differentiation is necessary to determine whether an increased or decreased dose of immunosuppressants is required.

Rejection is usually associated with fever, low urine output, a rapidly rising serum creatinine level, graft tenderness or enlargement and MAG3 scans that show reduced renal perfusion. Tacrolimus levels are usually low or within the trough reference range and on further reduction of the dose there is either no change or a worsening of renal function.

Tacrolimus toxicity is usually associated with an afebrile patient, low urine output, slowly or rapidly increasing creatinine levels, non-tender grafts and MAG3 scans that show reduced renal perfusion. Serum potassium levels may be high and the patient may be hypertensive. Tacrolimus levels are usually high (greater than 15–20 nanograms/mL) and reduction of the tacrolimus dose improves renal function.

The differentiation of the two is, however, often unclear and histological examination is frequently required. This may reveal renal tubular atrophy and interstitial scarring in the case of tacrolimus toxicity. Small blood vessels (arterioles) may show nodular thickening. The mechanism for tacrolimus nephrotoxicity is unclear, but one proposal is that the drug reduces renal perfusion by interfering with renal prostaglandin release, which may explain any accompanying hyperkalaemia. Initial studies suggested that co-administered synthetic prostaglandins of the E series, such as misoprostol, may protect against tacrolimus nephrotoxicity, but subsequent studies have not confirmed this.

Tacrolimus toxicity usually responds to a reduction in the tacrolimus dose. However, if it appears that the patient is exhibiting signs of toxicity even though the blood levels are not particularly high, then the intolerant patient may be switched to an alternative agent, e.g. sirolimus.

Further reading

Allen RDM, Chapman JR. *A Manual of Renal Transplantation*. Edward Arnold, Sevenoaks, 1994.

Andrews PA, Renal transplantation. *Br Med J* 2002; **324**: 530–534.

Bunn R, Ashley C. *Renal Drug Handbook*, 1st edn. Radcliffe Medical Press, Oxford, 1999.

Dupuis RE. Solid organ transplantation. In: *Applied Therapeutics: The Clinical Use of Drugs*, 7th edn. MA Koda-Kimble, LY Young, WA Kradjan *et al.*, eds. Lippincott Williams & Wilkins, Philadelphia, PA, 2001: 33.1–33.50.

Fahr A. Cyclosporin clinical pharmacokinetics. *Clin Pharmacokinet* 1993; **24**: 472–495.

Fellstrom B. Risk factors for and management of post-transplant cardiovascular disease. *BioDrugs* 2001; **15**: 261–278.

Halloran PF, Melk A. Tailoring therapy: balancing toxicity and chronic allograft dysfunction. *Transplant Proc* 2001; 33(suppl. 3A): 7S–10S.

Pascal M, Theruvath T, Kawai T *et al*. Strategies to improve long-term outcomes after renal transplantation. *N Engl J Med* 2002; **346**: 580–590.

Sperschneider H. A large multicentre trial to compare the efficacy and safety of tacrolimus with ciclosporin microemulsion following renal transplantation. *Transplant Proc* 2001; **33**: 1279–1281.

Tsunoda SM, Aweeka FT. Drug concentration monitoring of immunosuppressive agents. *BioDrugs* 2000; **14**: 355–369.

Yee GC, Stanley DL, Pessa GL *et al*. Effect of grapefruit juice on blood cyclosporin concentration. *Lancet* 1995; **345**: 955–956.

8

Duodenal ulcer

Linda J Dodds

Case study and questions

Day 1 Forty-eight-year-old Mr GE was admitted from casualty. He had a three-day history of intermittent stomach pains which had gradually become more severe. He also felt nauseated but had not been sick. Over the past 24 hours he had passed several loose stools that he described as dark and foul smelling, but he had not had frank diarrhoea or seen fresh blood. He described his pain as gnawing and generalised over his abdomen, and said that it was worse at night. He added that he had had several similar but much less severe bouts of pain and dyspepsia over the previous six months, but that these had responded to antacids purchased from his local pharmacy and had resolved in a couple of days.

Mr GE's regular therapy was atenolol 50 mg, which he had been taking for the past two years for hypertension. For the past 10 days he had also been taking diclofenac 50 mg three times daily for a knee injury sustained during a game of tennis. He said he was allergic to penicillin, having come out in a rash when treated with the drug in childhood. He admitted to smoking about 20 cigarettes a day and drinking 20 units of alcohol a week, mostly in connection with his job as a sales representative, but he denied any recent excessive alcohol intake.

On admission he was noted to be pale, sweating and shocked with a blood pressure of 120/60 mmHg and a pulse rate of 98 beats per minute. His abdomen was tender and a rectal examination revealed melaena. A provisional diagnosis of bleeding duodenal ulcer was made. Half-hourly observations were ordered and an endoscopy was arranged for later in the day so he was made nil by mouth. A venflon was inserted and intravenous saline written up to run in over eight hours, or until cross-matching was complete. He was prescribed:

- Ranitidine 50 mg intravenously every eight hours
- Metoclopramide 10 mg intramuscularly at once, then eight-hourly as required

Relevant serum biochemistry and haematology tests were as follows:

- Sodium 135 mmol/L (reference range 137–150)
- Potassium 3.8 mmol/L (3.8–5)
- Urea 7.2 mmol/L (2.5–6.6)
- Creatinine 93 micromol/L (80–150)
- Haemoglobin 10.3 g/dL (14–18)

- Mean cell volume (MCV) 73 femtolitres (78–94)
- Mean cell haemoglobin (MCH) 27 picograms (32–36)
- Haematocrit 0.31 (0.36–0.46)
- Liver function tests: within normal range

Q1 What might have precipitated Mr GE's gastrointestinal bleed?
Q2 What are the therapeutic aims for Mr GE?
Q3 Can drug therapy stop ulcer bleeding or prevent rebleeding?
Q4 Has the most appropriate drug therapy been prescribed for this patient?
Q5 Outline a pharmaceutical care plan for Mr GE.

His emergency endoscopy revealed global gastritis and a 1-cm ulcer crater in the duodenum adjacent to the antral mucosa. The ulcer base was clear and not actively bleeding. Samples of tissue were taken from the sump of the antrum, a CLOtest was performed and the result was positive.

Q6 What is a CLOtest and why has it been performed?
Q7 What is the significance of a positive CLOtest?
Q8 Does infection with *Helicobacter pylori* predispose to non-steroidal anti-inflammatory drug (NSAID)-induced damage to the gastrointestinal mucosa?
Q9 Is diclofenac an NSAID with a high risk of inducing a gastrointestinal bleed?

Day 2 Mr GE was looking and feeling much better. He had not vomited since admission and his abdominal pains had resolved, although he described his abdomen as 'tender'. He had received three units of whole blood and his haemoglobin had risen to 13.5 g/dL. His relevant biochemistry results were as follows:

- Sodium 133 mmol/L (135–150)
- Potassium 4.8 mmol/L (3.8–5.5)

- Urea 6.5 mmol/L (2.5–6.6)
- Creatinine 102 micromol/L (80–150)

In view of his progress he was allowed a light diet and oral therapy was prescribed.

Q10 What therapy would you recommend?

Mr GE was prescribed:

- Lansoprazole 30 mg orally every 12 hours
- Clarithromycin 500 mg orally every 12 hours
- Metronidazole 400 mg orally every 12 hours

Q11 What information would you discuss with Mr GE at this point in his care?

Q12 How would you monitor his therapy while he is in hospital?

Day 3 Mr GE was complaining of a strange taste in his mouth and loose stools. His blood pressure was 140/100 mmHg.

Q13 What action would you take?

His serum biochemistry results were all in the normal ranges and his haemoglobin was now 13.8 g/dL (14–18). The team decided that he could be discharged. Mr GE asked if something could be prescribed for his knee, which was not swollen, but was causing him pain when he walked. Examination suggested a ligament or tendon strain and he was referred for assessment by a physiotherapist.

Q14 What analgesia would you recommend for Mr GE?

Q15 Should Mr GE be prescribed iron therapy at discharge and, if so, in what form and dose?

Q16 How can you help prepare him for discharge?

Week 4 Mr GE attended at out-patient clinic. He had had no recurrence of his symptoms and was back at work. He said that he had reduced his alcohol intake but had not managed to stop smoking.

Q17 How can the effectiveness or otherwise of his treatment be monitored?

Q18 What action should be taken if he is still *H. pylori* positive?

Q19 Should maintenance therapy be prescribed to prevent relapse of his ulcer?

What might have precipitated Mr GE's gastrointestinal bleed?

A1 **The most probable factor responsible for precipitating his bleed was his recent consumption of a NSAID. Factors which may have predisposed Mr GE to peptic ulcer disease (PUD) are *H. pylori* infection, smoking, and (more controversially) stress and his alcohol intake.**

The potential for NSAIDs to induce mucosal damage is well recognised. Recent epidemiological studies as well as large case control studies and case reports have all demonstrated a link between NSAIDs and serious upper gastrointestinal tract disease, including peptic ulcer, bleeding and perforation. In the UK the gastrointestinal side-effects of this group of drugs probably account for around 1200 deaths per year. The complications may appear soon after the initiation of therapy, as in Mr GE's case. His risk of a NSAID-induced bleed may have been increased by the fact that he smokes and drinks alcohol. Other risk factors for NSAID-induced bleeds include being aged over 60, a previous history of PUD, concomitant use of steroids or anticoagulants and use of a high dose or two concurrent NSAIDs. In his age group meta-analysis has demonstrated that approximately one in 650 treated patients will suffer a gastrointestinal bleed. This will lead to death in one in 3800. The risk rises significantly with age. For example, in patients over 75, approximately one in 100 will suffer a bleed and in one in 650 this will lead to death.

NSAIDs also appear to increase the chance of complications such as bleeding in patients with underlying ulcer disease. NSAIDs lead to between a three- and 10–fold increase in ulcer complications, hospitalisation and death from ulcer disease. Mr GE's symptoms over the past few months are suggestive of underlying ulcer disease. A number of factors may have predisposed him to PUD. First, he may be infected with *H. pylori*. *H. pylori* is a Gram-negative microaerophilic organism which is found in the gastric mucosal surface of 85–100% of patients with a duodenal ulcer and 70–90% of patients with a gastric ulcer. There is substantial evidence that this organism contributes to the development of a duodenal ulcer in about 15% of the infected population, but its exact role in the pathogenesis of PUD is still being debated.

In addition, Mr GE smokes, and cigarette smoking has been demonstrated in controlled trials to impair ulcer healing and promote recurrence of ulcers. Many mechanisms have been suggested for this effect.

Other possible factors in his lifestyle which have been implicated to predispose to PUD include stress and a significant alcohol intake. Although, it has been difficult to study these risk factors under controlled conditions there is mounting evidence that stress may function as a cofactor with *H. pylori*, either by stimulating the production of gastric acid or promoting behaviour that causes a risk to health. Finally, genetic factors may determine susceptibility to PUD.

What are the therapeutic aims for Mr GE?

A2 (a) **Treat shock.**

(b) **Prevent ulcer rebleeding.**

(c) **Initiate ulcer healing.**

(d) **Ensure symptom control.**

Can drug therapy stop ulcer bleeding or prevent rebleeding?

A3 **Ulcer bleeding or rebleeding is most effectively controlled by endoscopic therapies; however, in patients who require endoscopic treatment of their ulcer, high-dose omeprazole infusion has been shown to reduce the risk of subsequent rebleeding substantially.**

Bleeding peptic ulcer is a medical emergency with an overall mortality rate of about 6% of patients admitted to hospital. Mortality and morbidity is highest in the elderly and in patients with continuing or recurrent bleeding or high transfusion requirements; however, bleeding from ulcers stops spontaneously in about 80% of patients, most of whom then go on to have an uneventful recovery.

Agents evaluated for the treatment of actively bleeding ulcers include acid suppressant drugs, somatostatin and antifibrinolytics.

(a) Acid suppressant drugs. Measures to prevent rebleeding have centred on optimisation of clot function. *In vitro* studies have demonstrated that a pH of greater than 6 is necessary for platelet aggregation, whilst clot lysis occurs when the pH falls below 6. As histamine H_2-receptor antagonists do not reliably increase gastric pH to greater than 6, trials have focused on proton pump inhibitor (PPI) use. A double-blind, placebo-controlled trial using an intravenous bolus of 40 mg omeprazole failed to demonstrate a reduction in mortality, rebleeding or transfusion requirements in treated patients, although some endoscopic evidence of a reduction in intragastric bleeding was reported. However, the study was criticised for using doses insufficient to neutralise gastric pH. Results have been more favourable in patients with actively bleeding ulcers who require endoscopic treatment. High-dose infusion of omeprazole after the endoscopic treatment (80 mg bolus, followed by 8 mg/h for 72 hours) reduced rebleeding within 30 days of treatment from 22.5% with placebo to 6.8% in the treated group. The length of hospital stay was also shortened in the treated group.

(b)   Somatostatin. High-dose intravenous somatostatin suppresses acid secretion and splanchnic blood flow and is theoretically an attractive therapy. However, although a meta-analysis of available trials showed some benefit, the quality of much of the data was poor and this drug is not routinely used for the management of bleeding peptic ulcers.

(c)   Antifibrinolytic agents. A meta-analysis of trials using tranexamic acid, which inhibits fibrinolysis, has demonstrated that the drug does not appear to reduce rebleeding, but does reduce the need for surgical intervention and may reduce mortality. However, the overall benefits are unclear and further trials are needed.

Has the most appropriate drug therapy been prescribed for this patient?

A4   **The therapeutic objectives that can be achieved by drug therapy have been met; however, an oral PPI should have been substituted for the parenteral ranitidine prescribed.**

(a)   Shock. Mr GE requires plasma expanders urgently, preferably whole blood. His low haemoglobin with haemodilution not yet complete and low haematocrit indicate acute blood loss, while his low MCV and MCH levels indicate an iron deficiency anaemia resulting from chronic blood loss. Sodium chloride 0.9% is an appropriate interim intravenous fluid as it expands the extracellular fluid volume. The addition of potassium to the saline is not advisable at this point as whole blood can contain large amounts of this ion from lysed cells.

(b)   Ulcer healing. Although the incidence of ulcer rebleeding is not reduced by conventional doses of ulcer-healing agents, it is vital that the process of ulcer healing is started as soon as possible. Mr GE could be classified from his symptom picture as having a moderate bleed. He has no serious co-morbidity and is under 60 years of age. Unless he is found to be still bleeding on endoscopy and to require endoscopic treatment, intravenous omeprazole to prevent rebleeding is not warranted. He is being observed and there is no reason that he cannot be allowed sips of fluid. The use of a parenteral H_2-receptor antagonist is no more effective than oral therapy. Furthermore, it is more expensive, requires more nursing time and carries more risks for the patient. All the parenteral H_2-receptor antagonists can cause confusion in susceptible patients. Mr GE is not vomiting and has been given a dose of metoclopramide for his nausea. He should instead receive a therapeutic dose of a PPI orally with sips of water. This will not affect his endoscopy and is thus preferable. A PPI is the drug of choice as it provides faster healing and better symptom relief than other available ulcer-healing agents. All PPIs exhibit similar healing rates and levels of side-effects. Mr GE is not likely to require any of the drugs known to interact with certain of the PPIs, so the product chosen should be governed by the hospital formulary.

(c) Symptom control. It is important to control Mr GE's symptom of nausea. Metoclopramide is an effective anti-emetic as it increases gastric emptying and also acts centrally at the chemoreceptor trigger zone to relieve vomiting. It is available in parenteral and oral formulations. After Mr GE has been endoscoped he should also be written up for adequate doses of a balanced antacid such as Maalox or Mucogel for ulcer pain, which is felt by some patients for up to 10 days after starting ulcer-healing therapy.

(d) Previous therapy. It is appropriate that his atenolol and NSAID therapy have been temporarily discontinued. Pain control for his knee injury will need to be reviewed before discharge while regular monitoring of his blood pressure will indicate when it is appropriate to restart his antihypertensive therapy.

Outline a pharmaceutical care plan for Mr GE.

A5 **The pharmaceutical care plan for Mr GE should include the following:**

(a) Ensure the most appropriate therapy is prescribed at the optimal dose.

(b) Monitor all therapy for efficacy and side-effects. Ensure desired therapeutic outcomes are met.

(c) Counsel Mr GE on his prescribed medicines and on other factors which might have a bearing on his disease outcome. In particular, encourage him to stop smoking.

(d) Facilitate his discharge from hospital.

(e) Ensure he understands what follow-up therapy and care will be required. If necessary, liaise with his GP and/or community pharmacist.

What is a CLOtest and why was it performed?

A6 **A CLOtest measures urease levels in tissue. It is used to detect the presence of the organism _H. pylori_ in gastric mucosa.**

A CLOtest is a sealed plastic slide holding an agar gel which contains urea and a pH indicator. A 2– to 3–mm biopsy specimen from the stomach (usually the sump of the antrum) is added to the slide. If the urease enzyme of _H. pylori_ is present, degradation of the urea causes the pH to rise and a corresponding change in the colour of the gel from yellow (negative) to purple (positive).

H. pylori is a highly motile Gram-negative bacteria that colonises the mucus layer of the stomach. It is one of the commonest pathogens in man, and it has been recognised as the principal cause of PUD and the main risk factor in the development of gastric cancer.

It is not known how the organism is usually acquired and its route of transmission is unknown, although gastro-oral or faeco-oral routes are probable. The prevalence of _H. pylori_ infection increases with age in the developed world, with infection rates of about 20% in Mr GE's age group in the UK. The prevalence is higher in developing countries, leading its acquisition to be linked with social deprivation.

Infection with _H. pylori_ initially induces an acute inflammatory gastritis which persists for life. A single patient may be infected with multiple strains of the organism (this is particularly common in the developing world) and the organisms in colonised hosts may mutate over decades of colonisation. Different strains are now being linked with different gastric diseases and in future genotyping could help identify people at risk of particular diseases. Some strains of _H. pylori_ appear to exert a protective effect against certain diseases (gastro-oesophageal reflux, Barrett's oesophagus, adenocarcinoma of the oesophagus and gastric cardia) leading to controversy over when to eliminate the organism.

Around 15% of infected individuals will go on to develop PUD or gastric cancer. It is thought that in patients with _H. pylori_-induced antral gastritis that there is a loss of regulatory feedback, together with an intact and undamaged acid-secreting gastric corpus, and that the consequent high acid load reaching the duodenum leads to duodenal gastric met-aplasia. These 'islands' of gastric metaplasia are then colonised by *H. pylori*, which leads to duodenitis and a high risk of duodenal ulcer. In patients with pangastritis, an inflamed corpus leads to the loss of acid-secreting cells, which leads in turn to an increased risk of gastric ulcer and gastric cancer.

A CLOtest has a high specificity (90–95%) and sensitivity (90–95%) for detecting the presence or absence of infection in the gastric mucosa. Its sensitivity is higher than other biopsy methods. However, it is recom-mended that multiple biopsy specimens be used to achieve the highest sensitivity, as infection is often patchy and up to 14% of infected patients do not have antral infection, but do have *H. pylori* elsewhere in the stomach.

A careful drug history should be taken from the patient before a CLOtest is performed. Antibiotics or bismuth salts taken in the three weeks prior to biopsy may suppress *H. pylori* growth making the organism difficult to detect and leading to a false negative result. In contrast, a false positive result can occur if the patient has achlorhydria, e.g. after taking high doses of an H_2-receptor antagonist or a PPI. Alternatively, PPIs can affect the pattern of *H. pylori* colonisation of the stomach and com-promise the accuracy of antral biopsy. For these reasons it is recom-mended that patients who have taken these drugs prior to endoscopy have multiple biopsies taken from the antrum and corpus for histology, plus either culture or urease testing.

What is the significance of a positive CLOtest?

A7   **It indicates that Mr GE is infected with *H. pylori*.**

Does infection with *H. pylori* predispose to NSAID-induced damage to the gastrointestinal mucosa?

A8   **There is now good evidence to suggest that the presence of *H. pylori* predisposes to NSAID-induced ulceration.**

NSAID administration can lead to a variety of gastrointestinal injuries, ranging from petechial haemorrhages to erosions and, occasionally, ulceration. However, the move from erosion to ulceration is not neces-sarily inevitable and endoscopic studies have shown that NSAID-induced erosions can appear and disappear over time, presumably as a result of adaptation and repair processes.

Investigations into the relationship between long-term NSAID use and *H. pylori* infection have concluded that NSAID-induced damage to the gastroduodenal mucosa does not increase susceptibility to *H. pylori* infection, but that ulcers are more likely to develop in long-term NSAID users who are infected with *H. pylori*, especially if they are smokers.

A recent meta-analysis has suggested that both *H. pylori* infection and NSAID use independently and significantly increase the risk of peptic ulcer and ulcer bleeding. In addition, there is a synergism for the development of peptic ulcer and ulcer bleeding between *H. pylori* infection and NSAID use. The presence of *H. pylori* infection has been shown to increase the rate of PUD in NSAID takers 3.5-fold in addition to the risk associated with NSAID alone, while the risk of ulcer bleeding with *H. pylori* and NSAID use separately was 1.8 and 4.6, respectively. This increased to 6.1 when both factors were present.

To try to establish whether eradication of *H. pylori* reduces the risk of NSAID-induced ulceration, a study of patients with a history of dyspepsia or PUD who were NSAID-naive but *H. pylori*-positive (via urea breath test) were randomised to either eradication therapy or PPI therapy alone for one week prior to commencement of the NSAID. Ninety percent of patients had *H. pylori* eradicated in the treatment group. After six months treatment with modified-release diclofenac 100 mg daily, 5 of 51 patients in the treated group and 15 of 49 of the group treated with omeprazole alone prior to therapy had ulcers. However, at the time of writing it remains unclear whether eradication of *H. pylori* reduces the risk of NSAID-induced ulceration other than in patients with known ulcer disease.

Is diclofenac an NSAID with a high risk of inducing a gastrointestinal bleed?

A9   **All NSAIDs carry a risk of inducing a gastrointestinal bleed, but diclofenac has been categorised as having a lower risk of causing a gastrointestinal bleed than all other NSAIDs studied except ibuprofen.**

Preclinical studies suggest two factors contribute to the pathogenesis of NSAID-associated ulcers. First, the inhibition of prostaglandin synthesis impairs mucosal defences and leads to erosive breach of the epithelial barrier. Secondly, acid attack deepens the breach into frank ulceration, whilst low pH encourages passive absorption of the NSAID so it is trapped in the mucosa.

A multicentre case control study in patients aged over 60 and living in the UK examined the risks posed by seven NSAIDs: ibuprofen, diclofenac, naproxen, piroxicam, ketoprofen, indometacin and azapropazone.

None of the NSAIDs studied were free of risk and the overall odds ratio for gastrointestinal bleeding was 4.5 (95% confidence interval 3.6–6.6). The odds ratio was lowest for ibuprofen, followed by diclofenac (4.2 95% confidence interval 2.6–6.8). The odds ratios were intermediate for indometacin, naproxen and piroxicam, and highest for azapropazone and ketoprofen. The risks were noted to increase as the drug dose increased. A further study, which was published about the same time, but used a different source of data, came to similar conclusions except with respect to the risks associated with ketoprofen.

The risk of admission for upper gastrointestinal bleed and perforation has been found to be constant during continuous NSAID exposure and in one study was found to persist after drug discontinuation.

What treatment would you recommend?

A10 **Mr GE requires therapy to eradicate his *H. pylori* infection and to ensure his ulcer is healed. He should receive proton pump-based triple therapy with lansoprazole 30 mg twice daily, metronidazole 400 mg twice daily and clarithromycin 500 mg twice daily for one week, followed by lansoprazole 30 mg daily for a further three weeks.**

The eradication of *H. pylori* can lead to a cure for patients with PUD. The National Institutes of Health consensus meeting in 1994 and the European Helicobacter Study Group in 1996 have recommended that the infection is eradicated in patients with active PUD and proven infection. Mr GE falls into this category.

Eradication of *H. pylori* is a challenging task. Although many antibiotics are bactericidal to the organism *in vitro*, even high-dose regimens have proved to be ineffective *in vivo*. Possible reasons for this are that bactericidal concentrations are not achieved in the gastric mucosa, the drugs are inactivated or ineffective at low pH, or a combination of these factors. To be effective, antibiotic therapy must thus be combined with either bismuth chelate or acid-suppressant therapy or both.

The rationale for the use of acid-suppressant therapy with antibiotics is to increase gastric pH, thus inducing a favourable environment for antibiotic activity. In addition, omeprazole has been observed to reduce antral colonisation by *H. pylori*, presumably by disturbing its environment, although the effect is only temporary and on cessation of therapy, colonisation returns to normal.

Many regimens have been evaluated for the eradication of *H. pylori*. Early dual therapies of omeprazole (40 mg daily) plus amoxicillin

(750 mg twice daily) or clarithromycin (500 mg three times daily), although fairly well tolerated, led to mean eradication rates of only 50–60%. Bismuth chelate can lyse *H. pylori* in 30–90 minutes *in vitro*; however, it is not clear whether the compound is bactericidal or bacteriostatic to the organism *in vivo*. If bismuth chelate is used as sole therapy, *H. pylori* eradication rates are low; however, when combined with antibiotics, eradication levels are much higher. The mechanism for this synergistic effect is unclear. Triple therapies of bismuth chelate plus two antibiotics (metronidazole 400 mg three times daily plus amoxicillin or tetracycline 500 mg four times daily) raises the eradication rate to approximately 80%; however, the regimen is very complex to take and the side-effects can be considerable and frequent (seen in 20–50% of patients) which means that non-compliance, whether intentional or non-intentional, can lead to treatment failure. The addition of a PPI to this regimen (quadruple therapy) increases the eradication rate to greater than 90%; however, side-effects and non-compliance remain significant issues, even in well-supported patients.

As a result, PPI-based triple therapy comprising a PPI plus two antibiotics has become the recommended first-line treatment for *H. pylori* eradication. It is simple, effective and much better tolerated than earlier regimes. A one-week course has a success rate of around 90%. As the drugs need only be taken twice or three times daily, compliance is easier. The PPI should be given at twice the therapeutic dose. The choice of antibiotic is usually amoxicillin 500 mg three times daily or 1 g twice daily, and either metronidazole 400 mg twice or three times daily or clarithromycin 250–500 mg twice daily. As Mr GE is allergic to penicillin, he should receive a regimen with metronidazole and clarithromycin, even though this is not ideal as treatment failure may induce resistance to one or both of the antibiotics. The components of the regimen could be prescribed separately or as a triple pack such as HeliMet to aid compliance. As Mr GE has recently haemorrhaged from his ulcer, after completion of the eradication therapy he should receive a further three weeks of PPI therapy. In uncomplicated PUD with proven *H. pylori* infection, eradication therapy alone would be deemed sufficient and no further antisecretory therapy would be necessary.

Resistance to metronidazole or clarithromycin can compromise the success rate of this regime, but if Mr GE takes the triple therapy as intended and if he is sensitive to metronidazole there is a greater than 90% chance that his infection will be eradicated. If he is resistant to metronidazole, the success rate will be lowered to 75%.

What information would you discuss with Mr GE at this point in his care?

A11 (a) **The rationale for an eradication regimen, followed by a healing regimen.**

(b) **The importance of compliance.**

(c) **Possible side-effects to his current therapy.**

(d) **The likelihood that his admission was precipitated by NSAID use and the need to avoid these drugs in the future (prescribed and over-the-counter) whenever possible.**

(e) **(General) The benefits of stopping smoking and reducing alcohol intake.**

It should be emphasised that this regimen offers the possibility of cure for his PUD and that non-compliance may lead to the development of antibiotic resistance which will make the organism much harder to eradicate in the future.

The advice regarding NSAID use is particularly important, as there is evidence that NSAIDs play an important role in the cause and relapse of PUD regardless of *H. pylori* status.

How would you monitor his therapy while he is in hospital?

A12 **For evidence of ulcer healing and side-effects of treatment.**

Symptom control provides the best guide to ulcer healing at this time. Antacid consumption should be monitored and the patient questioned directly.

It is important that Mr GE is able to complete his eradication regimen; however, each component of the regimen can cause a range of side-effects. Any unusual symptoms should be investigated. When interpreting biochemistry results it should be remembered that both clarithromycin and omeprazole can cause an increase in liver enzyme levels.

Finally, routine monitoring of his urea and electrolyte status and blood pressure control is still required.

What action would you take?

A13 **First, reassure Mr GE that these symptoms are side-effects of his eradication regime which will resolve when the regimen ends and, second, ensure his antihypertensive therapy is represcribed.**

Taste disturbance is a very common side-effect of clarithromycin therapy and is rarely sufficient to discontinue treatment.

Mr GE should be asked about the appearance of his stools to rule out possible further melaena, but it is most likely that his loose stools are the result of his antibiotic therapy. If this worsens, a low dose of codeine or loperamide could be considered.

His raised blood pressure indicates that his antihypertensive therapy should be restarted. There is no contra-indication to represcribing atenolol 50 mg daily, which was controlling his hypertension prior to admission.

What analgesia would you recommend for Mr GE?

A14 **Paracetamol 1 g up to four times daily, plus codeine 30–60 mg up to four times daily.**

Despite the fact that his injury probably has an inflammatory component, it is inadvisable to represcribe an NSAID. Nor does Mr GE fall into a category of patient to receive a cyclooxygenase (COX)-2 inhibitor. Furthermore, there is mounting evidence that some COX-2 inhibitors are not as safe as originally thought for patients with PUD.

Instead, simple analgesia should be tried. Paracetamol and codeine should be prescribed separately, and Mr GE encouraged to take the paracetamol regularly and the codeine only when he has breakthrough pain. This means that he will get the benefit of the full paracetamol analgesic effect and codeine in effective doses only when he really requires it. Codeine side-effects are thus minimised, although they might actually be beneficial whilst he is suffering from loose stools, and the use of subtherapeutic doses of paracetamol and codeine that can arise from the use of 'as required' combination therapy are unlikely.

Should Mr GE be prescribed iron therapy at discharge and, if so, in what form and dose?

A15 **Yes. Ferrous sulphate 200 mg twice daily for one month is appropriate.**

Although his haemoglobin result is now almost normal, his admission haematology demonstrated a microcytic, hypochromic picture indicating that he had been bleeding chronically. As a result, his iron stores are now likely to be depleted. Approximately 120 mg of elemental iron daily in divided doses should ensure adequate iron absorption and one month of therapy should be enough to replenish iron stores. If this form of iron is poorly tolerated, a formulation such as ferrous gluconate which contains less elemental iron per tablet could be tried, as gastrointestinal toxicity appears to be in direct proportion to the concentration of iron in the gut.

How can you help prepare him for discharge?

A16 (a) **By providing appropriate discharge medications and counselling for each item prescribed.**

(b) **By ensuring Mr GE is clear about his future therapy needs.**

(c) **By reinforcing the general counselling and advice provided earlier in his hospital stay.**

Non-compliance is an important reason for the failure of *H. pylori* eradication regimens. It is vital Mr GE understands the importance of completing his prescribed treatment. A medication record card plus any relevant information leaflets may help him cope after discharge. It is also vital that he understands how long each aspect of his treatment should continue and how further supplies of medication should be obtained.

A further opportunity should be taken to encourage lifestyle changes which will reduce his chance of relapse. In particular, it would be useful to discuss the benefits that would accrue from him stopping smoking and the strategies that could be used to help.

How can the effectiveness or otherwise of his treatment be monitored?

A17 **By performing a urea breath test at least four weeks after his eradication regimen is complete.**

Recurrent symptoms can indicate eradication failure or the presence of another disease such as gastro-oesophageal reflux. Also, duodenal ulcer can recur in about 5% of patients even after eradication and in the absence of reinfection or the use of NSAIDs. It is thus essential to establish whether eradication has been successful.

The usual definition of successful *H. pylori* eradication requires all tests for the organism to be negative at least one month after the end of treatment. This is particularly important for patients who have suffered complications, such as Mr GE. Earlier testing by any method may indicate suppression of the organism rather than its eradication.

Endoscopy is an invasive technique and is thus not usually performed unless the patient is in a clinical trial. However, it is the only method of ensuring ulcer healing has taken place. If performed, it should be remembered that samples for *H. pylori* taken after recent therapy with omeprazole or antibiotics can affect the accuracy of the CLOtest and other diagnostic measures for *H. pylori* detection, such as culture and histology, may be more appropriate.

If available, a non-invasive carbon-14 or carbon-13 urea breath test can be used to detect whether *H. pylori* recolonisation has occurred. However, this test does not indicate whether ulcer healing has occurred. In this test, labelled urea is swallowed by the patient. The urea reacts with urease produced by the organism to release ammonia and labelled bicarbonate which is absorbed into the blood stream. This is then exhaled as labelled carbon dioxide. At a fixed time a sample of air is collected and the result read on a scintillation counter (carbon-14 test). The carbon-14 test is a radioactive test and must thus be done in a hospital, but the carbon-13 test has the advantage of being non-radioactive and able to be performed in the GP's surgery with two breath samples taken at timed intervals sent away for analysis. This test also has slightly higher specificity and sensitivity than the carbon-14 test but is more expensive.

Serology using kits such as the Helisal whole-blood kit for the detection of *H. pylori* antibodies can also be used to monitor *H. pylori* eradication, but are not generally recommended. A drop of at least 50% in immunoglobulin antibody titre within three to six months is looked for. However, this is clearly only possible if pre-treatment antibody titres are available, which is not the case for Mr GE. Serology tests are both less specific and less sensitive than other non-invasive tests for *H. pylori*. This is particularly so for the fingerprick test available in some GP surgeries. Their accuracy when carried out in the laboratory further depends on the antigens used in the test, local validation of techniques and careful documentation of drugs taken by the patient.

What action should be taken if he is still infected with *H. pylori*?

A18 **A further attempt should be made to eradicate the organism.**

Antibiotic resistance is the major cause of failure of eradication. Widespread antibiotic use has resulted in an increase worldwide in the prevalence of antibiotic resistance to *H. pylori* with 11–70% of strains isolated in Western Europe resistant to metronidazole and up to 15% resistant to clarithromycin. Metronidazole resistance is most common in women and those living in developing countries, where it might rise to 80%. This is probably because these populations are more likely to have been exposed to the drug. In areas where there is known to be high resistance to metronidazole, increasing the length of eradication treatment to 10–14 days can improve the eradication rate. It has also been suggested that replacing the PPI with ranitidine bismuth citrate in this situation could also help as the bismuth chelate appears to reduce resistance to metronidazole therapy. This is a useful property as nitroimidazoles are valuable components of *H. pylori* eradication regimens because their bactericidal activity appears to be unaffected by low pH and the compounds achieve high concentrations in the gastric juices. This regimen would result in less acid suppression, but it would provide the additional antimicrobial action associated with bismuth. However hard evidence to support this strategy is lacking.

A survey in the UK reported in 2002 showed that only around 15% of Public Health Laboratories carry out routine culture and susceptibility testing for *H. pylori*. This may reflect difficulties associated with methods of assessing susceptibility to the organism and also around achieving consensus as to what defines resistance. However, this is likely to be resolved in the future and sensitivity testing may become a prerequisite to *H. pylori* eradication in the future.

In the meantime, if Mr GE is found still to be colonised with the organism eradication should be attempted again as it offers the best chance of a cure from his PUD which will otherwise follow a relapsing, remitting course over 10–20 years before 'burning out'. An attempt should be made to use an alternative antibiotic such as either metronidazole or clarithromycin plus tetracycline. The addition of ranitidine bismuth citrate and extension of the course of treatment should also be considered as discussed earlier. These strategies have led to improved success rates in prospective studies. If there is failure to eradicate again and compliance has been assured, culture and susceptibility testing will be necessary before a further attempt at treatment.

Should maintenance therapy be prescribed to prevent relapse of his ulcer?

A19 No.

Eradication of *H. pylori* and avoidance of NSAID therapy should have removed two important risk factors for relapse. Mr GE should be strongly encouraged to stop smoking and told to see his GP if symptoms recur.

Acknowledgement

I would like to thank Dr A Frank Muller (Consultant Physician, Kent and Canterbury Hospitals NHS Trust) for his helpful comments.

Further reading

Blaser MJ. *Helicobacter pylori* and gastric diseases. *Br Med J* 1998; **316**: 1507–1510.

British Society of Gastroenterology Clinical Practice Guidelines. Non-variceal upper gastrointestinal haemorrhage guidelines. *Gut* 2002; **51**(suppl. IV): 1–6.

Daneshmend TK, Hawkey CJ, Langman MJS *et al.* Omeprazole versus placebo for acute upper gastrointestinal bleeding: randomised double blind controlled trial. *Br Med J* 1992; **304**: 143–147.

De Boer WA, Tytgat GNJ. Treatment of *Helicobacter pylori* infection. *Br Med J* 2000; **320**: 31–34.

Garcia Rodriguez LA, Jick H. Risk of upper gastrointestinal bleeding and perforation associated with individual non-steroidal anti-inflammatory drugs. *Lancet* 1994; **343**: 769–772.

Harris A, Misiewicz JJ. Management of *Helicobacter pylori* infection *Br Med J* 2001; **323**: 1047–1050.

Huang JQ, Sridhar S, Hunt RH *et al.* Role of *Helicobacter pylori* infection and non-steroidal anti-inflammatory drugs in peptic ulcer disease – a meta-analysis. *Lancet* 2002; **359**: 14–22.

Langman MJS, Weil J, Wainwright P *et al.* Risks of bleeding peptic ulcer associated with individual non-steroidal anti-inflammatory drugs. *Lancet* 1994; **343**: 1075–1078.

Lau JYW, Sung JJY, Lee KC *et al.* Effect of intravenous omeprazole on recurrent bleeding after endoscopic treatment of bleeding peptic ulcers. *N Engl J Med* 2000; **343**: 310–316.

Logan RPH, Walker MM. Epidemiology and diagnosis of *Helicobacter pylori* infection. *Br Med J* 2001; **323**: 920–922.

MacDonald TM, Morant SV, Robinson GC *et al.* Association of upper gastro-intestinal toxicity of non-steroidal anti-inflammatory drugs with continued exposure: cohort study. *Br Med J* 1997; **315**: 1333–1337.

National Institute for Clinical Excellence. *Dyspepsia – Proton Pump Inhibitors 7.* NICE, London, 2000.

Scottish Intercollegiate Guidelines Network. *Which Patients with* H. pylori *should receive Eradication Therapy.* SIGN, Edinburgh, 1999.

Seager JM, Hawkey CJ. Indigestion and non-steroidal anti-inflammatory drugs. *Br Med J* 2001; **323**: 1236–1239.

9

Ulcerative colitis

Sandra Ross and Amanda Kemp

Day 1 Mr AJ, a 31-year-old male, was admitted with a three-week history of frequent bowel movements (about six per day) with some blood in the stool. Left-sided ulcerative colitis had been diagnosed 12 months earlier when colonoscopy had revealed the haemorrhagic and granular mucosa of the rectum and colon characteristic of this disease.

On examination no fever or tachycardia were noted. Colonic radiography appeared normal, with no evidence of colonic air, wall oedema or dilatation.

Stool cultures, to exclude potential enteric pathogens or *Clostridium difficile*, were negative.

Serum biochemistry and haematology results were as follows:

- Potassium 4.0 mmol/L (reference range 3.5–5.3)
- Sodium 138 mmol/L (137–145)
- Urea 6.2 mmol/L (2.5–6.6)
- Creatinine 62 micromol/L (80–150)
- Haematocrit 0.35 (0.36–0.46)

- Haemoglobin 12.8 g/dL (13–16)
- Albumin 29 g/L (32–50)
- Erythrocyte sedimentation rate (ESR) 19 mm/h (0–8)
- C-reactive protein (CRP) 22 mg/L (up to 10)

A diagnosis of mild left-sided ulcerative colitis was made.

Drug therapy at the time of admission was:

- Sulfasalazine 1 g twice daily
- Loperamide 2 mg when required

Q1 What are the therapeutic aims for Mr AJ?
Q2 What parameters will give an indication that these aims are being met?
Q3 Outline your pharmaceutical care plan for Mr AJ.
Q4 What is sulfasalazine's postulated mode of action in ulcerative colitis?

Q5 Mr AJ had been on maintenance therapy with sulfasalazine. Is sulfasalazine considered to be effective in the maintenance of remission?

Q6 Is oral sulfasalazine effective in the induction of remission?

Q7 Would you recommend that Mr AJ's dose of sulfasalazine be increased? Explain your answer.

Q8 What parameters should be monitored in order to detect toxicity with sulfasalazine?

On admission, prednisolone sodium metasulphobenzoate (Predenema) 20 mg at night was added to Mr AJ's regimen. His other therapy remained unchanged.

Q9 How effective are topical treatments in the induction of remission?

Q10 What factors govern the choice of topical steroid and the duration of treatment?

Q11 What side-effects are associated with the use of topical steroids? How can these be minimised?

Mr AJ was discharged a week later having shown symptomatic improvement. He now had bowel movements once each day and was producing formed motions with no blood. His discharge medication was:

- Sulfasalazine 1 g twice daily
- Predenema 20 mg at night

Q12 How should Mr AJ be counselled on his discharge medication?

Week 5 Mr AJ attended a routine out-patient appointment. He had remained well, so the Predenema was stopped. Mr AJ expressed concern about the possibility of sulfasalazine impairing his fertility as he and his wife hoped to start a family. Mesalazine was thus substituted for the sulfasalazine. He was advised that any impairment to his fertility would take up to two months to resolve.

Q13 What is mesalazine and how effective will it be compared to sulfasalazine in the maintenance of remission of ulcerative colitis?

Q14 What alternative aminosalicylates could have been considered?

Q15 What dose of mesalazine should be prescribed for Mr AJ to maintain remission?

Q16 Does mesalazine have a better side-effect profile than sulfasalazine? How should therapy be monitored?

Month 13, day 1 Mr AJ was admitted to the ward. His presenting complaints were watery, bloody diarrhoea, nausea and vomiting, abdominal pain and weight loss.

Over the past four months, Mr AJ described the following symptoms:

(a)   Worsening diarrhoea. On his best days, the frequency of opening his bowels was eight to 10 times a day; on his worst days he was unable to leave the toilet. His stools were very watery and bloody.
(b)   Nausea and vomiting: he was unable to keep food down.
(c)   Weakness and lethargy, increasing shortness of breath, dizzy spells and weight loss.
(d)   Colicky lower left-sided abdominal pain.

All of these symptoms had become worse over the last week.

On examination, Mr AJ looked unwell: he looked thin, dehydrated and anaemic. His pulse rate was 116 beats per minute.

His serum biochemistry and haematology results were:

- Haematocrit 0.26 (0.36–0.46)
- Haemoglobin 8.3 g/dL (13–16)
- Albumin 15 g/L (35–50)
- ESR 28 mm/h (0–8)
- CRP 101 mg/L (up to 10)

- Potassium 3.1 mmol/L (3.5–5.3)
- Sodium 137 mmol/L (137–145)
- Urea 8.1 mmol/L (2.5–6.6)
- Creatinine 64 micromol/L (80–150)

A diagnosis of severe ulcerative colitis was made.

Q17 What are the therapeutic aims for Mr AJ now?
Q18 What parameters can be monitored to assess Mr AJ's progress?

Blood was sent for cross-matching and intravenous saline with potassium was started. A plain abdominal x-ray was ordered. Samples of stool were sent for culture and a stool chart was commenced. Mr AJ was written up for hydrocortisone 100 mg intravenously three times daily.

Q19 Has appropriate intravenous fluid therapy been prescribed? Which other serum electrolyte would it be advisable to monitor at this point?
Q20 What is the rationale for the use of intravenous steroid therapy?
Q21 What biochemical monitoring should be carried out while Mr AJ is receiving hydrocortisone?
Q22 Should an antidiarrhoeal agent such as codeine phosphate be prescribed for Mr AJ?
Q23 What could be prescribed for Mr AJ's abdominal pain?
Q24 Would nutritional support aid Mr AJ's recovery?
Q25 How should Mr AJ's anaemia be treated?
Q26 Should an antibiotic be added to Mr AJ's treatment?

Month 13, day 3 An abdominal x-ray showed mucosal oedema throughout the colon with features indicating pancolitis.

Month 13, day 5 After 5 days of intravenous hydrocortisone therapy, Mr AJ was showing no clinical or radiological evidence of improvement. It was decided to start intravenous ciclosporin therapy and blood was sent for full blood count (FBC), urea and electrolytes, liver function tests (LFTs), serum magnesium and total cholesterol levels.

Mr AJ was written up for ciclosporin 160 mg daily (2 mg/kg) by continuous intravenous infusion. This was administered as ciclosporin 40 mg in 100 mL 0.9% sodium chloride over six hours, four times daily. The ciclosporin was tolerated by Mr AJ and consequently, after 24 hours, the dose was increased to 320 mg daily (4 mg/kg).

Q27 What is the rationale for the use of ciclosporin in Mr AJ?
Q28 Why was the intravenous ciclosporin given over six hours?
Q29 Why does Mr AJ need to be closely observed initially?
Q30 For how long should intravenous ciclosporin treatment be continued?
Q31 What monitoring is necessary during intravenous ciclosporin treatment?
Q32 What side-effects are possible with ciclosporin treatment?
Q33 Why was a serum cholesterol test done prior to initiating ciclosporin?

Month 13, day 10 A ciclosporin level was reported to be just above the upper limit of normal, at 403 nanograms/mL. The ciclosporin dose was thus reduced to 60 mg four times daily.

Month 13, day 11 Mr AJ was showing marked improvement, both clinically and radiologically.

Month 13, day 15 The ciclosporin and steroids were converted to oral regimens as follows:

- Ciclosporin 250 mg daily
- Prednisolone 40 mg daily

Q34 Why has the ciclosporin dose not been increased to reflect the decreased bioavailability of oral drug compared to the intravenous form?

Mr AJ was discharged on the above medication in addition to:

- Mesalazine 800 mg three times daily
- Ferrous sulphate 200 mg twice daily

Month 14   He was seen in clinic two weeks after discharge. His ciclosporin levels were found to be within the normal range, and he reported a major improvement in symptoms, with bowel movements reduced to once daily, formed motions.

Month 15–21   Over the next few months Mr AJ's dose of prednisolone was reduced by 5 mg each week and stopped. His ciclosporin therapy was continued for six months, then stopped and replaced by azathioprine at a dose of 1.5 mg/kg/day.

Q35 What is the rationale for prescribing azathioprine?
Q36 What maximum dose of azathioprine would you recommend and why? How should azathioprine therapy be monitored?

Month 27   Mr AJ remained in remission taking azathioprine and mesalazine.

What are the therapeutic aims for Mr AJ?

A1 **Induce and then maintain remission of his clinical symptoms and acute mucosal inflammation.**

What parameters will give an indication that these aims are being met?

A2 **An improvement in his clinical symptoms, together with a reduction in his ESR and CRP, and a rise in his serum albumin.**

Mr AJ's symptoms include up to six bowel movements a day with blood sometimes present in the stool, but no systemic signs such as fever, tachycardia or pain. These are consistent with mild distal colitis, i.e. mild disease limited to the rectum and left colon, which is generally amenable to topical therapies.

A reduction of ESR and of acute phase proteins generally accompanies a reduction in mucosal inflammation, but these parameters cannot be used as reliable markers of disease activity. In the absence of pathognomonic markers of disease activity, therapy is generally directed at relieving symptoms and inducing endoscopic evidence of mucosal regeneration.

For Mr AJ, a response to treatment will thus be indicated by: a reduction in the frequency of his bowel movements and the absence of blood in the stool, plus a reduction of his ESR and CRP. In addition, his serum albumin, which is low because of the leakage of protein from his inflamed mucosa (termed protein-losing enteropathy), should start to rise.

Outline your pharmaceutical care plan for Mr AJ.

A3 **The pharmaceutical care plan for Mr AJ should include the following:**

(a)   Ensure that optimal doses of drugs are used to prevent suboptimal therapy and to protect Mr AJ from toxicity.

(b)   Know the desired patient outcomes in order to monitor the effectiveness of treatment.

(c)   Establish toxicity monitoring parameters for each drug therapy to protect Mr AJ from potential harm due to drug-related adverse reactions.

(d)   Establish and provide the information he needs to aid his understanding of, and compliance with, his drug therapy.

What is sulfasalazine's postulated mode of action in ulcerative colitis?

A4   **An exact mechanism of action is unclear. Multiple sites of impact in the immune and inflammatory pathways that characterize ulcerative colitis have been postulated. These include: inhibition of prostaglandins, thromboxanes, leukotrienes and platelet-activating factor; inhibition of interleukin-1 and other cytokines; inhibition of immunoglobulin G production; and scavenging of reactive oxygen species.**

Sulfasalazine is a conjugate of 5-aminosalicylic acid (5-ASA) and sulfa-pyridine, linked by an azo bond. It is metabolised by colonic bacteria and azo-reduction to produce the sulpha and salicylate moieties in the colonic lumen. Most of the sulfapyridine is absorbed, acetylated by the liver, and excreted by the kidneys. 5-ASA is excreted mainly in the faeces after acetylation by colonic epithelium, bacteria or the liver, with only a small proportion of 5-ASA reaching the systemic circulation. The pharma-cologically active moiety for the treatment of ulcerative colitis is 5-ASA, with the sulphonamide component acting as a carrier to ensure its delivery to the colon.

Mr AJ had been on maintenance therapy with sulfasalazine. Is sulfasalazine considered to be effective in the maintenance of remission?

A5   **Yes.**

Sulfasalazine has been used routinely to maintain remission in ulcerative colitis. It drastically reduces the relapse rate (in one study the relapse rate during one year was 21% compared with 73% on placebo). Maintenance treatment is the main indication for oral sulfasalazine in ulcerative colitis.

Is oral sulfasalazine effective in the induction of remission?

A6   **Yes, but only in remission induction in mild disease (either distal or extensive).**

For patients with mild disease, induction of remission is achieved over six to eight weeks, with a gradual increase in dose from a starting dose of 500 mg once or twice daily. However, systemic steroids are more effective than sulfasalazine in moderate to severe disease, which must be treated aggressively in order to avoid surgery.

Would you recommend that Mr AJ's dose of sulfasalazine be increased? Explain your answer.

A7 **No. Although doses of up to 4 g daily have been shown to be more effective, this is at the expense of greatly increased side-effects.**

For this reason, 2 g a day is considered to be the optimum dose. At this dose side-effects are reported in about 30% of patients and necessitate drug discontinuation in 10%. The commonest dose-related side-effects are nausea and vomiting, abdominal pain, anorexia, headache, and impaired male fertility due to oligospermia and reduced sperm motility.

The incidence of side-effects is increased in slow acetylators. The enteric-coated formulation may be useful if gastrointestinal side-effects are troublesome.

What parameters should be monitored in order to detect toxicity with sulfasalazine?

A8 **FBC, LFTs and renal function.**

Idiosyncratic adverse reactions include skin rashes (including photosensitivity), agranulocytosis, thrombocytopenia, aplastic anaemia, hepatitis, nephrotic syndrome, neurotoxicity and fibrosing alveolitis.

Haematological and hepatic reactions occur mainly in the first few months of therapy: FBC and LFTs should thus be obtained at monthly intervals for the first three months, then less frequently.

Mr AJ should be reminded of the need to report immediately if he develops a sore throat, fever, malaise or non-specific illness. Sulfasalazine therapy should be stopped if there is suspicion, or laboratory evidence of, a blood disorder.

How effective are topical treatments in the induction of remission?

A9 **Topical steroids are as effective as oral treatment in distal colitis, providing rapid relief of rectal symptoms such as tenesmus and urgency, and improvement in the sigmoidoscopic appearance of the mucosa. However, topical mesalazine could also be considered.**

A recent Cochrane Review has shown topical mesalazine to be better than oral mesalazine and topical corticosteroids for patients with active distal colitis. Combination of oral and topical 5-ASA drugs is more effective than either drug alone for induction (and maintenance) of mild to moderate distal disease. Consequently, despite being more expensive, topical 5-ASA agents are being increasingly used first-line instead of topical steroids.

What factors govern the choice of topical steroid and the duration of treatment?

A10   **The choice of preparation will depend on the upper extent of disease, with suppositories or foam reaching about 15–20 cm and liquid enemas distributing to about 30–60 cm (to the splenic flexure) and sometimes as far as the ascending colon. The duration of treatment is dependent upon the severity of the disease.**

In the left-sided colitis of Mr AJ a liquid enema will be more effective because it spreads farther. The current choice lies between Predenema (prednisolone metasulphobenzoate) and Predsol (prednisolone sodium phosphate), both of which contain 20 mg prednisolone in 100 mL liquid. Theoretically Predenema would be preferable because it produces lower plasma steroid concentrations, but there is no evidence that this difference is important in normal usage, and both are equally effective clinically.

Patients with mild to moderate disease confined to the rectum and sigmoid colon prefer to use the 5-mL foam enemas such as Colifoam (hydrocortisone) or Predfoam (prednisolone metasulphobenzoate). Patients generally dislike anal administration of medicines and often have difficulty retaining the 100-mL enema.

Three to four week courses of once daily administration are usually necessary. In more severe exacerbations, enemas can be given twice daily for two to four weeks. The dose should then be reduced gradually over the next one to two months as improvement occurs.

What side-effects are associated with the use of topical steroids? How can these be minimised?

A11   **Occasionally systemic side-effects develop, such as fluid retention, mooning of the face or acne, but these only usually occur on long-term treatment.**

Poorly absorbed compounds such as prednisolone sodium phosphate and metasulphobenzoate were developed to have less effect on plasma cortisol, but plasma levels vary between the different preparations. More recent attempts to develop compounds with even lower systemic bio-availability have resulted in the development of budesonide enemas. These are reported to have equal efficacy to prednisolone sodium phosphate but to produce less suppression of plasma cortisol levels.

How should Mr AJ be counselled on his discharge medication?

A12 (a) **Sulfasalazine. Sulfasalazine causes orange discoloration of urine (and contact lenses). It should be taken with food and Mr AJ should tell his GP immediately if he develops a sore throat, a fever, bruising or feels generally unwell.**

(b) **Predenema. The enema should be administered once a day, at night. To do this the enema should be warmed to body temperature. Mr AJ should lie on his left side for its insertion, with one knee raised to his chest. The tip of the enema should be inserted rectally and the bag rolled up slowly in order to administer the liquid into his colon. He should wait for one minute before withdrawing the tip, then roll into the prone position for three to five minutes (to facilitate retention and proximal spread).**

What is mesalazine and how effective will it be compared to sulfasalazine in the maintenance of remission of ulcerative colitis?

A13 **Mesalazine is the name given to all enteric-coated and sustained-release preparations of 5-ASA, where 5-ASA is not joined to another compound. A recent meta-analysis, including 16 studies and 2479 patients, showed that relapse was less likely after six months of sulfasalazine than with 5-ASA (50% relapsed on 5-ASA compared with 43.6% with sulfasalazine). The difference was not statistically significant after one year. However, many clinicians prefer to use the 5-ASA drugs because they are better tolerated by patients.**

Enteric-coated mesalazine (Asacol) is coated with Eudragit-S, a pH-sensitive acrylic-based resin which dissolves when the luminal pH exceeds 7, releasing 5-ASA in the terminal ileum and colon.

Another enteric-coated mesalazine (Salofalk) is coated with the resin Eudragit-L which is released when the pH exceeds 6, beginning in the ileum and continuing through to the colon.

Ipocol is a recently launched brand of enteric-coated mesalazine for which there are very limited data available at the time of writing. Data from small *in vitro* dissolution studies suggest there may be inequivalence between Ipocol and Asacol. A trial comparing the clinical efficacy of the two drugs is ongoing. The *British National Formulary* for mesalazine states 'The delivery characteristics of enteric-coated mesalazine preparations may vary; these preparations should not be considered interchangeable'.

Sustained-release mesalazine (Pentasa) is a tablet consisting of granules coated with a semipermeable membrane which releases 5-ASA gradually at a pH between 6 and 7.5, and at a faster rate at a pH above 7.5.

What alternative aminosalicylates could have been considered?

A14   **Olsalazine or balsalazide.**

Olsalazine and balsalazide release 5-ASA after cleavage of an azo bond by colonic bacteria. Olsalazine consists of two azo-bonded 5-ASA molecules and balsalazide comprises 5-ASA bonded to an inert carrier, aminobenzoyl alanine. Some recent studies have suggested that balsalazide is more effective than mesalazine. A randomised, double-blind comparison of balsalazide 3 g daily and mesalazine 1.2 g daily for 12 months in 99 patients showed that balsalazide prevented more relapses in the first three months (10 versus 28%), although remission at 12 months was 58% in both groups.

What dose of mesalazine should be prescribed for Mr AJ to maintain remission?

A15   **400 mg three times daily.**

From various dose-ranging studies it has been concluded that for maintenance of remission at least 800 mg/day 5-ASA (equivalent to 2 g/day sulfasalazine) must be delivered to the colon, although the optimal dose may be nearer to 1000–1550 mg 5-ASA. A dose of 400 mg three times daily of Asacol is necessary to achieve colonic delivery of at least 800 mg 5-ASA; however, higher Asacol doses of 800 mg three times daily may be required in some patients for both induction and maintenance of remission.

Does mesalazine have a better side-effect profile than sulfasalazine?
How should therapy be monitored?

A16 **Yes. Patient tolerance of the new salicylates is better,
although they are not free from the more serious adverse
effects. FBC and renal function tests should be performed at
regular intervals.**

5-ASA compounds were developed in an attempt to avoid the adverse
effects thought to be due to the sulfapyridine moiety of sulfasalazine,
such as rash and blood dyscrasias. However, intolerance to 5-ASA drugs
occurs in about 10% of patients and serious adverse effects such as
aplastic anaemia, leucopenia, agranulocytosis and thrombocytopenia
have been reported.

The Committee on Safety of Medicines has made recommendations
based on evidence from spontaneous reporting and post-marketing surveillance that patients should be advised to report any unexplained
bleeding, bruising, purpura, sore throat, fever or malaise that occurs
during mesalazine treatment. A blood count should be performed and the
drug stopped immediately if a blood dyscrasia is suspected.

All 5-ASA drugs are potentially nephrotoxic and so regular testing of
renal function is also necessary.

What are the therapeutic aims for Mr AJ now?

A17 (a) **Induce and then maintain remission of his clinical
symptoms and acute mucosal inflammation.**

(b) **Correct his fluid and electrolyte imbalances.**

(c) **Treat his anaemia.**

Mr AJ now has signs and symptoms of severe disease. These are normally
defined as the passage of more than six bloody stools daily, plus at least
one of the following systemic disturbances: temperature greater than
37.5°C, pulse greater than 100 beats per minute, haemoglobin less than
10 g/dL and serum albumin less than 35 g/L.

Abdominal tenderness and pain are usual, while plain radiography
shows the presence of colonic air and oedema.

What parameters can be monitored to assess Mr AJ's progress?

A18   **The following parameters should indicate progress: reduction in diarrhoea and abdominal pain; rising serum albumin; no rectal blood loss; absence of fever; reduction in ESR and CRP; rising haemoglobin; normalisation of serum electrolytes; abdominal radiographic evidence of improvement.**

Has appropriate intravenous fluid therapy been prescribed? Which other serum electrolyte would it be advisable to monitor at this point?

A19   **Mr AJ's intravenous fluid therapy is appropriate provided it is monitored closely; however, it is advisable to monitor his serum magnesium level prior to initiating therapy.**

Blood transfusion is appropriate to compensate for Mr AJ's prolonged colonic blood loss which is demonstrated by his low haemoglobin plus low haematocrit.

Acute or chronic diarrhoea can cause depletion of sodium, potassium and chloride, as well as water. The ensuing dehydration will result in a raised blood urea, but the serum sodium may remain in the normal range because of mixed depletion of sodium and water. Appropriate therapy is thus isotonic sodium chloride solution – administration of water in the form of glucose 5% solution will further aggravate the reduction in extracellular fluid volume. Potassium should be replaced conservatively with careful monitoring of serum potassium levels, as Mr AJ is to receive whole blood, which can contain large amounts of potassium.

Prolonged diarrhoea can also deplete the body of magnesium. A potential complication in the replacement of potassium is the requirement for the body to be magnesium-replete before this is possible, magnesium being necessary for the functioning of the sodium–potassium pump which maintains the potassium concentration intracellularly. If Mr AJ is found to be magnesium-deficient, replacement using oral magnesium compounds such as magnesium hydroxide may be inappropriate, as these tend to cause diarrhoea which would be undesirable. Magnesium infusion is thus the preferred route. A typical regimen may be 16–24 mmol of magnesium per litre of sodium chloride 0.9% or glucose administered over 12–24 hours, repeated daily for five days.

What is the rationale for the use of intravenous steroid therapy?

A20   Intravenous corticosteroids are the drugs of choice for remission induction in severe attacks of ulcerative colitis.

It is standard practice to give seven days of intravenous steroid therapy equivalent to 200–300 mg hydrocortisone daily and then to switch to 40–60 mg oral prednisolone daily. Failure to respond during the initial seven days of therapy has, until recently, been taken as an indication for surgery.

The glucocorticoid properties of corticosteroids, i.e. immunosuppression and reduction of inflammation, are important in the therapy of ulcerative colitis. The multiple anti-inflammatory properties of steroids include direct lymphocytotoxicity, diminution of cytokine release and inhibition of arachidonic acid release from membranes.

Studies have shown that absorption of oral corticosteroids is impaired in acutely ill patients such as Mr AJ, so intravenous therapy is appropriate initially. Some centres use an alternative corticosteroid, methylprednisolone, which has less mineralocorticoid activity than hydrocortisone and so may cause less electrolyte disturbances.

What biochemical monitoring should be carried out while Mr AJ is receiving hydrocortisone?

A21   Serum sodium and potassium levels, and blood sugar measurements.

The mineralocorticoid properties of hydrocortisone may cause sodium and water retention and potassium depletion. In view of Mr AJ's diarrhoea-induced hypokalaemia, it is particularly important to monitor his serum potassium level. The glucocorticoid property of hydrocortisone may produce a rise in blood sugar so this parameter should also be monitored regularly.

Should an antidiarrhoeal agent such as codeine phosphate be prescribed for Mr AJ?

A22   No. The reduction in gut motility induced by such drugs may precipitate a state of toxic megacolon in a patient like Mr AJ.

Toxic megacolon is a life-threatening complication of inflammatory bowel disease in which the colon is very dilated. It carries the risk of gut perforation and haemorrhage. Other drugs reducing gut motility such as anticholinergics should also be avoided.

What could be prescribed for Mr AJ's abdominal pain?

A23 **Paracetamol may be tried; however, non-steroidal anti-inflammatory drugs should be avoided as prostaglandin inhibition may increase the mucosal inflammation. As discussed in Answer 22, opiates should be avoided wherever possible in order to prevent the development of toxic megacolon.**

Would nutritional support aid Mr AJ's recovery?

A24 **Total parenteral nutrition (TPN) is only necessary if the patient is malnourished.**

Unlike Crohn's disease, neither elemental diets nor TPN with bowel rest are of proven value in the treatment of ulcerative colitis. Generally, no food is allowed during an acute exacerbation, although the need for this is disputed. Patients who respond to treatment are usually allowed a light diet.

How should Mr AJ's anaemia be treated?

A25 **By further clinical investigations, then ferrous sulphate 200 mg twice daily, if appropriate.**

It is most likely that Mr AJ has an iron-deficiency anaemia resulting from his prolonged colonic blood loss; however, before treatment is started this must be confirmed by a blood film result that gives a microcytic, hypo-chromic picture with a low serum iron concentration.

However, it is usual practice to delay starting iron therapy until the acute flare has subsided because this can confuse the assessment of the bowel habit. Additionally, iron can precipitate relapse, especially in distal ulcerative colitis, by causing proximal constipation.

Should an antibiotic be added to Mr AJ's treatment?

A26 **No. In acute ulcerative colitis the addition of antibiotics to standard therapies is considered to confer no benefit.**

Despite strong evidence for the role of microbial factors in ulcerative colitis, apart from pouchitis, there is poor evidence for the efficacy of antibiotics.

Metronidazole was shown to be slightly more effective than sulfa-salazine in only one double-blind maintenance of remission trial in which patients were randomised to receive either metronidazole 600 mg/ day or sulfasalazine 2 g/day. In an earlier trial, metronidazole was shown to be ineffective in the treatment of acute ulcerative colitis.

Ciprofloxacin has been reported to be useful in inducing and maintaining remission in patients with moderate to severe ulcerative colitis refractory to conventional treatment; however, the trial was criticised for having an excess of smokers in the ciprofloxacin group (a known protective factor) and for including patients with suboptimal pre-entry therapy.

Evidence is emerging for the role of probiotics (live microorganisms which have a beneficial effect on health by altering the microbial environment). Trials to date, although small, support a role for probiotics as maintenance treatment in mild to moderate disease.

What is the rationale for the use of ciclosporin in Mr AJ?

A27 **For its immunosuppressant activity in an attempt to avoid colectomy.**

Ciclosporin impairs the activation of lymphocytes and macrophages by inhibiting the production of interleukin-2 and other cytokines. Previously, failure to respond to seven days treatment with hydrocortisone inevitably led to surgery. Several studies have demonstrated the success of ciclosporin in severe steroid-resistant ulcerative colitis patients. In an open study, colectomy was avoided in 73% of patients given intravenous ciclosporin after they had failed to respond to 10 days therapy with intravenous hydrocortisone. Results from a randomised, double-blind controlled trial in 20 patients who had failed to respond to seven days intravenous hydrocortisone, showed that nine out of eleven patients treated with ciclosporin at a dose of 4 mg/kg/day had a response within seven days, compared with none of the nine patients who received placebo. Although in some patients colectomy is only delayed and not avoided, over half of patients on this regimen avoid colectomy in the longer-term, and others are provided with time to prepare for elective colectomy. In 20 of 22 patients (91%) who avoided colectomy during their hospital admission, 53% had successfully avoided colectomy after a mean follow-up period of 39 months. A second study followed patients for five years after ciclosporin therapy and found that 62% of patients had avoided colectomy.

The rationale for giving ciclosporin intravenously rather than orally is based on studies documenting poor absorption of orally administered ciclosporin in patients with diarrhoea and inflammatory disease of the bowel.

Why was the intravenous ciclosporin given over six hours?

A28 **The maximum duration of stability of diluted ciclosporin injection is six hours because of its polyethoxylated castor oil content, which can cause phthalate stripping from PVC. Some centres favour a shorter two-hour infusion time.**

Why does Mr AJ need to be closely observed initially?

A29 **Because of the potential for anaphylaxis with intravenous ciclosporin therapy.**

Patients should be observed continuously during the first 30 minutes of the infusion because of the risk of anaphylaxis. This is due to the polyethoxylated castor oil component, and the reaction is manifested by symptoms of flushing, dyspnoea, hypotension and tachycardia.

For how long should intravenous ciclosporin treatment be continued?

A30 **For 10 days if proving to be effective.**

Intravenous ciclosporin therapy should be given in addition to intravenous hydrocortisone and dual therapy should be reviewed at five days and continued for 10 days if effective.

What monitoring is necessary during intravenous ciclosporin treatment?

A31 **Ciclosporin blood levels, renal function, hepatic function and blood pressure.**

The steady state ciclosporin blood levels should be checked twice weekly and should be within the range 250–400 nanograms/mL (from a whole-blood sample, as the use of plasma or serum samples is subject to inaccuracies resulting from the temperature-dependent uptake of ciclosporin by red blood cells. For further details of ciclosporin assays, see Chapter 7. The risk of nephrotoxicity, hepatotoxicity and other adverse effects increases with whole-blood ciclosporin concentration. Care with concurrent drug treatment is necessary because of potential effects on the cytochrome P450 enzyme system responsible for the metabolism of ciclosporin.

Plasma urea, creatinine and magnesium should be performed daily, with LFTs every two to three days.

Ciclosporin therapy can cause raised blood pressure and antihypertensive therapy should be started if Mr AJ's diastolic pressure increases above 90 mmHg.

Daily abdominal x-rays should be performed to monitor Mr AJ's response to treatment.

What side-effects are possible with ciclosporin treatment?

A32 **In addition to the effects on blood pressure and liver and kidney function already discussed, hirsutism, tremor, gingival hypertrophy, anorexia, nausea and vomiting, and hyperkalaemia have been reported. A burning sensation in the hands and feet may also occur, usually in the first week of therapy. The most common side-effect in patients not undergoing transplantation seems to be paraesthesia (e.g. tingling fingers) which is reported to be mainly subjective and does not require the drug to be stopped. Seizures have been reported rarely, in association with toxic blood levels of ciclosporin (and see Answer 33).**

Why was a serum cholesterol test done prior to initiating ciclosporin?

A33 **A low cholesterol (less than 3 mmol/L) in conjunction with ciclosporin therapy is associated with an increased risk of seizures.**

Why has the ciclosporin dose not been increased to reflect the decreased bioavailability of oral drug compared to the intravenous form?

A34 **To avoid high trough levels.**

The oral bioavailability of ciclosporin is only one-third that of the intravenous formulation. However, in ulcerative colitis, the initial oral maintenance dose is only slightly higher than the intravenous dose to avoid high trough levels, because the blood levels required for oral ciclosporin therapy are different from those required during the intravenous phase. The initial oral dose would be 5 mg/kg/day in two divided doses unless the intravenous dose has had to be reduced due to toxicity or high ciclosporin levels. The dose is then gradually titrated to achieve blood levels of 100–200 nanograms/mL (trough samples), if side-effects allow. Remission is usually sustained on 5–9 mg/kg/day.

These are lower doses than required following renal transplantation.

Mr AJ was in fact started on a dose of less than 5 mg/kg/day as he had had toxic levels on 4 mg/kg/day of intravenous therapy.

What is the rationale for prescribing azathioprine?

A35 **Azathioprine, an immunosuppressant drug, has been found to be an effective maintenance treatment both in patients with chronic active disease and those, such as Mr AJ, with fully remitted disease.**

Azathioprine is often used in patients with frequent relapses despite 5-ASA therapy and in those who are steroid-dependent in order to suppress acute symptoms. The slow onset of action of azathioprine led to trials of more potent immunosuppressive drugs such as ciclosporin for the treatment of acute, severe refractory disease. However, lower-dose oral ciclosporin regimens have not proved to be consistently effective for maintaining remission.

What maximum dose of azathioprine would you recommend and why? How should azathioprine therapy be monitored?

A36 **The dose should not exceed 2 mg/kg/day, as larger doses greatly increase the risk of bone marrow suppression. Liver function tests and full blood counts should thus be carried out regularly.**

At least 10% of patients are unable to tolerate azathioprine. Adverse effects which have been reported include nausea, vomiting, diarrhoea, abdominal pain, pancreatitis and cholestatic jaundice. A hypersensitivity reaction, characterised by fever, rigors, myalgia and arthralgia, is common.

Should Mr AJ be unable to tolerate azathioprine, its active metabolite 6-mercaptopurine may be tried. Despite a high rate of lymphoma and skin cancer seen in transplant recipients taking immunosuppressant drugs, surveys of non-transplant patients have reported a relatively low level of risk. In two studies investigating a total of 1381 patients followed for seven to nine years after starting therapy, azathioprine did not increase the risk of cancer compared with the general population.

However, the average duration of azathioprine therapy was only one to two years.

Acknowledgement

We would like to thank Dr Richard Long and Dr Kathy Teahon (Consultant Gastroenterologists, Nottingham City Hospital NHS Trust) for helpful advice and for reviewing this case study. Thanks also to Kirsty Maclean (formerly Medicines Evaluation Pharmacist, Amber Valley PCT, Southern Derbyshire) for assistance with the literature search.

Further reading

Abboudi ZH, Marsh JC, Smith-Laing G *et al*. Fatal aplastic anaemia after mesalazine (Letter). *Lancet* 1994; **343**: 542.

Anderson FH. The rectal approach to treatment in distal ulcerative colitis. *Lancet* 1995; **346**: 520–521.

Anon. A mesalazine enema for ulcerative colitis. *Drug Ther Bull* 1994; **32**: 38–39.

Anon. Maintenance drugs for inflammatory bowel disease. *Drug Ther Bull* 2001; **39**: 91–95.

Cohen RD, Stein R, Hanauer SB. Intravenous cyclosporin in ulcerative colitis: a five-year experience. *Am J Gastroenterol.* 1999; **94**: 1587–1592.

Committee on Safety of Medicines. *Curr Prob Pharmacovigilance* 1993; **19**: 6.

Committee on Safety of Medicines. *Curr Prob Pharmacovigilance* 1995; **21**: 5.

Courtney MG, Nunes DP, Bergin CF *et al*. Randomised comparison of olsalazine and mesalazine in prevention of relapses in ulcerative colitis. *Lancet* 1992; **339**: 1279–1281.

Farrell RJ, Peppercorn MA. Ulcerative colitis *Lancet* 2002; **359**: 331–340.

Ghosh S, Shand A, Ferguson A. Ulcerative colitis. *Br Med J* 2000; **320**: 1119–1123.

Green JR, Gibson JA, Kerr GD *et al*. and The ABACUS Investigator Group. Maintenance of remission of ulcerative colitis: a comparison between balsalazide 3 g daily and mesalazine 1.2 g daily over 12 months. *Aliment Pharmacol Ther* 1998; **12**: 1207–1216.

Hanauer SB. Inflammatory bowel disease. *N Engl J Med* 1996; **334**: 841–848.

Jarnerot G. New salicylates as maintenance treatment in ulcerative colitis. *Gut* 1994; **35**: 1155–1158.

Laidlaw ST, Reilly JT. Antilymphocyte globulin for mesalazine-associated aplastic anaemia (Letter). *Lancet* 1994; **343**: 981–982.

Lichtiger S, Present DH. Preliminary report: cyclosporin in the treatment of severe active ulcerative colitis. *Lancet* 1990; **336**: 16–19.

Lichtiger S, Present DH, Kornbluth A *et al.* Cyclosporin in severe ulcerative colitis refractory to steroid therapy. *N Engl J Med* 1994; **330**: 1841–1845.

Nilsson A, Danielsson Å, Lofberg R *et al.* Olsalazine versus sulfasalazine for relapse-prevention in ulcerative colitis: a multicenter study. *Am J Gastroenterol* 1995; **90**: 381–387.

Reynolds DJM, Aronson JK. ABC of monitoring drug therapy: cyclosporin. *Br Med J* 1992; **305**: 1491–1494.

Sninsky CA. New salicylates as maintenance treatment in ulcerative colitis (Letter). *Gut* 1995, **36**: 640.

Stack WA, Long RG, Hawkey CJ *et al.* Short- and long-term outcome of patients treated with cyclosporin for severe acute ulcerative colitis. *Aliment Pharmacol Ther* 1998; **12**: 973–978.

Sutherland LR, May GR, Shaffer EA. Sulfasalazine revisited: a meta-analysis of 5-aminosalicylic acid in the treatment of ulcerative colitis. *Ann Intern Med* 1993; **118**: 540–549.

Sutherland L, Roth D, Beck P *et al.* Oral 5–aminosalicylic acid for maintaining remission in ulcerative colitis (Cochrane Review). In: *The Cochrane Library 2*. Update Software, Oxford, 2003.

Thuluvath PJ. Mesalazine-induced interstitial nephritis. *Gut* 1994; **35**: 1493–1496.

Vincent F, Bensousan T-A, Whitmore SE *et al.* Cyclosporin in severe ulcerative colitis (Letter). *N Engl J Med* 1995; **332**: 127.

10

Alcoholic liver disease

Sarah Stoll

Day 1 Mrs CN, a 58-year-old retired pub landlady, was admitted to hospital by her GP with haematemesis and melaena. She had been feeling unwell over the last few days and had passed fresh blood when going to the toilet. On the morning of admission her husband said she had vomited about 500 mL of fresh blood. She was known to have liver cirrhosis and had been a heavy drinker for the past 15 years. She had recently been consuming about a bottle of vodka a day. Her drug history on admission was spironolactone 200 mg daily and chlorphenamine 4 mg three times a day. She also occasionally took ibuprofen for back pain, but had not taken any recently. On examination she was noted to smell of alcohol. She was pale and jaundiced, and appeared slightly confused. She had spider naevi on her face and upper body, and showed signs of muscle wasting. Ascites was noted. Her blood pressure was 90/50 mmHg and her pulse rate was 105 beats per minute. On admission she vomited another 500 mL of fresh blood and an emergency oesophago-gastro-duodenoscopy (OGD) was arranged.

Her laboratory results were:

- Sodium 131 mmol/L (reference range 130–145)
- Potassium 4.8 mmol/L (3.5–5.0)
- Urea 4.1 mmol/L (3.3–6.7)
- Bilirubin 65 micromol/L (3–20)
- Alkaline phosphatase 315 international units/L (30–130)
- Gamma glutamyl transferase 287 international units/L (1–55)
- Aspartate aminotransferase 110 international units/L (10–50)
- International normalised ratio (INR) 1.5 (0.9–1.2)
- Haemoglobin 6.8 g/dL (11.5–15.5)
- Creatinine 115 micromol/L (45–120)
- Platelets 105×10^9 L (150–450)
- Albumin 26 g/L (35–50)

Q1 What treatments should be given to Mrs CN to prepare her for the OGD?

Q2   What general pharmacokinetic and pharmacodynamic considerations
need to be taken into account when prescribing for Mrs CN?

Mrs CN was commenced on terlipressin. At endoscopy Mrs CN was found
to have three large oesophageal varices which were banded. There was
still generalised oozing from the oesophagus, but the exact source could
not be identified.

Q3   Outline a pharmaceutical care plan for Mrs CN.
Q4   What was the rationale for prescribing terlipressin?
Q5   What advice would you give the medical and nursing staff with regard
to using terlipressin in this patient?
Q6   What alternative treatments are there for acute variceal bleeding?

The 'nil by mouth' restriction was removed six hours after the procedure
and Mrs CN was prescribed the following additional therapies:

- Ciprofloxacin 500 mg orally twice daily
- Pabrinex (one pair of amps) intravenously three times daily
- Phytomenadione 10 mg intramuscularly once each day
- Lactulose 10 mL orally once each day
- Sucralfate 1 g orally four times daily
- Clomethiazole three capsules orally four times daily

Q7   What was the rationale for starting each of these drugs in Mrs CN?
Q8   What changes would you make to Mrs CN's prescriptions?

Day 5   Mrs CN had been stabilised and was transferred to a medical
ward. She was, however, complaining of back pain and had requested
ibuprofen as she said she had found it to be effective in the past.

Q9   What advice would you give regarding the treatment of Mrs CN's
back pain?

Day 10   Mrs CN was told that she would be started on a new tablet to
help prevent her having another variceal bleed.

Q10   What was the new tablet likely to be and how should it be
monitored?

Day 15   Mrs CN was ready for discharge home and said she was keen to
abstain from alcohol.

Q11   What pharmacological treatments can be given to help Mrs CN
abstain from alcohol?

Month 3 Mrs CN was readmitted to hospital from clinic with abdominal distension and bilateral ankle swelling. She was complaining of abdominal discomfort and pruritus. Her weight was now 68 kg compared to 62 kg at her last admission. On examination she was jaundiced and had signs consistent with chronic liver disease. Her abdomen was grossly distended and she was found to have a moderate amount of ascites present. On admission she was taking spironolactone 100 mg daily, chlorphenamine 4 mg three times a day, lactulose 20 mL twice daily. She had also recently started taking Gaviscon 10 mL four times a day for indigestion.

Her serum biochemistry results were:

- Sodium 133 mmol/L (reference 130–145)
- Potassium 4.2 mmol/L (3.5–5.0)
- Urea 2.8 mmol/L (3.3–6.7)
- Bilirubin 54 micromol/L (3–20)
- Creatinine 75 micromol/L (45–120)

- Albumin 30 g/L (35–50)
- Alkaline phosphatase 300 international units/L (30–130)
- Gamma glutamyl transferase 255 international units/L (1–55)

Q12 Do you agree with the choice of chlorphenamine for Mrs CN's pruritus?

Q13 What are the pharmacological options for treating Mrs CN's ascites and how should they be monitored?

Q14 What non-pharmacological options are available if Mrs CN fails to respond to drug treatment?

Day 1 Mrs CN had her spironolactone dose increased to 200 mg daily. She also had a diagnostic paracentesis performed.

Day 2 Mrs CN's weight was still 68 kg so her dose of spironolactone was increased again to 200 mg twice daily. Her diagnostic paracentesis result showed a polymorphic nuclear count above 250/mm^3.

Q15 What infection is Mrs CN suffering from and what treatment should be given?

Day 4 Mrs CN's weight had been falling over the past few days and was now down to 63 kg. Her biochemistry results were:

- Sodium 128 mmol/L (reference 130–145)
- Potassium 5.2 mmol/L (3.5–5.0)

- Creatinine 110 micromol/L (45–120)
- Urea 8.2 mmol/L (3.3–6.7)

Q16 How should Mrs CN's diuretic therapy be adjusted?

Days 5–13   Mrs CN began to feel better and she no longer had any abdominal pain. Her weight stabilised at 62 kg and her biochemistry results normalised with the adjustments made to her diuretic therapy.

Day 14   Mrs CN was discharged home on the following medications:

- Lactulose 20 mL orally twice a day
- Spironolactone 200 mg orally daily
- Norfloxacin 400 mg orally daily
- Colestyramine 4 g orally twice a day
- Mucogel 10 mL orally three times a day when required
- Propranolol 40 mg orally twice a day

Q17   What medication counselling points should be covered with Mrs CN before discharge?

What treatments should be given to Mrs CN to prepare her for the OGD?

A1 (a) **Colloids and blood (packed red cells) for fluid resuscitation.**

(b) **Fresh frozen plasma (FFP) and vitamin K for correction of coagulopathy.**

(c) **Terlipressin for treatment of potential gastric or oesophageal varices.**

(d) **Midazolam as premedication for her endoscopy.**

Mrs CN needs urgent fluid resuscitation as she has suffered large blood loss, and as a consequence has low blood pressure and a high pulse rate. The circulating volume needs to be monitored carefully, preferably via a central venous catheter. Care needs to be taken not to fluid overload Mrs CN otherwise further bleeding may be provoked. Volume replacement should be started with colloids such as Gelofusine, whilst transfusions are being prepared. Crystalloid fluids containing sodium chloride should be avoided as they can aggravate fluid retention in patients with chronic liver disease. Blood and coagulation factors (FFP) should be administered as required. Terlipressin should be started as it can reduce the incidence of active bleeding at the time of endoscopy and improves bleeding control in patients admitted with bleeding varices. Care needs to be taken with the dosing of midazolam as a premedication for OGD as patients with liver disease are more sensitive to the cerebral effects of sedatives. The metabolism of midazolam is likely to be reduced in Mrs CN as she has reduced liver blood flow and poor synthetic function. Over-sedation may cause respiratory depression with a risk of aspiration and can precipitate encephalopathy in these patients.

What general pharmacokinetic and pharmacodynamic considerations need to be taken into account when prescribing for Mrs CN?

A2 **It is known that Mrs CN has cirrhosis of the liver and this will affect the pharmacokinetics of any drug that is hepatically metabolised. The pharmacodynamic consequences of liver disease will make her more susceptible to adverse effects from a number of drug therapies.**

Cirrhosis is defined as fibrosis resulting in disruption of the normal architecture of the liver. There is also a reduction in hepatic cell mass with a corresponding decrease in the functional capacity of the liver. This is reflected in Mrs CN's low serum albumin level of 26 g/L (35–50) and prolonged INR.

The presence of liver disease will influence pharmacokinetic parameters such as absorption, metabolism, volume of distribution and the extent of hepatic extraction of a drug, but it is not possible to predict quantitatively the extent to which these variables will be affected in any one individual. In cirrhosis of the liver a reduction in intrahepatic blood flow plus the development of portal systemic shunts which divert blood from the liver to the systemic circulation result in an increased bioavailability of drugs that are highly extracted on the first pass through the liver (flow-limited drugs). Peak plasma concentrations of such drugs will be increased and their half-life will be prolonged. This may necessitate a reduction in dose and/or lengthening of the dosage interval.

The reduced functional capacity associated with cirrhosis will cause an increase in the bioavailability of drugs with a high extraction ratio, owing to a reduction in first-pass metabolism. Reduced functional capacity and therefore delayed elimination from the systemic circulation will also prolong the half-life of drugs with low hepatic extraction (capacity-limited drugs) which are dependent on the functional capacity of the liver for their clearance. In such cases, adjustment of the dosing interval will be necessary to avoid toxicity on repeated dosing.

Mrs CN's reduced albumin level will result in reduced plasma protein binding of drugs, which in turn will increase the concentration of free, active drug. In the presence of reduced hepatic blood flow, the bioavailability of drugs with a high hepatic extraction will be increased. For drugs that are poorly extracted by the liver at first pass, bioavailability will depend on the capacity of the liver to metabolise that drug. If liver function is not impaired, the increase in free drug concentration due to reduced protein binding will only be temporary, as a new equilibrium will develop.

In clinical practice it is important to account for pharmacodynamic variations associated with liver disease as they can affect a patient's response to therapy. In patients with liver disease cerebral sensitivity to drugs with sedative and hypnotic effects is increased. Drugs with cerebral depressant activity should be prescribed with caution in severe liver disease, as there is a risk of precipitating hepatic encephalopathy. Care should also be taken when prescribing drugs that can cause constipation, as constipation can also precipitate encephalopathy in liver patients. An alternative agent causing less constipation should be used, or lactulose can be co-prescribed. Drugs which may cause gastric irritation or an increase in bleeding tendency should be avoided, e.g. non-steroidal anti-inflammatory drugs (NSAIDs). NSAIDs can also cause deterioration in liver function, precipitate renal failure, and cause fluid retention and are therefore contra-indicated in patients with hepatic cirrhosis.

Outline a pharmaceutical care plan for Mrs CN.

A3 The pharmaceutical care plan for Mrs CN should include the following:

(a) Ensure appropriate drug therapy is prescribed in doses appropriate to Mrs CN.

(b) Monitor Mrs CN's prescriptions for drugs which may be contra-indicated or cause a deterioration in her condition.

(c) Ensure that the method of administration of parenteral therapy is appropriate.

(d) Monitor the outcomes of any prescribed drug therapy for efficacy and toxicity.

(e) Counsel Mrs CN on all aspects of her drug therapy.

(f) Counsel Mrs CN on her discharge medication and the likely duration of each therapy. Liaise with relatives/carers on the importance of continued medication and arrangements for resupply where appropriate.

What was the rationale for prescribing terlipressin?

A4 Terlipressin has been shown to reduce bleeding and improve survival in patients with bleeding oesophageal varices.

In cirrhosis the normal liver architecture is destroyed by fibrosis which results in an increased resistance to blood flow within the portal blood system and portal hypertension. In normal individuals portal venous pressure is 7–12 mmHg; in portal hypertension this may increase to 30 mmHg or more. Increased portal pressure leads to the development of porto-systemic collateral vessels, especially in the region of the stomach and oesophagus. These collateral veins become distended, forming varices, which may bleed if the pressure in the portal venous system increases. Bleeding varices can result in massive haemorrhage and are associated with a mortality of up to 50% on the index bleed and 30% for subsequent bleeds.

Terlipressin is a synthetic analogue of vasopressin. It works by reducing blood flow to varices through vasoconstriction of blood vessels.

It has a biphasic action: the intact molecule has an immediate vasocon-
stricting effect which is followed by a delayed effect caused by the slow
transformation of terlipressin *in vivo* to lysine vasopressin. A meta-
analysis of the three studies involving terlipressin showed a significant
improvement in the rate of bleeding control and survival for patients
treated with terlipressin compared to placebo.

What advice would you give the medical and nursing staff with regard
to using terlipressin in this patient?

A5 **Terlipressin should be administered as an initial 2 mg
intravenous bolus. Repeated intravenous injections of
1–2 mg should then be given every four to six hours until
haemostasis is achieved. The patient's blood pressure, serum
sodium, potassium and fluid balance should be checked and
side-effects monitored whilst she is on therapy.**

Terlipressin's side-effects include coronary vasoconstriction and increases
in arterial blood pressure, and it should therefore be used with extreme
caution in patients with a history of ischaemic heart disease. Although
the coronary side-effects are less than with vasopressin, glyceryl trinitrate
should be administered concurrently with terlipressin or an alternative
agent, such as octreotide, should be used in patients with ischaemic heart
disease. Other side-effects include, ischaemic colitis, abdominal cramps
and headaches. Therapy should be continued until haemostasis is achieved. It is licensed to be given for up to 72 hours but five days treatment
may be required to prevent early rebleeding.

What alternative treatments are there for acute variceal bleeding?

A6 **(a) Other vasoactive agents which include vasopressin,
somatostatin, octreotide and lanreotide.**

Vasopressin was the first drug to be used to treat variceal bleeding and has
been reported to be effective in approximately 50% of cases. Glyceryl
trinitrate (40–400 micrograms/min by infusion or as a patch) has been
used with vasopressin to help reduce coronary vasoconstriction, which is
a side-effect of this therapy. The use of vasopressin has now virtually been
abandoned because of its severe side-effects.

Somatostatin is a vasoactive peptide hormone that causes selective
splanchnic vasoconstriction and decreases portal pressure. It is free from
any of the systemic adverse effects associated with vasopressin but it is not

available in the UK. Octreotide is a derivative of somatostatin, but is more potent and has a longer duration of action. Octreotide, administered as an infusion at 25 micrograms/h, has been shown to be as effective as balloon tamponade in controlling bleeding in the acute situation and preventing rebleeding post-injection sclerotherapy. However, in a large randomised clinical trial octreotide was not shown to improve survival or control of bleeding when compared to placebo. Octreotide is not licensed for the treatment of bleeding oesophageal varices.

A new somatostatin analogue, lanreotide, could potentially cause more aggressive lowering of portal pressure but the results of clinical trials assessing its efficacy are awaited at the time of writing.

(b) Endoscopic sclerotherapy or band ligation.

Emergency endoscopy should be performed to identify the source of bleeding and sclerotherapy or band ligation may be carried out. Sclerotherapy involves injection of a sclerosant, usually 5% ethanolamine oleate, in 1–2 mL boluses into the varix. Tissue adhesives and bovine thrombin have also been used to control bleeding gastric varices. Sclerotherapy performed at the time of endoscopy controls acute bleeding in more than 90% of patients (in 60% of cases, variceal bleeding will stop spontaneously). Banding or endoscopic variceal ligation may be undertaken in acutely bleeding patients and has been shown to be as successful as sclerotherapy at controlling acute bleeding.

(c) Balloon tamponade.

Balloon tamponade controls bleeding by reducing inflow at the gastro-oesophageal junction. It is effective in up to 90% of cases. It involves the insertion of a four-lumen tube (Sengstaken–Blakemore tube) through the mouth and into the stomach. The tube has an inflatable gastric balloon, an inflatable oesophageal balloon, and tubes through which to aspirate the stomach and oesophagus. Inflation of the gastric balloon is effective in controlling bleeding in most cases. Inflation of the oesophageal balloon should be considered as a last resort, due to the tendency of this strategy to cause oesophageal ulceration and perforation. Balloon tamponade is indicated in massive bleeding or as a bridge to other treatments.

(d) Transjugular intrahepatic porto-systemic shunt (TIPS).

TIPS has been shown to be highly effective in the management of uncontrolled bleeding oesophageal varices when the first-line therapies have failed. The main problems are the limited availability of this procedure, development of encephalopathy in up to 30% of patients and occlusion of the shunt in up to 25% of cases. TIPS has largely replaced the surgical procedures which were performed in the past, such as oesophageal transection and portacaval shunts.

What was the rationale for starting each of these drugs in Mrs CN?

A7   (a)   **Ciprofloxacin is used as antibiotic prophylaxis in patients with variceal bleeding as it has been shown to decrease the rate of infection and can improve survival.**

Bacterial infections occur in 35–66% of cirrhotic patients who have a variceal bleed. Antibiotic prophylaxis should always be given as it has been shown in trials to decrease infection rates and improve survival. A seven-day course of antibiotic therapy is recommended. A number of different antibiotics have been shown to be of benefit in clinical trials, but oral quinolones tend to be the drugs of choice. Broad-spectrum intravenous antibiotics are used in very sick patients and in those patients who are perceived to be at risk of aspiration pneumonia post-endoscopy.

(b)   **Pabrinex is given to provide high doses of vitamins B and C. It contains thiamine (vitamin B$_1$) which is given to prevent the development of Wernicke–Korsakoff syndrome.**

Alcohol-dependent people tend to have an inadequate food intake, and a diet that is high in carbohydrate and low in protein, vitamins and minerals. In addition, absorption of nutrients such as vitamins may be impaired due to alteration of active transport and absorption in the intestinal mucosa. Pabrinex provides a source of high doses of vitamins B and C, including 250 mg of thiamine. Administration of thiamine is important as thiamine deficiency can result in the development of Wernicke–Korsakoff syndrome. The acute component is Wernicke's encephalopathy, which is characterised by mental confusion, ataxia and ophthalmoplegia. Early administration of thiamine can reverse this encephalopathy and prevent the development of the irreversible amnesic syndrome, Korsakoff's psychosis.

(c)   **Phytomenadione (vitamin K$_1$) is given in an attempt to correct the patient's coagulopathy.**

The liver is responsible for the production of vitamin K-dependent clotting factors. Administration of vitamin K will help to correct a patient's INR if the patient is vitamin K deficient due to malabsorption or inadequate dietary intake. However, this approach is often ineffective because the liver is unable to produce clotting factors due to underlying liver damage.

(d)   Lactulose is given to prevent encephalopathy.

Acute or chronic encephalopathy is seen in patients with decompensated cirrhosis. It is thought to be associated with raised plasma concentrations of ammonia and other nitrogenous toxins and can be precipitated by a number of factors, including constipation, gastrointestinal bleeding, diarrhoea and vomiting, infection, alcoholic binges, sedative and opiate drug therapy, electrolyte abnormalities, uraemia, dietary protein excess, surgery, and acute worsening of liver disease.

Following a gastrointestinal bleed there is an increased nitrogen load on the gastrointestinal tract which can result in increased ammonia production by intestinal bacteria. This means that Mrs CN is at increased risk of encephalopathy. Lactulose is a disaccharide which is converted to lactic, acetic and formic acids by intestinal bacteria, thus changing the pH of the gut contents from 7 to 5. The acidic pH reduces the absorption of non-ionised ammonia and creates an environment more suitable for the growth of weak ammonia-producing organisms, such as *Lactobacillus acidophilus*, rather than proteolytic ammonia-producing organisms such as *Escherichia coli*. The osmotic laxative effect of lactulose also speeds intestinal transit and so prevents constipation, reducing the time available for the absorption of potentially toxic nitrogenous compounds.

(e)   Sucralfate is given as a mucosal protectant and helps to treat any ulceration caused by endoscopic banding.

(f)   Clomethiazole is prescribed for treatment of alcohol withdrawal.

Chronic excessive alcohol consumption can result in the development of withdrawal symptoms when a patient stops drinking. The symptoms can range from irritability, sweating, hypertension and tremor, to confusion, hallucinations, convulsions and dysrhythmias. Clomethiazole, a compound structurally related to thiamine, has hypnotic, sedative, anxiolytic and anticonvulsant properties. It can be given to prevent or control the symptoms of alcohol withdrawal.

What changes would you make to Mrs CN's prescription?

A8   **(a)   The phytomenadione should be given intravenously rather than intramuscularly.**

Intramuscular injections should be avoided in patients with liver disease as they can lead to the development of a haematoma at the injection site in patients with a coagulopathy. Konakion MM is the intravenous product. It can be administered either as a 20–30 min intravenous infusion diluted with 55 mL of 5% glucose, or as a slow injection (at a maximum rate of 1 mg/min). A dose of 10 mg daily for three days is usually given.

(b)   The lactulose dose should be increased to a starting dose of at least 15 mL twice daily.

High-dose lactulose therapy is used to prevent encephalopathy. The dose of lactulose should be titrated to produce two soft motions a day without diarrhoea.

(c)   Chlordiazepoxide could be considered as a substitute for clomethiazole. Both drugs should be given on an 'as-required' basis for 24 hours to assess the patient's requirements. The total dose administered over the 24 hours should then be divided by four to give a six-hourly dose, which should be prescribed in a reducing regimen over six days.

Problems that have been documented with clomethiazole are a risk of respiratory depression, hypothermia, hypotension, coma and even death. Clomethiazole is particularly dangerous in an out-patient setting, where the patient may continue to drink alcohol. There is no specific antidote to clomethiazole and there is thus a trend to switch to chlordiazepoxide, a long-acting benzodiazepine, due to its equivalent efficacy and greater safety.

What advice would you give regarding the treatment of Mrs CN's back pain?

A9   Paracetamol should be given instead of ibuprofen as it is safer in patients with liver disease. If paracetamol alone is ineffective, dihydrocodeine can be added in.

Ibuprofen should be avoided in Mrs CN as NSAIDs can cause gastric bleeding and ulceration. This is a particular problem for Mrs CN as she has a prolonged prothrombin time and therefore is at an increased risk of bleeding. NSAIDs may also lead to renal and hepatic impairment, and can cause fluid retention, which is a problem in liver patients who have ascites.

Paracetamol is the drug of choice and this should be prescribed for Mrs CN initially. If paracetamol alone is not sufficient to control her pain then a weak opiate such as dihydrocodeine should be added in. Dihydrocodeine, like all other opiates, can cause sedation and constipation which may precipitate encephalopathy. It should be started at the lowest possible dose and titrated up according to her response.

What was the new tablet likely to be and how should it be monitored?

A10 **The new tablet is likely to be propranolol which is used as first-line therapy in secondary prevention of variceal bleeding. It should be started at a dose of 40 mg orally twice daily. The dose should then be titrated to the patient's blood pressure and pulse, which should be monitored whilst they are on treatment.**

Propranolol, a non-selective beta-blocker, reduces portal pressure by decreasing splanchnic blood flow and the hyperdynamic circulation associated with cirrhosis. It has been shown in trials to reduce the risk of rebleeding from varices. It has also been shown to be of benefit in reducing the risk of the first variceal bleed in patients with cirrhosis who have moderate to large varices. It is started at a low dose as it is metabolised by the liver and undergoes extensive first-pass metabolism. The dose should be titrated to achieve a 25% reduction in pulse rate. However, the pulse rate should not be allowed to fall below 55 beats per minute. Ideally portal pressure studies, which look at the pressure in the portal vein, should be performed to see if a patient has responded to propranolol therapy. The aim is to reduce the portal pressure below 12 mmHg, as the patient is then no longer at risk of bleeding from their varices. Although most trials have involved propranolol, nadolol, another non-selective beta-blocker, can also be used.

What pharmacological treatments can be given to help Mrs CN abstain from alcohol?

A11 **Disulfiram, acamprosate or naltrexone.**

Disulfiram is used as an adjunct in the treatment of alcohol dependence. Whilst taking this medication patients are prevented from drinking alcohol by the extremely unpleasant side-effects that occur after the ingestion of even the smallest amounts of alcohol (including that contained in some oral medicines). The reactions, which include facial flushing, palpitations, headache, arrhythmias, hypotension and collapse, occur because acetaldehyde accumulates when patients taking disulfiram drink alcohol. Because of its powerful interaction with alcohol, disulfiram is reserved for patients who have undergone several unsuccessful treatments for alcoholism and have suffered multiple relapses. Acamprosate is a gamma-aminobutyric acid receptor antagonist which is used to help maintain abstinence from alcohol by reducing cravings. It should be used in combination with counselling. Treatment should be initiated as soon as possible after the alcohol withdrawal period and maintained if the patient relapses. The recommended treatment period for acamprosate is one year. The most common side-effect with acamprosate is diarrhoea, which occurs in about 10% of patients.

Naltrexone is another agent which has been used to maintain abstinence from alcohol, although it is not licensed for this indication. It is similar to acamprosate in that it has significant anti-craving effects which reduce alcohol consumption. The main side-effects are headache and anxiety, which occur in about 10% of patients. Both naltrexone and acamprosate are effective in preventing full-blown relapses in patients who return to drinking after achieving abstinence.

Do you agree with the choice of chlorphenamine for Mrs CN's pruritus?

A12 **Antihistamines such as chlorphenamine are relatively ineffective (apart from their sedative effect) and should not be used as first-line therapy for pruritus. Colestyramine and colestipol are anion-exchange resins which are the usual first-line therapy.**

Bile salts under the skin are one of the factors that cause itching in liver patients. Anion exchange resins are used to bind bile salts in the gut and to help prevent itching by stopping the bile salts being absorbed. Ursodeoxycholic acid is also frequently used in cholestatic liver disease, and long-term use has been shown to improve pruritus. Other drugs such as rifampicin, ondansetron, naltrexone and naloxone are sometimes used if patients fail to respond to first-line agents.

What are the pharmacological options for treating Mrs CN's ascites and how should they be monitored?

A13 **Diuretics are the drug treatments used for treating ascites. Spironolactone is the diuretic of choice. Loop diuretics are sometimes added to spironolactone therapy as they have a synergistic effect. Amiloride is a suitable alternative for patients who develop gynaecomastia on spironolactone therapy.**

Ascites is the presence of free fluid in the peritoneal cavity. The precise mechanism by which ascites develops is unclear. Contributing factors include portal hypertension, reduced oncotic pressure and activation of the renin–angiotensin–aldosterone system. Spironolactone is a specific antagonist of aldosterone and is the drug of choice for the treatment of ascites. Spironolactone is initially prescribed at a dose of 100 mg daily, and should be effective after two or three days of treatment. The aim is to induce a negative fluid balance, which can be assessed by daily monitoring of the patient's weight and fluid balance. The rate of fluid loss from the vascular compartment should not exceed the rate at which fluid can be relocated from the ascitic compartment and weight loss should not exceed 0.5 kg/day (1 kg if peripheral oedema is also present). Excessive diuresis may result in hypovolaemia, electrolyte disturbances including hyponatraemia and uraemia, and a risk of precipitating hepatic encephalopathy and renal impairment. Spironolactone may also cause hyperkalaemia and close monitoring of serum electrolytes is essential throughout treatment. Measurement of sodium and potassium concentrations in the urine is sometimes used to indicate the effectiveness of spironolactone and a urinary sodium to potassium ratio of greater than 1 should be aimed for. If necessary, the dose of spironolactone may be increased by increments of 100 mg to a maximum of 400 mg daily. Dose escalation should be stopped if the serum sodium falls below 130 mmol/L or if the creatinine level rises to more than 130 micromol/L. Furosemide, at a starting dose of 40 mg a day, may be added to the regimen if the response to spironolactone alone is poor.

What non-pharmacological treatments are available if Mrs CN fails to respond to drug treatment?

A14 **Paracentesis, a Leveen Shunt or TIPS can be used to relieve ascites in patients who have diuretic-resistant ascites or tense ascites.**

A patient is usually termed 'diuretic resistant' if they have failed to respond to 400 mg of spironolactone a day plus 160 mg of furosemide. Diuretic-resistant ascites has a one-year mortality of 25–50%. Paracentesis (removal of ascites via a cannula inserted into the peritoneal cavity through the abdominal wall) may be indicated to remove ascites if the patient does not respond to diuretics. During paracentesis a large volume of ascites can be drained, and there is a risk of hypovolaemia, renal failure and encephalopathy. These complications can be largely overcome by simultaneously infusing albumin at the time of fluid removal. One bottle of 20% albumin is usually infused for every 1 L of ascites drained. If the volume of fluid removed is less than 5 L other colloidal solutions such as HAES-steril can be substituted instead of albumin. A Leveen Shunt is at least as effective as paracentesis in the control of refractory ascites, but due to the numerous complications associated with its use it is reserved for patients who are not eligible for transplantation or those who cannot have paracentesis because of surgical scars. TIPS is the only treatment which relieves portal pressure and it may be of benefit in selected patients.

What infection is Mrs CN suffering from and what treatment should be given?

A15 **Mrs CN is suffering from spontaneous bacterial peritonitis (SBP) which is diagnosed by an ascitic polymorphic nuclear count above 250/mm^3. A third-generation cephalosporin or agent with a similar spectrum of activity should be initiated. The antibiotic should be continued for a minimum of five days. Mrs CN should then be commenced on norfloxacin 400 mg daily as prophylaxis against further episodes of SBP.**

SBP is an infection of the ascites that occurs in the absence of any clear source of infection. Most cases (70%) of SBP are caused by normal gut flora. *Escherichia coli* accounts for almost half of these cases. Gram-positive bacteria account for 20% of cases and enterococci account for 5%. A third-generation cephalosporin or co-amoxiclav are effective treatments for SBP. They should be given for at least five days and on average a seven or eight day course is required for SBP resolution. Long-term prophylaxis with norfloxacin should be initiated as soon as possible after the antibiotics for the acute event have been completed.

How should Mrs CN's diuretic therapy be adjusted?

A16 **Mrs CN should stop her spironolactone until her serum sodium returns to above 130 mmol/L and her spironolactone should then be cautiously recommenced at a dose of 100 mg daily.**

Mrs CN's weight has dropped by 5 kg in two days, which exceeds the maximum recommended weight loss of 1 kg/day for patients who have ascites plus peripheral oedema. Over-diuresis has also resulted in her serum sodium falling below 130 mmol/L. Her spironolactone dose was increased too quickly from 100 to 300 mg on the first day. Dose increases should be in increments of 100 mg every few days with the patient's weight and electrolytes being carefully monitored.

What medication counselling points should be covered with Mrs CN before discharge?

A17   Mrs CN should be told the indication of each of her drugs, how to take them and any important side-effects. She should be told to use paracetamol for her back pain and to avoid NSAIDs.

(a)   Lactulose. This is a laxative that helps prevent encephalopathy. She needs to take it regularly at the prescribed dose as it has a delayed action of about 48 hours. The lactulose should be taken at a dose to produce two or three soft stools a day. Care needs to be taken to avoid diarrhoea as this can cause electrolyte disturbances and precipitate encephalopathy.

(b)   Spironolactone. This is a diuretic to reduce her ascites which she should take in the morning. If she develops gastrointestinal disturbances the daily dose can be divided.

(c)   Norfloxacin. This is an antibiotic to prevent reinfection of her ascites.

(d)   Colestyramine. This is an anion-exchange resin used to treat pruritus. To overcome the unpleasant taste it can be incorporated into various foods and drinks to make it more palatable (a handbook is available from the manufacturer). It can take up to seven days for the colestyramine to take its effect. It must be taken one hour before or four to six hours after her other tablets. As colestyramine can cause constipation, she must ensure she is taking the appropriate dose of lactulose to counteract this side-effect.

(e)   Propranolol. This is a beta-blocker given to prevent her from having another variceal bleed. Mrs CN should be warned that if she feels faint or dizzy whilst on this medication she should contact her doctor, as it may be a sign that the dose needs to be reduced.

(f)   Mucogel. Mucogel has been prescribed for her indigestion instead of Gaviscon. This preparation is better for her as it does not contain as much sodium. Gaviscon contains 3 mmol/5 mL and could worsen Mrs CN's ascites.

(g)   Mrs CN should be told not to take any NSAIDs for pain relief but to use paracetamol instead.

Acknowledgements

I would like to thank Mrs Gillian Cavell (Clinical Services Manager, King's College Hospital), Dr Rachael Harry (Specialist Registrar, Liver Unit,

King's College Hospital) and Helen Williams (Senior Clinical Pharmacist, King's College Hospital) for their assistance in preparing this chapter.

Further reading

Aldersley MA, O'Grady JG. Hepatic disorders – features and appropriate management. *Drugs* 1995; **49**: 84–89.

Bernard B, Nguyen KE, Opolon P *et al.* Antibiotic prophylaxis for the prevention of bacterial infections in cirrhotic patients with gastrointestinal bleeding: a meta-analysis. *Hepatology* 1999; **29**: 1665–1661.

Burroughs AK. Management of chronic liver disease. *Med Int* 1994; **22**: 485–494.

Cornish JW, O'Brien CP. Pharmacotherapies to prevent relapse: disulfiram, naltrexone and acamprosate. *Medicine* 1999; **27**: 26–28.

D'Amico G, Pagliaro L, Bosch J. The treatment of portal hypertension: a meta-analytic review. *Hepatology* 1995; **22**: 332–354.

Dillon JF, Simpson KJ, Hayes PC. Oesophageal variceal haemorrhage: a practical approach. *Br J Hosp Med* 1994; **52**: 348–352.

Finlayson NDC. Drugs and the liver. *Med Int* 1994; **22**: 455–460.

Garcia-Tsao G. Spontaneous bacterial peritonitis. *Gastroenterol Clin North Am* 1992; **21**: 257–275.

Harry R, Wendon J. Management of variceal bleeding. *Curr Opin Crit Care* 2002; **8**: 164–170.

Kennedy PTF, O'Grady J. Diseases of the liver – chronic liver disease. *Hosp Pharmacist* 2002; **9**: 137–144.

McCormack G, McCormick PA. A practical guide to the management of oesophageal varices. *Drugs* 1999; **57**: 327–335.

Mills PR. Clinical assessment of liver disease. *Med Int* 1994; **22**: 421–424.

Mowat C, Stanley A. Review article: spontaneous bacterial peritonitis-diagnosis, treatment and prevention. *Aliment Pharmacol Ther* 2001; **15**: 1851–1859.

Naik P, Lawton J. Pharmacological management of alcohol withdrawal. *Br J Hosp Med* 1993; **50**: 265–269.

Parks RW, Diamond T. Emergency and long-term management of bleeding oesophageal varices. *Br J Hosp Med* 1995; **54**: 161–168.

Sanchez-Fueyo A, Rhodes J. Ascites. *Medicine* 1999; **27**: 75–76.

Vale A. Alcohol withdrawal. *Medicine* 1999; **27**: 18–19.

Welch S, Strang J. Basic management of problem drinkers. *Medicine* 1999; **27**: 16–18.

Williams SGJ, Westaby D. Management of variceal haemorrhage. *Br Med J* 1994; **308**: 1213–1217.

11

Asthma

Helen Bates and Helen Thorp

Case study and questions

Day 1 Mr SN, a 24-year-old insurance salesman, was admitted at 11 a.m. via ambulance from his place of work. On admission he was severely short of breath, drowsy and unable to speak more than a couple of words at a time.

Mr SN had been complaining of flu-like symptoms and a hacking cough over the past few days. That morning he had started to complain of increasing difficulty in breathing. He had been seen to use his inhalers several times and then had suddenly collapsed at his desk. He had fallen off his chair and appeared to be having a fit. His limbs had jerked for about a minute, after which he lay unconscious until coming round in the ambulance. The paramedic had diagnosed an asthma attack and a fit of some sort, although with no lasting neurological deficit. He had administered a 2.5-mg dose of nebulised salbutamol via a nebuliser, with some improvement in shortness of breath, and also 35% oxygen via a face mask.

Mr SN was able to confirm that he had a past medical history of asthma and epilepsy.

On examination, Mr SN was tachypnoeic (respiratory rate of 28 breaths per minute) and tachycardic (140 beats per minute). His blood pressure was 150/95 mmHg with no paradoxus. On auscultation the chest was almost silent. His peak expiratory flow rate (PEFR) was unrecordable. Chest x-ray showed no areas of consolidation and excluded a diagnosis of pneumothorax. Arterial blood gases after 15 minutes of 35% oxygen in the ambulance were:

- pO_2 6.7 kPa (reference range 12.0–14.6)
- pCO_2 3.7 kPa (4.5–6.0)
- pH 7.47 (7.35–7.45)
- HCO_3 22 mmol/L (22–27)

Neurological observations were normal, as was his temperature (36.6°C). His white cell count was 6.5×10^9/L (4–10×10^9/L).

Mr SN was immediately given 60% oxygen via a high-flow mask and an intravenous sodium chloride 0.9% drip was started. He was moved to an acute medical ward and the following drugs were prescribed:

- Intravenous hydrocortisone 200 mg immediately, then 100 mg six-hourly
- Salbutamol 5 mg nebulised six times a day
- Ipratropium 500 micrograms nebulised six times a day   } with 6 L oxygen/min
- Intravenous cefotaxime 1 g three times a day
- Intravenous aminophylline 250 mg immediately followed by 1 g in 1 L normal saline to run over 24 hours

Q1 What important signs and symptoms of acute severe asthma does Mr SN exhibit?

Q2 Outline a pharmaceutical care plan for Mr SN.

Q3 Did the treatment received by Mr SN comply with current guidelines regarding the management of acute severe asthma?

Q4 Would you recommend any adjustments or alterations to Mr SN's prescribed therapy?

Q5 Which parameters would you want to monitor during the acute phase of Mr SN's asthma attack?

The patient's mother arrived on the ward and she was able to expand on Mr SN's past medical history and the events which had resulted in him being admitted into hospital.

The family had a history of atopy with Mr SN's father and his two brothers all having asthma. Following a motorbike accident at age 17 years he had developed generalised epilepsy, although this was well controlled with sodium valproate 500 mg three times daily and he had not had a fit for about five years. His mother said that Mr SN had been well up until the last few days when he had complained of feeling 'flu-y' and had suffered from a barking cough, especially during the night. He also sometimes found it difficult to catch his breath, especially after exercise. He had bought some cough medicine with no real effect and so had seen his GP who had prescribed a brown inhaler. She commented that Mr SN had been quite annoyed about this because he said he got no relief from it and so he had stopped using it.

Q6 Was it appropriate for Mr SN's GP to prescribe a beclometasone dipropionate (BDP) inhaler?

By 8 p.m. Mr SN was feeling better and was able to give a history. He could remember feeling very short of breath that morning, and using both his salbutamol and his new BDP inhaler several times with no effect. He said that he had been using his salbutamol inhaler at least 10 times a day in the last week or so. His GP had given him a BDP inhaler as well but Mr SN could not understand why because it did not seem to be helping at all, so he had left it in a drawer at work and had not bothered with it until this morning. His PEFR was now 140 L/min. Mr SN had never monitored his PEFR at home. Sodium valproate 500 mg three times daily was added to his prescription. His arterial blood gases were:

- pO_2 10.7 kPa (12.0–14.6)
- pCO_2 4.7 kPa (4.5–6.0)
- pH 7.44 (7.35–7.45)
- HCO_3 23 mmol/L (22–27)

Q7 Was Mr SN correct to administer several doses of his inhalers as his attack worsened?

Q8 What is a PEFR and what is its role in the management of an asthmatic patient?

Q9 Can a 'normal' PEFR be predicted for Mr SN?

Day 2   On the ward round a regular steroid inhaler was started. His pre-nebuliser PEFR was 120 L/min compared to 220 L/min 15 minutes after his 6 a.m. nebulised therapy. It was therefore decided to continue ipratropium and aminophylline for at least another 12 hours. Following continuous administration of 60% oxygen his arterial oxygen concentration was 13 kPa (12.0–14.6) so the oxygen prescription was changed to 'when required'. Mr SN was now on the following:

- Intravenous hydrocortisone 100 mg six-hourly
- Salbutamol 5 mg nebulised six times daily
- Ipratropium 500 micrograms nebulised six times daily } using a compressor
- Fluticasone metered-dose inhaler (MDI) 250 micrograms/puff, one puff twice daily
- Intravenous aminophylline 1 g over 24 hours
- Sodium valproate enteric-coated (EC) 500 mg three times daily
- 60% oxygen when required.

The theophylline level was 23 mg/L (10–20 mg/L).

Q10 What alterations would you recommend be made to Mr SN's therapy now?

Q11 How can the pharmacist contribute to optimising the administration of inhaled therapy?

Q12 Is there any advantage in using inhaled fluticasone over beclometasone or budesonide in Mr SN?

Q13 What key counselling points should be covered with Mr SN during his hospital stay?

Q14 Would there be any advantage in using a spacer with the inhaled steroid?

Later that afternoon the house officer rang to say that the intravenous aminophylline was being discontinued and he wanted to prescribe an equivalent oral dose.

Q15 What advice would you offer?

Day 3 Mr SN felt much better, almost back to his normal self. His PEFR was coming up but still showed quite a difference between pre- and post-nebuliser therapy (255 and 325 L/min, respectively). A neurology opinion concluded that Mr SN had had a fit as a result of the hypoxia he had experienced and that there was no lasting deficit. An out-patient follow-up was arranged as a precaution. His prescription remained unchanged. On the ward round, the senior house officer asked whether salmeterol therapy would benefit Mr SN.

Q16 What are the roles of long-acting beta$_2$-agonists (LABAs) and leukotriene antagonists in the treatment of asthma?

Q17 Would you recommend that either be prescribed for Mr SN?

Day 5 Mr SN's PEFR continued to improve and stabilised around 500 L/min. He felt completely back to normal and was eager to go home.

Q18 Is it appropriate that Mr SN be allowed home now?

Day 7 Mr SN was allowed to go home after being back on his inhaled bronchodilator for 48 hours. A self-management plan was discussed with him before he left. His discharge prescription was:

- Salbutamol MDI 100 micrograms/ puff, two puffs four times daily and when required
- Fluticasone MDI 250 micrograms/ puff, one puff twice daily via spacer
- Prednisolone 40 mg each morning for seven more days then stop
- Sodium valproate EC 500 mg three times daily
- Peak flow meter and chart

Q19 What are the key elements of a self-management plan for an asthma patient?

Q20 How would you counsel Mr SN on his discharge medication?

Q21 How should Mr SN's pharmaceutical care be continued over the next few months?

What important signs and symptoms of acute severe asthma does Mr SN exhibit?

A1 **Tachypnoea, tachycardia, an unrecordable peak expiratory flow rate (PEFR), a near silent chest and severe hypoxia despite 35% oxygen therapy.**

The British Thoracic Society (BTS) has published guidelines on the management of acute severe asthma which aim to alert doctors to the importance of recognizing the key features of the condition and to respond appropriately with optimum treatment. These guidelines are summarised in the latest *British National Formulary* (BNF).

Many, if not most, hospital admissions for acute severe asthma are preventable, as are most asthma deaths (currently around 1500 per annum in the UK). The severity of an attack is often underestimated by the patient, his relatives and/or his doctors, largely because of failure to make objective measurements. In many cases the patient will have been deteriorating over the preceding few days; this is typically seen as a reduction in PEFR measurement, an increase in diurnal variation of the PEFR (particularly morning 'dipping'), and an increase in symptoms such as shortness of breath and cough.

Mr SN exhibited several features of a severe life-threatening asthma attack. First, his PEFR was unrecordable. Patients often say they are too short of breath to perform a PEFR and then, when encouraged, produce a reasonable result. A PEFR should always be taken, even if it is unrecordable, as this is a valuable clinical indicator of attack severity. However, this should not delay urgent therapy. A silent chest indicates poor air entry into the lungs (as a result of bronchoconstriction) and is another feature of asthma of life-threatening severity. Despite 35% oxygen therapy, Mr SN was hypoxic on admission, although he had not progressed to retaining CO_2, which can result from exhaustion and failing respiratory effort; instead his pCO_2 was slightly low, denoting hyperventilation.

Outline a pharmaceutical care plan for Mr SN.

A2 **The pharmaceutical care plan for Mr SN should include the following:**

(a) Checking appropriate selection of drug therapy, as outlined in the current BTS guidelines.

(b)   Monitoring administration of each drug to ensure maximum bene-
       fit to Mr SN.
(c)   Advising on therapeutic drug monitoring for intravenous
       aminophylline.
(d)   Looking at outcome parameters, e.g. PEFR.
(e)   Giving consideration to maintenance therapy once he is over the
       acute attack.
(f)   Counselling on all aspects of his therapy.

> Did the treatment received by Mr SN comply with current guidelines
> regarding the management of acute severe asthma?

A3   **Yes.**

The current BTS guidelines give recommendations on the appropriate
prescriptions for acute severe asthma. Mr SN's therapy should be compared with them.

(a)   High concentration oxygen set at a high flow rate. Oxygen therapy
       does not aggravate carbon dioxide retention in acute severe asthma,
       thus 24% or 28% oxygen is inappropriate. Mr SN remained hypoxic
       despite 35% oxygen in the ambulance so it was vital that a higher
       percentage be administered on admission. The 60% oxygen started
       in casualty was appropriate.
(b)   Intravenous hydrocortisone. High doses of systemic steroids are
       essential in acute severe asthma in order to damp down the inflam-
       matory process occurring within the airways. This results in a
       reduction in the oedema and hypersecretion of mucus, which in
       turn helps to relieve bronchoconstriction. There is no real difference
       clinically between giving intravenous hydrocortisone (3–4 mg/kg or
       a standard 100–200 mg for an adult patient) and oral prednisolone
       (40–50 mg), but the intravenous route may be preferable at first as
       the patient may be so breathless that he has difficulty swallowing.
(c)   Nebulised bronchodilators. Salbutamol 5 mg or terbutaline 10 mg
       should be given immediately and repeated on a four to six-hourly
       basis. Mr SN is currently receiving 60% oxygen via a high-flow mask
       and ideally this should not be interrupted for the administration of
       the nebuliser. The nebulised fluid should consist of at least 2 mL
       solution, and ideally 4–5 mL as there is a 'dead' volume of approx-
       imately 1 mL which is retained in the nebuliser chamber. The
       driving gas in this instance should be oxygen at a flow rate of at
       least 6 L/min. This minimum flow rate is essential to obtain the

optimum droplet size in the aerosolised liquid. Under optimum conditions nebulisation will take about 10 minutes to complete. Ipratropium may be added to the beta$_2$-agonist if there are life-threatening features present. By blocking vagal tone, ipratropium produces bronchodilation via a different mechanism than a beta$_2$-agonist and the two agents together may produce an additive effect.

(d)   Intravenous aminophylline. The current BTS guidelines state that, in acute asthma, the use of intravenous aminophylline is not likely to result in any additional bronchodilation compared to standard care with inhaled bronchodilators and steroid tablets. They recommend use of intravenous aminophylline only after consultation with senior medical staff. Given that Mr SN showed clinical signs of life-threatening asthma, the decision was taken to use intravenous aminophylline. A loading dose may be given if a patient's condition is deteriorating, but otherwise the maintenance infusion can be started immediately. However, a loading dose should *only* be given if the patient does not already take an oral theophylline preparation: dangerous toxicity may result if a patient on regular oral therapy is given an inappropriate loading dose. The loading dose is usually 5 mg/kg given in a suitable volume over 20 minutes. This allows time for drug distribution into the extracellular space, and so avoids a transient dangerously high peak concentration. If the patient's weight is not known, then a standard dose of 250 mg (small patient) or 500 mg (large patient) is usually given. A 24-hour maintenance infusion should then follow. This is usually made up as a 1 mg/mL solution and infused at 0.5 mg/kg/h. If the weight is not known then a standard dose of 750 mg (small patient) or 1500 mg (large patient) is given over 24 hours. Therapeutic efficacy, and absence of toxicity, should be checked by monitoring Mr SN clinically and by checking his serum theophylline level. As he has received a loading dose he is effectively at steady state once loading is complete and levels may be measured within the first few hours of starting his maintenance infusion. Convulsions can occur with theophylline toxicity; this is especially important to monitor for in Mr SN, who is epileptic.

(e)   Intravenous magnesium. The current BTS guidelines state that a *single* dose of intravenous magnesium sulphate has been shown to be safe and effective in acute severe asthma and should be considered in life-threatening or near-fatal asthma. The dose is 1.2–2 g as an intravenous infusion over 20 minutes.

Would you recommend any adjustments or alterations to Mr SN's prescribed therapy?

A4 **Yes. The use of intravenous cefotaxime is inappropriate and should be challenged.**

The routine prescribing of an antibiotic is often the 'gut reaction' of a doctor faced with an acutely ill patient; however, this is only appropriate if the patient shows clear signs of having a chest infection. Mr SN is apyrexial, has a normal white cell count, and has no signs of consolidation on the chest x-ray. Furthermore, if he did show signs of chest infection, the most likely organisms would typically be 'community' in origin, i.e. *Streptococcus pneumoniae* or *Haemophilus influenzae*. First-line use of ampicillin, amoxicillin or erythromycin would be more appropriate if antibiotic therapy was required. (Note that erythromycin can interact with theophyllines to increase the latter's serum concentration.)

Which parameters would you want to monitor during the acute phase of Mr SN's asthma attack?

A5 (a) **PEFR before and after nebulised or inhaled beta$_2$-agonist therapy throughout his hospital stay.**

(b) **Arterial blood gases.**

(c) **Blood theophylline level, aiming for a concentration of 10–20 mg/L (55–110 micromols/L).**

(d) **Blood potassium level. Steroids, beta$_2$-agonists and aminophylline can all cause hypokalaemia.**

(e) **Blood glucose level. This may be elevated by corticosteroids in susceptible individuals.**

(f) **Pulse and respiratory rate.**

Was it appropriate for Mr SN's GP to prescribe a beclometasone inhaler?

A6 **Yes.**

Mr SN was starting to show signs of uncontrolled asthma with recent onset of night-time symptoms and worsening of daytime symptoms. Such patients are at significant risk of developing acute severe asthma. According to the BTS guidelines, Mr SN had previously been managed at Step 1, i.e. occasional use of relief bronchodilators. With the onset of this exacerbation of his symptoms, moving to Step 2 was the logical action for his GP to take. Step 2 is the addition of regular inhaled anti-inflammatory agents plus inhaled bronchodilators when required. The current guidelines recommend a starting dose of 400 micrograms daily of BDP (or equivalent) in adults. It is clear, however, that Mr SN was not counselled on his new therapy and had failed to understand that his asthma was deteriorating and that it was thus important to use his new inhaler regularly. His GP should perhaps also have initiated regular PEFR monitoring. In addition, a short course of oral steroids may have been valuable in preventing this acute episode.

Was Mr SN correct to administer several doses of his inhalers as his attack worsened?

A7   **Yes.**

The BTS guidelines (as summarised in the BNF) recommend that if a nebuliser is not available, then administration of two puffs of a beta$_2$-agonist inhaler 10–20 times via a spacer should be initiated in order to deliver a high dose. Use of repeated doses of a steroid inhaler in similar circumstances will not be helpful, as this will act too slowly to be of any benefit in the acute situation. However, it is clear that Mr SN did not recognize the severity of his condition and had not sought urgent medical attention. One of the elements of a self-management plan (see later) should address this issue.

What is a PEFR and what is its role in the management of an asthmatic patient?

A8   **The PEFR is the maximum flow rate which can be forced during an expiration. Changes in PEFR are an important indicator of an asthmatic patient's clinical status.**

It is important that the patient is encouraged to produce the maximal force of expiration that he can manage, otherwise inaccurate values may be recorded. PEFR monitoring can easily be undertaken by the patient at home using a PEFR meter (prescribable on FP10) and provides a useful self-assessment tool. Measurements should be undertaken twice a day, before inhaled therapy, and the results recorded on a chart (FP10 10) which can then be reviewed by the doctor. Patients should be taught to recognize signs of deteriorating asthma, namely a sustained reduction in PEFR value and/or a 25% or greater diurnal variation between morning and evening values, with the lower reading occurring characteristically in the morning (morning 'dipping'): such changes are often the first signs that a patient's asthma is becoming uncontrolled.

Can a 'normal' PEFR be predicted for Mr SN?

A9   **It is not possible to a predict a 'normal' PEFR for an asthmatic patient.**

The 'predicted normal' PEFR for a non-asthmatic person is related to height, age and sex, and can be obtained from various 'predicted normal' PEFR charts. However, an asthmatic patient of the same height, age and sex may have a best PEFR considerably lower than the values in the chart. It is thus important for asthmatic patients to establish their own record of monitoring so that comparisons to their own best recording can be made. In the interim, the 'predicted normal' PEFR can be used as a level to aim for.

What alterations would you recommend be made to Mr SN's therapy now?

A10   (a)   **Change his steroid therapy from the intravenous to the oral route.**

(b)   **Adjust the dose of intravenous aminophylline to bring it into the therapeutic range and thus avoid the development of symptoms of toxicity.**

Mr SN is now much improved after 24 hours in hospital. He no longer needs to be given intravenous steroids and should be converted to a once-daily dose of prednisolone (40–50 mg) in the morning; in fact, this change could have taken place the previous evening.

Mr SN's plasma theophylline level is slightly high, although he is not showing any symptoms of theophylline toxicity. It is possible to calculate a dose to bring the theophylline level into the therapeutic range using the formula:

$$\frac{S \times F \times \text{dose}}{T} = C_{\text{pss av.}} \times Cl$$

where S = salt factor (0.79 for aminophylline), dose = dose (in mg), F = bioavailability factor, T = dosage interval (in hours), $C_{\text{pss av.}}$ = average plasma concentration at steady state and Cl = clearance.

In this case *F* is a constant (with a value of 1) because the drug is being given intravenously, therefore:

$$\frac{0.79 \times 1 \times 1000 \text{ mg}}{24} = 23 \text{ mg/L} \times Cl$$

thus *Cl* = 1.43 L/h (for this patient).

To give an average theophylline concentration of 15 mg/L then:

$$\frac{0.79 \times 1 \times \text{dose}}{24} = 15 \times 1.43$$

thus dose = 652 mg/24 h. This could be rounded down to 650 mg for ease of administration.

The need for continued nebulised ipratropium and intravenous aminophylline should also be reviewed as these two drugs can often be discontinued once the patient has recovered significantly from the acute event.

How can the pharmacist contribute to optimising the administration of inhaled therapy?

A11 **The pharmacist can have a key role in the selection of the most appropriate inhaler device for each individual patient and in counselling on its correct use.**

If a patient is to get maximum benefit from therapy, it is crucial that he understands, and is competent to use, his particular device. Inhaler counselling requires patience and tact. The BTS guidelines comment that in adults an MDI with or without a spacer is as effective as any other hand held inhaler and so it is standard practice to try an MDI first. Some patients have great difficulty coordinating their inhalation with the triggering of the MDI. As such, use of a spacer device will not only get round this difficulty but also improves lung deposition of the drug by up to 100% compared to an MDI alone. Spacers are especially suitable for inhaled steroids as these tend to be given twice daily and so the spacer can be kept at home. However, for 'when required' bronchodilators, using a spacer may prove both cumbersome and also make the patient feel conspicuous. This can be a particular problem in adolescent patients. Thus a range of breath-activated devices can be demonstrated to the patient and the choice tailored individually. The Further reading section at the end of this chapter includes references which contain detailed information on the use and selection of inhaler devices, and it is essential that the pharmacist is familiar with all the devices available.

Is there any advantage in using inhaled fluticasone over beclometasone or budesonide in Mr SN?

A12 **To date, no significant clinical advantages of fluticasone over conventional inhaled steroids have been demonstrated. The choice of inhaled steroid needs to be made on an individual patient basis, taking into consideration the risk-benefit ratio and choice of inhaler device.**

Fluticasone propionate (FP) is a synthetic trifluorinated glucocorticoid licensed for the prophylactic management of all grades of asthma. It is promoted as being more potent than the conventional inhaled steroids BDP and budesonide, with a lower risk of systemic side-effects.

In animal models of inflammation, FP has been shown to be twice as potent an anti-inflammatory agent as BDP, and probably budesonide, on a weight-for-weight basis. As such, most of the available studies have compared an FP dose which is half the amount of BDP. Over study periods ranging from four weeks to one year, FP and BDP (at equipotent doses) have been shown to be, on the whole, equivalent in terms of efficacy [improvements in PEFR, forced expiratory volume in one second (FEV_1), forced vital capacity (FVC), symptom scores and rescue medication] and tolerability. In moderate to severe asthma in adults over a period of a year, both drugs improved lung function; however, FP showed a statistically significant increase in improvement in PEFR in the first three months. Furthermore, 2% of patients taking FP compared with 10% of those on BDP experienced a severe exacerbation during the study. There was no significant difference between the two treatments in terms of other variables such as, for example, symptom-free days or nights, and use of rescue medication. Large meta-analyses suggest that equipotent doses of inhaled steroids show, on the whole, no significant differences in terms of a variety of subjective and objective measurements of asthma severity.

There is increasing concern that the wider use of long-term inhaled steroids in both adults and children may result in typical steroid side-effects such as skin and bone thinning, and growth retardation in children. These systemic side-effects are thought to result from the absorption of active drug from the gut and lower respiratory tract. Up to 90% of any inhaled drug is swallowed and thus available for absorption. FP undergoes almost complete first-pass hepatic metabolism and so oral bioavailability is negligible. Lung absorption is thought to be the main source of its systemic activity, therefore increasing lung deposition (i.e. with an increased dose) can increase systemic activity.

There is little evidence that inhaled steroids in conventional doses cause major systemic steroid side-effects; however, adrenal suppression has been shown to occur at doses above 1.5 mg/day of BDP and budesonide, and 0.75 mg/day of FP. The Committee on Safety of Medicines (CSM) has raised concerns that very high doses of FP may lead to a higher risk of systemic adverse effects. They advise that doses greater than 1 mg/day of FP should be prescribed only in patients with severe asthma. In children, slow lower-leg growth rates have been demonstrated in some small-scale studies, but it is still not clear how this translates into adulthood. Asthmatic children tend to have a slower pre-pubertal growth velocity and later onset of puberty, regardless of steroid treatment. Adult studies have looked at reduction in bone mineral density in patients on inhaled steroids but there have been conflicting conclusions. There are many variables that can complicate studies, e.g. previous exposure to oral steroids, age, smoking status and activity levels.

Recent studies have shown that the dose–response curve is relatively flat for all the inhaled steroids. As such, increasing the dose may not significantly improve asthma symptoms but may increase the risk of systemic side-effects. For example, one recent study showed that in patients with mild-to-moderate asthma, similar symptom control was achieved with 200 micrograms/day FP and 500 micrograms/day.

In summary, BDP and budesonide have a proven track record in the management of asthma and most asthmatic patients can be adequately controlled with a conventional dose of one or the other, titrated to response. Treatment appears to be safe even when continued in the long-term and for these patients FP probably offers no advantages. The use of high-dose inhaled steroids in chronic asthma is currently controversial because they may increase the risk of systemic adverse effects. Where higher doses are used initially, they should be reviewed regularly, every one to three months, and reduced gradually once good control is achieved to the minimum effective dose.

The consultant's rationale for the use of FP in Mr SN was that he had previously failed on BDP therapy. However, proper compliance with one of the conventional steroids would probably have achieved as good a response as with FP.

What key counselling points should be covered with Mr SN during his hospital stay?

A13 **It is essential to ensure that Mr SN is counselled as follows:**

(a) **To understand and recognise the condition of asthma, including how and why the symptoms arise.**

(b) **To identify and avoid any personal trigger factors.**

(c) **On the difference between various asthma treatments, specifically the concept of 'preventers' and 'relievers'.**

(d) **For each agent prescribed: how it works, the rationale behind its prescription, the dose, frequency and any adverse effects commonly associated with its use. The importance of compliance with regular 'preventer' therapy should be emphasised.**

(e) **How to recognise the warning signs of worsening asthma and how to manage them in the context of a self-management plan.**

(f) **How to use a peak flow meter and record the values obtained, and why this is important.**

All counselling should be tailored to a level to suit the individual patient.

There are many reasons why patients may be non-compliant, quite apart from the problem of an individual using an inappropriate technique for the inhalation of drugs. Increasing both the patients' and their relatives' understanding of asthma and of the drugs prescribed gives most individuals the confidence to cope extremely well with the disease.

Mr SN needs to be provided with a lot of information and this cannot all be done in one session. Helpful written information, e.g. the National Asthma Campaign booklets, are widely available and the pharmacist should use this in collaboration with other health care professionals' counselling time to reinforce some of the often complex information provided to the patient.

Would there be any advantage in using a spacer with the inhaled steroid?

A14 **Yes. Although the side-effects associated with inhaled steroids are much less of a concern than with oral steroids, the use of a spacer may help avoid such effects.**

Asthma is a chronic inflammatory condition and anti-inflammatory treatment is required by most patients. Steroids reduce airway inflammation and hyperactivity and inhaled steroids are the mainstay in the prevention of further acute episodes in patients such as Mr SN. At the time of writing, the BTS guidelines introduce standard dose (400 micrograms BDP daily or equivalent) anti-inflammatory agents at Step 2 of asthma management.

As discussed earlier, the incidence of systemic effects with inhaled steroids is rare, and appears to be related to total daily dose. Suppression of the hypothalamic–pituitary axis is extremely unusual in adults receiving less than 1500 micrograms/day of inhaled BDP/budesonide, or 750 micrograms/day FP; however, the use of a spacer device does reduce oropharyngeal impaction and the subsequent swallowing of steroid, thereby in theory reducing the risk of systemic side-effects in the long-term. It will also reduce local side-effects associated with inhaled steroids, such as oral candidiasis, sore throat and hoarse voice, which are related to the amount of steroid deposited in the mouth and the frequency of exposure. Mouth rinsing after the use of a steroid inhaler may also further reduce these side-effects.

Although the devices are bulky, twice daily dosing is now common practice, so the devices do not have to be carried around with the patient. Once they appreciate the advantages, most patients can be persuaded to accommodate the device into a 'toothbrushing' routine.

What advice would you offer?

A15 **There is no indication to convert Mr SN to oral theophylline at this stage.**

Oral theophylline should initially be considered in patients who need to move up to Step 3–4 of the BTS guidelines to control their asthma, i.e. when inhaled steroid has failed to produce adequate control. This commonly occurs when night-time symptoms are disproportionately prominent despite otherwise good control. Although a sustained-release theophylline is one option at this stage, current evidence supports the use of an inhaled LABA as the first-line choice (see Answer 16).

The house officer should be advised to reduce the aminophylline infusion rate slowly over the next few hours.

What are the roles of LABAs and leukotriene antagonists in the treatment of asthma?

A16 **LABAs (salmeterol/formoterol) are synthetic, sympatho-mimetic amines. They are structurally and pharmacologically similar to the short-acting beta$_2$-agonist salbutamol and are**

licensed for the treatment of reversible airway obstruction in patients requiring long-term regular bronchodilator therapy. Leukotriene antagonists (montelukast/zafirlukast) selectively block the action of leukotrienes on the respiratory tract, resulting in both an anti-inflammatory and a bronchodilator action. Evidence supports their use as potential add-on agents in asthma uncontrolled by inhaled steroids and LABAs.

LABAs have a prolonged duration of action of 12 hours compared with four to six hours for salbutamol. They are not a replacement for inhaled steroids, nor for sodium cromoglicate in children. Neither should they be used for the relief of acute attacks. An important counselling point to discuss with patients receiving LABAs is the differences between them and salbutamol; it is vital that all patients know they should use a short-acting beta$_2$-agonist for the relief of acute symptoms.

Several randomised controlled trials have compared the addition of salmeterol to standard-dose inhaled steroid versus a high-dose inhaled steroid alone. These have shown that a combination of salmeterol and standard-dose inhaled steroid is more effective in terms of a variety of measurements of asthma control, including objective measures of lung function, symptom scores and use of short-acting beta$_2$-agonists for symptom relief. As such, the current BTS guidelines recommend that a LABA be added at Step 3, leaving the inhaled steroid dose unchanged in the first instance.

Leukotriene antagonists are more effective than placebo but current evidence does not support their use in place of inhaled steroids. Small benefits have been seen when leukotriene antagonists are added to an inhaled steroid regimen. In a small study in aspirin-allergic asthmatics, improvements in pulmonary function and symptoms were observed when montelukast was added to inhaled steroids. Cysteinyl leukotrienes are particularly important mediators in aspirin-sensitive asthmatics and leukotriene antagonists may therefore have a role in such patients. Use of a leukotriene antagonist is one option for add-on therapy at Step 4 of the current guidelines.

Would you recommend that either be prescribed for Mr SN?

A17   No.

Mr SN requires an initial treatment period with inhaled steroids (Step 2 BTS guidelines). Only if Mr SN's symptoms are uncontrolled (e.g. if he suffers from frequent exacerbations, requires excessive relieving broncho-dilators, is limited in activity or develops nocturnal symptoms) should treatment be stepped up to achieve better control. The next stage, Step 3, is to add a LABA to standard-dose inhaled steroids (see Answer 16). There is little evidence to support the addition of a leukotriene antagonist at this stage especially as Mr SN does not report any aspirin allergy which may favour their inclusion. At every stage it is necessary to check that the patient still uses the chosen inhaler device effectively and that lifestyle changes have not occurred which may need to be accommodated.

Whenever a new therapeutic agent is added to a patient's regimen it is important that its benefits are assessed over a suitable period of time, preferably by using PEFR records and symptom diaries. Additional treatments should only be continued if they provide objective or significant subjective improvement. If these cannot be demonstrated, the agent should be withdrawn and an alternative choice then assessed. Poly-pharmacy should be avoided wherever possible.

Is it appropriate that Mr SN be allowed home now?

A18 **No. Patients should not usually be discharged from hospital until their symptoms have cleared and lung function has stabilised or returned to its normal or best level.**

A guide to this stage is when the peak expiratory flow is above 75% of the predicted or best value, diurnal variability is below 25% and there are no nocturnal symptoms. Patients should also have been using inhaled therapy in place of nebulised drugs for at least 24 hours before discharge.

Mr SN is obviously feeling better and it would be appropriate, from his monitored parameters, to discuss changing him back to standard inhaler devices at this time.

What are the key elements of a self-management plan for an asthmatic patient?

A19 **There are three key elements to a self-management plan:**
   (a)   Monitoring of symptoms, PEFR and drug usage, *leading to*
   (b)   The taking of prearranged action by the patient, *according to*
   (c)   Written guidance.

A self-management plan should be initiated prior to discharge, then developed and confirmed over the weeks following discharge. The plan should be carefully individualised for, and discussed with, the patient. The key points to be included are when to initiate or increase inhaled steroids, when to self-administer steroid tablets (when the peak flow falls below the level previously agreed for that individual) and to seek urgent medical attention when treatment is not working.

The exact level for action in an individual patient must be revised in the light of experience and records of peak flow monitoring.

How would you counsel Mr SN on his discharge medication?

A20 **Mr SN should by now have received extensive counselling from the members of the multidisciplinary team caring for him in the hospital, the pharmacist being one such contributor (see Answer 13). There are, however, some specific points related to his medication that should be discussed at discharge.**

(a)   It should be emphasised that Mr SN is being asked to use his reliever (salbutamol) regularly four times a day and also when required for an initial short period of time following discharge. However, this regular use of his reliever may be reviewed after a suitable period. If Mr SN responds well to the steroid inhaler, he may only need to use his reliever intermittently and prophylactically, e.g. before exercise.

(b)   It should be explained that the spacer used with his FP (preventer) may be used with the salbutamol reliever during an acute exacerbation. Patients often feel more confident knowing that they can use the spacer to deliver one to two puffs up to 10–20 times if symptoms warrant it. This advice must be given in conjunction with Mr SN's self-management plan and he must be clear at which point he needs to seek further assistance. Use of a high-dose reliever is not a substitute for seeking urgent medical attention.

(c)   The need to complete the course of oral steroids. Patients such as Mr SN should be discharged taking prednisolone for a minimum of a week. This should be explained in light of the co-prescription of inhaled steroids. Any worries regarding the safety or adverse effects from short courses of oral steroids should be addressed. A reserve course of oral steroids may be incorporated into Mr SN's self-management plan.

(d)   Sodium valproate EC is being continued in order to control Mr SN's epilepsy. The tablets should be swallowed whole and not chewed.

How should Mr SN's pharmaceutical care be continued over the next few months?

A21 **By ensuring good communication between secondary and primary health carers, continual assessment of his condition, and by reinforcing counselling as necessary.**

Good communication with Mr SN's GP is essential. Information supplied to his GP should include PEFRs on admission and discharge, details of treatment to be continued at home, and a copy of any self-management plan discussed in the hospital. All patients should be followed up in a hospital clinic within one month of discharge, in addition to earlier follow-up by the GP.

Community and hospital out-patient pharmacists are in an ideal position to offer reinforcement of counselling to patients such as Mr SN when they return for repeat inhaler prescriptions.

Mr SN is currently being managed according to Step 2 of the BTS guidelines but continual assessment of his asthma control is essential, not only to ensure stepping up of treatment when necessary, but also to review stepping down when possible. The BTS guidelines emphasise the importance of considering stepping down treatment in well-controlled patients. They comment that this is often not implemented, leaving some patients over-treated. In particular, patients should be maintained on the lowest possible dose of inhaled steroid – reduction should be considered every three months, decreasing the dose by approximately 25–50% each time.

Acknowledgements

The authors gratefully acknowledge the British Thoracic Society for their kind permission to reproduce various elements of the current guidelines in this chapter.

Further reading

Anon. Chlorofluorocarbon-free metered-dose inhalers: update. *WeMeReC Bull* 2001; **8**(4): 1–2.
Anon. Chronic asthma. *MeReC Bull* 2002; **18**: 1–5.
Anon. Drugs used in the treatment of diseases of the respiratory system. In: *British National Formulary*, current edn. British Medical Association/ Royal Pharmaceutical Society of Great Britain, London.
Anon. Inhaler devices for asthma. *Drug Ther Bull* 2000; **38**(2): 9–14.

Anon. Leukotriene antagonists: new drugs for asthma. *MeReC Bull* 1999; **10**(1): 1–4.

Anon. Reminder: fluticasone propionate (Flixotide): use of high doses (>500 micrograms/twice daily). *Curr Prob Pharmacovigilance* 2001; **27**: 10.

Anon. The use of inhaled corticosteroids in adults with asthma. *Drug Ther Bull* 2000; **38**(1): 5–8.

Anon. The use of inhaled corticosteroids in childhood asthma. *Drug Ther Bull* 1999; **37**(10): 73–77.

Barnes J. Scientific rationale for inhaled combination therapy with long-acting beta$_2$-agonists and corticosteroids. *Eur Respir J* 2002; **19**: 182–191.

British Guideline on the Management of Asthma. *Thorax* 2003; **58**(suppl. 1): i1–i94.

Charlton I, Charlton G, Broomfield J *et al*. Evaluation of peak flow and symptoms only self-management plans for control of asthma. *Br Med J* 1990; **301**: 1355–1359.

Gibbs KP, Portlock JC. Asthma. In: *Clinical Pharmacy and Therapeutics*, 2nd edn. R Walker, C. Edwards, eds. Churchill Livingstone, Edinburgh, 1999: 347–368.

Royal Pharmaceutical Society of Great Britain Respiratory Disease Task Force. *Practice Guidance on the Care of People with Asthma and COPD. Appendix 5 – Inhaler Technique and Choice of Device*. Royal Pharmaceutical Society of Great Britain, London, 2000: 48–54.

Various authors. Respiratory disorders. *Medicine* 1999; **27**(8–11): 1–178.

12

Chronic obstructive pulmonary disease

Peter Bramley and Susan Brammer

Day 1 Sixty-five-year-old Mr LT was admitted to a medical ward via casualty. He had suffered increasing dyspnoea and wheeze over the past five days. He had a cough productive of yellow sputum and swelling of the ankles. His wife said he had become too breathless to speak or eat and today had been delirious. He could not walk further than from the chair to the toilet.

His current drug therapy was:

- Co-amilofruse 5/40 three tablets once daily
- Beclometasone dipropionate 100-microgram metered-dose inhaler (MDI), two puffs twice daily
- Salbutamol respirator solution, one 2.5 mg nebule up to four times a day when required
- Simple Linctus, 5 mL when required

Mr LT's wife admitted that her husband had not used his beclometasone inhaler for some months because 'it did not help'. He was using bottled oxygen from two to four hours every day, whereas he used to use it only 'in an emergency'.

Mr LT had been a heavy smoker, but had stopped completely two years earlier. He lived with his wife in a bungalow and had retired from his job as a factory storekeeper at the age of 60.

On examination he was centrally cyanosed. His chest was initially silent, but after one dose of salbutamol 2.5 mg by nebulisation coarse crackles could be heard at the right base. He was diagnosed as having a right basal pneumonia with deterioration of his obstructive airways disease. An arterial blood sample was sent for analysis of blood gases, with the patient breathing 35% oxygen by face mask.

Mr LT's blood gas results were:

- Blood pH 7.16 (reference range 7.32–7.42)
- PaCO$_2$ 11.21 kPa (4.5–6.1)
- PaO$_2$ 10.23 kPa (12–15)
- Standard bicarbonate 29.2 mmol/L (21–25)

In view of Mr LT's serious condition non-invasive ventilation (NIV) was thought to be appropriate. This was started on the ward. Unfortunately he did not tolerate the face mask and so was transferred to the intensive care unit for mechanical ventilatory support. He was sedated (propofol 120 mg by intravenous bolus) and given a muscle relaxant (atracurium 40 mg by intravenous bolus) to enable tracheal intubation and commencement of intermittent positive pressure ventilation (IPPV). For maintenance sedation, propofol (variable dose continuous intravenous infusion of 0.3–4.0 mg/kg/h) was written up, supplemented by the opiate alfentanil (variable dose continuous intravenous infusion 1–5 mg/h). A central venous catheter was inserted via the right subclavian approach. An arterial catheter was inserted into the left radial artery for arterial blood gas sampling. Mr LT also underwent urinary catheterisation.

Mr LT was thought to be fluid-depleted and was prescribed 1 unit of polygeline intravenous infusion to be given over 30 minutes, followed by 2 L of glucose/saline infusion, each litre to be given over eight hours.

The following drug therapy was written up:

- Aminophylline 500 mg in 500 mL 5% glucose infusion twice daily, each dose to be given by continuous intravenous infusion over 12 hours
- Salbutamol 2.5 mg every four hours via a nebuliser
- Ipratropium bromide 500 micrograms every four hours via a nebuliser
- Hydrocortisone 100 mg intravenously every six hours
- Ceftriaxone 2 g intravenously once daily

Serum biochemistry and haematology results were:

- Sodium 141 mmol/L (137–150)
- Potassium 5.2 mmol/L (3.5–5.0)
- Urea 5.4 mmol/L (2.5–6.6)
- Haemoglobin 17.7 g/dL (14–18)
- Haematocrit 0.57 (0.36–0.46)
- White blood cells (WBC) 18.1 × 10^9/L (4–11 × 10^9)

Q1 What do Mr LT's history, symptoms and blood gases indicate about his respiratory disease?

Q2 What are the immediate therapeutic priorities for Mr LT?

Q3 Outline the key elements of a pharmaceutical care plan for Mr LT.

Q4 Has the most appropriate sedative therapy been chosen for Mr LT? How is the dose of propofol titrated?

Q5   Do you agree with the choice of agents to treat Mr LT's respiratory condition? Comment on the doses prescribed.

Q6   What would you tell a nurse who had never administered salbutamol or ipratropium by nebuliser before?

Q7   What are the likely explanations for Mr LT's abnormal haematology and serum biochemistry results?

Day 2 Very few rhonchi could be heard on examination of Mr LT's respiratory system, and his blood gases were satisfactory. Urinary output was good (75–100 mL/h) and a positive fluid balance had been achieved overnight. A repeat chest x-ray still showed some increased shadowing at the right base. The patient was noted to be shaking, and in response to this observation it was suggested on the ward round that the salbutamol dose should be reduced to 2.5 mg by nebuliser every six hours.

Q8   Could Mr LT's drug therapy be causing his tremor?

Q9   Is the suggested change in treatment appropriate? If not, what recommendations would you make?

Mr LT's salbutamol dosage was reduced as suggested. Aminophylline was continued by the intravenous route and the infusion rate unchanged.

It was decided to raise Mr LT's level of consciousness by gradually decreasing the rate of propofol infusion. The dose of hydrocortisone was reduced to 100 mg four times daily.

Day 3 Only scattered rhonchi could now be heard in both lungs. Bowel sounds were present, and so nasogastric feeding was started. Mr LT was apyrexial, conscious and alert.

Day 4 Mr LT was improving rapidly and the ventilation mode was changed to synchronised intermittent mandatory ventilation (SIMV) with a reduced mandatory rate to accelerate weaning. The propofol infusion was stopped at 9 a.m. and Mr LT was extubated at 12 noon. His serum theophylline concentration was reported to the ward as 15.8 mg/L (10–20). His intravenous aminophylline therapy was stopped and oral aminophylline liquid at a dose of 500 mg twice daily was prescribed.

Q10 How does reducing the mandatory mechanical ventilation rate help the weaning process?

Q11 Can drug therapy be helpful in the weaning process?

Q12 What action would you take after noting Mr LT's theophylline level and the change in prescribed aminophylline therapy?

Day 5   Mr LT's condition continued to improve, with no breathlessness or wheezing, minimal coughing and sputum production, and no cyanosis. Oxygen 28% was continuously administered through a face mask. Regular peak flow measurements were recorded, before and after bronchodilators, at 6 a.m., 2 p.m. and 6 p.m.

Day 6   Mr LT was transferred to a general medical ward. It was noted that he still had some tremor, mild pitting oedema bilaterally and some evidence of right ventricular strain on the ECG. He had a good urine output and was managing well without a catheter. His peak expiratory flow rate was 100 L/min before nebulised salbutamol and 120 L/min 10 minutes after the 6 a.m. dose. He was changed from intravenous hydrocortisone to oral prednisolone at a dose of 30 mg once daily.

Day 7   Mr LT was changed from intravenous ceftriaxone to oral cefaclor 500 mg every eight hours.

Day 8   Theophylline 400 mg slow-release tablets, one twice daily was written up: the theophylline level was to be measured in a few days.

Day 11   Since a degree of cor pulmonale was present, with ankle oedema and ECG abnormalities (large P waves and right axis deviation), Mr LT was restarted on co-amilofruse 5/40 at a dose of one tablet each morning.

Q13 Is this treatment appropriate for Mr LT's cor pulmonale? What alternative therapies could be prescribed?

Day 12   A pre-dose serum theophylline level was reported as 19.6 mg/L (10–20). Mr LT was noted to have a significant tremor.

Q14 Would you recommend any change in his theophylline dosage?

Day 14   Mr LT's respiratory condition was greatly improved and his ankle swelling had diminished significantly on co-amilofruse 5/40. He was discharged on the following medication:

- Co-amilofruse 5/40, one in the morning
- Prednisolone 10 mg once daily, reducing to nil over one week
- Theophylline 300 mg slow-release tablets one twice daily
- Salbutamol 2.5 mg four times daily via a nebuliser
- Ipratropium 500 micrograms four times daily via a nebuliser

He was given an out-patient appointment in six weeks.

Q15 Would there be any advantage in continuing Mr LT's oral steroid therapy long-term? Would inhaled steroid therapy be more appropriate?
Q16 What changes might be made to his bronchodilator therapy?
Q17 What points would you discuss with Mr LT when counselling him on his take-home medication?

Day 56   Mr LT attended the out-patient department. He was reasonably well, able to walk around the house, dress and wash himself. He was still short of breath on exertion, with some ankle oedema and a few rhonchi at both bases. He was warned he might need antibiotics should he get another chest infection. He was written up for beclometasone dipropionate 250 micrograms by metered-dose inhaler, two puffs twice daily, and shown how to use a peak flow meter. He was told to use the peak flow meter daily until his follow-up appointment in two weeks.

Q18 Would you recommend that Mr LT receive continuous antibiotic prophylaxis? If so, which agents would you recommend and at what dose?

Day 70   Mr LT's peak flow readings had improved since the last appointment, but he was now suffering from oral thrush. He was prescribed amphotericin, one lozenge five times daily for two weeks.

Q19 What measures would you suggest to reduce the risk of Mr LT suffering from oral thrush again?

What do Mr LT's history, symptoms and blood gases indicate about his respiratory disease?

A1 **Mr LT's rapidly increasing dyspnoea and general disability over the past few days suggest that his respiratory condition has deteriorated because of an acute event. His productive cough and discoloured sputum make a chest infection the most likely cause. His increasing use of oxygen, together with his symptoms of cyanosis, show that his lungs are failing to provide efficient gaseous exchange and that he is in respiratory failure.**

This can be confirmed by the blood gas results. Mr LT was given 35% oxygen on admission, before the first blood gases were measured. Usually a lower oxygen concentration (24%) is commenced, in order to avoid inhibiting the hypoxic ventilatory drive often present in chronic obstructive pulmonary disease (COPD) patients. The high oxygen concentration administered to Mr LT initially may have contributed to Mr LT's carbon dioxide retention. There is little point raising the PaO_2 above 8–9 kPa, as the increase in oxygen saturation achieved will not be worthwhile (from about 90 to 95%) when balanced against the risk of raising the $PaCO_2$.

Mr LT's $PaCO_2$ is markedly raised, which means that he has Type 2 (ventilatory) failure, where alveolar ventilation is insufficient to prevent a rise in $PaCO_2$. This is in contrast to Type 1 (oxygenation) failure, where the PaO_2 falls below 8 kPa, but a rise in $PaCO_2$ is counteracted by increased respiratory muscle drive. This relatively poor response to hypoxia puts Mr LT in the 'blue bloater' category of COPD patients. It should, however, be noted that he has emphysematous changes. The classical association of emphysema solely with the 'pink puffer' category of COPD patient is now known to be incorrect.

Accumulation of carbon dioxide leads to respiratory acidosis with a low blood pH. When this becomes a chronic condition, as in Mr LT's case, the kidneys compensate by excreting more hydrogen ions into the urine at the expense of potassium ions and returning more bicarbonate ions to the circulation, thus causing a rise in plasma bicarbonate.

What are the immediate therapeutic priorities for Mr LT?

A2 **The immediate therapeutic aims are:**

(a) Correction of acute respiratory failure.

(b) Treatment of infection.

Outline the key elements of a pharmaceutical care plan for Mr LT.

A3 **The pharmaceutical care plan for Mr LT should include the following:**

(a) Advise medical staff on:

  (i) Choice of antibiotics and formulary restrictions.
  (ii) Dosage regimens of bronchodilators.
  (iii) Therapeutic drug monitoring of aminophylline/theophylline.
  (iv) Treatment options for cor pulmonale.

(b) Advise nursing staff on:

  (i) Administration of intravenous antibiotics.
  (ii) Administration of nebulised bronchodilators.

(c) Monitor Mr LT's therapy for efficacy and toxicity of antibiotics, bronchodilators and diuretics.
(d) Monitor theophylline serum concentration measurements.
(e) Review therapy prescribed for his acute condition, assessing the suitability of each drug for long-term maintenance therapy.
(f) Assess the suitability of the patient's own drugs (PODs) belonging to Mr LT for use in hospital, and remove those no longer appropriate, after discussion with the patient or his relatives.
(g) Counsel Mr LT on the use of his medication with particular emphasis on his inhaled therapy.
(h) Ensure that the PODs are still current and suitably labelled before discharge, and check that any medicines at home are still appropriate for his use.
(i) Consider issuing a Patient Medication Record to the patient, his carer, his GP and/or a community pharmacist of his choice.
(j) Consider non-drug factors which may be important, e.g. if he is still smoking, would referral to a smoking cessation clinic be appropriate?
(k) Consider whether the patient is suitable for long-term oxygen therapy.
(l) Consider referral to a local Pulmonary Rehabilitation Programme.

Has the most appropriate sedative therapy been chosen for Mr LT? How is the dose of propofol titrated?

A4 **Mr LT's sedative therapy is appropriate, but vecuronium may have been a more appropriate muscle relaxant for him. The dose of propofol should be titrated according to his response.**

The sedatives chosen for Mr LT were the most appropriate at the time of writing. Propofol was used for both intubation and maintenance in this case. Propofol is a short-acting anaesthetic agent which is now licensed for sedation during intensive care for periods of up to three days. It causes appreciable respiratory depression at sedative doses, but is associated with significantly less accumulation than the other agents available, and so rapid recovery occurs. This results in a shorter weaning time. The drug is highly lipophilic and is distributed rapidly from the blood into the tissues (half-life 30 minutes). A slow terminal elimination half-life of five hours is thought to result from the slow return of propofol from poorly perfused tissue, but this third phase of elimination does not appear to affect recovery time.

A short-acting water-soluble benzodiazepine such as midazolam would have been a suitable alternative sedative for intubation. This drug also causes significant respiratory depression, but this is not an important consideration for Mr LT, as the decision to ventilate him mechanically has already been made. Benzodiazepines also produce amnesia of the intubation procedure. As a single dose, it is doubtful whether midazolam has any advantage over diazepam; however, in a situation such as Mr LT's, repeat doses can be required, and multiple doses of diazepam would be associated with a higher risk of drug accumulation and prolonged action.

When intubation has been accomplished the choice of sedative depends on the condition of the patient. In Mr LT a combination of propofol and the short-acting opiate alfentanil was used for maintenance as it was anticipated that he would only be ventilated for a short time. An alternative regimen for longer-term ventilation would be midazolam with morphine or fentanyl. This would be an effective and less expensive regimen, but could result in a longer weaning time in the case of morphine due to increased accumulation, particularly in older patients.

The maintenance dose of propofol usually required for continuous sedation is 0.3–4.0 mg/kg/h. The dose should be titrated according to Mr LT's response. He should be calm but easily rousable (sedation scoring systems are available). The initial rate is set according to age and weight, and then adjusted by increments of 10–20 mg/h, at regular intervals, until the patient is in the desired state.

Alfentanil infusion is used to supplement the action of propofol, and provides analgesia and suppression of respiratory activity in the ventilated patient. It is licensed for periods of use of up to four days. Bolus doses of 0.5–1.0 mg of alfentanil may be given to increase the level of sedation/analgesia during stressful or painful procedures such as physiotherapy. Midazolam may also be used in this way.

Finally, atracurium, a short-acting non-depolarising muscle relaxant, was used during initiation of IPPV to relax the vocal chords and enable intubation to take place. As it is associated with some histamine release it can exacerbate COPD; vecuronium, which is not associated with histamine release would theoretically have been a better choice for Mr LT. It may also be necessary to add a muscle relaxant to the maintenance sedative regimen of propofol and alfentanil if this combination does not permit synchronisation of the patient to the ventilator.

Do you agree with the choice of agents to treat Mr LT's respiratory condition? Comment on the doses prescribed.

A5 **(a) Antibiotic therapy.**

An antibiotic with a narrower spectrum of activity would have been more appropriate.

The cause of Mr LT's acute respiratory failure is infection, so treatment with an appropriate antibiotic is very important. Sputum and blood samples should be sent for culture and sensitivity, but the most likely causative organisms are *Haemophilus influenzae* or *Streptococcus pneumoniae*. Ampicillin, amoxicillin, erythromycin or trimethoprim would therefore usually be adequate; however, up to 10% of *H. influenzae* strains are now resistant to ampicillin and amoxicillin, and, bearing in mind the severity of Mr LT's condition, the use of these agents is probably not appropriate without a sensitivity report. Co-amoxiclav at a dose of 1.2 g eight-hourly would have been a more suitable alternative for Mr LT, as it is effective against penicillinase-producing bacteria that are resistant to amoxicillin. In a patient with a severe, community-acquired pneumonia such as Mr LT, the British Thoracic Society (BTS) guidelines recommend a combination of a broad-spectrum, beta-lactamase antibiotic such as co-amoxiclav, cefuroxime or ceftriaxone, together with a macrolide antibiotic, such as erythromycin or clarithromycin. This would then cover for Legionnaire's disease and other atypical organisms.

Use of a macrolide would also be appropriate if Mr LT had recently returned from a foreign holiday. Additionally, penicillin-resistant pneumococci are becoming much more common, particularly in certain parts of Europe, South Africa and South America, and recent travel to these areas could justify the use of ceftriaxone.

A urine test is available for pneumococcal and legionella antigens, which could have confirmed or eliminated the presence of these organisms in 15 minutes.

(b)   Bronchodilator therapy.

It was appropriate to prescribe three bronchodilators for Mr LT, but a loading dose of aminophylline should have been given.

Much of the airways obstruction of COPD is not reversible by bronchodilator therapy as it is caused by mucus plugs and bronchiolar inflammation; however, some patients, like Mr LT, have a reversible component and will obtain benefit from bronchodilators. Patients with COPD often have hypertrophy of bronchial smooth muscle and hyper-reactive airways. Although only small objective improvement can be measured, e.g. by peak flow measurement, this may be significant in someone with extremely poor respiratory function.

The mode of action of $beta_2$-agonists is to increase smooth-muscle cell cyclic adenosine monophosphate levels and stabilise mast cells. Salbutamol or terbutaline in nebulised form is acceptable. The maximum recommended dose for nebulised salbutamol is 5 mg four times daily, but because in severe airways obstruction the quantity of drug reaching the site of action may be limited, a smaller dose given more frequently can be more successful.

Ipratropium bromide is an anticholinergic agent, which blocks the cholinergic reflex that causes bronchospasm. It is particularly useful in combination with $beta_2$-agonists in COPD patients, producing slightly greater bronchodilation than either agent alone. The onset of action of ipratropium is slower than for the $beta_2$-agonists and the duration of action is longer. The peak effect is noted between one and two hours after the dose. The maximum recommended dose of nebulised ipratropium is 500 micrograms four times daily and in view of its longer duration of action than salbutamol there is unlikely to be any advantage in giving the drug more frequently than this. Rationalisation of the use of ipratropium nebules in this way can also result in a significant cost-saving.

In addition to causing relaxation of bronchial smooth muscle, there is some evidence that theophylline may have other beneficial actions in COPD. It is thought to act as a respiratory stimulant, reduce respiratory muscle fatigue, improve right ventricular performance and increase mucociliary clearance. Another advantage is that, unlike the other two bronchodilators in the regimen, intravenous aminophylline does not depend on penetration of the obstructed bronchioles to exert its effect. Although clinical evidence for these properties is inconclusive, intra-venous aminophylline should be added to the bronchodilator therapy of a COPD patient like Mr LT who has severe acute respiratory failure.

However, the aminophylline dosage regimen prescribed for Mr LT was not optimal. He was given an arbitrary maintenance dose (MD) of 42 mg/h. As he was not taking oral theophylline or aminophylline before admission, he should have received a loading dose (LD) in order to achieve a therapeutic concentration rapidly. The normal half-life of theophylline in adults is eight hours and so steady state without a LD can only be achieved after approximately 32 hours. With a suitable LD of 5 mg/kg (or worked out by pharmacokinetic calculation) administered over 20–30 minutes, a therapeutic concentration would have been ach-ieved far more rapidly. After loading is completed, the MD should be started. Ideally the MD should be determined using pharmacokinetic calculation which takes into account those factors which affect theophyl-line clearance, such as smoking history.

The plasma concentration of theophylline should then be mon-itored to maintain therapeutic levels between 10 and 20 mg/L. As no LD was given, the earliest time usefully to measure Mr LT's plasma concentra-tion is 12–20 hours after starting the infusion, which represents twice the normal half-life. Even at this time, the concentration can only be a guide as to whether the dose is too high or too low, as steady state will not have been reached. If a LD had been given, it would have been worthwhile to check the level after six to eight hours and to adjust the dose up or down if necessary.

(c) Corticosteroid therapy.

The use of intravenous and oral corticosteroids in the short-term in Mr LT's condition is normal practice, and makes theoretical sense as inflam-mation plays a significant part in the airways obstruction. However, there is still a lack of good evidence of benefit and after the first few days the role of steroids becomes even more controversial. The dose of hydro-cortisone prescribed for Mr LT is one commonly used and should be reduced as his condition improves, with a change to prednisolone as soon as he can take oral medication.

What would you tell a nurse who had never administered salbutamol or ipratropium by nebuliser before?

A6 **(a)   Volume of nebulised solution.**

Nebulisers have a dead volume, usually of just under 1 mL, which will not be available to the patient, so the larger the fill volume, the greater the fraction of drug released. However, increasing the volume increases the time for nebulisation. In hospital a volume of 4–5 mL is an acceptable compromise, producing an administration time of 15–30 minutes. As Mr LT is written up for 2.5 mg salbutamol (one 2.5 mL nebule) and 500 micrograms ipratropium (one 2 mL nebule) every four hours, it is convenient to mix the two in the nebuliser, making a total volume of 4.5 mL. This is common practice on wards, although the stability of the two solutions combined has not been fully evaluated. Unpublished work carried out on the stability of the mixture using the preserved formulations suggested that they would be compatible when mixed in this way, but both formulations are now preservative-free, which could theoretically affect the results. Where the volume of fluid is insufficient and dilution is required, sodium chloride 0.9% (e.g. Normasol sachets) should be used, as hypotonic solutions may provoke bronchospasm.

A combination product, Combivent nebules, is available, containing ipratropium bromide 500 micrograms plus salbutamol 2.5 mg, in 2.5 mL saline. This product may be used as an alternative where the dose of each drug prescribed is equivalent, bearing in mind the above considerations. The need for these drugs to be prescribed together should be considered carefully in each case, however, particularly in long-term maintenance therapy.

(b)   Driving gas.

The driving gas may be air or oxygen at a rate of 6–8 L/min. In patients with COPD who may have low oxygen tolerability the driving gas should be air; however, as Mr LT is ventilated and on 35% oxygen already, the choice is not so critical and oxygen is acceptable as a driving gas. An alternative approach would be to use air as the driving gas for administration of bronchodilators and administer supplementary oxygen, when required, via nasal cannulae.

(c)   Administration in ventilated patients.

The ventilator itself affects the delivery of nebulised drug. With some ventilators, connecting the nebuliser to the inspiratory arm of the tubing leads to a proportion of the drug being drawn back into the ventilator during the expiratory phase because the nebulised drug is continually fed into the tubing by the driving gas. Some ventilators have a synchronised nebuliser cycle, which electronically opens a valve to allow the nebulised drug to pass into the inspiratory arm only during the inspiratory phase. When the ventilator does not have this facility, the patient may be disconnected from the machine and 'bagged' while the drug is administered, to prevent loss of drug into the machine. In some situations however, bagging may be dangerous. If the patient is on high levels of peak end expiratory pressure (PEEP) it is not advisable, unless the bagging circuit has a PEEP valve. Also there is a high risk of barotrauma if the patient is hyperinflated.

Administration of nebulised drug via the ventilator tubing takes longer than in a non-ventilated patient because the ventilator delivers less breaths per minute than a patient breathing spontaneously.

What are the likely explanations for Mr LT's abnormal haematology and serum biochemistry results?

A7   **Mr LT has a raised haematocrit and white blood cell count. Secondary polycythaemia occurs as a response to chronic hypoxia, causing a raised haemoglobin and also a raised haematocrit, which is an indicator of red cell volume. The raised white blood cell count indicates that Mr LT has an infection. Mr LT's raised serum potassium concentration is likely to be a result of his respiratory acidosis, which is caused by accumulation of carbon dioxide.**

Sodium conservation by the kidney and the sodium pump at the cell wall both involve the exchange of sodium for potassium or hydrogen, the latter two ions being in free competition. In acidotic states there is an excess of hydrogen ions in the blood and so they are cleared in preference to potassium at these two sites. The clearance of potassium is consequently reduced and hyperkalaemia results.

Could Mr LT's drug therapy be causing his tremor?

A8   **Yes.**

Salbutamol is known to cause a fine tremor of skeletal muscle, along with other manifestations of sympathetic stimulation such as an increase in heart rate and peripheral vasodilation. These effects particularly occur when large doses are inhaled. Aminophylline can also cause tremor, but in most cases only at plasma concentrations above the therapeutic range.

> Is the suggested change in treatment appropriate? If not, what recommendations would you make?

A9 **Yes. If the doses of both drugs are changed simultaneously, it will be impossible to determine which is causing the problem. It is appropriate to reduce Mr LT's salbutamol dose as suggested and to measure his serum theophylline level.**

If a serum theophylline concentration were available it would give a clearer indication of what is causing Mr LT's tremor. In the absence of a level, pharmacokinetic calculation indicates that it is unlikely that Mr LT's theophylline concentration is above the therapeutic range, so a reduction in salbutamol dose would be a reasonable response to his symptom of tremor. However, if Mr LT's serum theophylline level is found to be in the toxic range, an appropriate adjustment in intravenous infusion rate can be determined by pharmacokinetic calculation.

> How does reducing the mandatory mechanical ventilation rate help the weaning process?

A10 **On admission to the intensive care unit the mandatory ventilation rate on Mr LT's ventilator would have been adjusted to allow him to maintain his 'normal' PaCO$_2$. This value would be well above the normal physiological range in view of Mr LT's damaged lungs. Reducing the SIMV rate allows him to take spontaneous breaths through the ventilator as his sedation is reduced, avoiding competition with the mechanical breaths.**

> Can drug therapy be helpful in the weaning process?

A11 **Yes. Although respiratory stimulants have fallen from general use in recent years, they have a limited place in the treatment of respiratory failure.**

It is important that a patient's clinical situation is assessed carefully before the decision to use this type of drug is made. If, during weaning, Mr LT (a 'blue bloater') failed to respond to a reduced level of sedation by increasing his spontaneous respiratory rate, then a trial of respiratory stimulant could be indicated. However, in a patient who is already fighting for breath (a 'pink puffer'), further respiratory stimulation could actually lead to a dangerous situation where more carbon dioxide is produced metabolically than the compromised lungs can eliminate. Before resorting to drug therapy, the use of NIV would now be considered when difficulty in weaning occurs.

The only useful respiratory stimulant available at present in the UK is doxapram. Other alternatives, such as nikethamide, are now considered too toxic. Doxapram is thought to act principally on the peripheral chemoreceptors to produce an increase in tidal volume and, to a lesser extent, an increase in respiratory rate. The dose is between 1.5 and 4.0 mg/min by continuous intravenous infusion, depending on the condition and response of the patient. An interaction, presenting as agitation and increased skeletal muscle activity, has been reported between doxapram and aminophylline.

> What action would you take after noting Mr LT's theophylline level and the change in prescribed aminophylline therapy?

A12 **As the plasma concentration is in the middle of the therapeutic range conversion to an equivalent oral regimen is appropriate; however, the prescription for aminophylline liquid requires some adjustment.**

The infusion has been running for over 48 hours at a constant rate so steady state has been achieved and, as it is a continuous intravenous infusion, the sampling time is not critical. As always, when interpreting drug level data the result should also be judged in the light of the patient's clinical response: if the current dose had been ineffective or toxicity had occurred, a change of dose should have been considered even if the reported level was in the therapeutic range.

In converting Mr LT to an oral liquid formulation for administration via the nasogastric tube, the prescriber has not considered the effect of a change of formulation and route on the plasma concentration. In addition, there is no oral liquid form of aminophylline so theophylline must be prescribed and the salt factor taken into account. The patient has received 1000 mg of aminophylline (a combination of theophylline and ethylenediamine) in 24 hours:

$$1000 \text{ mg aminophylline} = 1000 \times 0.8 \text{ (salt factor)}$$
$$= 800 \text{ mg theophylline}$$

The bioavailability of the infusion and oral liquid is assumed to be the same.

Furthermore, a twice-daily dosage regimen is not appropriate. The peak concentration of theophylline after an oral liquid dose will occur after about one hour. In order to avoid toxic peak or subtherapeutic trough concentrations, smaller doses should be given more often, i.e. three to four times daily. A suitable regimen would be 200 mg four times daily. As theophylline liquid is available in a concentration of 60 mg in 5 mL, a more convenient dose would be 180 mg (i.e. 15 mL) four times daily.

When calculating a convenient dose for Mr LT, it is advisable to round the dose downwards, because in some patients theophylline exhibits zero-order kinetics in the upper half of the therapeutic range and a small increase in dose may produce a large increase in plasma concentration.

Is this treatment appropriate for Mr LT's cor pulmonale? What alternative therapies could be prescribed?

A13 **Yes, providing that Mr LT's serum potassium level is first checked. Treatment of the respiratory failure, supplementation with oxygen, and diuretic therapy are the mainstays of the treatment of cor pulmonale. Other drugs, e.g. vasodilators, may be helpful as second-line agents.**

Cor pulmonale is fluid retention and heart failure associated with diseases of the lung. It is initiated by pulmonary artery hypertension, which produces a high afterload and consequently right ventricular hypertrophy. There is no intrinsic abnormality of the heart and initially there may be sufficient functional reserve to maintain cardiac output at normal values; however, the right ventricle eventually fails to compensate for the hypertension and venous pressure becomes elevated. There is also evidence that the oedema associated with COPD may be partly due to poor water handling by hypoxic kidneys and may occur without raised atrial pressure, i.e. before pulmonary hypertension has occurred.

It is now believed that pulmonary hypoxic vasoconstriction, rather than anatomical damage to the capillary bed, causes the rise in pulmonary artery pressure. Erythrocytosis, occurring as a response to hypoxia and causing a rise in haematocrit, increased resistance to flow and an increase in red cell clumping, can also play a part. As hypoxia is the causative factor, treatment of Mr LT's respiratory failure is vital. Episodes of frank heart failure frequently appear during infective episodes. Supplementation with oxygen reduces hypoxia and there is now good evidence that long-term oxygen therapy reduces mortality, morbidity and frequency of hospital admission in such patients. Long-term treatment is only considered in patients with persistent daytime hypoxaemia [PaO_2 < 7.3 kPa (12–15)] and the oxygen must be given for at least 15 hours a day.

Diuretic therapy will reduce oedema, improve peripheral circulation and may improve gaseous exchange in the lungs if pulmonary congestion is present. It should be remembered that, as Mr LT recovers from the acute exacerbation of his pulmonary disease, the cor pulmonale is also likely to improve and his diuretic requirement may thus decrease.

The potency of a loop diuretic will be valuable in the acute treatment of Mr LT's cor pulmonale. In addition, as he had a raised serum potassium on admission, the greater capacity of loop diuretics for lowering potassium levels acutely may be a further advantage. During long-term use, however, thiazides have a greater potential for causing hypokalaemia and as patients with COPD tend to have low total body potassium, a loop diuretic would also appear to be more appropriate as long-term therapy. Furthermore, a potassium-sparing diuretic can be added to the treatment to avoid exacerbation of this problem. Spironolactone has traditionally been used in severe heart failure and is theoretically appropriate as raised aldosterone levels are frequently present owing to hepatic congestion. Amiloride is a suitable alternative, but before either of these drugs is prescribed for Mr LT it is important to check that his serum potassium has returned to normal. Whichever diuretics are chosen, it is important that their effect on Mr LT's electrolyte balance is monitored.

Digoxin is thought to be of little value in cor pulmonale unless atrial fibrillation needs to be controlled. Pulmonary vasodilators are theoretically useful additions to therapy, but are not yet of proven value; hydralazine, calcium-channel blockers and angiotensin-converting enzyme inhibitors (ACEIs) are examples.

Although ACEIs are first-line therapy in many forms of heart failure, there is no evidence of their benefit in cor pulmonale. This group of drugs is beneficial in patients who have left ventricular failure, which is not the case in cor pulmonale, where left ventricular function is usually not severely impaired. If there is a more complex aetiology, such as a history of ischaemic heart disease, there may be a place for an ACEI.

Would you recommend any change in his theophylline dosage?

A14   **Yes. Mr LT's dose of slow-release theophylline should be reduced to 300 mg twice daily, given every 12 hours.**

The serum theophylline sample was taken on the third day after changing to slow-release tablets, so steady state had been reached. As the level is from a pre-dose or trough sample it is likely that the peak theophylline concentration is above 20 mg/L. This observation, combined with Mr LT's continued tremor, which is a side-effect associated with high serum theophylline levels, leads to the recommendation for dosage reduction. A suitable dose could be more accurately determined by pharmacokinetic calculation. His serum theophylline level should then be checked at his first out-patient appointment or preferably earlier by his GP. The sample should ideally be taken eight hours post-dose, giving a mean steady-state concentration for a 12-hourly regimen, but this is unlikely to be practicable in an out-patient setting and the actual time of sampling must be taken into account when interpreting the result.

Would there be any advantage in continuing Mr LT's oral steroid therapy long-term? Would inhaled steroid therapy be more appropriate?

A15 **No. Continuation of Mr LT's systemic corticosteroid therapy indefinitely would not be appropriate at this point. A formal trial of oral or inhaled steroids is, however, warranted.**

It is not possible to predict which COPD patients will benefit from long-term systemic steroid therapy. A formal trial should thus be carried out when Mr LT has recovered from this acute exacerbation of his condition. The following regimen is recommended by the BTS: high-dose oral prednisolone (30 mg daily) should be given for two weeks, combined with measurement of lung function before and afterwards using forced expiratory volume in one second (FEV_1). Significant reversibility is demonstrated by an increase in FEV_1 of more than 200 mL *and* a 15% increase over the baseline value.

Alternatively a six-week course of inhaled corticosteroid (beclometasone 500 micrograms twice a day or equivalent), may be used. Only COPD patients who demonstrate reversibility in such a trial should receive long-term inhaled corticosteroid therapy. There is some evidence that continuing inhaled corticosteroids long-term may reduce the decline in lung function or reduce the number of acute exacerbations in some patients, but this is by no means conclusive.

Prior to admission Mr LT had been prescribed a beclometasone inhaler, but he had not used it for several months because he felt it did not help. This is a common observation by patients with COPD (and asthma), but is very misleading. On further questioning it can frequently be established that the patient did not realise that regular, continuous therapy was required for benefit, and he or she had stopped using it because no immediate relief was obtained on a 'when required' basis. A formal trial of corticosteroids is therefore warranted for Mr LT before long-term steroid therapy is initiated.

What changes might be made to his bronchodilator therapy?

A16 **Mr LT could have been changed from nebulised to inhaler therapy before discharge, to simplify his treatment at home. The use of tiotropium as an alternative to ipratropium in his bronchodilator regimen, could also be considered.**

The change should be made at least a few days before discharge, so that the effect on respiratory function can be determined. Ipratropium has a longer duration of action than salbutamol and comparative studies suggest that anticholinergic drugs are as effective or more effective than beta$_2$–stimulants in COPD. Because of this it would be logical to prescribe regular ipratropium therapy for Mr LT, with salbutamol added on a 'when required' basis to supplement this if necessary. However, since Mr LT already has a nebuliser at home, it may be that inhaler therapy is no longer considered to be effective for him.

If it is considered that inhaled ipratropium combined with supplementary use of salbutamol is no longer adequate for Mr LT, there is now evidence that the new long-acting anticholinergic agent, tiotropium may be more effective. It would therefore be appropriate to substitute tiotropium for ipratropium at this stage (continuing 'when required' salbutamol) before resorting to long-term nebulised therapy.

There is now also good evidence that tiotropium is more effective than salmeterol in COPD. As yet there is no evidence that the combination of salmeterol and tiotropium is more effective than tiotropium alone, but in theory this combination could be the final inhaled regimen to assess before long-term nebulised therapy is commenced.

It should also be noted that current evidence suggests that nebulised therapy is no more likely to be effective in COPD than inhaled therapy, unless inhaled therapy cannot be effectively administered.

Reversibility testing to bronchodilators is detailed in the BTS guidelines for management of COPD. As for steroid trials, these tests should be performed when the patient is clinically stable and free from infection, and the same improvement in FEV$_1$ values as detailed for steroids indicates reversibility, but a negative response does not preclude symptomatic improvement from bronchodilators. Patients who show a positive response are more likely to respond to a trial of steroids.

What points would you discuss with Mr LT when counselling him on his take-home medication?

A17 (a) **Salbutamol and ipratropium.**

The nebulised therapy is the most complex part of his treatment and must be explained to Mr LT in detail, if he is to continue using it long-term, with emphasis on the importance of using the correct fill volume and flow rate of gas. It should be stressed that oxygen cylinders are not a suitable supply of gas for nebulised therapy due to the low flow rate generated by the prescribable flow heads. If possible, Mr LT should be observed using his own equipment. He must also know who to contact if the machine breaks down.

(b) **Prednisolone.**

The tailing-off of the prednisolone dose should be explained, ensuring that Mr LT understands that he is to stop taking this drug after one week. In addition, in view of Mr LT's previous belief that steroids were of no benefit, he must be counselled before starting any formal trial of inhaled or oral steroids. This counselling should cover the importance of taking or using steroids regularly and the delay in obtaining useful effect with this type of medication.

(c) **Co-amilofruse 5/40.**

The dose should be taken regularly in the morning and Mr LT should continue taking these tablets until told otherwise.

(d) **Theophylline.**

The tablets should be swallowed whole, at regular intervals and preferably after food with a cold drink. The concept of sustained release should be explained. Mr LT should realise that this therapy will continue indefinitely and that he will need occasional blood tests to check that the dose is right for him. He should be aware that a number of other medicines, including some antibiotics, affect the level of theophylline and he should remind his doctor that he is on theophylline when his treatment is changed. This is also important when buying over-the-counter medicines.

(e) **General.**

If, in the future, Mr LT is given a course of antibiotics to take when required, he must understand when to start treatment, e.g. when his sputum is discoloured, and at what point to get medical help.

Would you recommend that Mr LT receive continuous antibiotic prophylaxis? If so, which agents would you recommend and at what dose?

A18 No. This hospital admission was Mr LT's first serious acute exacerbation due to infection; however, if he has further severe infective episodes, this option should be considered.

There is no general agreement as to the ideal drug for prophylactic antibiotic therapy, but wide-spectrum antibiotics such as amoxicillin, cefaclor and doxycycline, which have activity against *S. pneumoniae* and *H. influenzae*, have been prescribed at the normal therapeutic dose for mild to moderate infections, e.g. amoxicillin 250 mg three times daily. Evidence for clinical benefits of prophylaxis, such as a reduction in the number of exacerbations or a reduction in the rate of decline in pulmonary function, is distinctly lacking. Prophylaxis has become less popular and should be reserved for patients who experience frequent exacerbations, defined as four or more per year. There are several strategies that may be adopted. Patients may be given daily antibiotics throughout the winter months or for four days per week, changing to a broader-spectrum agent such as co-amoxiclav when acute infection occurs. Alternatively, patients may be supplied with a seven to 10 day course of antibiotic to start at the first sign of a 'chest cold'.

Finally, Mr LT is in the group of patients highly vulnerable to influenza and he should be vaccinated annually. Pneumococcal pneumonia is also a significant risk and COPD patients should receive the pneumococcal vaccine at least once.

What measures would you suggest to reduce the risk of Mr LT suffering from oral thrush again?

A19 Mr LT should use a spacer device with his inhaler and rinse out his mouth after each dose.

This problem is caused by deposition of the steroid in the mouth and throat. Two measures may reduce the risk of it recurring. First, Mr LT can rinse out his mouth with water after each administration, although the benefits of this measure are not proven. Secondly, most of the drug that stays in the mouth is deposited when the inhaler is fired: if a spacer device is used, this deposition occurs in the device itself. Using a spacer device should also help to overcome Mr LT's poor inhaler technique, which probably contributed to this problem in the first place. When counselling on these points, Mr LT should also be instructed to use the steroid inhaler 10 minutes after a dose of salbutamol, to improve steroid penetration.

Further reading

Anon. Inhaled corticosteroids: their role in chronic obstructive pulmonary disease. *MeReC Bull* 2000; **11**: 21–24.

British Thoracic Society. Guidelines for the management of chronic obstructive pulmonary disease. *Thorax* 1997; **52**(suppl 5): S1–S28.

British Thoracic Society. Guidelines for the management of community acquired pneumonia. *Thorax* 2001; **56**(suppl. IV): IV1–IV63.

Hvizdos KM, Goa KL. Tiotropium bromide. Adis New Drug Profile. *Drugs* 2002; **62**: 1195–1203.

Mandell G, Bennett J, Dolin R. *Principles and Practice of Infectious Diseases*, 5th edn. Churchill Livingstone, London, 2000.

Stoller JK. Acute exacerbations of chronic obstructive pulmonary disease. *N Eng J Med* 2002; **346**: 988–994.

Winter ME. *Basic Clinical Pharmacokinetics*, 4th edn. Applied Therapeutics, Vancouver, WA, 2003.

Koda-Kimble MA, Young LY, Kradjan WA *et al.*, eds. *Applied Therapeutics: The Clinical Use of Drugs*, 7th edn. Lippincott Williams & Wilkins, Philadelphia, PA, 2001.

13

Pulmonary tuberculosis

Ruth Bednall, Railton Scott and Robert Horne

Case study and questions

Day 1 Mr AQ was admitted via A & E. He was a 65–year-old Bengali man, who had been resident in the UK for three years. He was a widower and lived with his 28-year-old daughter, her husband and their two children (aged two and three years). Mr AQ's understanding of English was limited and his medical history was taken with the help of his daughter, who had accompanied him to the hospital.

Mr AQ presented with a four-week history of cough, which had become productive in the past two weeks, night sweats and lethargy. These symptoms had worsened over the past week. He did not smoke cigarettes or drink alcohol.

The patient's past medical history included asthma and Type 2 diabetes mellitus. He had recently been prescribed gliclazide for his diabetes as his blood sugar control had not returned to normal following a course of oral corticosteroids prescribed for an acute exacerbation of his asthma.

On examination Mr AQ was thin, feverish and pale. His temperature was 38.5°C. His blood pressure was 120/70 mmHg, and his pulse was 80 beats per minute and regular. He complained of chest pain which was exacerbated by cough.

His medication history was as follows:

- Salbutamol 100-microgram metered-dose inhaler (MDI) two puffs when required
- Beclometasone dipropionate 100-microgram MDI two puffs twice daily
- Gliclazide 160 mg once daily
- Paracetamol 500 mg tablets, one to two daily when required

His serum urea, electrolytes, haemoglobin and liver function tests (LFTs) were all within the normal ranges, and his random blood sugar was 4.0 mmol/L. Examination of his respiratory system was as follows:

trachea, central; expansion, right = left; dull to percussion on the left apex; slight expiratory wheeze. A chest x-ray was performed and showed bilateral apical shadowing which was more marked on the left than the right. There was evidence of calcification in both right and left apices. Sputum, blood and urine samples were sent for microbial examination, and a Mantoux 1 in 10 000 test was ordered.

A diagnosis of pulmonary tuberculosis (TB) was made based on Mr AQ's chest x-ray and clinical presentation.

Q1 Given the presentation of the case was a diagnosis of pulmonary TB reasonable?
Q2 Can any potential triggers for the post-primary infection be identified?
Q3 Was the correct Mantoux test chosen? How would you recommend the test be carried out?
Q4 Was it appropriate to start treatment before the results of microbiological culture were known?

Mr AQ, who weighed 62 kg, was prescribed:

- Rifampicin 600 mg daily
- Isoniazid 300 mg daily
- Pyrazinamide 2 g daily

Q5 Outline a pharmaceutical care plan for Mr AQ.
Q6 Was the antitubercular therapy prescribed for Mr AQ appropriate?
Q7 Were the prescribed doses correct? How should the drugs be given?
Q8 Would you recommend additional therapy at this stage?
Q9 What tests will be required to monitor Mr AQ's treatment?

Day 2 Ethambutol 900 mg was added to Mr AQ's drug chart. He still had a low-grade fever but his appetite had improved and he was now eating regularly and well. He was managing to take his medication as prescribed. It was noted by nursing staff that his blood sugars were starting to creep upwards.

Q10 What may be the reason for the sustained increase in Mr AQ's blood sugar readings?
Q11 What changes would you recommend to his treatment regimen if he should become unable to tolerate oral medication?

Day 3 Mr AQ's condition was stable. His fever remained low grade and was not causing undue distress or discomfort. His intake of food and fluids was excellent and his blood sugars were now within an acceptable range as his gliclazide had been increased to 240 mg daily (160 mg in the morning and a further 80 mg at night).

A palpable induration of 12 mm diameter was recorded at the site of his Mantoux test, indicating a positive response to tuberculin purified protein derivative (PPD) 1 in 10 000.

Q12 What is the significance of the positive Mantoux test?

Q13 What other skin tests are used in the diagnosis of TB? What are their advantages and disadvantages?

Q14 Should Mr AQ's grandchildren and their mother be allowed to visit at this stage?

Q15 Is prophylactic treatment indicated for Mr AQ's grandchildren? If so, which agent(s) and dosage regimen would you recommend?

Q16 Mr AQ's daughter is two months pregnant. Which, if any, prophylactic agent(s) should she receive?

Day 5 Mr AQ was 'feeling fine'. His temperature was now settling. His blood sugar, electrolytes and blood count remained within normal limits; however, the results of his LFTs were as follows:

- Alanine aminotransferase (ALT) 78 units/L (reference range 7–35)
- Aspartate aminotransferase (AST) 80 units/L (7–40)
- Alkaline phosphatase 47 units/L (25–90)
- Bilirubin (total) 12 micromol/L (< 17)
- Bilirubin (direct) 2 micromol/L (< 6)

Mr AQ was not jaundiced and clinical signs of hepatic disease were absent.

Q17 What might have caused Mr AQ's abnormal LFTs? What action would you recommend?

Day 12 Mr AQ continued to improve steadily. His LFTs had returned to within normal limits. It was decided that he should be discharged in three days time if his current progress was maintained.

Q18 For how long is antitubercular treatment likely to be necessary?

Q19 What are the major points you would want to convey to Mr AQ during his discharge counselling?

Q20 What general measures could you adopt to encourage Mr AQ's compliance?

Q21 If it was suspected at a later date that Mr AQ was not complying with his treatment regimen, what alternative strategies would you recommend? What additional monitoring may be necessary?

Given the presentation of the case, was a diagnosis of pulmonary TB reasonable?

A1 **Yes. There are several important diagnostic features which are supported by the patient's recent medical history.**

It is first important to distinguish between TB infection and disease. Primary infection usually occurs when droplets of infected sputum are inhaled into the lungs. When first exposed, the host lacks acquired immunity and the bacteria may spread rapidly from the lungs to the lymph, and possibly to other tissues such as the kidney and joints.

Widespread symptomatic infection is usually prevented by the development of acquired resistance to the mycobacterium. Macrophages engulf the bacteria and later coalesce to form clumps or tubercules, which may become calcified. Primary infection therefore rarely produces any symptoms except perhaps a fever or mild illness and may even go unnoticed. An exception is in infancy, when infection may be fatal if it becomes disseminated or uncontrolled.

Primary infection may be followed by post-primary disease if the subject becomes reinfected or the primary disease is reactivated. The likelihood of this depends on the patient's age, general health, nutritional and immune status, and on the virulence of the organism.

In adults post-primary disease most commonly surfaces in the lungs, but may focus on other organs (such as the kidneys, lymph nodes or joints), or it may be disseminated (miliary TB). It should be noted that adult Asian and African immigrants in Britain often present atypically, e.g. with tuberculous meningitis.

Can any potential triggers for the post-primary infection be identified?

A2 **Yes. Mr AQ's past medical history includes Type 2 diabetes mellitus, which acts as an increased clinical risk factor. In addition, a recent exacerbation of Mr AQ's asthma was treated with a course of oral prednisolone and corticosteroid use is also considered to act as an increased clinical risk factor, as steroids may suppress cell-mediated immunity.**

Was the correct Mantoux test chosen? How would you recommend the test be carried out?

A3 **The correct Mantoux test was chosen, as it was strongly suspected that Mr AQ was tuberculin-sensitive. The test involves the intradermal injection of a small quantity of tuberculin PPD into the volar surface of the arm.**

Previous or current infection with *Mycobacterium tuberculosis* produces an allergic type IV response, which results in a zone of induration (localised skin thickening due to oedema) at the site of intradermal injection. The size of the zone of induration depends on the degree of hypersensitivity. In the UK, a zone of induration greater than 5 mm in diameter, measured 72 hours after injection of 10 units of tuberculin PPD, is usually recognised as a positive result.

Tuberculin PPD is available in three strengths. For the Mantoux test, the amount injected is always 0.1 mL. The usual test dose is 10 units, or 0.1 mL of a 1 in 1000 dilution (100 units/ml). If there is any doubt about the zone size, a higher dose of 100 units (0.1 mL of a 1 in 100 dilution) may be given after two days. In order to avoid a severe local reaction and tissue damage, a person who is thought to be tuberculin-sensitive should be given a low dose of 1 unit (0.1 mL of a 1 in 10 000 dilution).

The test should be applied as follows. After cleaning the skin of the volar surface of the arm with alcohol, 0.1 mL of the tuberculin PPD test solution should be injected intradermally, using a needle number 25 or 26. The result should be read 72 hours later. Only areas of induration should be measured; erythema should be ignored. Young children should usually be given half the adult dose.

Was it appropriate to start treatment before the results of microbiological culture were known?

A4 **Yes. Mr AQ has sufficient clinical features to suggest that the diagnosis of active pulmonary TB is accurate. Prompt treatment with the appropriate antituberculants is therefore indicated at this stage.**

A delay in starting active treatment while awaiting confirmation via sputum and skin testing is not justified. As the mycobacterium is a slow growing organism, culture results and sensitivities often take several weeks to obtain. Swifter results are possible if DNA testing of the mycobacterium is carried out, although this is not available in all centres. It should also be borne in mind that the results of Mr AQ's chest x-ray indicated possible previous TB infection.

Changes to therapy may be made if, following culture, resistance to specific drugs is established.

Outline a pharmaceutical care plan for Mr AQ.

A5   **Mr AQ's pharmaceutical care plan should be considered in two halves. First the acute care plan and secondly that required for discharge.**

(a)   Acute care plan. In the acute stage the pharmacist should ensure that therapy to treat active problems is appropriate.

   (i) Ensure the choice and dose of antituberculars is appropriate.
   (ii) Monitor for efficacy (temperature chart, sputum results, red discolouration of body fluids caused by rifampicin).
   (iii) Monitor for side-effects.
   (iv) Assess the patient's and his relatives' understanding of his disease and its treatment.
   (v) Diabetes – monitor blood glucose levels and review the dose of gliclazide.
   (vi) Asthma – monitor peak expiratory flow rate, check inhaler technique, check understanding of purpose of inhalers.
   (vii) Overall, assess Mr AQ's understanding of his diseases and treatments.

(b)   When planning for discharge the following should be addressed:

   (i) Long-term concordance with TB treatment. For therapy to be effective Mr AQ must complete the entire course. For much of the time Mr AQ will feel quite well and, as with many chronic illnesses, the motivation to continue to take the medication may recede. Careful education of the patient and his family needs to be undertaken to ensure that therapy is continued as long as necessary.
   (ii) Mr AQ's ongoing supply of medication in the community needs to be ensured In particular sufficient take home medication must be supplied to allow him time to obtain further supplies from his GP.
   (iii) Advice may need to be provided to his GP on what monitoring will be required (e.g. LFTs, urea and electrolyte checks).

(iv)   Mr AQ will need to be provided with appropriate education on the management of his asthma and diabetes.

As with all care, every member of the health care team providing care to this patient should be involved with the pharmaceutical care given, and in order to achieve maximal benefit from pharmaceutical interventions, the outcomes of drug therapy should be recorded and evaluated. and any alterations deemed beneficial should be implemented.

Was the antitubercular therapy prescribed for Mr AQ appropriate?

A6   **No. Current guidance from the British Thoracic Society recommends that four drugs be used as standard initial therapy in order to ensure that resistant strains are treated effectively. Mr AQ should be prescribed rifampicin, isoniazid, pyrazinamide plus ethambutol.**

Combination therapy is required in order to minimise the risk of treatment failure due to existing or emergent bacterial resistance and to widen the scope of attack to maximise bacterial kill.

Isoniazid is the most potent bactericidal agent and is active against large numbers of growing bacteria. Along with rifampicin it also prevents the emergence of drug resistance by suppressing resistant mutants within the bacterial population.

Rifampicin and pyrazinamide are most effective at killing 'bacterial persisters', which are slowly metabolising organisms that exist in a semi-dormant state. Failure to eradicate these could result in re-emergence of the disease.

Ethambutol and streptomycin are weaker antitubercular drugs but are nevertheless worthwhile additions to therapy if resistance is suspected. Ethambutol may be omitted if the patient is thought to be at low risk for resistance to isoniazid. This would be defined as a previously untreated white patient known to be HIV-negative. Positive HIV status, previous therapy (note Mr AQ's old x-ray changes), other ethnic groups and recent arrivals in the UK are all risk factors for resistance. As such, Mr AQ requires ethambutol to be added to his drug chart.

In circumstances where multidrug resistant strains have been identified, old drugs such as protionamide, para-aminosalicylic acid, cycloserine and thioacetazone may be considered. These are unlicensed preparations which require named patient supply.

Were the prescribed doses appropriate? How should the drugs be given?

A7 **The prescribed doses are appropriate with the addition of ethambutol 900 mg daily. Initially, all the drugs prescribed for Mr AQ should be given as a single daily dose to ensure maximal plasma concentrations.**

Similar doses and regimens are used to treat most other forms of TB. Reference to the urea and electrolyte and LFT results indicates that Mr AQ does not need to have any of the drug doses adjusted to compensate for impaired hepatic or renal function. The doses of rifampicin, isoniazid and pyrazinamide are therefore appropriate for Mr AQ's age and weight. Ethambutol should be commenced at a dose of 900 mg once daily.

Rifampicin is best absorbed on an empty stomach and, together with isoniazid, should be given half to one hour before breakfast, with a full glass of water. When advising on drug administration, it should be remembered that rifampicin may stain body fluids orange/red. It is therefore important to inform Mr AQ and all those caring for him of this harmless, but potentially distressing, effect.

Pyrazinamide tablets (500 mg) are large and Mr AQ may find them difficult to swallow. This drug may also irritate the gastric mucosa and, for this reason, it is often prescribed in three or four divided doses, with or immediately after food. Although Mr AQ is at present eating little, his pyrazinamide should initially be given as a single daily dose at the same time as the rifampicin and isoniazid. If he complains of gastric irritation, the pyrazinamide dose could then be changed to 500 mg four times a day, taken with milk, at least one hour after the dose of rifampicin.

It should also be remembered that Mr AQ's increased appetite and improved health could result in an increase in his body weight. The drug doses may thus need to be adjusted accordingly as treatment progresses.

Would you recommend additional therapy at this stage?

A8 **Yes. Pyridoxine 10 mg daily should be prescribed.**

Isoniazid may cause a reversible peripheral neuritis, which is attributed to an effect of isoniazid on vitamin B_6 (pyridoxine) metabolism – isoniazid interferes with enzymatic reactions in which pyridoxal phosphate acts as a coenzyme.

Isoniazid is eliminated mainly by hepatic acetylation. The population is split into slow and fast acetylators, slow acetylators being more prone to isonazid-induced neuritis. Acetylator status is genetically determined and there are clear ethnic differences: Orientals and Innuits are predominantly fast acetylators, and may therefore require larger doses of isoniazid, whereas in Caucasians and Asians there are roughly equal proportions of fast and slow acetylators. Although the acetylator status of an individual can be demonstrated by a laboratory test, widespread testing is not justified when prophylaxis can be so easily and safely administered to all individuals. For the majority of patients, prophylaxis with low doses of pyridoxine, such as 10 mg daily is enough to reduce the incidence of isoniazid-induced neuritis from 20% to less than 1%. However, some sources, particularly in the US, recommend higher doses of 50–100 mg pyridoxine daily. As Mr AQ also suffers from Type 2 diabetes, in which there is an increased chance of developing peripheral neuritis, there may be some justification for using a pyridoxine dose at the higher end of the dosage range.

What tests will be required to monitor Mr AQ's treatment?

A9 **Regular hepatic and renal function tests, and regular eye tests.**

(a) Liver function tests (LFTs). Rifampicin, isoniazid and pyrazinamide may all produce hepatotoxicity which can range in severity from mild subclinical alterations in LFTs, to more serious reactions producing clinical jaundice or, rarely, fatal hepatitis.

Experts are divided as to when LFTs should be monitored. Routine LFTs should be performed before treatment is started and during the initial few weeks of treatment. Thereafter, regular monitoring of LFTs is usually only necessary if the patient is over 50, regularly consumes large quantities of alcohol, has existing liver disease, or is receiving other hepatotoxic drugs. As Mr AQ is over 50 and is taking isoniazid, his LFTs should be monitored weekly for the first four weeks and monthly for three months afterwards.

(b) Renal function tests. The elimination of each of the four drugs used to treat Mr AQ is to some extent dependent upon his renal function. As Mr AQ's renal function on starting treatment was normal, standard doses of his prescribed drugs were justified. The dose of isoniazid should, however, be reduced in severe renal impairment. Reduced renal elimination of rifampicin may be compensated for by increased biliary excretion. In renal failure the dose of ethambutol should be reduced and therapeutic drug levels monitored (therapeutic range 3–5 mg/L).

(c) Eye tests. Ethambutol affects the optic nerves and defects in vision may occur during therapy. These include loss of red/green colour vision and visual field defects such as tunnel vision. These side-effects are dose-dependent and usually reversible on withdrawal of the drug. Patients prescribed ethambutol need to be able to describe vision defects. Eye tests should be done prior to starting therapy and six-monthly thereafter. Macular thresholds should be checked prior to commencing and during therapy.

What may be the reason for the sustained increase in Mr AQ's blood sugar readings?

A10 **There are two possible factors: Mr AQ is eating regularly and well or it is possible that his rifampicin, a potent inducing agent of the cytochrome P450 enzyme system, is interacting with his sulphonylurea antidiabetic agent gliclazide, with a resulting reduction in antidiabetic effect.**

Although there is considerable inter-individual variation, the enzyme-inducing effect of rifampicin has been noted as early as two days after the start of treatment.

Mr AQ's blood sugar levels should be monitored on a regular basis. Once his dietary intake has stabilised, it may prove necessary to increase his dose of gliclazide for as long as he remains on the rifampicin therapy.

What changes would you recommend to his treatment regime if he should become unable to tolerate oral medication?

A11 **Rifampicin and isoniazid may be given by intravenous and intramuscular injection, respectively. Pyrazinamide is only available in tablet form. No intravenous alternative can be sourced and if NG/PEG (nasogastric/percutaneous endoscopic gastrostomy) administration of a 'specials' formulation is not possible, then an alternative parenteral drug, e.g. streptomycin, should be substituted. Ethambutol is available in intravenous form (100 mg/10 mL) but this is an unlicensed product and has to be obtained on a named patient basis.**

What is the significance of the positive Mantoux test?

A12 **A positive response to the Mantoux test demonstrates hypersensitivity to tuberculoproteins, which usually indicates**

that the subject has been previously infected with *M. tuberculosis* or has received a Bacillus Calmette-Guérin (BCG) vaccination. It is impossible to differentiate between these two.

It is likely that the degree of tuberculin sensitivity after infection is related to the size of the infecting dose, the virulence of the organism and the subject's immune status. A negative response usually indicates the absence of infection and that the subject is suitable for BCG vaccination.

In some cases, a negative response to tuberculin testing may occur in someone who is strongly suspected of being infected with *M. tuberculosis*. Possible explanations for this are:

(a)   1–3% of patients infected with *M. tuberculosis* are negative tuberculin reactors.
(b)   If the test is performed within six weeks of infection, hypersensitivity may not have had time to develop.
(c)   The test has been incorrectly performed or read.
(d)   A higher concentration of tuberculin may be necessary.
(e)   The person may be taking immunosuppressant drugs such as corticosteroids, which may suppress the subject's sensitivity to tuberculin.
(f)   The person is suffering from a disease that may suppress tuberculin sensitivity. Such diseases include some cancers, such as Hodgkin's lymphoma, leukaemia, bronchial carcinoma (sensitivity may be unaffected if the cancer is not far advanced) and sarcoidosis.
(g)   The infection may be with an atypical mycobacterium. In this case the patient may show a weakly positive response to tuberculin PPD testing. This is particularly important in immunocompromised patients or those with HIV disease, in whom atypical infections are commonplace.
(h)   Tuberculin sensitivity seems to diminish with time, and elderly people previously infected with *M. tuberculosis* may be tuberculin-negative unless they have active lesions.

What other skin tests are used in the diagnosis of TB? What are their advantages and disadvantages?

A13   **The Heaf test, Imotest and Tine test.**

The Mantoux test is the most commonly used tuberculin PPD test in the UK. Alternative tests include:

(a)   The Heaf test. An apparatus is used which consists of six pre-set
      needles (2 mm for adults and older children, 1 mm for children
      under three years old). A drop of tuberculin is placed on the
      patient's arm. The apparatus (Heaf gun) is placed over the thin film
      of tuberculin formed and the needles are released while holding the
      patient's arm taut. The test can be read after three days, but the
      results are usually still visible after a week. This is convenient when
      groups of people are being tested. The size of the zone of palpable
      induration indicates the grade of positivity. It is recommended that
      the Heaf test apparatus is sterilised after each use by dipping the end
      in methylated spirits and flaming. This test has become less popular
      in recent years because of the theoretical risk of transmission of HIV
      or viral hepatitis.
(b)   The Imotest (Servier). This is similar to the Heaf test but has the
      advantage of being a disposable plastic unit.
(c)   The Tine test. This is a disposable plastic unit with four prongs. The
      test must be carefully applied and read in order to avoid false results.
      Some physicians argue that the Tine test produces inconsistent
      results, but others maintain that if it is carefully applied it provides
      a simple and reliable screening test.

> Should Mr AQ's grandchildren and their mother be allowed to visit at
> this stage?

A14 **Mr AQ has active pulmonary TB and so must be considered a
likely infection risk. Before visiting can be permitted, Mr
AQ's household contacts should be given a Mantoux test and
a chest x-ray to ascertain whether or not they are infected
with *M. tuberculosis*.**

This is particularly important in the case of young children, because in
this group primary disease is more likely to lead to miliary TB or
tuberculosis meningitis. Prompt treatment is then essential in order to
avoid the high degree of mortality and morbidity associated with these
conditions. However, it has been established that Mr AQ has been living
in close contact with his immediate family members for some considerable time. It is therefore probable that any infection will have already
been passed on to these immediate family members. Mr AQ is sick and in
a strange and frightening environment. His command of English is poor.
A visit from his daughter and grandchildren could prove immensely
therapeutic. Further information and improved communication may also
result from this visit. It may be an ideal time to begin the process of
counselling and education.

Is prophylactic treatment indicated for Mr AQ's grandchildren? If so, which agent(s) and dosage regimen would you recommend?

A15 **Preventative treatment is warranted if the tuberculin sensitivity of the child indicates that he or she is at risk of developing active disease. For example, if the results of the tuberculin testing are clearly positive with a normal chest x-ray and the absence of clinical symptoms.**

Owing to the high incidence of the disease in Asian families in the UK and the severe nature of the disease in children, Mr AQ's grandchildren should undergo tuberculin testing. The Imotest should be used. The reaction produced is graded on a scale of 1–4, according to the tuberculin sensitivity of the individual. Subsequent management depends on the results. If the reaction is graded 0–1, BCG vaccination should be offered. If the child has been previously vaccinated, a follow-up chest x-ray should be taken in three months' time. If the reaction is graded 2–4, a chest x-ray should be taken and prophylaxis with isoniazid 5–10 mg/kg/day for six to 12 months should be prescribed. In this case the child should be followed up with chest x-rays for two years.

Mr AQ's daughter is two months pregnant. Which, if any, prophylactic agents should she receive?

A16 **The decision must be based on the results of tuberculin testing and on the interpretation of her clinical picture.**

The decision to administer any drug during the first trimester of pregnancy is complicated by the fact that safety can never be guaranteed and that there is a lack of correlation between drug effects in humans and those observed in animal studies. It is rarely possible to give a 'black or white' verdict of 'safe or not safe' during pregnancy. In deciding to use an anti-infective agent during pregnancy, the potential teratogenic effects of the drug must be balanced against the risks to mother and foetus of withholding treatment. Most authorities now consider that the use of isoniazid, pyrazinamide and ethambutol during the first trimester can be justified providing there are good clinical indications. The use of rifampicin is more controversial – large doses of the drug are teratogenic in rats and the drug manufacturers consider it to be contra-indicated during the first trimester; however, the World Health Organization states that 'There is no evidence that the doses of rifampicin used in clinical practice have a teratogenic effect'. Streptomycin is best avoided because of the risk of ototoxicity to the foetus.

The decision to treat Mr AQ's daughter should therefore depend on the results of tuberculin testing and her clinical picture. A positive test and normal chest x-ray would indicate the need for preventative treatment with isoniazid, 300 mg as a single daily dose for six to 12 months. Clinical evidence of active disease would warrant treatment with normal adult doses of isoniazid, pyrazinamide, ethambutol and rifampicin. Extra pyridoxine, e.g. a dose of 50–100 mg daily, should be given with the isoniazid, as pregnant women have an increased requirement for this vitamin.

What might have caused Mr AQ's abnormal LFTs? What action would you recommend?

A17   **It seems likely that Mr AQ's drug therapy has caused his abnormal LFTs, but no action is required at present.**

Ethambutol is not associated with changes in LFTs; however, isoniazid, rifampicin and pyrazinamide are potentially hepatotoxic. It is often difficult to attribute hepatitis directly to drug treatment, or to decide which antituberculant is responsible, as the drugs are nearly always given in combination.

Isoniazid may produce hepatocellular damage that resembles hepatitis (elevated serum levels of ALT and AST, but little change in alkaline phosphatase and bilirubin). This is usually mild and subclinical and disappears even if therapy is continued. However, a proportion of people (0.1–1%) develop acute hepatic injury, which in about 10% of these patients progresses to a chronic active hepatitis. The exact mechanism is unknown, but is thought to have an autoimmune basis and be linked with the production of a toxic metabolite. Pre-existing liver disease, alcoholism and age over 50 are predisposing factors. The reaction usually occurs between two and 12 months after starting treatment.

Rifampicin may produce two types of liver damage: dose-related cholestasis resulting from interference with the uptake and excretion of bilirubin or idiosyncratic hepatocellular damage. The latter reaction usually occurs three to five weeks after starting treatment. It is rare, but may pose a risk in patients who are alcohol-dependent, elderly or have pre-existing liver disease.

The hepatitis produced by pyrazinamide is dose-related and is limited if doses are kept below 40 mg/kg/day.

In the absence of a clinical explanation, Mr AQ's abnormal LFTs may be attributed to his drug treatment. Mild, transient elevations in LFTs are common during the first two months of antitubercular therapy.

Treatment should be stopped if there is clinical evidence of liver damage, such as jaundice, hepatic enlargement, anorexia and malaise. If clinical signs are absent, it will, in most cases, be safe to continue treatment. Exceptions to this rule of thumb include those who consume large amounts of alcohol, elderly patients, the very young or those with pre-existing liver disease. Large, defined as more than three to four times normal, or persistent elevations in ALT or AST serum levels may necessitate a break in therapy.

Mr AQ's LFTs are only slightly raised. His treatment should thus be continued with careful monitoring of his LFTs. If they continue to increase or if he develops clinical signs of liver damage, **all** of his antituberculars should be stopped, as it is not possible to identify the agent responsible for his abnormal results, although his normal serum bilirubin result indicates that rifampicin therapy is probably not the cause. The antituberculars should then be reintroduced one at a time, each drug being given for about a week before another is added. This should be accompanied by regular monitoring of LFTs and close clinical supervision, so that the drug responsible may be identified by a recurrence in symptoms. The offending drug could then be omitted from the regimen or replaced by streptomycin.

For how long is antitubercular treatment likely to be necessary?

A18   The treatment of TB is usually split into two phases: an initial intensive phase and a 'consolidation' phase.

The British Thoracic Society currently recommends treatment for pulmonary TB with four drugs (isoniazid, rifampicin, pyrazinamide plus ethambutol) for the initial two months, followed by four months treatment with two drugs (usually rifampicin and isoniazid). Four drugs should be continued until culture results are available if this takes longer than the two months of the initial phase of therapy.

Mr AQ has made a rapid recovery. He should receive isoniazid, rifampicin, pyrazinamide and ethambutol for a further six weeks. The duration of the next phase of treatment is debatable: preliminary data from a relatively recent trial seemed to support the efficacy of short-course treatments (i.e. a second phase of four months); therefore, until further evidence is available, Mr AQ is likely to receive isoniazid and rifampicin for a further four months. For the second phase the dose of rifampicin and isoniazid can be reduced to 450 and 300 mg daily, respectively.

What are the major points you would want to convey to Mr AQ during his discharge counselling?

A19 **(a)   The importance of compliance.**

It is better for him to stop taking the whole drug regimen than to regularly omit one or two drugs, as the latter strategy might lead to the development of resistance to the remaining agent(s). This would preclude future use of these drugs and necessitate the inclusion of more toxic second-line agents such as cycloserine, capreomycin and protionamide.

(b)   The need to continue therapy until told otherwise.

In order to 'keep the disease at bay', he must continue treatment even though he may feel well.

(c)   When and how to take his medicines.

All four drugs may be taken together, with a full glass of water, about an hour before breakfast. To lessen the risk of gastric irritation, the pyrazinamide dose can be split into 500 mg every six hours, but if this is likely to lessen compliance, it should be taken as a single dose of 2 g in the morning.

(d)   He should always give his doctor or pharmacist a list of the drugs he is taking.

This is to prevent interactions which may occur between rifampicin and many other drugs such as corticosteroids and oral hypoglycaemic agents.

What general measures could you adopt to encourage Mr AQ's compliance?

A20 **(a)   A combination preparation of rifampicin and isoniazid may be convenient.**

(b)   Encourage a drug-taking routine by fitting medication into activities of daily living.

(c)   As Mr AQ's English is limited, he should be counselled while his daughter is present as translator. She and her husband may then be willing to supervise and help with the administration of Mr AQ's treatment regimen, particularly if compliance seems likely to be a problem.

(d)   After the dosage regimen is explained, Mr AQ should be asked to repeat what he has been told, as a check that he has understood the instructions.

(e)   Tablet bottles should be labelled clearly in simple English and Mr AQ provided with a Bengali translation as a written reminder, if one can be obtained from a member of the hospital staff. Certain pharmaceutical companies have produced information leaflets for non-English-speaking patients.

Educational interventions may be more effective if they build on the patient's existing ideas about his illness and treatment. Ideally the pharmacist should begin by eliciting the patient's views about his illness and treatment. This is necessary because research has shown that people form coherent beliefs about their illness and treatment which may conflict with the 'medical view' and influence their adherence to treatment. For example, Mr AQ may see his TB as a serious, but short-term, illness which is currently making him feel unwell. His hospitalisation and distressing symptoms provide him with a clear rationale for taking medication which he hopes will fight the infection, reduce his symptoms and make him feel better. However, after a few weeks at home his symptoms are likely to be far less severe, if present at all. In this situation Mr AQ may feel that his medicine has 'done the trick' and is no longer necessary. Despite instructions on the label to 'finish the course' he may decide to stop his medication in the belief that this instruction is over-cautious. Equally, Mr AQ might be concerned about the possibility of 'dangerous side-effects' occurring if the treatment is taken for longer periods.

By listening to the patient's own ideas and then providing clear explanations which build on these and correct any problematic misconceptions, the pharmacist may be able to provide the patient with a rationale for adhering to long-term treatment recommendations.

If it was suspected at a later date that Mr AQ was not complying with his treatment regimen, what alternative strategies would you recommend? What additional monitoring may be necessary?

A21   Directly observed therapy (DOT) may be a suitable approach to improving compliance. Traditionally DOT has been provided as an intermittent, supervised drug regimen, with the drugs being given twice or three times a week under full out-patient supervision. However, it is becoming accepted practice that any suitably trained, responsible individual can supervise therapy and a willing member of the patient's

**family supervising therapy at home may be far more
appropriate than twice weekly visits to the hospital. Indeed
in the case of Mr AQ it may well be appropriate to introduce
DOT at the start of treatment rather than wait for a problem
to occur. In this way no time is wasted in weeks of
suboptimal therapy and the risk to the general public of
further spread of the disease can be reduced.**

The rifampicin dose should not exceed 600 mg twice weekly, as high-dose intermittent use is associated with an increased incidence of a flu-like syndrome (in about 1% of patients) and thrombocytopenia. Platelet counts should be monitored and therapy changed to 300 mg daily if thrombocytopenia occurs. The isoniazid dose should be adjusted to 15 mg/kg twice a week, pyrazinamide to 3 g twice a week and pyridoxine to 50 mg twice a week.

Further reading

Barnes P, Barrows S. Tuberculosis in the 1990s. *Ann Intern Med* 1993; **119**: 400–410.

Bednall R, Dean G, Bateman N. Directly Observed Therapy for the treatment of tuberculosis – evidence based dosage guidelines. *Respir Med* 1999; **93**: 759–762.

Chan ED, Iseman MD. Current medical treatment for tuberculosis. *Br Med J* 2002; **325**: 1282–1286.

Davidson P. Managing tuberculosis in pregnancy. *Lancet* 1995; **346**: 199.

Dodds L. Interactions with antitubercular drugs. *Pharm J* 1988; **240**: 182.

Dole E. Beyond pharmaceutical care. *Am J Hosp Pharm* 1994; **51**: 2183–2184.

Girling DJ. The hepatic toxicity of antituberculosis regimens containing isoniazid, rifampicin pyrazinamide. *Tubercle* 1978; **59**: 13–32.

Guillebaud J. *Contraception – Your Questions Answered*, 3rd edn. Churchill Livingstone, Edinburgh, 1999.

Horne R. One to be taken as directed: reflections on non-adherence (non-compliance). *J Soc Admin Pharm* 1993; **10**: 150–156.

Horne, R. Compliance, adherence and concordance. In: *Pharmacy Practice*. K Taylor, G Harding, eds. Taylor & Francis, London, 2001: 165–184.

Iseman MD. Treatment of multidrug resistant tuberculosis. *N Engl J Med* 1993; **329**: 784–791.

Jessa F. Are TB patients misunderstood? *Hosp Pharm Pract* 1994; April: 159–160.

Joint Tuberculosis Committee of the British Thoracic Society Chemotherapy and Management of Tuberculosis in the United Kingdom. Recommendations 1998. *Thorax* 1998; **53**: 536–548.

Marshall P. Patient compliance with TB treatment. *Pharm J* 1988; **240**: 183.

Snider DE Jr, Castro KG. The global threat of drug resistant tuberculosis. *N Engl J Med* 1998; **388**: 1689–1690.

14

Epilepsy

Alison Issott

Year 1 10-year-old Miss SL was brought to her GP's surgery by her mother who was concerned by her daughter's behaviour. She said that her daughter had jerky movements of the shoulders and arms that usually occurred around breakfast time. On questioning, her doctor discovered that Miss SL did not lose consciousness with these movements and that, over the past year, she had also occasionally had periods when she seemed to 'blank out' for a few seconds. The GP referred Miss SL to a consultant neurologist who made a diagnosis of juvenile myoclonic epilepsy and started Miss SL on sodium valproate 200 mg twice daily.

Q1 What is epilepsy and what are the main types of seizure?
Q2 Do you agree with the choice of therapy for Miss SL?
Q3 What are the therapeutic aims of drug therapy?
Q4 Why is monotherapy generally preferred for the treatment of epilepsy?

Over the next few months Miss SL returned to her GP who gradually increased the dose of sodium valproate to 400 mg twice daily. Miss SL's condition improved on this dose and her jerks reduced to one a month.

Q5 Outline a pharmaceutical care plan for Miss SL.
Q6 What general points should be discussed with patients starting anti-epileptic drug treatment?
Q7 What adverse effects of sodium valproate therapy should Miss SL be warned about?
Q8 How should Miss SL's sodium valproate therapy be monitored?

Year 4 Miss SL, now 14, had been noticing worsening myoclonic jerks. She was admitted to the paediatric ward of the local hospital after she experienced an 'attack' that her mother described as a worsening of the jerks that had thrown her to the floor and resulted in a loss of consciousness. The house officer added carbamazepine 100 mg four times daily to her therapy of sodium valproate 400 mg twice daily.

Q9 Was the house officer right to prescribe carbamazepine for Miss SL?
Q10 Comment on the dose of carbamazepine?

After discharge, Miss SL struggled to remember to take her midday dose and so her GP changed her medication to a modified-release carbamazepine preparation.

Q11 What must be considered when changing plain carbamazepine to a modified-release preparation?

Over the next few months Miss SL was delighted that her myoclonic spasms improved but her mother noticed that her absences had increased.
    Her GP thus increased the dose of sodium valproate to 500 mg three times daily and on her next visit to the neurology clinic her carbamazepine was stopped.

Q12 Would it have been better to use a long-acting preparation of sodium valproate?

Year 8   Now 18 years old, Miss SL attended her GP's surgery when she discovered that she was 10 weeks pregnant. The pregnancy was unplanned and she had not been taking any form of contraception; however, she had decided that she wanted to go ahead and have the baby. She asked whether she could stop taking her medication whilst she was pregnant.

Q13 What are the risks to a baby born to an epileptic woman?
Q14 What is the current thinking regarding discontinuation of antiepileptic drugs during pregnancy?

Her GP was concerned that Miss SL was taking sodium valproate but was unsure how to proceed with managing her pregnancy. He therefore prescribed folic acid therapy and referred her to the neurologist.

Q15 Why is Miss SL's GP concerned about her taking sodium valproate therapy during her pregnancy?
Q16 What dose of folic acid should be prescribed and for how long?

Q17 What options does the neurologist have for managing Miss SL during her pregnancy?

The neurologist decided to change Miss SL's medication from sodium valproate to lamotrigine and so he prepared a treatment plan for her GP to follow. He also telephoned the Belfast Pregnancy Register to inform them of Miss SL's pregnancy.

Q18 Is lamotrigine safe in pregnancy?
Q19 What are the main side-effects associated with lamotrigine therapy?
Q20 How should the change from sodium valproate to lamotrigine therapy be managed?
Q21 What is the Belfast Pregnancy Register?

The GP agreed to manage the change in Miss SL's medication and saw her regularly. She had no problems with the change apart from feeling increasingly tired, which she attributed to her pregnancy. She was worried about whether her baby would be born healthy. At week 36 of her pregnancy, she was prescribed oral vitamin K.

Q22 Why was vitamin K prescribed and what dose would you recommend?

At week 40, Miss SL gave birth to a healthy baby boy. She asked about future contraception.

Q23 What general advice would you give to Miss SL after her baby has been born?
Q24 What would you advise her and her GP about future contraception needs?

What is epilepsy and what are the main types of seizure?

A1 **Epilepsy can be defined as a continuing tendency towards epileptic seizures. A seizure is defined as a sudden, brief, abnormal discharge of cerebral neurones which is accompanied by motor, sensory, autonomic or behavioural symptoms. Many different terms have been used to describe the various types of epilepsy; however, most neurologists now use the classification produced by the International League against Epilepsy. In this classification seizures are divided into two types: generalised and partial (or focal).**

An abbreviated version of the classification is as follows:

(a)   Generalised seizures:

  (i)   Absence seizures (petit mal): brief episodes of unconsciousness with little or no motor accompaniment.
  (ii) Myoclonic seizures: single or multiple sudden or uncontrollable jerks.
  (iii) Tonic/clonic seizures (grand mal): unconsciousness and generalised tonic/clonic convulsions.

(b)   Partial seizures (seizures beginning locally):

  (i)   Simple partial seizures: without impairment of consciousness. Symptoms may be motor, sensory, aphasic, cognitive etc., depending on the anatomical site of seizure discharge.
  (ii) Complex partial: may have simple partial onset, followed by impaired consciousness, or impairment of consciousness at onsct. A prodrome is commonly experienced.

Partial seizures are often associated with secondary generalised tonic/clonic seizures.

Juvenile myoclonic epilepsy (JME) is an idiopathic generalised epileptic syndrome characterised by myoclonic jerks, generalised tonic/clonic seizures and sometimes absence seizures.

Do you agree with the choice of therapy for Miss SL?

A2 **Yes. JME is the most common primary generalised epilepsy. Sodium valproate is usually the drug of choice for first-line treatment of primary generalised absences and myoclonic seizures.**

Seizure classification has some importance in determining groups of drugs which will be of most value for the treatment of specific seizure types. Some anti-epileptic drugs are more effective than others in certain forms of epilepsy, depending on their mode of action.

There are three basic mechanisms for the action of antiepileptic drugs:

(a) Suppression of sodium influx. The antiepileptic drug binds to the sodium channels when they are in the inactive state, thus prolonging the inactive state which in turn decreases the ability of the neurons to fire at high frequency. Seizures that depend on high-frequency discharge are therefore suppressed. Carbamazepine and phenytoin exert their main action in this way and are particularly effective in limiting the spread of a discharge from a focus.

(b) Suppression of calcium influx. The antiepileptic drug acts by inhibiting the influx of calcium ions through T-type calcium channels. These calcium channels generate T-currents which usually play a minimal role in action potential generation, but in some neurons in the hypothalamus, T-currents cause action potentials. Absence seizures are caused by increased firing of hypothalamic neurons and, thus, drugs that act by this mechanism are preferred for absence seizures. Sodium valproate and ethosuximide act in this way.

(c) Potentiation of gamma-aminobutyric acid (GABA). GABA is an inhibitory neurotransmitter that is widely distributed in the brain and causes a general decrease in neuronal excitation. Antiepileptic drugs potentiate GABA, either by acting directly on the GABA receptors (e.g. phenobarbital), by promoting GABA release (e.g. gabapentin) or by inhibiting the enzyme that degrades GABA (e.g. vigabatrin).

The choice for Miss SL would be a drug that helped to reduce absence seizures, but also suppressed seizures caused by the high frequency discharge of neurons.

Sodium valproate suppresses high-frequency neuronal firing by blocking sodium channels. It also suppresses calcium influx through T-type calcium channels. It is therefore more effective in the treatment of absences than phenytoin or carbamazepine. In addition, about 25% of children with absence seizures will go on to have tonic/clonic seizures, so it is best to prescribe a drug like sodium valproate which will control both types of seizure.

Sodium valproate and lamotrigine are considered the drugs of choice for primary generalised seizures, and should be prescribed if there is doubt around the classification of seizure type. Both drugs are also effective for absence and myoclonic seizures, and either would have been a suitable choice for Miss SL.

For partial and secondary generalised seizures, carbamazepine, sodium valproate, lamotrigine and oxcarbazepine are regarded as first-line treatments. It has been suggested that there is little difference in effectiveness between phenytoin, sodium valproate, phenobarbital and carbamazepine, so it is important to consider the differences in toxicity and dosage regimens when choosing a drug.

What are the therapeutic aims of drug therapy?

A3   **To suppress seizures with the minimum of side-effects.**

A diagnosis of epilepsy is usually considered when an individual has had two or more seizures in a short interval, although initiation of anti-convulsant treatment after a single seizure may be considered (depending on individual circumstances such as age, type of seizure or implications of further fits on social and/or employment prospects). When anticonvulsants are prescribed the overall aim is to suppress seizures completely without producing troublesome side-effects, in a regimen that is as simple as possible. This then allows the patient to live as normal a life as possible.

Why is monotherapy generally preferred for the treatment of epilepsy?

A4   **To minimise side-effects, maximise compliance and facilitate therapy monitoring.**

As with most drug therapy, the administration of more than one drug to a patient increases the likelihood of adverse reactions and produces a potential for drug interactions. In addition, patient compliance may be reduced with the prescribing of increased numbers of drugs.

In the treatment of epilepsy there is no evidence that the use of several drugs in low dosage will produce additive therapeutic effects without additive toxicity. In addition, the interpretation of plasma levels of drugs becomes more difficult when two or more drugs are given concurrently, as most therapeutic ranges have been determined using monotherapy. Two drugs may, however, be useful in patients with mixed seizure types, such as myoclonic jerks and tonic/clonic fits appearing together.

In general, therapy should be initiated with one drug and the dose adjusted until seizures are controlled and/or levels within the therapeutic range are achieved. If seizures are not controlled despite adequate plasma levels, the dose of the ineffective drug should be gradually reduced and an alternative agent introduced.

Outline a pharmaceutical care plan for Miss SL.

A5   **Patients with epilepsy have a chronic condition which may have a fluctuating course. This will have a very significant effect on their social and working lives and they will usually have to take long-term drug therapy.**

The key elements of a pharmaceutical care plan for a patient such as Miss SL should include:

(a)   Contributing to the choice of an optimum drug regimen.
(b)   Preparing and contributing to a monitoring strategy for the drug therapy chosen. Monitoring may include therapeutic drug monitoring and/or the recording of seizures experienced.
(c)   Providing patient education and counselling, including expected outcomes of treatment and potential side-effects.
(d)   Helping to arrange how further supplies of medication will be obtained.
(e)   Helping ensure concordance with therapy.

What general points should be discussed with patients starting anti-epileptic drug treatment?

A6   **(a)   The aims of drug treatment, in particular the balance between optimum clinical effect in terms of elimination of seizures and the incidence of adverse effects.**

(b)   The name(s), doses, general actions, common adverse effects of the drug(s) prescribed.

(c)   The importance of strict compliance if treatment failure is to be avoided. Simplified regimens, divided pillboxes, diary cards and other measures may be of value.

(d)   The need to avoid running out of medication.

(e)   The need for regular medication, even during periods of illness. Missed doses or abrupt drug withdrawal can cause treatment failure and seizure recurrence or an increase in seizure frequency. Missed doses should be taken as soon as possible, but not doubled up when the next dose is due.

(f)   Advice to report any possible side-effects to a doctor or pharmacist.

(g)   If the patient is 'of child-bearing potential', she should be advised of the risks of pregnancy and encouraged to use contraception appropriately.

(h)   If the patient is able to drive (s)he should be advised to notify the DVLA. Further information is available on www.dvla.gov.uk/at_a_glance.

The patient should also be made aware of the British Epilepsy Association (New Anstey House, Gateway Drive, Yeadon, Leeds LS19 7XY) or a local branch or support group. The British Epilepsy Association can be found on-line as Epilepsy Action at www.epilepsy.org.uk. Helplines are also available: Freephone helpline 0808 800 5050 or e-mail helpline@ epilepsy.org.uk.

What adverse effects of sodium valproate therapy should Miss SL be warned about?

A7   **Miss SL should be counselled on a number of potential adverse effects.**

Advice should include:

(a)   How to recognise the signs of blood and liver disorders. Thrombocy-topenia and liver damage are very rare but serious side-effects of sodium valproate therapy and so should be carefully monitored for.

(b)   The possibility that the drug may increase her appetite and hence lead to weight gain.

(c)   The possibility of hair loss. Although there may be some hair loss in the early stages of treatment, she can be reassured that it will regrow without the need to stop therapy.

(d)   That sodium valproate can cause nausea, tremor and irregular periods.

How should Miss SL's sodium valproate therapy be monitored?

A8   Primarily by clinical monitoring for efficacy and side-effects. Regular liver function tests should be performed, especially during the first six months of therapy.

Plasma valproate concentrations are not a useful index of efficacy and so routine valproate blood level monitoring is not necessary; however, monitoring of drug concentration may be desirable if Miss SL shows signs of toxicity or if her compliance is in question.

If a blood level is required for a patient on a short-acting preparation, the trough concentration should be measured. The use of the long-acting preparation makes the measurement of plasma levels less dependent on the time of sampling.

Blood levels may be necessary for patients on phenytoin and, to a lesser extent, carbamazepine therapy, where the kinetics are not linear and the patient may experience toxicity with small dose changes. Nevertheless, even with phenytoin, dose changes should be made more on the basis of clinical response than on the blood level.

As liver damage is a rare, but serious, side-effect of sodium valproate therapy, liver function tests should be monitored, especially in the first six months of treatment.

Was the house officer right to prescribe carbamazepine for Miss SL?

A9   No. Carbamazepine may worsen primary generalised epilepsy by precipitating myoclonic seizures and aggravating absences.

Carbamazepine acts by the suppression of high-frequency neuronal discharge in and around seizure foci by delaying recovery of sodium channels from their inactive state. However, it also causes a reduction in GABA, thus removing the inhibition of general neuronal excitation across the brain. This can lead to aggravation of primary generalised epilepsy.

Comment on the dose of carbamazepine.

A10   Introducing carbamazepine at a dose of 100 mg four times daily may cause problems with compliance and also increased side-effects.

Carbamazepine has a number of adverse effects which may be a problem for some patients. The most common of these are nausea, headache, drowsiness, sedation, ataxia and diplopia. These can be minimised by introducing the drug at a low dose (e.g. 100 mg twice daily) and increasing in increments of 200 mg every one to two weeks until optimal clinical effects are obtained.

Carbamazepine induces liver enzymes which increase its own metabolism and that of some other drugs. The half-life of carbamazepine after a single dose is 24–36 hours. This falls to 10–20 hours on chronic dosing, thus, dose requirements are likely to increase with time as carbamazepine clearance increases. The full effect of this enzyme induction may not be seen for up to one month after the start of therapy.

What must be considered when changing plain carbamazepine to a modified-release preparation?

A11 **The use of a modified-release preparation (e.g. Tegretol Retard) smoothes out the plasma concentration curve and eliminates some of the side-effects seen two to three hours after a conventional dose. However, the modified-release formulation is 20–30% less bioavailable than an equivalent dose of standard preparations. For this reason some physicians recommend increasing the dose of carbamazepine when changing to the modified-release formulation, although this is not recommended in the *British National Formulary* (BNF). For example, a total daily dose of carbamazepine 800 mg would be changed to a total daily dose of Tegretol Retard 1000 mg.**

The bioavailabilty of carbamazepine differs by 85–100% between different formulations. It is therefore important that, when the drug is prescribed for epilepsy, it is prescribed by brand name to avoid fluctuations due to differences in bioavailability.

Would it have been better to use a long-acting preparation of sodium valproate?

A12 **Using a long-acting modified-release preparation of sodium valproate could aid compliance. In addition, the modified-release formulation reduces peak concentrations and ensures more even plasma concentrations throughout the day.**

In patients where control has been achieved, the long-acting preparation (Epilim Chrono) is interchangeable with the conventional preparation on an equivalent daily dosage basis, and should be given in one or two divided doses.

What are the risks to a baby born to an epileptic woman?

A13   **All mothers with epilepsy have an increased risk of giving birth to babies with congenital abnormalities regardless of whether or not they are taking an antiepileptic drug. Malformations include cleft lip and palate, cardiac defects (ventricular septal defects), neural tube defects, and urogenital defects.**

The risk of congenital malformations in the general population is 2–3%, with the risk to infants of epileptic mothers significantly higher. The risk of malformations in any individual pregnancy in women with epilepsy taking a single antiepileptic drug is about 4–6%.

Premature births and low birth weight is also more common in epileptic women, while still births and neonatal deaths are twice that of the general population. There is also a higher risk of mental retardation, learning disabilities and epilepsy in infants born to epileptic mothers.

The aetiology of congenital malformations is multifactorial and so epileptic patients should also be advised to avoid alcohol and smoking, and to have a balanced diet before and during pregnancy.

What is the current thinking regarding discontinuation of antiepileptic drugs in pregnancy?

A14   **A risk analysis is needed for each patient. The decision to discontinue therapy must balance the risk to the foetus from the side-effects of the antiepileptic drug against the risk to the foetus from the mother falling during a seizure. In general it is considered more risky to the foetus for medication to be changed during pregnancy than to continue with the antiepileptic preparation throughout pregnancy.**

When seizures are absences or simple partial, the prospective mother often chooses to stop all medication, but when the seizures are tonic/clonic, it is usual to continue with one drug at modest dosage.

Withdrawal of treatment for patients like Miss SL with JME is not usually possible without seizures recurring and life-long therapy is generally required.

The frequency of seizures may change during pregnancy. A third of patients will have an increase, whilst the rest will have no change or a decrease. This change in seizure frequency is possibly due to the physiological changes and stress associated with pregnancy. Increased steroid hormone levels, sleep deprivation and metabolic changes are also thought to play a part. The physiological changes occurring during pregnancy can also influence the kinetics and pharmacological actions of drugs through a variety of mechanisms including:

(a)   Alterations in gastrointestinal function which affect the rate and extent of drug absorption.
(b)   Increased renal elimination.
(c)   Variable changes in hepatic metabolism and elimination.
(d)   Greater plasma volume in the later stage of pregnancy resulting in an increased volume of distribution.
(e)   Alterations in plasma protein and plasma free fatty acid concentrations causing changes in drug binding.

Patients with epilepsy who are not pregnant can have their drug treatment successfully withdrawn, although there is a significant failure rate (seizures may occur in 12–36% of patients). The decision to discontinue therapy in an individual patient will be influenced by their medical history, their social and employment situation, their age and their personal preference. The possibility of seizure recurrence, with consequent effects on driving and employment, is obviously an important factor to consider.

Drug withdrawal may be considered after a seizure-free period of two to three years and studies have indicated the factors which identify patients who are likely to remain seizure-free after drug withdrawal. In addition, the relative risks of drug continuation versus the risks associated with drug withdrawal should be considered. If a decision is made to withdraw drug treatment it should be done gradually over three to six months to prevent precipitation of rebound seizures.

Why is Miss SL's GP concerned about her taking sodium valproate therapy during her pregnancy?

A15 **Sodium valproate is specifically associated with neural tube defects and about one in 100 women taking valproate during pregnancy will give birth to a child with spina bifida or anencephaly. It is thus recommended that screening is carried out at the end of the first trimester.**

Higher doses of sodium valproate are associated with an increased risk of malformation, including neural tube defects, orofacial defects, congenital heart abnormalities and hypospadias.

What dose of folic acid should be prescribed and for how long?

A16 **Folic acid 5 mg daily should be prescribed until week 16.**

Folic acid is given to prevent the occurrence of neural tube defects in the foetus. The need for prophylactic folic acid therapy should be discussed when a female patient becomes fertile, so that ideally treatment with folic acid can be commenced pre-conception.

It is now accepted that all women should take 400 micrograms folic acid daily from pre-conception and throughout the first trimester of pregnancy; however, women taking antiepileptic drugs are at greater risk of having a child with neural tube defects and, in addition certain anti-epileptic drugs, including sodium valproate, phenytoin and carbamazepine are folic acid antagonists, and women taking these have been shown to have low folate levels during pregnancy. For these reasons epileptic mothers require a higher level of folic acid than the general population and should be prescribed a dose of 5 mg daily.

What options does the neurologist have for managing Miss SL during her pregnancy?

A17 **There are a number of options available for managing Miss SL during her pregnancy:**

   (a) Keep her on sodium valproate and monitor her closely.

   (b) Keep her on sodium valproate, but reduce the dose and monitor her closely.

   (c) Change her from sodium valproate to lamotrigine therapy.

   (d) Change her from sodium valproate to levetiracetam therapy.

If the decision is made not to change the drug therapy, the foetus is at greater risk of developing neural tube defects. Reducing the dose of sodium valproate may lessen the risks to the foetus from neural tube defects, but it may also increase the risk of harm from a fall caused by seizure.

Changing to lamotrigine will reduce the risk of neural tube defects but as it will not stop Miss SL's myoclonic jerks there is still a danger to the foetus from falls caused by a seizure. Levetiracetam is a newer, effective, well-tolerated broad-spectrum antiepileptic drug with few interactions. Although it is not licensed for use in pregnancy it is growing in popularity and is considered safe by many neurologists.

Miss SL is at week 10 of her pregnancy. As most neural tube defects occur in the first trimester, there is probably little reason for changing Miss SL's therapy at this point in her pregnancy.

Is lamotrigine safe in pregnancy?

A18 **Lamotrigine is considered to be the drug of choice in women of child-bearing age as its teratogenic profile is better than other antiepileptic drugs and the risk of major malformations is reduced.**

As lamotrigine is a weak folate inhibitor there is a theoretical risk of malformation; however, no teratogenic effects are reported in the manufacturer's data sheet. There is as yet insufficient evidence on which to base advice on the safety of lamotrigine in pregnancy and the data sheet advises that it should only be used if benefit outweighs risk.

What are the main side-effects associated with lamotrigine therapy?

A19 **The main side-effect of lamotrigine is adverse skin reactions, usually occurring within the first eight weeks of therapy and increased by the concomitant prescribing of sodium valproate. These are usually self-limiting but may occasionally be severe and associated with systemic illness.**

Side-effects increase in the presence of sodium valproate which inhibits the major route of elimination of lamotrigine (glucuronidation). Clearance of lamotrigine is halved and the plasma concentration of a given dose is doubled. Any change from sodium valproate to lamotrigine as monotherapy therefore has to be carefully managed.

The BNF advises that hepatic, renal and clotting parameters should be monitored closely during lamotrigine therapy, while the Committee for Safety in Medicine has advised that prescribers should be alert for symptoms associated with aplastic anaemia or bone marrow depression.

How should the change from sodium valproate to lamotrigine therapy be managed?

A20 **Lamotrigine should be added in gradually to the regimen whilst maintaining the dose of sodium valproate (rash is less likely to occur if lamotrigine is started at low dose and increased slowly). Miss SL should be advised to follow the**

dosage regimen carefully, report any rashes or other side-
effects and report any change in fit type or frequency
(myoclonic jerks are likely to increase as sodium valproate is
withdrawn).

A sample cross-over regimen is as follows:

Dose titration schedule for switching from sodium valproate to lamotrigine monotherapy		
Week	Lamotrigine	Sodium valproate
1–2	25 mg alternate days	maintenance dose
3–4	25 mg/day	maintenance dose
5–6	50 mg/day	maintenance dose
7–8	75 mg/day	maintenance dose
9–10	100 mg/day*	maintenance dose
Continue	Increase by 25 mg every two weeks if required**	Reduce by 200–500 mg every two weeks

* The dose of lamotrigine may be increased to 200 mg/day (by 25 mg every two weeks before withdrawal of sodium valproate).
** Lamotrigine therapy should not exceed 300 mg/day when used as add-on therapy to sodium valproate.

This would mean that Miss SL would be at week 25 of her pregnancy by
the time the substitution has taken place.

What is the Belfast Pregnancy Register?

A21 **The Belfast Pregnancy Register was set up to monitor the
safety of drugs in epilepsy. The recording of successful births
and problems associated with certain drug regimens can
help build up a picture of drug safety to inform epileptic
mothers of risks in the future.**

Pregnant women with epilepsy should be encouraged to register their
details as soon as possible. The register can be contacted on: 01232
894968 or 0800 3891248.

Why was vitamin K prescribed and what dose would you recommend?

A22 **It was prescribed to help prevent neonatal haemorrhage and early haemolytic disease of the newborn. A dose of 10 mg daily would be appropriate.**

Infants born to epileptic mothers are at increased risk of neonatal haemorrhage, particularly if the mother is taking an enzyme inducing epileptic drug (phenytoin, primidone, phenobarbital and carbamazepine). Vitamin K deficiency is associated with early haemolytic disease of the newborn and, as vitamin K crosses the placenta, it is recommended that the mother takes oral vitamin K from 36 weeks gestation until delivery. There is some debate in the literature about what dose of vitamin K should be prescribed. Currently 10–20 mg daily is recommended.

If a mother is taking enzyme-inducing antiepileptic drugs, then her infant is also at increased risk of late haemolytic disease of the newborn and should be given vitamin K intramuscularly at birth.

What general advice would you give to Miss SL after her baby has been born?

A23 **Advice should be given regarding breast-feeding, safe practice in caring for her child and remaining seizure-free.**

All antiepileptic drugs pass into breast milk to varying degrees. Breast feeding is usually encouraged as it enables the infant to withdraw more slowly from the antiepileptic drugs that it has been exposed to during pregnancy. In Miss SL's case, lamotrigine passes into breast milk in concentrations of about 40–45% of the plasma concentration, but no adverse effects have been reported. However, the infant should be monitored for side-effects such as anaemia, bruising or infection suggestive of bone marrow failure.

Miss SL should be given extra support in learning to care for her new baby, with safe practice encouraged to reduce the risks to the infant from her suffering a fall during a seizure. Advice should be given on safe ways of carrying the baby up stairs, changing, feeding and bathing.

Miss SL's medication should now be reviewed, especially as there was a change of medication during her pregnancy.

What would you advise her and her GP about future contraception needs?

A24 **Many pregnancies in patients with epilepsy are not planned and Miss SL should be given advice on the need for future contraception. Lamotrigine (and also sodium valproate, levetiracetam, gabapentin and tiagabine) do not alter the efficacy of oral contraceptives and so Miss SL can be advised to use a standard dose.**

Many antiepileptic drugs (e.g. phenytoin, phenobarbitone, primidone and carbamazepine) are potent inducers of liver microsomal enzymes that metabolise oestrogen and progestogen. This leads to a reduction in the effectiveness and an increased risk of contraceptive failure with standard doses of oral contraceptives. Patients taking enzyme-inducing antiepileptic drugs should thus be prescribed appropriate doses of contraceptives. The following considerations apply:

Combined oral contraceptives should be prescribed with a minimum daily oestrogen dose of 50 micrograms, increasing to 80–100 micrograms if breakthrough bleeding occurs. Tri-cycling (i.e. taking three or four packets of a monophasic preparation without a break followed by a short tablet-free interval of four days) is also recommended as an option.

The oral progestogen-only pill is not recommended, as efficacy cannot be guaranteed due to the increased metabolism of progestogen.

Depot progesterone (Depo-Provera) may be prescribed concurrently with enzyme-inducing drugs, but needs to be given every 10 weeks instead of every 12 weeks to ensure adequate levels of progesterone for contraception.

Intra-uterine devices can be used with antiepileptic drugs, and some specialists prefer the use of the intra-uterine progestogen-only system (Mirena) for their epileptic patients.

If emergency contraception is required for a patient taking an enzyme-inducing antiepileptic drug, it is recommended that the standard dose be increased by 50%.

Further reading

Anon. Epilepsy and pregnancy. *Drugs Ther Bull* 1994; **32**: 49–51.
Anon. Managing childhood epilepsy. *Drugs Ther Bull* 2001; **39**: 12–16.
Bar-Oz B, Nulman I, Koren G et al. Anticonvulsants in pregnancy: a critical review. *Paediatr Drugs* 2000; **2**: 113–126.
Browne T, Holmes G. Epilepsy. *N Engl J Med* 2001; **344**: 1145–1151.

Chadwick D, Orme M, Appleton B. *The Management of Epilepsy in General Practice*. Alden Press, Oxford, 1991.

Commission on Classification and Terminology of the International League Against Epilepsy. Proposal for classification of epilepsies and epileptic syndromes. *Epilepsia* 1989; **30**: 389–399.

Costs and Options in Epilepsy. Medicom UK, Esher, 2000: 4–22.

Devinsky O, Cramer J. Safety and efficacy of standard and new anti-epileptic drugs. *Neurology* 2000; **55**(suppl. 3): S5–S10.

Hernandez Diaz S, Werler MM, Walker AM *et al*. Folic acid antagonists during pregnancy and the risk of birth defects. *N Engl J Med* 2000; **343**: 1609–1614.

Holmes LB, Harvey EA, Coull BA *et al*. The teratogenicity of anticonvulsant drugs. *N Engl J Med* 2001; **344**: 1132–1138.

Macdonald RL, Kelly KM, Antiepileptic drug mechanisms of action. *Epilepsia* 1993; **34**(suppl. 5): S1–8.

Marson AG, Williamson PR, Hutton JL *et al*. Carbamazepine versus valproate monotherapy for epilepsy (Cochrane Review). In: *Cochrane Library 2*. Update Software, Oxford, 2001.

Perucca E, Gram L, Avanzini G *et al*. Antiepileptic drugs as a cause of worsening seizures. *Epilepsia* 1998; **39**: 5–17.

Scottish Intercollegiate Guidelines Network. *Diagnosis and Management of Epilepsy in Adults*. SIGN, Edinburgh, 2001.

Scottish Obstetrics Guidelines and Audit Project. *The Management of Pregnancy in Women with Epilepsy*. SOGAP, Edinburgh, 1997.

Yerby M. Quality of life, epilepsy, advances and the evolving role of anticonvulsants in women with epilepsy. *Neurology* 2000; **55**(suppl. 1): S21–S31.

15

Parkinson's disease

Robert C A Hirst

Day 1 (1995) Mr LN, a 67-year-old retired bookmaker, was admitted to the neurology ward. His presenting complaints included difficulty in getting up from chairs and initiating walking.

Eighteen months earlier he had noticed that his self-winding wrist-watch, which he wore on his right wrist, was consistently losing time. When moved to his left wrist the watch kept perfect time. Friends had pointed out that he had developed a limp, dragging his right foot. These symptoms had worsened over the following 18 months, and he had also developed a resting tremor in his right hand and leg.

His GP suspected Parkinson's disease and referred Mr LN to a neurologist for confirmation of the diagnosis.

Q1 What are the main symptoms of Parkinson's disease?
Q2 Is it possible to make a definitive diagnosis of idiopathic Parkinson's disease (IPD)?
Q3 What biochemical defects are thought to be present in a patient such as Mr LN?
Q4 Outline a pharmaceutical care plan for Mr LN.
Q5 Which drugs are usually considered for the initial treatment of patients with idiopathic Parkinson's disease and what are their modes of action?

Day 2 Mr LN was started on Sinemet Plus, one tablet three times daily.

Q6 Do you agree with this choice?
Q7 How should Mr LN's levodopa therapy be adjusted to optimise his response?
Q8 How can the adverse effects of levodopa be minimised?

Day 13   The dose of levodopa had been gradually increased over the preceding days to two tablets of Sinemet Plus three times daily and Mr LN was discharged on this dose.

Month 63 (2001)   Mr LN was admitted for reassessment.

Day 1 (of readmission)   Mr LN's therapy and symptoms had remained unchanged until recently when he had started to notice shaking of his arms occurring about one hour after each dose of Sinemet Plus. This shaking lasted for about 45 minutes before stopping. Mr LN also complained of painful dystonic cramps at night, which caused him to wake early most mornings. He had attempted to counter this by taking an extra Sinemet Plus tablet shortly before going to bed, which sometimes helped. His wife added that he was becoming profoundly immobile up to two hours before his Sinemet doses were due during the day.

On examination he was found to have a mask-like face and a resting tremor of both hands and legs. 'Cog-wheel' rigidity was found in all four limbs. He had difficulty initiating speech and his voice was very quiet. He struggled to rise from his chair, and had a characteristic 'parkinsonian shuffle' when walking. When his shoulders were pulled forward from standing he staggered forward and had to be supported to stop him falling.

Mr LN complained of occasional falls and was not confident to leave the house. He relied on his wife to do everything for him. He admitted to being depressed about his condition.

There was no other medical history of note. All routine laboratory tests were within normal ranges. His drug therapy was two Sinemet Plus tablets at 8 a.m., 2 p.m. and 7 p.m. and, occasionally, one Sinemet Plus tablet at 11 p.m.

Q9   Which of the long-term complications of levodopa therapy is Mr LN suffering from?

Q10   What alterations to Mr LN's drug therapy would you recommend in order to try to minimise these effects?

Q11   How could you monitor and assess Mr LN's response to these changes?

Q12   Can you suggest any non-drug management that might benefit Mr LN?

Day 2   Mr LN's drug therapy was changed to one Sinemet Plus tablet at 7 a.m., 10 a.m., 1 p.m., 4 p.m., 7 p.m. and 10 p.m. In addition, he was prescribed one Sinemet CR tablet at 10 p.m. A tablet of Madopar dispersible 62.5 mg was prescribed on the 'as required' side of the drug chart to be given upon waking in the morning. The nursing staff were asked to complete an hourly 'on–off' chart. Part of the chart for days one and five are shown below:

Time	Day 1	Day 5
7 a.m.	off	off (dose)
8 a.m.	off (dose)	on (dyskinesia)
9 a.m.	on (dyskinesia)	on
10 a.m.	on (dyskinesia)	off (dose)
11 a.m.	on	on (dyskinesia)
12 noon	off	on
1 p.m.	off	on (dose)
2 p.m.	off (dose)	on (dyskinesia)
3 p.m.	on (dyskinesia)	on

Mr LN's mobility and dyskinesias were improved; however, he remained depressed about his condition.

Q13 Would an oral dopamine agonist benefit Mr LN?
Q14 Would Mr LN benefit from an antidepressant?
Q15 If so, which would you choose?

Day 8 It was decided to start Mr LN on cabergoline. He was prescribed 1 mg at night for one week and discharged on 2 mg at night. The GP was requested to increase the dose by 1 mg per week, according to response, to a maximum dose of 4 mg at night.

Day 70 Mr LN was admitted as an emergency by his GP, having developed visual and auditory hallucinations over the previous week. He was hearing voices talking about him, threatening to kill him. He was also seeing insects crawling up the walls and burrowing into his skin. On examination he was clearly distressed and very frightened. His medication on admission was one Sinemet Plus tablet six times a day, one Sinemet CR tablet at night, cabergoline 4 mg at night and occasionally one Madopar 62.5 mg dispersible tablet upon waking.

Q16 Which drugs might have contributed to Mr LN's symptoms?
Q17 What adjustments would you recommend be made to Mr LN's medication?

Day 74 The recommendations were carried out. Mr LN's visual hallucinations improved; however, he was still experiencing distressing auditory hallucinations and the control of his Parkinson's symptoms had deteriorated, such that he was experiencing frequent 'off' periods.

Q18 What course of action would you suggest to improve Mr LN's symptoms?

Mr LN was started on quetiapine 25 mg at night. The dose was increased over the next 10 days to 50 mg twice daily. His dopaminergic therapy was adjusted to one Sinemet Plus tablet six times daily, one Sinemet CR tablet at night, cabergoline 1 mg at night and one Madopar 62.5 mg dispersible tablet upon waking. His hallucinations resolved, and acceptable control of his Parkinson's disease symptoms was achieved. He was discharged on this regimen.

Q19 What is the long-term outlook for Mr LN?

What are the main symptoms of Parkinson's disease?

A1 **The main symptoms found in patients with Parkinson's disease are tremor, rigidity, bradykinesia (slowness of movement), akinesia (loss of movement) and postural abnormalities.**

Onset of Parkinson's disease is usually insidious and progression is slow. Many patients first notice a resting tremor. This usually initially affects the hands and may be unilateral. The tremor disappears on movement and during sleep and may be worse under stress. The patient is usually over 50 years old on presentation.

Rigidity manifests as an increased resistance to passive movement and is classically termed 'cog-wheel' rigidity, with a ratchet-like phenomenon felt at the wrist on passive movement of the hand.

Bradykinesia is reflected in immobile features and a fixed, staring appearance. Together with the rigidity, it is responsible for the typical abnormalities of gait: difficulty in starting and finishing steps, resulting in shuffling; a stooped head; flexed neck, upper extremities and knees; and a lack of normal arm swing.

Loss of postural reflexes leads to postural imbalance and sometimes to frequent falls. Other common symptoms include micrographia, drooling of saliva, constipation, difficulty in swallowing and speech alteration. Symptoms increase in number and severity as the disease progresses.

Is it possible to make a definitive diagnosis of idiopathic Parkinson's disease (IPD)?

A2 **Currently the only way of making a definite diagnosis of IPD is by post-mortem study of the brain.**

IPD is the most common cause of parkinsonism, accounting for approximately 75% of cases presenting to neurologists. Other causes of parkinsonian signs include other neurodegenerative diseases such as progressive supranuclear palsy (PSP) and multiple system atrophy (MSA), intoxication with heavy metals, treatment with therapeutic drugs (neuroleptics, metoclopramide), and chronic cerebrovascular disease.

The definitive diagnosis of Parkinson's disease is based on characteristic neuropathologic findings of Lewy bodies and neuronal loss in the substantia nigra and other brainstem nuclei. Studies have shown that only 65–75% of patients diagnosed as having early Parkinson's disease had the characteristic findings at post-mortem.

Currently there are no established diagnostic tests available to support a diagnosis of IPD, but they may be available soon. They include positron emission tomography scanning using the tracer [^{18}F]fluorodopa, and single photon emission computed tomography using dopaminergic tracers to image the brain.

It is important to try to exclude other causes of parkinsonism before commencing treatment. PSP and MSA respond poorly to conventional levodopa therapy, and any drugs which may be causing the symptoms should be stopped or substituted for a more suitable alternative.

What biochemical defects are thought to be present in a patient such as Mr LN?

A3   **Several biochemical defects are thought to be present in patients with Parkinson's disease.**

A combination of cholinergic (excitatory) and dopaminergic (inhibitory) mechanisms acting in the striatal tracts of the basal ganglia of the brain are thought to be responsible for the smooth control of voluntary movements. Imbalances in the neurotransmitters lead to movement disorders. In patients with Parkinson's disease, dopamine concentrations in the three major parts of the basal ganglia are reduced to a fraction of normal. Compensatory mechanisms operate and symptoms are not noted until a severe loss of dopaminergic neurons has occurred. The severity of some symptoms, such as bradykinesia, has been found to correlate with striatal dopamine levels; however, abnormalities of other neurotransmitters, including noradrenaline (norepinephrine), 5-hydroxytryptamine (serotonin) and gamma-aminobutyric acid, have also been reported. The full relevance of these changes is as yet unclear.

Outline a pharmaceutical care plan for Mr LN.

A4   **The goals of symptomatic drug treatment are to help the patient to keep functioning independently for as long as possible, and to achieve this with the minimum of adverse effects.**

Patients with Parkinson's disease have a chronic deteriorating condition which will result in life-long drug therapy of increasing complexity.

A long-term pharmaceutical care plan would include:

(a)   Involving Mr LN in the choice of appropriate initial therapy.

(b)   Ensuring the development of appropriate treatment outcome meas-
       ures and a suitable treatment monitoring programme.

(c)   Ensuring that the patient understands the role of drugs in the
       symptomatic treatment of the disease and their possible adverse
       effects.

(d)   Ensuring the patient and carers understand the importance of
       compliance and timing of drug doses.

(e)   Anticipating problems such as the potential for nausea and vomit-
       ing with levodopa preparations and offering appropriate advice on
       prevention.

(f)   Counselling the patient and carers about drugs which should be
       avoided in Parkinson's disease. These include medicines which act
       as dopamine antagonists, such as metoclopramide and the older
       antipsychotics (e.g. chlorpromazine, haloperidol).

(g)   As the disease progresses and more drugs are added, medicine taking
       may become problematic and advice on methods for improving and
       maintaining adequate compliance should be given.

(h)   As most patients with IPD will be elderly, the general considerations
       given to elderly patients should also be applied.

As treatment may continue for many years and become increasingly
complex, continuity of pharmaceutical care is an issue and consideration
should be given to a personal, individualised patient record that can be
used by pharmacists involved with the patient at various stages in the
disease.

The Parkinson's Disease Society (0207 931 8080; www.parkinsons.
org.uk) publishes a helpful booklet on drug use in IPD which is of value
to patients and carers and can be used as a counselling aid. Patients with
IPD now have a life expectancy which is near to normal, so treatment,
help and support may be necessary for over 20 years. Non-
pharmacological considerations include education on the disease itself,
advice on diet, exercise programmes and other areas such as driving,
alcohol intake and recreational activities.

Which drugs are usually considered for the initial treatment of patients
with idiopathic Parkinson's disease, and what are their modes of action?

A5   **Initial drug therapy will usually be chosen from the
          following: levodopa preparations, a dopamine agonist, an
          anticholinergic drug (e.g. trihexyphenidyl, orphenadrine,
          benzatropine) or selegiline.**

There is still considerable debate about the best choice of therapy for
initiation of treatment in patients with IPD, and also around when to

start symptomatic treatment. Some experts advocate early treatment to provide patients with maximal clinical benefit at the start of their illness. Others prefer to delay initiation of treatment to minimize the risk for development of long-term complications of levodopa therapy. Most Parkinson's disease specialists start treatment when a patient's symptoms begin to interfere with their lifestyle. What constitutes this will vary from patient to patient, but may include impairment in managing activities of daily living, threatened loss of employment, or gait disturbance with a risk of falling.

When a decision is made to initiate treatment the age of the patient, the degree and type of symptoms and the patient's expectations will influence drug choice. Patients should be made aware that drug treatment can provide symptomatic relief, but there is at present no way of halting the progression of the disease. Levodopa is the most effective drug in the treatment of Parkinson's disease. Virtually all patients will experience meaningful benefit; however, it can cause significant short and long-term adverse effects, and there is a growing body of evidence and opinion among experts that most patients should be started on a dopamine agonist instead.

The rationale for early use of dopamine agonists is that they provide similar benefits to levodopa in early disease, and are significantly less likely to lead to the development of motor complications, particularly dyskinesias. Studies directly comparing levodopa with the dopamine agonists ropinirole, pramipexole and cabergoline as initial therapy for Parkinson's disease have been published and appear to confirm this theory. It is thus generally recommended to initiate therapy with a dopamine agonist in patients who require dopaminergic therapy but who still have relatively mild symptoms. Patients with more severe symptoms, and those over 70 (in whom the development of motor complications is less likely) should probably be started on a levodopa preparation.

Anticholinergic drugs are now rarely used for the treatment of Parkinson's disease. They provide some relief of tremor, but are of little value in the treatment of other features such as rigidity and bradykinesia. In addition, adverse effects are common. They include peripheral effects such as dry mouth, blurred vision and constipation, as well as potentially serious central effects including confusion and hallucinations. Their use is best reserved for younger patients (under 60), in whom resting tremor is the predominant feature. Anticholinergic drugs are thought to act by correcting the relative central cholinergic excess brought about by dopamine deficiency. Anticholinergics are considered to have more effect on tremor and rigidity than on bradykinesia and they act synergistically with levodopa preparations.

Selegiline selectively inhibits monoamine oxidase B, one of the two enzyme systems which break down dopamine. The action of endogenous dopamine is thus augmented. Selegiline has a mild anti-parkinsonian effect and is sometimes used either alone in early disease, or later, to potentiate the action of levodopa preparations. It is widely believed to possess neuroprotective properties in early disease, but this is yet to be proved.

Dopamine deficiency cannot be rectified by the administration of dopamine, because dopamine does not cross the blood–brain barrier. Levodopa does cross the blood–brain barrier and is converted to dopamine in the basal ganglia. Levodopa is thus thought to act primarily by increasing brain dopamine concentrations. If levodopa is administered alone, over 95% of a dose is decarboxylated to dopamine peripherally, which results in reduced amounts being available to cross the blood–brain barrier and problematic peripheral side-effects, such as nausea, vomiting, anorexia, and postural hypotension. Levodopa is therefore now almost always administered with a dopa-decarboxylase inhibitor, either carbidopa or benserazide. These dopa-decarboxylase inhibitors do not cross the blood–brain barrier and so smaller daily doses of levodopa can be administered, thereby reducing the incidence of peripheral side-effects. Levodopa therapy is particularly helpful in controlling symptoms of bradykinesia or akinesia.

Do you agree with this choice?

A6   **Yes.**

In 1995 most of the dopamine agonists now in routine clinical use were not available, so realistically the choice of initial therapy for Mr LN was between an anticholinergic and a levodopa preparation. Given his age and the nature of his symptoms, an anticholinergic drug would have been less suitable than Sinemet.

How should Mr LN's levodopa therapy be adjusted to optimise response?

A7   **It was appropriate to start Mr LN on a low dose of levodopa/dopa-decarboxylase inhibitor therapy, e.g. Sinemet Plus (100 mg levodopa plus 25 mg carbidopa) three times a day. This dose should be increased gradually until optimal effects are achieved.**

Levodopa and dopa-decarboxylase inhibitors are marketed in the UK as Sinemet (levodopa plus carbidopa: co-careldopa) and Madopar (levodopa plus benserazide: co-beneldopa). There are six Madopar preparations and six Sinemet preparations available in a variety of levodopa strengths and formulations (standard, dispersible and controlled release). The potential for confusion among clinicians and pharmacists is considerable, and care must be taken to ensure that the patient receives the intended preparation.

At the start of levodopa therapy the effects of a dose usually last for four to eight hours, so the tablets may be prescribed three times daily. The dose should be increased by one tablet every two to three days until optimum effects are seen or adverse effects occur. If daily doses of less than 70 mg carbidopa are used, the peripheral decarboxylase will not be saturated and Mr LN will be more likely to suffer from nausea and vomiting. For this reason there are low-levodopa Sinemet preparations containing 25 mg carbidopa plus 100 mg levodopa. There are also pre-parations containing 10 mg carbidopa plus 100 mg levodopa that are suitable when higher levodopa doses are needed. This is not a problem with benserazide preparations. Most patients are initially controlled on 400–800 mg levodopa daily.

How can the adverse effects of levodopa be minimised?

A8 **The peripheral side-effects of levodopa are significantly reduced by combining levodopa with a dopa-decarboxylase inhibitor (see Answer 5); however, peripheral side-effects may still occur.**

Levodopa therapy is thus best started at a low dose and the daily dosage increased gradually. In addition, ensuring that the drug is taken with or after food can reduce the incidence of nausea and vomiting still further. Using domperidone, a dopamine antagonist that does not cross the blood–brain barrier, can also reduce nausea and vomiting. Doses of 10–20 mg domperidone one hour before levodopa preparations are effective.

Which of the long-term complications of levodopa therapy does Mr LN appear to be suffering from?

A9 **End-of-dose akinesia and dyskinesias.**

Initial treatment with levodopa leads to sustained improvement through-out the day. Most patients will show a slow improvement in response during the first 18–24 months of treatment. Symptoms are then adequately controlled for three to five years. Unfortunately, after long-term treatment (over five years) only about 25% of patients continue to have a good, smooth response. The main complications that develop are fluctuations in response, dyskinesias, psychiatric side-effects and partial or substantial loss of efficacy.

Fluctuations in response initially consist of end-of-dose deterioration or end-of-dose akinesia. End-of-dose akinesia is the term used when the therapeutic effects of a dose of levodopa are lost. This commonly occurs first thing in the morning (after the longest dosage interval) or just before or after a dose during the day, when the effect of the previous dose wears off and before the next dose is taken or effective. Patients may become immobilised and unable to do anything except wait for the next dose. After prolonged treatment, gradual deterioration in symptoms may begin between one and three hours after a dose.

Long-term levodopa therapy is also associated with the 'on–off' phenomenon. The patient develops a sudden loss of effectiveness (off) when 'freezing' occurs, which may last for only one minute or for up to several hours before normal function returns (on).

Dyskinesias (abnormal movements) can occur in 60–90% of patients and are usually dose-related. They are generally worse when the response to a dose of levodopa is maximal, and have been correlated with high levodopa plasma levels. They are therefore commonly seen after a dose has been taken. Symptoms include grimacing, gnawing and involuntary rhythmic jerking movements.

What alterations to Mr LN's therapy would you recommend in order to try to minimise these effects?

A10 **Increase the frequency of levodopa administration to three-hourly and reduce the amount of levodopa given with each dose.**

The most common approach to response fluctuation is to reduce each individual dose of levodopa and to increase the frequency of administration. This approach can reduce end-of-dose akinesia, but care must be taken to ensure a clinical response is maintained.

End-of-dose bradykinesia or akinesia is thought to be caused by a progression of the underlying disease or an unexplained occurrence of symptoms of dopamine deficiency after an initial response to each dose. Although there is no change in the plasma half-life of levodopa, it appears that the pharmacological half-life is reduced. End-of-dose akinesia has been shown to be corrected by levodopa infusion; however, this is not a genuine therapeutic option, as levodopa must be infused in large volumes, due to its acidity, and it also commonly causes thrombophlebitis. The initial approach taken to minimise the end-of-dose effect is therefore to try to decrease the levodopa dosage interval.

Modified-release versions of co-careldopa (Sinemet) and co-beneldopa (Madopar) are available which result in a more prolonged and constant plasma level of levodopa. Both preparations lead to delayed action and lower peak concentrations than standard levodopa, and the risk of dose failure may be higher. Patients may still need to take controlled-release preparations every three or four hours and may need doses of standard preparations to produce optimal clinical effects, especially with the first dose of the day.

Dyskinesias may occur at the time of peak benefit, at the beginning or end of a dose, or both (diphasic), or during 'off' periods. A reduction in levodopa dose may benefit peak dose dyskinesias, as may the partial replacement of levodopa with a dopamine agonist. Diphasic dyskinesias may also be helped by partial levodopa replacement with dopamine agonists. 'Off' period dyskinesia may be improved by administering a fast-acting (e.g. dispersible) preparation or, for those occurring in the early morning, by administering a controlled-release preparation last thing at night.

Another approach may be to add the catechol-O-methyltransferase (COMT) inhibitor entacapone. This works by inhibiting the peripheral metabolism of levodopa by the enzyme COMT, thereby increasing its availability to the brain. Entacapone is licensed for use as an adjunct to levodopa in Parkinson's disease; studies have shown that its use can significantly reduce 'off' time and increase 'on' time in patients with 'wearing off' episodes. It should be given at a dose of 200 mg with each dose of levodopa, up to 10 times daily.

Complications of entacapone include new-onset or worsening of existing dyskinesias, which may necessitate a 15–30% reduction in the levodopa dose, and diarrhoea. Urine may be coloured orange. The large size of the tablets may cause problems for patients with swallowing difficulties.

A reasonable approach for Mr LN would be to give his present total daily dose of 600–700 mg of levodopa in six, rather than three, aliquots and to add a dose of controlled-release levodopa at bedtime to try to improve his night-time symptoms.

How could you monitor and assess Mr LN's response to these therapy changes?

A11 **By charting his mobility regularly.**

Some neurology wards use mobility charts on which an indication of a patient's mobility can be recorded at suitable intervals. Such charts can be a valuable aid to the manipulation of drug administration in order to optimise therapy. One version of a scoring system is described below. In addition to a score, a brief description of the patient's condition may be added.

State	Description
On	No rigidity, mobilizing
Off	Rigid, with or without tremor
	Unable to mobilise or only with assistance
On with dyskinesia	No rigidity, mobilising but with involuntary movements

Can you suggest any non-drug management that might benefit Mr LN?

A12 **Mr LN may benefit from some remedial therapy such as speech and language therapy, physiotherapy or occupational therapy.**

The role of these therapies is to maintain the maximum level of functional mobility and capacity to perform activities of daily living (ADLs). Early therapeutic intervention cannot reverse the course of Parkinson's disease, but it can delay potential deformity and functional decline.

Physiotherapy for Parkinson's disease patients addresses the functional limitations caused by rigidity and bradykinesia. It may include an exercise program that focuses on maintaining flexibility, balance and strength.

Occupational therapy focuses on finding solutions to difficulties patients encounter performing ADLs. Specialist adaptive equipment may be provided if necessary.

Mr LN and his relatives should also be made aware of the existence of the Parkinson's Disease Society, which can provide education and general advice.

Would an oral dopamine agonist benefit Mr LN?

A13 **Probably.**

Dopamine agonists act directly on post-synaptic dopaminergic receptors and therefore act independently of the degenerating dopaminergic neurons.

A total of six oral dopamine agonists are available in the UK. Bromocriptine, lisuride, pergolide and cabergoline are all derivatives of ergot. The newer agents ropinirole and pramipexole are non-ergot derivatives.

As discussed earlier, there is a growing body of evidence supporting the use of dopamine agonists as initial therapy of PD. However, they have been more commonly used as adjuncts to levodopa when it alone is inadequate or high doses cannot be tolerated. The ergot derivative dopamine agonists all have similar efficacy. Cabergoline has the advantage of a very long elimination half-life (around 60 hours) and can be given once daily.

The acute side-effects of dopamine agonists are similar to those of levodopa. Most Parkinson's disease experts initiate treatment with a low dose and titrate gradually to the desired clinical response. Domperidone can be used to minimise peripheral dopaminergic effects during the first few weeks of treatment. Rare long-term side-effects of dopamine agonists include erythromelalgia and retroperitoneal fibrosis. The non-ergot derivative drugs may be less likely to cause these problems.

Would Mr LN benefit from an antidepressant?

A14 **Probably.**

Depression is very common in Parkinson's disease. Approximately 40% of patients suffer from depression at least once during the course of their disease. Depression in Parkinson's disease is characterised by feelings of guilt, helplessness, remorse and sadness. It is independent of age, disease duration, severity of symptoms or cognitive impairment.

Ensuring adequate Parkinson's disease treatment should be the first step before considering more specific antidepressant therapy. This has been achieved in Mr LN, so a trial of an antidepressant would be reasonable.

If so, which would you choose?

A15 **A tricyclic antidepressant (TCA) or selective serotonin reuptake inhibitor (SSRI) antidepressant could be prescribed for Mr LN.**

TCAs (e.g. amitriptyline, dosulepin) are effective in Parkinson's disease; however, they are associated with anticholinergic effects and orthostatic hypotension, which may limit their usefulness.

The SSRIs (e.g. fluoxetine, sertraline, citalopram) have also been shown to be effective in Parkinson's disease. They are free of the anticholinergic effects associated with the tricyclics and theoretical concerns that they may worsen parkinsonian symptoms have not been borne out by recent studies.

Which drugs might have contributed to Mr LN's symptoms?

A16 **All the drugs prescribed for Mr LN can cause the psychiatric complications described.**

Levodopa causes a variety of psychiatric symptoms, including hallucinations. Dopamine agonists such as cabergoline can cause central nervous system effects such as hallucinations and confusion. These psychiatric complications are especially common in elderly patients. In addition, progression of the disease itself may contribute to these symptoms.

What adjustments would you recommend be made to Mr LN's therapy?

A17 **Reduce his dose of cabergoline.**

The psychiatric complications of most anti-parkinsonian drugs are dose related and often respond to a reduction in dosage.

It is generally recommended to reduce or eliminate anti-parkinsonian drugs in the following order, corresponding to their relative propensity to cause psychiatric problems versus degree of anti-parkinsonian activity: anticholinergics, amantadine, selegiline, dopamine agonist, levodopa.

Mr LN's dose of cabergoline should be reduced to the point of improving hallucinations without drastically worsening his parkinsonism, if possible. It should be gradually reduced as sudden withdrawal of dopaminergic agents may precipitate a neuroleptic malignant syndrome. The levodopa dose should only be reduced if hallucinations persist after elimination of all other anti-parkinsonian agents.

What course of action would you suggest to improve Mr LN's symptoms?

A18   **Add a low dose of an 'atypical' antipsychotic drug.**

Haloperidol and chlorpromazine are effective antipsychotics but are not recommended for Parkinson's patients because of their capacity to block striatal dopamine D_2-receptors and exacerbate parkinsonism.

The newer, 'atypical' antipsychotics (e.g. clozapine, olanzapine, risperidone, quetiapine) are relatively free of D_2-receptor blocking potential. In principle they should improve psychotic features without worsening parkinsonism. The best studied of these is clozapine, which has been shown to reduce hallucinations in Parkinson's patients without worsening parkinsonism. However, the potential for clozapine to cause agranulocytosis (1–2% of patients) and the consequent rigorous monitoring requirements often deter its use. Olanzapine and risperidone have proved less effective than clozapine in comparative studies, and also worsened parkinsonism.

Quetiapine appears to be the most promising agent. In one study, 20 of 24 patients initiated on quetiapine for drug-induced psychosis in Parkinson's disease experienced marked improvement in psychosis without worsening of parkinsonism. A starting dose of 12.5 mg at bedtime is recommended and the dose titrated at three- to five-day intervals until the desired effect is achieved.

What is the long-term outlook for Mr LN?

A19   **It is likely that Mr LN's condition will start deteriorating again after two to two and a half years, as the duration of efficacy of cabergoline when added to levodopa therapy is usually around this length of time. Apomorphine therapy could then be considered.**

Apomorphine is a potent dopamine agonist licensed for the treatment of refractory motor fluctuations ('off' periods) in IPD. The drug cannot be given orally and must be administered subcutaneously. It may be given as a continuous subcutaneous infusion or as single injections. It causes severe nausea and vomiting so three days' pre-treatment with domperidone (20 mg three times daily) is used to minimise this. Domperidone therapy may be continued until tolerance to this side-effect develops. Apomorphine is effective within five to 10 minutes and patients may remain in the 'on' state for up to 60 minutes. During this time an oral dose of medication should have taken effect. Many patients are helped by up to five injections a day, although up to 10 may be needed in some patients. If the number of injections needed is high, then continuous infusions of apomorphine should be considered. If the nausea and vomiting can be overcome, apomorphine therapy is generally well tolerated. Bruising, nodules or abscesses may form at the site of an infusion so the site should be changed daily.

The development of novel pharmacological and surgical approaches to the management of both early and advanced Parkinson's disease offers considerable hope for the future. Surgical techniques such as deep brain stimulation and pallidotomy are available in specialist centres for the treatment of severe, drug-resistant IPD, while for the management of early disease much work is focusing on the development of neuro-protective strategies, interventions to protect or rescue vulnerable dopaminergic neurons and to slow down or stop disease progression.

Further reading

Elble RJ. Tremor and dopamine agonists. *Neurology* 2002; **58**(suppl. 1): S57–S62.

Fernandez HH, Friedman JH, Jacques CC *et al.* Quetiapine for the treatment of drug-induced psychosis in Parkinson's disease. *Mov Disord* 1999; **14**: 484–487.

Friedman JH, Factor SA. Atypical antipsychotics in the treatment of drug-induced psychosis in Parkinson's disease. *Mov Disord* 2000; **15**: 201–211.

Giron LT, Koller WC. Methods of managing levodopa-induced dyskinesias. *Drug Safety* 1996; **14**: 365–374.

Hibble JP. Long-term studies of dopamine agonists. *Neurology* 2002; **58**(suppl. 1): S42–S50.

Jankovic J. Levodopa strengths and weaknesses. *Neurology* 2002; **58**(suppl. 1): S19–S32.

Koller WC. Treatment of early Parkinson's disease. *Neurology* 2002; **58**(suppl. 1): S79–S86.

Korczyn AD, Nussbaum M. Emerging therapies in the pharmacological treatment of Parkinson's disease. *Drugs* 2002; **62**: 775–786.

Lang AE, Lozano AM. Parkinson's disease – first of two parts. *N Engl J Med* 1998; **339**: 1044–1053.

Lang AE, Lozano AM. Parkinson's disease– second of two parts. *N Engl J Med* 1998; **339**: 1130–1143.

LeWitt PA. New drugs for the treatment of Parkinson's disease. *Pharmaco-therapy* 2000; **20**(1 part 2): 265–325.

Olanow CW, Watts RL, Koller WC. An algorithm (decision tree) for the management of Parkinson's disease (2001): treatment guidelines. *Neurology* 2001; **56**(suppl. 5): S1–S88.

16

Stroke

Derek Taylor

Day 1 Mr DF, a 62-year-old-man, was admitted to hospital after collapsing and experiencing a brief loss of consciousness three hours earlier. On admission, he was fully conscious and apyrexial. He had lost voluntary movement in both his left arm and leg. His blood pressure was 160/100 mmHg.

His previous medical history included hypertension, for which he had been prescribed bendroflumethiazide 2.5 mg daily for six years. He had also been on carbamazepine 400 mg twice a day for epilepsy for 10 years. He lived at home with his wife, and smoked 15 cigarettes per day and occasionally drank alcohol.

His serum biochemistry results were:

- Sodium 137 mmol/L (reference range 135–145)
- Potassium 4.9 mmol/L (3.5–5.0)
- Urea 4.7 mmol/L (2.5–7.0)
- Creatinine 95 micromol/L (50–130)

A diagnosis of ischaemic stroke was made. Mr DF was prescribed aspirin 300 mg orally and transferred to the Acute Stroke Unit. A computed tomography (CT) scan was ordered.

Q1 What risk factors did Mr DF have for developing a stroke?
Q2 What is the rationale for ordering a CT scan?
Q3 When should aspirin be administered if benefit is to be obtained and what dose should be given?
Q4 Should Mr DF be prescribed prophylaxis against peptic ulceration?
Q5 What other agents, apart from aspirin, have been shown to be of benefit in the treatment of ischaemic stroke?
Q6 Would Mr DF be a suitable candidate for a thrombolytic agent?
Q7 What metabolic parameters should be monitored closely?
Q8 What supportive treatment does Mr DF require?

Q9 Should the carbamazepine therapy be discontinued?

Q10 How should Mr DF's hypertension be managed?

Day 3   Mr DF was still experiencing loss of movement and hemiplegic pain in his left arm and leg. He also had difficulty swallowing and was therefore referred to the physiotherapist, speech and language therapist and dietitian. A nasogastric tube was inserted.

Q11 Outline a pharmaceutical care plan for Mr DF.

Q12 How would you recommend his pain be managed?

Q13 What other complications associated with his stroke might Mr DF experience?

Q14 What problems might occur when administering Mr DF's medication via the nasogastric tube?

Q15 What advice would you give to the nursing staff to overcome these problems?

Day 9   Mr DF was transferred to a rehabilitation ward. His blood pressure was 150/100 mmHg and he was therefore prescribed perindopril 2 mg daily. His serum cholesterol level was 5.2 mmol/L.

Q16 Should Mr DF be started on warfarin?

Q17 What are the alternative antiplatelet agents to aspirin?

Q18 What is the rationale for the initiation of an angiotensin-converting enzyme inhibitor (ACEI)?

Q19 Should a statin be prescribed for Mr DF?

Day 23   Mr DF's swallow reflex had partially returned. Therefore, he was started on a puréed diet during the day and given fluids overnight via the nasogastric tube.

Day 44   Mr DF had regained most of his limb function and his swallow reflex had almost fully returned. His nasogastric tube was therefore removed and he was discharged home on a soft diet.
     His medication on discharge was:

- Aspirin 75 mg orally daily
- Bendroflumethiazide 2.5 mg orally daily
- Carbamazepine suspension 400 mg twice a day
- Amitriptyline 50 mg tablet at night
- Perindopril tablets 4 mg daily

Q20 What lifestyle changes would you recommend?

Q21 How could the pharmacist contribute to Mr DF's discharge?

What risk factors did Mr DF have for developing a stroke?

A1 **Hypertension, smoking and gender.**

Hypertension is the major risk factor for stroke. Current trial data suggest that lowering blood pressure by 5–6 mmHg diastolic and 10–12 mmHg systolic for two to three years may reduce the annual risk of stroke from 7 to 4.8%. Smoking increases the risk of stroke by around 50% and men are 25–30% more likely to have a stroke than women.

Other risk factors, which are not present in Mr DF, include alcohol abuse, drug abuse, cardiovascular disease (especially atrial fibrillation), diabetes mellitus, migraine headaches and previous transient ischaemic attacks.

What is the rationale for ordering a CT scan?

A2 **To differentiate between an ischaemic stroke and a haemorrhagic stroke.**

Approximately 85% of strokes are the result of an infarct in the brain (ischaemic) with the remaining 15% being due to intracerebral or sub-arachnoid haemorrhage. A haemorrhagic stroke must be excluded by brain imaging before the prescribing of thrombolytics or anticoagulants can be considered in appropriate patients.

When should aspirin be administered if benefit is to be obtained and what dose should be given?

A3 **Aspirin 300 mg orally should be given within 48 hours.**

The rationale for aspirin treatment in the acute phase of ischaemic stroke is to prevent further occlusion of blood supply to surrounding areas of brain tissue. A dose of 300 mg of aspirin should be administered as soon as possible after the onset of stroke symptoms if a diagnosis of haemorrhage is considered unlikely. The initial diagnosis of an ischaemic stroke is a clinical decision, and studies have shown that aspirin may be administered before a brain scan has been undertaken. However, a brain scan must always be undertaken before commencing anticoagulation or thrombolysis, due to the significantly increased risk of intracerebral haemorrhage.

This use of aspirin is supported by two large studies of the treatment of acute ischaemic stroke: the International Stroke Trial (IST) and the Chinese Acute Stroke Trial (CAST). In the IST, those patients treated with aspirin 300 mg daily for 14 days had significantly fewer recurrent ischaemic strokes (2.8 versus 3.9%, $2p < 0.001$) and no significant excess of haemorrhagic strokes (0.9 versus 0.8%) within 14 days, compared with placebo. However, the reductions in deaths within 14 days (9.0 versus 9.4%) and the numbers of patients dead or dependent after six months (62.2 versus 63.5%, $2p = 0.07$) were not significant. In the CAST, those patients treated with aspirin 160 mg/day for up to four weeks (started within 48 hours of stroke onset) showed a small, but significant reduction in recurrent ischaemic stroke rate (1.6 versus 2.1%, $2p = 0.01$) and a non-significant increase in haemorrhagic strokes (1.1 versus 0.9%, $2p > 0.1$) after four weeks, compared with placebo. Overall mortality in the CAST, after four weeks, was shown to fall from 3.9 to 3.3% ($2p = 0.04$).

The authors concluded that when the results of these two studies are combined, aspirin started early in hospital produces a small, but definite net benefit, with about nine fewer deaths or non-fatal strokes per 1000 patients in the first few weeks ($2p = 0.001$) and about 13 fewer dead or dependent per 1000 patients at six months ($2p < 0.01$).

In line with the evidence from these trials, aspirin should be administered at a dose of 300 mg daily for at least the first 14 days after an ischaemic stroke. After this period of time, the dose may be reduced to 75 mg daily for secondary prevention of further thromboembolic events.

Should Mr DF be prescribed prophylaxis against peptic ulceration?

A4   **No.**

Mr DF does not have a history of peptic ulcer disease. The incidence of major gastrointestinal bleeds with aspirin, at the doses used for cardiovascular protection, is 2–3%. There is still some debate over the relative risk to benefit ratio (for gastrointestinal bleeds) between using higher doses (above 300 mg) and lower doses (below 150 mg) of aspirin.

If prophylaxis is required, a maintenance dose of a proton pump inhibitor (PPI) may be prescribed, e.g. lansoprazole 15 mg daily. The current UK National Institute for Clinical Excellence guidelines recommend the use of low-dose PPI therapy for patients with a history of ulcers but not for those patients with a history of dyspepsia.

What other agents, apart from aspirin, have been shown to be of benefit in the treatment of ischaemic stroke?

A5 **Thrombolytic agents.**

The rationale behind the use of thrombolytics in the acute phase of an ischaemic stroke is to accelerate reperfusion of the affected area in the brain. However, there is still much debate over the effectiveness of thrombolysis, as a result of the very conflicting results of several published trials. The use of thrombolytics in the treatment of acute ischaemic stroke is also dependent on patients reaching hospital as soon as possible, and the availability of out-of-hours CT scanning to confirm the diagnosis.

In the National Institute of Neurological Disorders and Stroke rt-PA Stroke Study Group Trial, patients who received alteplase (0.9 mg per kg to a maximum dose of 90 mg) within three hours of ischaemic stroke onset were shown to have a significantly better outcome (no or minimum disability) at three months, than those who received placebo. There was, unfortunately, no significant reduction in mortality at three months (17% in the alteplase group and 21% in the placebo group; $p = 0.30$). Trials with streptokinase have been stopped early due an increased incidence of early death in patients, usually due to cerebral haemorrhage.

The use of heparin was not shown to be of any benefit in the treatment of acute ischaemic stroke by the results of the IST. In this trial, subcutaneous heparin 5000 international units twice daily and 12 500 international units twice daily were compared with placebo. Heparin therapy produced a non-significant reduction in mortality within 14 days (9.0 versus 9.3%) compared with placebo. Patients receiving heparin had significantly fewer recurrent ischaemic strokes within 14 days (2.9 versus 3.8%, $2p = 0.005$) but this was offset by a similar size increase in haemorrhagic strokes (1.2 versus 0.4%, $2p < 0.00001$). When compared with the low-dose heparin regime, heparin 12 500 international units twice daily was associated with significantly more transfused or fatal extracranial bleeds, more haemorrhagic strokes, and more deaths or non-fatal strokes within 14 days (12.6 versus 10.8%, $2p = 0.007$). Perhaps as a result of this, at six months the number of patients dead or dependent was identical to placebo after six months (62.9%).

Would Mr DF be a suitable candidate for a thrombolytic agent?

A6 **No.**

Mr DF did not present to hospital until three hours after the onset of his symptoms. The Royal College of Physician's National Clinical Guidelines for Stroke state that thrombolytic treatment with a tissue plasminogen activator (tPA) should only be given if the following criteria are met: tPA is administered within three hours of onset of stroke symptoms, haemorrhage has definitely been excluded (by CT scan), and the patient is in a specialist centre with appropriate experience and expertise in thrombolytic use.

What metabolic parameters should be monitored closely?

A7   **Mr DF's state of hydration, blood glucose level and temperature.**

(a)   Hydration. His fluid balance, urea, creatinine and sodium levels should be monitored closely. Excessive hydration can result in hyponatraemia, which can force fluid into neurones and therefore exacerbate damage from ischaemia. Hyponatraemia can also lead to seizures, which may further affect the damaged neurones.

(b)   Blood glucose level. Hypoglycaemia may lead to significantly worse clinical outcomes. It is therefore important that Mr DF's blood glucose levels be kept within the normal range.

(c)   Temperature. Any pyrexia, e.g. linked with infection, should be controlled with paracetamol, fan and treatment of the underlying cause.

What supportive treatment does Mr DF require?

A8   **He requires assessment of his level of consciousness, swallow reflex, pressure sore and venous thromboembolism risk, nutritional status, cognitive impairment, moving and handling needs, and bladder and bowel management needs.**

A multidisciplinary assessment using a formal procedure or protocol should be undertaken and documented in the notes within five working days of his admission. Mr DF's swallowing reflex should be assessed within 24 hours of admission and his nutritional status, cognitive impairment and moving and handling needs all within 48 hours.

Dysphagia is common and occurs in about 45% of all stroke patients admitted to hospital. It is associated with more severe strokes and worse outcome. The presence of aspiration may be associated with an increased risk of developing pneumonia after stroke. Malnutrition is also common and is found in about 15% of all patients admitted to hospital, increasing to about 30% a week after admission.

Venous thromboembolism often occurs in the first week of a stroke, most often in immobile patients with paralysis of the leg, but its impact after stroke is still unclear. Studies have shown that deep-vein thrombosis (DVT) occurs in up to 50% of patients with hemiplegia but clinically apparent DVT probably occurs in fewer than 5%. Similarly, although autopsy has identified pulmonary embolism (PE) in a large percentage of patients who die, clinically evident PE occurs in only 1–2% of patients. To minimise the risk of venous thromboembolism, it is recommended that compression stockings should be worn by stroke patients with weak or paralysed legs, once the patient's peripheral circulation, sensation and the state of their skin have been assessed. These stockings should be full-length in patients with hemiparesis. Mobilisation and optimal hydration should also be maintained as far as possible from the outset. Prophylactic anticoagulation should not be routinely used in either the acute or rehabilitation phases as it increases the risk of cerebral haemorrhage; however, if a venous thromboembolism has been clinically diagnosed, anticoagulant treatment should be started.

Most patients presenting with moderate to severe stroke are incontinent at presentation and may still be incontinent on discharge. This is a major burden on carers and may impede rehabilitation. Management of both bladder and bowel problems must therefore be seen as an essential part of the rehabilitation process.

Should the carbamazepine therapy be discontinued?

A9 **No.**

Seizures may occur in up to 20% of stroke patients and with his history of epilepsy and the dangers of fitting in the acute post-stroke phase, Mr DF should be continued on his carbamazepine therapy. He should be changed to the same dose given as suspension.

How should Mr DF's hypertension be managed?

A10 **Mr DF should be maintained on his bendroflumethiazide. There should be no further attempts to reduce blood pressure in the acute phase of his stroke, unless his blood pressure continues to increase.**

Caution should be exercised in acutely controlling Mr DF's blood pressure, because decreasing the blood pressure too rapidly will compromise cerebral blood flow and expand the region of ischaemia and infarction, whereas hypertension will place him at greater risk for cerebral haemorrhage, especially if a thrombolytic agent is used. However, one study which compared treated and untreated patients who were hypertensive in association with an acute stroke failed to demonstrate any difference in outcome between the groups. The aim is to maintain a systolic blood pressure, in the acute phase, of less than 180 mmHg and a diastolic pressure of less than 110 mmHg.

A parenteral beta-blocker or nitroprusside can be used to achieve this target, if required, but if there is a clinical deterioration in neurological function associated with the reduction in blood pressure, the infusion rate of the antihypertensive should be slowed or discontinued. Maintenance therapy can then be initiated with an appropriate oral agent.

Outline a pharmaceutical care plan for Mr DF.

A11   The pharmaceutical care plan for Mr DF should include the following:

(a)   Antiplatelet therapy

(i)   Ensure antiplatelet agent is continued daily at the current dose.

(ii)   Monitor for signs of gastric irritation.

(b)   Dysphagia

(i)   Determine his swallow reflex after liaison with speech and language therapist.

(ii)   Assess suitable alternative formulations if an enteral feeding tube in place.

(iii)   Check timing of medication doses if on an enteral feed.

(c)   Hypertension

(i)   Regular monitoring of blood pressure.

(ii)   Aim for a target blood pressure (in the rehabilitation phase) of below 140/85 mmHg.

(iii)   Do not increase doses or prescribe new doses of antihypertensives until at least seven days after the initial stroke.

(d)   Aggravating drug therapy. Centrally acting drugs should be avoided if possible as they may compromise memory and cognition.

(e)   Monitor other parameters

   (i)   Urea and electrolytes.
   (ii)   Blood glucose.
   (iii)   Temperature.

How would you recommend his pain be managed?

A12 **If the pain is genuinely a hemiplegic pain, a low dose of amitriptyline should be prescribed.**

It is very important that the correct cause of the pain is diagnosed. Other possible causes of post-stroke limb problems may be muscular, spasticity or joint-related. These types of pain may respond to careful manipulation and physiotherapy. Appropriate medication, such as paracetamol, baclofen or intra-articular injections may also be prescribed for each of these problems respectively.

   If the pain is of a central origin, a low dose of amitriptyline, e.g. 25 mg at night, may be prescribed. This should be titrated at 25 mg intervals every week, according to response. The patient should be monitored closely for any signs of central nervous system suppression and therapy should not be commenced until the patient is medically stable. Alternative options include carbamazepine (which Mr DF is already on) or gabapentin.

What other complications associated with his stroke might Mr DF experience?

A13 **Agitation, delerium, stupor, coma, cerebral oedema, pneumonia, pulmonary oedema, deep vein thrombosis, arrhythmias and depression.**

Pneumonia, pulmonary oedema, deep vein thrombosis and arrhythmias after an ischaemic stroke may be related to further infarction, haemorrhage or cerebral oedema. Pneumonia and deep vein thrombosis are further exacerbated by inactivity, hence the need to mobilise Mr DF as soon as possible.

   Stroke patients often experience psychological reactions, the most common of which is depression, which occurs in 40–50% of patients. If this depression interferes with recovery and rehabilitation, a selective serotonin reuptake inhibitor may be prescribed.

What problems might occur when administering Mr DF's medication via the nasogastric tube?

A14 **Carbamazepine may bind to the feeding tube and interact with the enteral feed.**

The first option when selecting alternative formulations for administration is to use a commercially available oral solution or dispersible tablet. If this is not an option, the next step is to crush and fully disperse the contents of the tablet or capsule. This should not be done with enteric-coated or modified-release preparations as it may result in changes in bioavailabilty with dangerous peaks or troughs, or blockage of the tube.

Carbamazepine suspension may bind to the material of the enteral tubing or interact with the enteral feed itself. Both of these effects may alter the bioavailabilty and clinical effectiveness of the medication.

What advice would you give to the nursing staff to overcome these problems?

A15 **The feed should be stopped at least one hour before the dose. The carbamazepine suspension should be diluted with at least 30–60 mL of water and the tube flushed with at least an equal volume after the dose. The enteral feed should not be restarted until two hours after the dose.**

Should Mr DF be started on warfarin?

A16 **No.**

Anticoagulation should only be considered for patients in valvular or non-valvular atrial fibrillation. It should not be started until intracerebral haemorrhage has been excluded by brain imaging, and usually only after 14 days have elapsed. Meta-analysis of several trials into the use of warfarin have suggested a relative risk of stroke in patients receiving warfarin of 0.33 compared with placebo. This means that only one-third as many strokes occurred in patients receiving warfarin compared with those receiving placebo. There also appears to be a relative risk for deaths from causes other than stroke of 0.57 in patients receiving warfarin compared with placebo.

What are the alternative antiplatelet agents to aspirin?

A17 **Dipyridamole or clopidogrel.**

The European Stroke Prevention Study 2, compared the efficacy of low-dose aspirin, modified-release dipyridamole and the two agents combined for the prevention of ischaemic stroke in patients with prior stroke or transient ischaemic attacks. Risk of stroke (after 24 months) was reduced by 18% with aspirin (25 mg twice daily) alone (p = 0.013), 16% with modified release dipyridamole (200 mg twice daily) alone (p = 0.039) and 37% with the combination (p < 0.001). The authors therefore concluded that when aspirin and dipyridamole are co-prescribed the protective effects against stroke appear to be additive and significantly greater than either agent prescribed singly.

Clopidogrel, a thienopyridine derivative, is an antiplatelet drug, which appears to be modestly superior to aspirin in reducing the incidence of thromboembolic events. In the CAPRIE trial, clopidogrel 75 mg daily showed a relative risk reduction of 8.7% (p = 0.043) versus aspirin 325 mg daily.

The Royal College of Physicians Stroke Guidelines state that clopidogrel 75 mg daily or low-dose aspirin and modified-release dipyridamole are possible first-line alternatives to aspirin alone. However, in aspirin-intolerant patients clopidogrel and modified-release dipyridamole alone may be used. Aspirin intolerance is defined as those patients who are allergic to aspirin or those patients who have a history of peptic ulcer disease. A history of simple dyspepsia, due to taking aspirin on an empty stomach, is not a contra-indication to low-dose aspirin therapy.

What is the rationale for the initiation of an ACEI?

A18 **To reduce the risk of Mr DF suffering a further stroke.**

The management of Mr DF's hypertension should now be a priority with a target blood pressure of below 140/85 mmHg aimed for; however his blood pressure should only be reduced gradually and additional anti-hypertensives are not normally prescribed until at least seven days after a stroke as a sudden drop in blood pressure could impair cerebral perfusion, which may impair consciousness or result in further infarction.

In the PROGRESS study the combination of an ACEI (perindopril) and a thiazide diuretic (indapamide) produced a stroke risk reduction of 43% compared with placebo in both hypertensive and non-hypertensive patients. As Mr DF is already on bendroflumethiazide and was still hypertensive on day 9, it was decided to prescribe perindopril 2 mg daily and titrate the dose upwards slowly as needed.

There is still debate as to whether the reduction in stroke risk observed in the trial is a class effect, or unique to perindopril, or just as a result of aggressive lowering of blood pressure. In the HOPE study, ramipril reduced the risk of stroke by 33% in high-risk patients with vascular disease or diabetes and one other risk factor. The resultant cardiovascular benefit was greater than that attributable to a decrease in blood pressure. However, HOPE was not specifically designed to examine the prevention of further strokes after an initial stroke.

Should a statin be prescribed for Mr DF?

A19 No.

The Royal College of Physicians Stroke Guidelines state that a statin should be considered for all patients with a history of ischaemic heart disease and a cholesterol greater than 5.0 mmol/L following stroke. This statement is supported by the results of the CARE study, in which pravastatin 40 mg daily significantly reduced the incidence of stroke and transient ischaemic attacks after myocardial infarction in patients with average serum cholesterol levels. In the Heart Protection Study, simvastatin 40 mg daily for five years prevented further thromboembolic events in 70 out of 1000 patients who had a history of coronary disease. These results were irrespective of serum cholesterol level.

However, as Mr DF did not have a history of ischaemic disease, it was decided not to prescribe him a statin.

What lifestyle changes would you recommend?

A20 Smoking cessation, reduction of alcohol intake, weight reduction and moderate regular exercise.

Mr DF should be advised about the availability and use of nicotine replacement therapy. A reduction in alcohol intake, regular, moderate exercise and dietary advice may also reduce his cardiovascular risk.

How could the pharmacist contribute to Mr DF's discharge?

A21 The pharmacist can contribute to the discharge by providing pharmaceutical advice and support to the patient and their carers. There should also be effective liaison with his GP and community pharmacist.

The pharmacist can contribute to Mr DF's discharge in the following ways:

(a) Counselling. Mr DF should be given both written (patient information leaflets and a reminder chart) and verbal information regarding the purpose and use of his medicines. The importance of long-term antiplatelet therapy and good control of his blood pressure and cholesterol level should be stressed to him.

Early treatment of acute stroke appears to be the most important factor in determining optimal outcome, therefore, Mr DF and his carers should be carefully instructed to seek urgent medical attention if he experiences any weakness or paralysis, speech impairment, numbness, blurred or sudden loss of vision or altered level of consciousness.

(b)   Compliance assessment. This must be assessed in the light of any existing impairment of his manual dexterity or cognitive function as a result of the stroke. Mr DF still has some restriction in movement in his arm, which may impair the opening of his medication containers. The use of any compliance aids must be with the consent of Mr DF and his carers.

(c)   Liaison with his GP and community pharmacist. Information regarding medication changes (i.e. the prescribing of aspirin, perindopril and amitriptyline), alternative formulations of medicines (i.e. the carbamazepine suspension), nutritional products and compliance aids should be communicated to the patient's GP and community pharmacist.

(d)   Liaison with patient support groups. Mr DF should be given contact information for organisations that provide support and information to both patients and carers, e.g. The Stroke Association, Different Strokes and The National Stroke Association.

Further reading

Bhatt DL, Hirsch AT, Ringleb PA. Reduction in the need for hospitalisation for recurrent ischaemic events and bleeding with clopidogrel instead of aspirin. CAPRIE investigators. *Am Heart J* 2000; **140**: 67–73.

CAST (Chinese Acute Stroke Trial) Collaborative Group. CAST: randomised placebo-controlled trial of early aspirin use in 20 000 patients with ischaemic stroke. *Lancet* 1997; **349**; 1641–1649.

Diener HC, Cunha L, Forbes C *et al.* European Stroke Prevention Study 2. Dipyridamole and acetylsalicylic acid in the secondary prevention of stroke. *J Neurol Sci* 1996; **143**: 1–13.

Heart Outcomes Prevention Evaluation Study Investigators. Effects of an angiotensin-converting-enzyme inhibitor, ramipril on cardiovascular events in high-risk patients. *N Engl J Med* 2000; **342**: 145–153.

Intercollegiate Working Party for Stroke. *National Clinical Guidelines for Stroke.* Royal College of Physicians, London, 2000.

International Stroke Collaborative Group. The International Stroke Trial (IST): a randomised trial of aspirin, subcutaneous heparin, both, or neither among 19 435 patients with acute ischaemic stroke. *Lancet* 1997; **349**: 1569–1581.

Plehn JF, Davis BR, Sacks FM *et al.* Reduction of stroke incidence after myocardial infarction with pravastatin: the Cholesterol and Recurrent Events (CARE) study. The CARE Investigators. *Circulation* 1999; **99**: 185–188.

PROGRESS Collaborative Group. Randomised trial of a perindopril-based blood-pressure lowering regimen among 6105 individuals with previous stroke or transient ischaemic attack. *Lancet* 2001; **358**: 1033–1041.

The National Institute of Neurological Disorders and Stroke rt-PA Stroke Study Group. Tissue plasminogen activator for acute ischemic stroke. *N Engl J Med* 1995; **333**: 1581–1587.

17

Schizophrenia

Carol Paton

Day 1   Mr MB, a 22-year-old man, was visited at home by a psychiatrist at the request of his GP.

Mr MB's mother had become increasingly concerned about him isolating himself in his room. He only ever went out to visit the library, where he selected books on various religious and philosophical themes. Mr MB no longer watched television with his family, as he said that it 'wound him up', and he had not been out with his friends for several months. He had not been to work for two weeks. He told his mother that there was not a job for him anymore; however, she later discovered that his attendance and timekeeping had been deteriorating over a period of weeks, and then he had failed to attend at all. She said that he 'refused to discuss the matter sensibly with her'. As Mr MB had always been a reasonably outgoing and sociable young man, this behaviour was very out of character for him.

Mr MB's mental state examination revealed that he was an unkempt young Caucasian man, wearing his pyjamas under his trousers. He appeared slightly over-aroused. His speech was of a normal rate, but very disjointed, e.g. 'I have books in my room – it's special, the moon – God controls it – do you know him – he controls life – the forces can win'. The content of his speech mainly concerned religion and philosophy, and how they affect us all. His mood was euthymic and somewhat incongruous. Mr MB said that he could feel something was going on 'out there'. He also said that he had heard people talking about him in the street and occasionally he heard a single male voice saying 'go to your room, it is safe there'. He said that he had seen cosmic rays. His orientation and cognition were grossly intact.

After some discussion, Mr MB accepted the offer of a few days in hospital 'for a rest'. On admission, his routine physical examination and baseline bloods were unremarkable. His urine screen was positive for nicotine and cannabis.

Q1   Which of Mr MB's symptoms are consistent with a psychotic illness?
Q2   What is the significance of Mr MB's positive urine screen for cannabis?
Q3   Outline a pharmaceutical care plan for Mr MB.
Q4   Would you recommend treatment with an antipsychotic at this time and, if so, which one would you recommend?

Mr MB was prescribed risperidone. The dose was titrated against response up to 4 mg taken as a single dose at bedtime.

Q5   Was the dose appropriate?
Q6   What is meant by 'response' and over what time course does this usually occur?

Week 4   Mr MB's symptoms had improved. He still felt that spiritual matters were important, but was less preoccupied by them. He refused to stay in hospital any longer and, as he was not 'sectionable', he was discharged home. He was given a supply of risperidone 4 mg tablets and was noted to be ambivalent about taking medication.

He did not attend for out-patient follow-up. His mother said that he was living at home and 'doing OK'.

Month 7   Mr MB was brought to the ward by his brother. He had developed an interest in martial arts and had punched a hole in his bedroom wall 'in order to defend himself'. A mental state examination revealed systematised paranoid delusions surrounding a plot to steal his soul. He also admitted to his thoughts being interfered with by an outside agent who removed thoughts from his head and inserted it's own.

Mr MB refused to stay in hospital and punched out at a nurse who tried to prevent him from running off. It was decided to place him under Section 2 of the Mental Health Act.

Q7   What is the scope and purpose of Section 2 of the Mental Health Act 1983?
Q8   How should Mr MB's acutely disturbed behaviour be dealt with?
Q9   What medication would you recommend for Mr MB and why?

Mr MB was given haloperidol 5 mg and lorazepam 2 mg intramuscularly. Fifteen minutes later his head was tipped to the side and his eyes fixed upwards towards the ceiling.

Q10 What is happening to Mr MB and what would you recommend should be done?

Mr MB was sensitive to extrapyramidal side-effects (EPSEs) with typical antipsychotics and refused to take risperidone again as he said it 'didn't agree' with him. He was therefore prescribed olanzapine Velotabs 10 mg at night, increased to 20 mg over the next five weeks. His urine screen was negative for drugs of abuse.

Mr MB remained very symptomatic although no longer aggressive. He still believed that someone was out to get him and his thinking continued to be muddled. Nursing staff suspected that Mr MB was not taking his medication (by taking a sip of water and spitting the Velotab back into the cup). The consultant decided to prescribe a depot antipsychotic.

Q11 What is the main advantage of administering a depot antipsychotic to Mr MB?
Q12 Which depot antipsychotic would you recommend and why?

Mr MB's Section 2 was converted to a Section 3, which is a treatment order lasting a maximum of six months in the first instance. Mr MB accepted risperidone depot, but over the next two months his mental state remained virtually unchanged. He was then prescribed zuclopenthixol depot 200 mg every two weeks. Again, little response was apparent. Trifluoperazine 10 mg daily was added to his prescription. Mr MB protested by refusing his injection. A second-opinion doctor was requested to visit Mr MB for the purposes of Section 58 of the Mental Health Act.

Q13 Why has a second opinion been requested?
Q14 What role can the pharmacist play in this process?
Q15 Can anything be done to change Mr MB's attitude towards antipsychotic drugs?

The trifluoperazine was discontinued. Over the next two months, the zuclopenthixol dose was increased to 600 mg/week. Mr MB became slightly less suspicious, but was still very unwell. Sulpiride 600 mg/day was added to his prescription.

Q16 What are the risks associated with high-dose and combination antipsychotics?

After a lengthy discussion with Mr MB and his family it was agreed that there was little point in pursuing the above prescription and Mr MB should be offered treatment with clozapine.

Q17 Why has clozapine been prescribed for Mr MB and is its use appropriate at this time?

Q18 How should treatment with clozapine be initiated and monitored?

Q19 How should treatment with clozapine be optimised?

Q20 What side-effects might you anticipate and how would you deal with them?

Q21 What further options are available if Mr MB fails to respond to clozapine?

Which of Mr MB's symptoms are consistent with a psychotic illness?

A1 **Formal thought disorder, probable delusional ideas, auditory and visual hallucinations, and poor self care and social isolation.**

(a) Formal thought disorder.

This is the term used to describe the abnormal construction (form) of speech that occurs in psychotic illness. In milder forms, occasional derailment may be all that is seen. This is when the line of thought jumps from one topic (rail) to another and the connection is not easily understood by the listener. Other terms commonly used to describe this phenomenon include loosening of associations, tangential thinking and knight's move thinking (as in a game of chess). In more severe cases, such as Mr MB's, the conversation may change themes several times within the same sentence and eventually the speech becomes completely incomprehensible. This is sometimes described as schizophrenic word salad. Formal thought disorder occurs in various forms in many psychiatric syndromes and its presence is by no means diagnostic of schizophrenia.

(b) Delusions.

A delusion is a culturally inappropriate belief that is held firmly despite any logical argument to the contrary. Delusions can take many forms. There are three pieces of evidence in Mr MB's presentation that are suggestive of delusional ideas.

He no longer watches television. This may be due to *delusions of reference*: Mr MB may interpret the content of a television programme to be directly related to himself, e.g. the presenter may be speaking directly to him or making comments about him. Many people with schizophrenia are unable to watch television or listen to the radio because they are troubled by delusions of reference (also called ideas of reference).

The content of Mr MB's speech is concerned entirely with religion and philosophy. Although there is insufficient evidence to be sure, Mr MB may think that his presence is central to the situation that he is describing. This is an example of a *grandiose delusion*.

Mr MB says that he can 'feel something going on out there'. This phenomenon can be described as both an abnormal perception and a delusional idea. It is usually called a *delusional perception*.

(c) Hallucinations.

A hallucination is a perception for which no stimulus exists. Any of the senses can be affected, although auditory hallucinations are the most common. Mr MB describes three types of hallucination.

Second-person auditory hallucinations, where he hears a single voice speaking directly to him. The particular voice that Mr MB is hearing is giving him an instruction. This is called a command hallucination. People with schizophrenia may find it difficult to resist these 'commands' and acting upon them is not uncommon.

Third-person auditory hallucinations, where he hears other people talking about him. These are also called commentary hallucinations and of all the abnormal perceptions, they are the most predictive of schizophrenia.

Visual hallucinations. Mr MB says that he has seen cosmic rays.

(d) Poor self-care and social isolation.

In schizophrenia, symptoms abnormal by their presence such as hallucinations and delusions are referred to as positive symptoms. Symptoms abnormal by their absence, such as lack of self-care, poverty of speech, social isolation or blunting of emotional response, are referred to as negative symptoms (and sometimes, where their presence dominates the clinical picture, as the defect state). Mr MB has negative symptoms in that his self-care is poor and his social interactions limited.

The above description has only touched the surface of abnormalities that can be found in the mental state. Each case of psychotic illness is different and many phenomena not described above can be present. No individual symptom described above is diagnostic of schizophrenia. For a more complete understanding of psychopathology, terminology and the way in which symptoms are grouped together to reach a diagnosis, further reading is strongly recommended. The *Oxford Textbook of Psychiatry* gives an excellent account of psychopathology. The diagnosis of schizophrenia is described in the International Classification of Diseases (ICD–10) or the Diagnostic and Statistical Manual of Mental Disorders (DSM-IV).

What is the significance of Mr MB's positive urine screen for cannabis?

A2 **Acute psychotic episodes can be precipitated by cannabis. It can also exacerbate symptoms in patients with schizophrenia. Mr MB should be discouraged from using cannabis in the future.**

Although there is good evidence that cannabis may contribute to the presentation of psychotic illness, the relationship is complex. People with schizophrenia are six times more likely to develop a problem with substance misuse compared with the general population. The most frequently misused drug is cannabis. Cannabis may cause an acute toxic psychosis characterised by euphoria, fragmented thoughts, paranoia, hyperacusia, depersonalisation, derealisation, and auditory and visual hallucinations, particularly if large quantities are consumed. Symptoms usually resolve within a week of abstinence. The literature in this area consists mainly of uncontrolled studies and case reports, so the incidence of these reactions has not been accurately quantified.

There is little evidence to suggest that chronic psychotic illness develops after cannabis use and large observational studies have failed to identify any individual symptoms or symptom clusters that would separate cannabis-induced psychosis from schizophrenia. However, the role of cannabis in precipitating an episode of psychosis in a patient who is predisposed should not be discounted. Cannabis use may be a 'life event stressor' in these individuals.

Cannabis use is widespread. In one study in the UK, 60% of university students claimed to have used the drug at least once. With such widespread use, the fact that its use is illegal, together with the large number of non-standard preparations that are available means that attempts to make qualitative and quantitative associations between cannabis use and psychotic symptoms will continue to be fraught with difficulty.

Cannabis has a very long half-life and, in chronic users, can be detected in the urine for four weeks or more after consumption. A positive urine screen (which is usually qualitative) cannot confirm acute intoxication. The situation is further complicated by the fact that cannabis may ameliorate the negative symptoms of schizophrenia as well as some of the side-effects of antipsychotic drugs and may be used as 'self-medication' for these purposes. Cannabis use in some patients may post-date rather than pre-date the emergence of psychotic symptoms.

Although the use of cannabis in those with psychotic illness should be discouraged, the exact role that it plays in each clinical presentation must be determined from the individual circumstances of that case.

Mr MB's symptoms are of at least several weeks duration and his presentation is suggestive of a primary psychotic illness, but as this is his first episode, the possible role of cannabis should not be excluded. Mr MB should be discouraged from using cannabis in the future as it may predispose him to further episodes and/or exacerbate his psychotic symptoms.

Outline a pharmaceutical care plan for Mr MB.

A3   **The pharmaceutical care plan for Mr MB should include the following:**

(a)   The decision to administer any drugs at all should be discussed with the multidisciplinary team.

(b)   The anticipated effects and side-effects of antipsychotics should be discussed with Mr MB. This must be done sensitively with regard to his mental state and level of insight.

(c)   Mr MB's views about drug choice should be respected if possible.

(d)   The antipsychotic dose should be titrated against both clinical symptoms and side-effects. The aim is to prescribe one antipsychotic at a therapeutic (not high) dose.

(e)   The effect of Mr MB's mental health act status on the multidisciplinary team's ability to medicate him should be constantly reviewed.

Would you recommend treatment with an antipsychotic at this time and, if so, which one would you recommend?

A4   **Yes, treatment with an antipsychotic is appropriate at this time, but the choice of drug is a matter for negotiation with the patient and should be determined by consideration of a number of factors. For Mr MB a typical or atypical antipsychotic would be appropriate depending on his views and the views of his psychiatrist. In the absence of any previous drug history or physical pathology, risperidone is a reasonable first choice.**

Mr MB has well documented psychotic symptoms which are of sufficient severity to interfere markedly with his ability to function normally. The potential benefits of antipsychotics therefore outweigh the risks in his case.

Three main factors influence the choice of antipsychotic drug:

(a)   Previous response to treatment. If there is a history of a previous good response to any individual antipsychotic, it is logical to use the same drug again. Similarly, previous poor response or a history of adverse reactions would mitigate against the use of an individual drug. For Mr MB this is the index episode, so no useful information is available in this respect.

(b)   The clinical presentation. This requires consideration of both the severity of the illness and the predominant symptoms. Mr MB is a young man with a florid psychotic illness. However, he has come into hospital voluntarily and is not an immediate danger to himself or others. There is no need to select a drug that is available in a parenteral form.

(c)   Physical pathology and anticipated side-effect profile. All antipsychotics have in common the ability to block dopamine receptors, but they vary in the degree to which they block other central neurotransmitter pathways. Sometimes this difference can be clinically relevant. For example, cholinergic blockade is associated with dry mouth, blurred vision, constipation and urinary retention. It is obviously unwise to administer antipsychotics which have significant anticholinergic effects to patients who have narrow angle glaucoma or prostatism. Alpha-adrenergic blockade is associated with postural hypotension. The elderly are particularly at risk. Blockade of histamine receptors is associated with sedation. Sometimes this can be desirable, sometimes not. The relevant potencies of antipsychotics at dopamine, serotonin, alpha-adrenergic, histaminergic and cholinergic receptors is well documented and can be found in several standard texts. EPSEs are a major problem with typical antipsychotics. Acute dystonias are painful and frightening. Akathisia (inner restlessness) is felt by many patients to be intolerable. Pseudo-parkinsonism can interfere with activities of daily living and tardive dyskinesia (which can be irreversible) is very stigmatising. Atypical antipsychotics are relatively free from these motor side-effects but tend to cause more weight gain than the older drugs. Clozapine and olanzapine may also cause impaired glucose tolerance, frank diabetes and unfavourable lipid profiles. The distinction between typical and atypical drugs is not a clear one. The original definition of atypicality was a lack of potential to cause EPSEs or raise serum prolactin, yet the atypical antipsychotics risperidone and amisulpride cause prolactin related side-effects and risperidone causes EPSEs in doses above 6 mg/day. It is more useful clinically to think of all antipsychotic drugs as being on several spectrums: those that can produce severe EPSEs to those that cause none, those that can lead to enormous weight gain to those that cause less weight gain, those that are very sedative to those that are not sedative etc. Drug choice should be negotiated between Mr MB, his psychiatrist and pharmacist. Such discussion is central to achieving the objectives of the National Service Framework for Mental Health ('patients should be consulted about their treatment' and 'all patients who might benefit from treatment with an atypical antipsychotic should be offered one') and addressing the criticisms outlined in the National Schizophrenia Fellowship's report, *A Question of Choice* (where over 25% of patients said that no-one had ever discussed their medicines with them).

Was the dose appropriate?

A5 **The optimal dose for many antipsychotic drugs has been determined in randomised controlled trials. Often this dose is considerably less than the licensed maximum dose for the drug. It is important to be aware of these optimal doses and not titrate the dose too rapidly. This will only lead to an increased side-effect burden.**

For example, the majority of patients respond to risperidone 6 mg/day or less or haloperidol 10 mg/day or less. Higher doses have not been shown to confer any benefit in either the speed or magnitude of response.

Mr MB has been prescribed risperidone 4 mg, an 'optimal dose'.

What is meant by 'response' and over what time course does this usually occur?

A6 **The aims of antipsychotic treatment are to treat positive and negative symptoms, and normalise social functioning. The time course of response to antipsychotics is poorly documented although most therapeutic gain tends to be seen in the first six weeks.**

(a)   Positive symptoms. Antipsychotics are most effective at treating positive symptoms such as delusions and hallucinations, both of which are present in Mr MB. The onset of this effect is variable. Improvements can sometimes be seen after four or five days treatment, but can take much longer. Psychotic symptoms should not be expected to disappear suddenly, but rather to 'melt away'. Delusions often change in quality from being overvalued ideas to being of no importance at all, although they may be remembered as having been true in the past.

As a general rule of thumb, the longer a delusion has been held, the longer it will take to go. Untreated psychotic symptoms of many months or sometimes years duration can be very difficult to treat in clinical practice. This is the most powerful argument for early intervention with antipsychotics. In addition, approximately one-third of patients with schizophrenia will have repeated episodes of acute illness. These repeated episodes can be progressively more difficult to treat, with a worsening post-treatment baseline after each episode. This is a powerful argument for maintenance treatment. Unfortunately there is no way of identifying those who are at risk of having subsequent episodes.

(b)   Negative symptoms. Negative symptoms such as poverty of speech, emotional blunting, lack of volition, etc., are less successfully treated by antipsychotics. Primary enduring negative symptoms are particularly difficult to treat. By virtue of their side-effects, typical antipsychotics can produce secondary negative symptoms such as akinesia and an expressionless face. It is important not to confuse the lack of EPSEs seen with atypical antipsychotics with their ability to treat negative symptoms.

(c)   Social functioning. Improved socialisation can take many months and may never be completely achieved.

A 'response' to antipsychotics in clinical trials can be as little as a 20% reduction in the Brief Psychiatric Rating Scale, a scale used to quantify psychotic symptoms. By definition, many patients who are classified as 'responders' have residual symptoms.

Approximately 30% of patients will fail to 'respond' to typical or atypical antipsychotics. The management of these patients is discussed in more detail in Answer 17.

What is the scope and purpose of Section 2 of the Mental Health Act 1983?

A7   **Section 2 of the Mental Health Act 1983 involves a compulsory admission to hospital for a maximum of 28 days for the purpose of assessment and treatment of mental disorder.**

Section 2 is used when an individual who is thought to suffer from mental disorder refuses to come into hospital voluntarily and admission is considered to be in the best interests of the patient or the public. Application to invoke Section 2 can be made by the patient's nearest relative or a social worker. Two independent medical recommendations are required, one of which must be by a psychiatrist who has been approved for the purpose (so called, 'Section 12 approved'). The patient has the right of appeal, when he can present his case to the Mental Health Review Tribunal.

How should Mr MB's acutely disturbed behaviour be dealt with?

A8 **De-escalation strategies should be tried first. These include 'talking down' and offering Mr MB voluntary 'time out' in a room on his own with an open door and staff nearby. This may be followed by voluntary oral, then enforced parenteral medication. In extreme cases seclusion may be used.**

Acute behavioural disturbance can occur in the context of psychiatric illness, physical illness, substance abuse or personality disorder. Psychotic symptoms are common and the patient may be aggressive towards others secondary to persecutory delusions or auditory, visual or tactile hallucinations.

With skilled handling, only a small proportion of 'incidents' require enforced parenteral medication. A balance must be drawn between building a trusting relationship with the patient and maintaining the safety of the ward environment. All psychiatric in-patient units should have guidelines for the treatment of behavioural emergencies as they will otherwise be dealt with by junior (inexperienced) doctors on call. This is at best unfair and at worst potentially dangerous. Pharmacists have a key role to play in developing local guidelines and re-enforcing their content.

What medication would you recommend for Mr MB and why?

A9 **The principal objective is to calm Mr MB which will be best achieved by the combination of a parenteral antipsychotic and a benzodiazepine. Haloperidol 5 mg intramuscularly or olanzapine 10 mg intramuscularly plus lorazepam 2 mg intramuscularly would be a suitable choice.**

Rapid tranquillisation (RT), the use of drugs to rapidly control disturbed behaviour, is required at this point. The common clinical practice of RT is not underpinned by a strong evidence base. Patients who require RT are usually too disturbed to give informed consent and therefore cannot be included in randomised controlled trials. The largest randomised controlled trials to date were the licensing studies conducted with intramuscular olanzapine. Olanzapine was at least as effective as haloperidol and associated with less motor side-effects. However, the majority of patients who were recruited to this study were only mildly or moderately behaviourally disturbed. The efficacy of intramuscular olanzapine in the management of real clinical emergencies has yet to be evaluated.

In clinical practice, the combination of a modest dose of an anti-psychotic and a benzodiazepine has been shown to achieve the best control of disturbed behaviour.

Parenteral chlorpromazine is best avoided because of the association between low-potency phenothiazines, QTc prolongation and sudden cardiac death. It must be remembered that all antipsychotics have the potential to prolong the QTc interval in vulnerable patients and that QTc prolongation is a risk factor for torsades de pointes, a potentially fatal cardiac arrhythmia. Risk factors for developing QTc prolongation include genetic vulnerability, ischaemic heart disease, hypokalaemia, autonomic arousal and co-prescribing of metabolic inhibitors of antipsychotics. Pimozide, sertindole, thioridazine and droperidol are associated with the highest risk.

The slow onset of action of Clopixol Acuphase makes it unsuitable for use in RT. Its long duration of action (72 hours) raises ethical questions around its enforced administration to informal patients. This is not an issue for Mr MB.

Care should always be taken when administering intramuscular injections to a struggling patient as vasodilation secondary to autonomic arousal may lead to inadvertent bolus intravenous administration.

It is essential to perform regular physical observations in all patients post-RT. As a minimum, temperature and BP should be recorded. Patients who are asleep should be subject to 'constant observation' until they are ambulatory again.

What is happening to Mr MB and what would you recommend should be done?

A10 **Mr MB is experiencing a type of acute dystonic reaction called an oculogyric crisis. This is both painful and frightening and should be dealt with by the immediate administration of Intramuscular or intravenous procyclidine. One 10 mg dose is usually sufficient, although it can be repeated if required.**

What is the main advantage of administering a depot antipsychotic to Mr MB?

A11 **Compliance can be assured.**

Non-compliance and partial compliance with antipsychotic drugs is common in in-patient settings. One study found that 10% of in-patients had no trace of prescribed medication in their blood despite the existence of signed administration records.

Which depot antipsychotic would you recommend and why?

A12 **Mr MB experienced an acute dystonic reaction with haloperidol. Ideally he should receive risperidone depot due to its reduced propensity to cause motor side-effects. If Mr MB refuses risperidone depot, any of the others could be used, however if this is the case, a test dose would be essential.**

The nature of Mr MB's objections to oral risperidone are unclear. It is important to clarify if he experienced intolerable side-effects or just objected to taking any medication at all.

If the latter is found to be the case (as is likely), risperidone depot should be prescribed at a dose of 25 mg every two weeks. A test dose is not required as Mr MB has tolerated oral risperidone. Mr MB should also be prescribed oral risperidone in liquid form for the first three weeks of treatment although he may refuse to take it.

The pharmacokinetics of risperidone depot are very different to those of conventional depots. The risperidone is contained in microspheres which need to be suspended in diluent immediately prior to administration. The microspheres slowly dissolve releasing the active drug into the intramuscular site over a period of weeks. The first injection does not give therapeutic plasma levels until three weeks after administration. Thereafter the drug has to be administered every two weeks to maintain therapeutic levels.

If Mr MB had experienced side-effects with oral risperidone such as headaches or nausea, a typical antipsychotic in depot form could be used. Conventional depot antipsychotics are virtually indistinguishable with respect to efficacy or side-effects. Whichever one is chosen, a 'test dose' should be administered. This allows Mr MB to be observed for EPSEs and any allergic (local) reaction to the depot oil. Systemic (anaphylactic) reactions to depot antipsychotics have not been documented.

Why has a second opinion been requested?

A13 **Mr MB is refusing his injection and more than three months of his Section 3 have elapsed.**

When patients are detained under Section 3 of the Mental Health Act 1983, medication can be administered against their will for the first three months only. After this time, medication can only be enforced if a Section 58 (Form 39) has been completed by a second-opinion doctor who is a representative of the Mental Health Act Commission. The completed Form 39 should be attached to the patient's prescription chart and the drugs prescribed should be strictly in accordance with the permission that it gives. Future changes in drug therapy may require a further visit from the second-opinion doctor.

What role can the pharmacist play in this process?

A14 **In order to comply with Section 58, the second-opinion doctor must consult with two professionals who are involved in the clinical care of the patient. The first is usually the key nurse. The Mental Health Act states that the second person should be 'neither a doctor nor a nurse'. As an understanding of drug therapy is required, pharmacists are in an ideal position to fulfil this role. The Mental Health Act is currently under review. It is likely that the new Act will expand the role of pharmacists further.**

Can anything be done to change Mr MB's attitude towards antipsychotic drugs?

A15 **Mr MB is not accepting of the need to take medication. There is much to be gained from trying to work with him on this issue. Psychoeducation to address the nature of his illness and the likely effects and side-effects of medication is a priority. His views should be listened to and accommodated if at all possible. This approach, which has been called 'compliance therapy', has been shown to improve attitudes towards medication, increase compliance and delay readmission to hospital.**

What are the risks associated with high-dose and combination antipsychotics?

A16 **High-dose antipsychotics may be associated with sudden cardiac death. They carry a high risk of motor side-effects. Combinations of typical and atypical antipsychotics are particularly illogical as the patient may experience two different sets of side-effects simultaneously.**

It is unlikely that high-dose and combination antipsychotics confer significant therapeutic benefit to the majority of patients who receive them, although the evidence from studies that examine this issue is not incompatible with individual patients deriving benefit occasionally. This is where the problem lies in clinical practice: the majority of psychiatrists claim to treat many such patients.

A recent audit conducted by the Royal College of Psychiatrists Research Unit found that 20% of all in-patients who were prescribed antipsychotics could potentially receive a high (i.e. greater than the *British National Formulary* maximum) dose. 'As required' prescribing was a major source of 'high-dose' prescriptions and in the majority of cases there was no record in the patient's notes that a high dose had been prescribed. Monitoring for physical side-effects, particularly QTc prolongation, in these patients was poor. Antipsychotic polypharmacy was found in 48% of patients and 60% of those who were prescribed an atypical drug were prescribed a typical one in addition.

Patients receiving high-dose and combination antipsychotics are invariably disabled by a plethora of side-effects including EPSEs, sedation, anticholinergic side-effects, postural hypotension and potential QTc prolongation leading to life-threatening cardiac arrhythmias. As can be seen from the above audit, these side-effects often go unnoticed.

An excellent review of the evidence for the efficacy of high-dose antipsychotics and the risks associated with their use is to be found in the Royal College of Psychiatrists consensus statement. This statement also gives good practical guidelines on how to review treatment and document the clinical decision to use high-dose antipsychotics. It is both essential reading and a good audit tool for examining local practice.

Why has clozapine been prescribed for Mr MB and is its use appropriate at this time?

A17 **Mr MB has treatment-resistant schizophrenia. Clozapine is the only antipsychotic that has superior therapeutic efficacy in this situation and its use is thus indicated for Mr MB at this time.**

Mr MB's symptoms have failed to respond to three different antipsychotics given in adequate doses for adequate periods of time. His symptoms are disabling and his quality of life poor. His illness can, therefore, be described as treatment-resistant schizophrenia. The excellent study by Kane *et al.* demonstrated the superior efficacy of clozapine in otherwise treatment-resistant schizophrenia, with 30% of patients responding after six weeks of treatment. Follow-up studies have shown that double this number will show worthwhile therapeutic benefit if treatment is continued for six months to one year. These findings have been replicated by several groups.

Clozapine, therefore, offers Mr MB the best chance of relief from his symptoms.

How should treatment with clozapine be initiated and monitored?

A18 **Clozapine is associated with a 3% risk of neutropenia and haematological monitoring is a mandatory condition of treatment. This is coordinated by the Clozapine Patient Monitoring Service (CPMS). Mr MB should be registered with the CPMS. Depot antipsychotics should be discontinued and oral antipsychotics used during the change over period. Treatment with clozapine can be initiated once the CPMS receives satisfactory haematological results. The dosage should be titrated gradually upwards as described in the product data sheet and Mr MB should be observed for side-effects.**

Mr MB is currently receiving zuclopenthixol depot 600 mg/week and sulpiride 600 mg/day. It is routine clinical practice to omit the depot for one dosage interval before starting clozapine. In Mr MB's case this would mean starting clozapine 12.5 mg at night seven days after his last depot injection was administered and reducing the dose of sulpiride over the next few weeks as the clozapine dose is increased. There are no set rules for the duration of this cross-over period as it will be determined by Mr MB's mental state and ability to tolerate increasing doses of clozapine. Most patients can be successfully switched to clozapine monotherapy within four weeks.

When treatment is initiated, patients should be monitored for postural hypotension (due to alpha-adrenergic block), sedation (due to histaminergic block), tachycardia (due to cholinergic block) and fever (can be due to agranulocytosis, but is usually unexplained and benign and settles despite continued treatment).

Weekly blood counts, to monitor white cells, neutrophils and platelets, are performed for the first 18 weeks of treatment as this is the period of maximum haematological risk. Thereafter, fortnightly monitoring is required. If the haematological profile remains stable throughout the first year, the patient can move on to monthly monitoring.

For patients who are clinically stable, defined as stable mental state plus monthly monitoring, the option exists to be cared for through shared care protocols when GPs can prescribe continuing treatment and community pharmacies supply the clozapine. Full details of this system are available through the CPMS.

Whichever system is used, clozapine can only be dispensed on receipt of satisfactory haematological results. No blood, no drug.

How should treatment with clozapine be optimised?

A19 **The dose should be titrated up to 300–400 mg/day unless limited by side-effects. If there is no response after several weeks, a trough serum level should be measured. If the serum concentration is less than 350 micrograms/L, the dose should be increased to achieve a level over this threshold. If there is still no response, the dose should be increased to the maximum tolerated (up to 900 mg/day). It is important to remember that only 50% of eventual responders show therapeutic gains in the first six weeks. Clozapine should be prescribed for six months to one year before concluding that Mr MB has not responded.**

What side-effects might you anticipate and how would you deal with them?

A20 **Excess sedation, hypersalivation, postural hypotension, hypertension, tachycardia, nausea, constipation, nocturnal enuresis, weight gain, impaired glucose tolerance, diabetes and seizures can all occur. Myocarditis and cardiomyopathy have also been reported. EPSEs are extremely rare.**

Some of these side-effects are dose related, others are idiosyncratic. Dose-related side-effects are obviously best dealt with by slowing the rate of dosage titration or decreasing the dose. If this is not clinically possible or the problematic side-effect is not dose related, the following approaches can be useful:

(a) Excess sedation. This sometimes responds to alterations in the timing and distribution of the daily dose, e.g. early morning hang-over may be reduced by giving the last dose of the day at 8 p.m. Care must be taken to distinguish true drug-induced sedation from the lack of volition often seen in schizophrenia, or simple inactivity due to boredom.

(b) Hypersalivation. Simple measures such as propping up the pillows at night can sometimes resolve the problem. Hyoscine (Kwells) or pirenzepine often help. Pirenzepine is widely prescribed for hyper-salivation as it does not cross the blood–brain barrier and cause central side-effects; however, it must be imported for use in the UK as it has been discontinued.

(c)   Tachycardia. If persistent, beta-blockers may help. This is also a useful strategy in clozapine-induced hypertension.

(d)   Nausea. The aetiology of clozapine-induced nausea is poorly under-stood. Pragmatically, domperidone, ranitidine or a proton pump inhibitor often help.

(e)   Nocturnal enuresis. If restricting evening fluids fails to correct the problem and nocturnal seizures are not implicated, oxybutynin often helps. In severe cases, desmopressin may be used.

(f)   Weight gain. This should be anticipated and steps taken to prevent it. The mechanisms of antipsychotic weight gain are poorly under-stood and once the weight has been gained it is very difficult to lose. Obesity increases the risk of cardiovascular disease, some cancers, diabetes and osteoarthritis.

(g)   Diabetes. This requires evaluation of risk versus benefit in each case. There is no guarantee that the diabetes will resolve if clozapine is discontinued.

(h)   Seizures. These occur in 5% of patients who receive doses of cloza-pine in excess of 600 mg/day. Sodium valproate is effective. A dose of at least 1000 mg/day is usually required.

(i)   Sensitivity myocarditis and cardiomyopathy. It is important to be aware of these very rare side-effects. A high degree of vigilance should be shown if the patient displays any symptoms or signs suggestive of new onset cardiovascular disease.

What further options are available if Mr MB fails to respond to clozapine?

A21   **There are no other antipsychotics either currently available or in development that are as effective overall as clozapine. Various strategies have been used to augment response to clozapine. These include the addition of sulpiride, lamotrigine, valproate and benzodiazepines. It is essential to consult the primary literature before embarking upon any of these routes.**

Further reading

Allison DB, Mentore JL, Heo M et al. Anti-psychotic-induced weight gain: a comprehensive research synthesis. Am J Psychiatry 1999; **156**: 1686–1696.

American Psychiatric Association. Diagnostic and Statistical Manual of Mental Disorders, 4th edn. American Psychiatric Association, Washington DC, 1994.

American Psychiatric Association. Tardive Dyskinesia: A Task Force Report. American Psychiatric Association, Washington, 1992.

American Psychiatric Association. Practice guidelines for the treatment of patients with schizophrenia. Am J Psychiatry 1997; **154**: 1–49.

Ashton HC. Pharmacology and effects of cannabis. Br J Psychiatry 2001; **178**: 101–106.

British Medical Association and Royal Pharmaceutical Society of Great Britain. British National Formulary. British Medical Association and Royal Pharmaceutical Society of Great Britain, London, 2002.

Chong SA, Remmington G. Clozapine augmentation: safety and efficacy. Schizophrenia Bull 2000; **26**: 421–440.

Cree A, Mir S, Fahy T. A review of the treatment options for clozapine-induced hypersalivation. Psychiatr Bull 2001; **25**: 114–116.

Department of Health. National Service Framework for Mental Health. Department of Health, London, 1999.

Dursan SM, McIntosh D, Milliken H. Clozapine plus lamotrigine in treatment resistant schizophrenia. Arch Gen Psychiatry 1999; **56**: 950.

Geddes J, Freemantle N, Harrison P et al. Atypical anti-psychotics in the treatment of schizophrenia: systematic overview and meta-regression analysis. Br Med J 2000; **321**: 1371–1376.

Gelder M, Gath D, Mayou R. Oxford Textbook of Psychiatry, 4th edn. Oxford Medical Publications, Oxford, 2001.

Harrington M, Lelliott P, Paton C et al. The results of a multi-centre audit of the prescribing of anti-psychotic drugs for in-patients in the United Kingdom. Psychiatr Bull 2002; **26**: 414–418.

Johns A. Psychiatric effects of cannabis. Br J Psychiatry 2001; **178**: 116–122.

Kane J, Honigfeld G, Singer J et al. Clozapine for the treatment resistant schizophrenic. Arch Gen Psychiatry 1988; **45**: 789–796.

Keck P, Cohen B, Baldessarini R et al. Time course of anti-psychotic effects of neuroleptic drugs. Am J Psychiatry 1989; **146**: 1289–1299.

Kemp R, Kirov G, Everitt B et al. Randomised controlled trial of compliance therapy. Br J Psychiatry 1998; **172**: 413–419.

Killian JG, Kerr K, Lawrence C et al. Myocarditis and cardiomyopathy associated with clozapine. Lancet 1999; **354**: 1841–1845.

Mir S, Taylor D. Atypical anti-psychotics and hyperglycaemia. Int Clin Psychopharmacol 2001; **16**: 63–73.

National Institute for Clinical Effectiveness. Guidelines for the Use of Atypical Anti-psychotics in Schizophrenia. NICE, London, 2002.

National Schizophrenia Fellowship. *A Question of Choice*. National Schizo-phrenia Fellowship, London, 2001.

Overall JE, Gorham DR. The Brief Psychiatric Rating Scale. *Psychol Rep* 1962; **10**: 799–812.

Paton C, Morrison P. Should community mental health nurses be trained in recognising and treating anaphylaxis. *Mental Health Pract* 1999; **2**: 18–20.

Paton C, Okocha C. Anti-psychotic drugs: old and new. *New Med* 2001; **1**: 45–50.

Paton C, Banham S, Whitmore J. Benzodiazepines in schizophrenia. *Psychiatr Bull* 2000; **24**: 113–115.

Paton C, Lelliott P, Harrington M *et al*. Patterns of antipsychotic and anti-cholinergic drug prescribing for hospital inpatients. *J Psychopharmacol* 2003; **17**: 223–229.

Pilowsky L, Ring H, Shine P *et al*. A survey of emergency prescribing in a general psychiatric hospital. *Br J Psychiatry* 1992; **160**: 831–835.

Reilly J, Ayis S, Ferrier IN *et al*. QTc interval abnormalities and psychotropic drug therapy in psychiatric patients. *Lancet* 2000, **355**: 1048–1052.

Reilly JG, Thomas SHL, Ferrier IN. Recent studies on ECG changes, anti-psychotic use and sudden death in psychiatric patients. *Psychiatr Bull* 2002; **26**: 110–112.

Rifkin A, Doddi S, Karajgi B *et al*. Dosage of haloperidol for schizophrenia. *Arch Gen Psychiatry* 1991; **48**: 166–170.

Taylor D. Depot anti-psychotics revisited. *Psychiatr Bull* 1999; **23**: 551–553.

Taylor D, Paton C. *Case Studies in Psychopharmacology*, 2nd edn. Martin Dunitz, London, 2002.

Thompson C for the Royal College of Psychiatrists Consensus Panel. Con-sensus statement on the use of high dose anti-psychotic medication. *Br J Psychiatry* 1994; **164**: 448–458.

World Health Organization. *The ICD–10 Classification of Mental and Behav-ioural Disorders – Clinical Descriptions and Diagnostic Guidelines*. WHO, Geneva, 1992.

Wright P, Birkett M, David SR *et al*. Double-blind, placebo controlled compar-ison of intramuscular olanzapine and intramuscular haloperidol in the treatment of acute agitation in schizophrenia. *Am J Psychiatry* 2001; **158**: 1149–1151.

18

Depression

Stuart Gill-Banham

Day 1 Miss CT, a 35-year-old female, made an appointment to see her GP because she felt run-down and generally unable to cope. She said she felt tired all day long, yet at night she could not sleep. Concentrating on any task had become difficult and she felt everything was getting on top of her. Frequently she would be reduced to tears when faced with a task and she dreaded having to go out, as she felt quite panicky when she left the house. She had not felt 100% for the last few months, since she had split up with her partner. She denied ever having felt like this in the past, although she had been extremely saddened by the sudden death of her mother when she was 14 years old. The GP prescribed fluoxetine 20 mg daily plus diazepam 2 mg twice daily for just two weeks.

Q1 Are Miss CT's presenting symptoms typical of depression?
Q2 Is this depressive episode purely a reaction to the end of her relationship or could it be due to other factors?
Q3 In what ways can depression be treated?
Q4 Is the combination of fluoxetine and diazepam appropriate?

Week 3 Miss CT had been concerned that she would become addicted to the medication so after two weeks she had stopped both the fluoxetine and diazepam as she was feeling slightly better. However, her mood had quickly deteriorated and so she returned to her GP.

Q5 Are antidepressants addictive and how long should they be prescribed for?

The GP persuaded Miss CT that antidepressants are not addictive and she restarted the fluoxetine plus a further two-week course of diazepam.

Q6 Outline a pharmaceutical care plan for Miss CT.

Week 12   Miss CT was still experiencing poor concentration and feeling unable to cope with daily activities. When her GP saw her he noticed that she had lost a considerable amount of weight and had an unkempt appearance. Miss CT was adamant that she has been taking the fluoxetine regularly every day.

Q7   What treatment options are available to the GP now?

The GP decided to try Miss CT on venlafaxine 37.5 mg twice daily.

Q8   Was the starting dose of venlafaxine appropriate?
Q9   How should venlafaxine therapy be monitored?

Week 20   The dose of venlafaxine had reached 225 mg daily. It had been higher than this, but Miss CT could not tolerate the associated severe nausea, so the dose had had to be reduced. Miss CT described herself as 50% better. She was now able to leave her house without feeling panicky and she no longer felt like crying as much as before. However, she still lacked motivation and her appetite remained poor.

Q10 What options are there to improve Miss CT's mood further?

The GP decided to try to augment her antidepressant therapy with lithium.

Q11 Is this appropriate treatment for Miss CT?
Q12 What baseline checks need to be performed before lithium is started and how frequently should lithium levels be monitored?
Q13 What points should be covered when counselling Miss CT about her lithium therapy?
Q14 How long should treatment with lithium and venlafaxine be continued?
Q15 What other treatment options could be considered if Miss CT fails to respond to this therapy?

Are Miss CT's presenting symptoms typical of depression?

A1 **It is difficult to say exactly which symptoms of depression are typical due to the varied ways in which the illness can present. However, Miss CT does display some key symptoms of a depressive illness.**

Depression is a syndrome characterised by persistent low mood, anhedonia, a lack of interest in usual daily activities and a lack of energy. In addition to these key symptoms a wide range of accompanying symptoms can be present. Accompanying symptoms can be psychological (e.g. anxiety, increased sense of guilt, pessimism or suicidal thoughts and plans), physical (e.g. disturbed sleep, early morning wakening, tiredness, lack of energy, loss of appetite and increased sensitivity to pain), cognitive (e.g. impaired concentration and memory) and psychomotor (e.g. agitation, physical slowing or refusal of food and drink). In order to make a diagnosis of mild depression at least four symptoms, two of which need to be key symptoms, need to have been present for at least the preceding two weeks. Moderate depression is diagnosed when six symptoms are present. Again, two need to be key symptoms. Severe depression is diagnosed when eight symptoms are present, at least three of which have to be key symptoms.

Depressive symptoms are more common than most people realise. Up to 10% of the population will experience some form of depressive illness at some time in their life. Women are more than twice as likely as men to develop depression, in part as a result of an increased readiness to admit what their true feelings are.

The key symptoms displayed by Miss CT were low mood, poor sleep, lack of energy, poor concentration and severe anxiety, which was impairing her daily routine. Frequently depression is not diagnosed when patients seek medical help, especially when they present with predominantly physical complaints. Depression ratings scales, which are formal sets of questions that can be used to give a numerical score to symptom severity, can be helpful in the diagnosis of depression. Such rating scales should not be seen as providing a black and white answer to the question of whether somebody is depressed; rather they serve as a guide to indicate when an individual's underlying problem might be depressed mood.

Is this depressive episode purely a reaction to the end of Miss CT's relationship or could it be due to other factors?

A2 **Although a depressive episode is frequently triggered by a stressful life event, it is not possible to say that one event is solely responsible. Several factors, such as genetic predisposition, previous experiences and childhood upbringing, can influence how an individual handles life events and in turn the likelihood of a stressful event leading to an episode of depression.**

The degree to which somebody has a predisposition to depression is determined by a combination of genetic factors along with their upbringing and previous life experiences. Studies comparing rates of depression in identical and non-identical twins have found depression is nearly twice as likely in the brother or sister of an identical twin with depression compared with a non-identical twin. Genetic predisposition could exert its influence upon the biochemical structure of the brain or its influence could be subtler, by altering individual character traits. Along with genetic factors early life experiences, particularly parental discord or abuse, can influence the degree of predisposition faced by an individual.

Regardless of an individual's predisposition to depression, some life events may be more likely than others to cause depression. Events that lead to feelings of entrapment or humiliation are thought to be particularly important.

For Miss CT the break-up of her relationship was a significant factor, but it may not have been the cause of her depression. In her personal history she had coped with the loss of her mother at an early age. It is impossible to say how this influenced her upbringing, but it could have affected the way she coped with stressful events. Although the relationship ended about the same time as the depressive episode started it might have been the emerging depressive illness that caused the relationship to end.

In what ways can depression be treated?

A3 **A range of options are available to treat depression including psychological therapy, drug therapy and electroconvulsive therapy (ECT).**

Deciding which treatment option is the most appropriate depends upon the severity of the depressive episode, and the preferences of both the doctor and the patient. Drug therapy is not necessarily the best option for mild depressive episodes. Studies of mild depression frequently fail to demonstrate that antidepressants have a significant effect, largely as a result of high placebo response rates. Many patients prefer non-drug approaches to managing depression; they particularly value practical support and problem solving approaches. Additional non-drug therapies may include dynamic psychotherapy, which examines interpersonal dynamics and how these may contribute to an individual's predisposition to experiencing depression, or cognitive therapy, which examines how an individual interprets adverse events and how this may make depression more likely. The availability of non-drug therapies can be limited as they require a greater level of support than can sometimes be offered.

A wide range of antidepressant drugs are available and they are classified according to either their mechanism of action, e.g. selective serotonin reuptake inhibitors (SSRIs) or monoamine-oxidase inhibitors (MAOIs), or according to their chemical structure, e.g. tricyclic anti-depressants (TCAs). Many of the more recently introduced antidepres-sants cannot be classified in any of these groups and are placed in groups of their own, e.g. venlafaxine, a selective noradrenaline (norepinephrine) and serotonin reuptake inhibitor, or reboxetine, a selective noradrenaline reuptake inhibitor. Classifying antidepressants in this way causes con-fusion, as it implies some agents have a unique mechanism of action when this is not the case. For example, venlafaxine is not the only antidepressant to block the reuptake of both noradrenaline and serotonin as several TCAs have an effect on both of these neurotransmitters.

Antidepressants from different therapeutic classes differ little in their overall effectiveness. Studies which have directly compared different antidepressants have found the response rates achieved to be comparable. However, individual patient response to antidepressants and tolerance of side-effects can vary considerably.

Different classes of antidepressants have quite distinct side-effect profiles. The TCAs predominantly cause sedation, dry mouth, blurred vision, constipation and weight gain. SSRIs predominantly cause head-aches, nausea, diarrhoea and initial weight loss, although when patients start to respond to the antidepressant effect, weight gain is produced.

Selecting the most appropriate antidepressant for an individual is largely based upon a consideration of the likely response and the side-effects which may be seen.

ECT has been found to be effective in cases of severe depression, especially when psychotic symptoms are present. Due to its rapid onset of action patients can improve after just one session. ECT is a treatment option when the patient is refusing fluids and so is in grave danger of harm.

Is the combination of fluoxetine and diazepam appropriate?

A4   **Fluoxetine is a reasonable choice for first-line antidepressant and combining it with a short benzodiazepine course could have many advantages. Care is needed to ensure that any potential benefits of this combination are not outweighed by the risks of addiction or tolerance to the benzodiazepine.**

All antidepressants are equally effective in treating depression. Choice of antidepressant therefore relies upon considering response to previous treatment, potential side-effects, the likelihood of an intentional overdose, the age and physical condition of the patient, whether there are any other concurrent drug therapies and the personal preferences of the prescriber. Miss CT is young fit and healthy, and has never been treated with an antidepressant before, so the choice will largely be based upon the potential side-effects.

It is widely believed that SSRIs are better tolerated than TCAs, although evidence from clinical trials is not necessarily as conclusive as popular belief. Whether SSRIs are better tolerated is not as important as the fact that when patients are prescribed an SSRI they are more likely to receive an effective dose than if they are prescribed a TCA. Another potential benefit of prescribing an SSRI as first-line therapy is their safety in overdose. It is estimated that the average number of deaths from overdose with TCAs is 34 per million prescriptions, whereas for SSRIs the figure is two deaths per million prescriptions.

In deciding which SSRI to use it needs to be remembered that studies have failed to demonstrate any single agent to be more effective than another. As the main SSRIs have similar side-effect profiles, then the choice is based upon an individual prescriber's experiences and preferences or on cost considerations.

Addition of a benzodiazepine to antidepressant therapy has numerous potential benefits, particularly when anxiety symptoms predominate. It is likely that Miss CT's anxiety is a symptom of her depression, so if the depression is treated then the anxiety will resolve. However, depression can take between two and four weeks to respond to an antidepressant and during this time the anxiety may become worse, particularly as fluoxetine, in common with other SSRIs, can cause an initial increase in anxiety. A recent review by the Cochrane collaboration found that adding a benzodiazepine to an antidepressant improved the initial antidepressant response and reduced the likelihood of therapy being discontinued. A benzodiazepine such as diazepam will quickly reduce anxiety symptoms and by the end of the two-week course there will hopefully be some response to the antidepressant. Use of the benzodiazepine should be restricted to less than four weeks' duration in order to minimise the risk of tolerance and addiction.

Are antidepressants addictive and how long should they be prescribed for?

A5 **Contrary to popular belief, antidepressants are not addictive but sudden discontinuation can produce a withdrawal reaction. The minimum length of time they should be prescribed for is six months after all symptoms have been resolved. Continuous therapy may need to be considered for patients who have had multiple episodes of depression.**

One of the major concerns that patients have when prescribed an antidepressant is that they are addictive and by taking them they may become dependent upon them for life. This simply is not true. Antidepressants are not addictive and needing to take them for long periods to treat depression should not be confused with being dependent upon them. A useful analogy is to compare treatment of depression with the treatment of any physical illness. For many patients with a physical condition medication is needed to control symptoms of that disease. When the medication is stopped the symptoms may return but this is not the same as dependence. It is true that many antidepressants if stopped abruptly will produce withdrawal symptoms such as anxiety, flu-like aches and pains or irritability but this should not be seen as evidence of addiction because there is not a physical craving for the antidepressant. Withdrawal symptoms can be avoided by gradually reducing doses of an antidepressant before it is stopped. For Miss CT the risk of any withdrawal reaction is minimal as fluoxetine has one of the longest half-lives of any antidepressant so hardly ever causes a withdrawal reaction.

Despite antidepressants being non-addictive, patients tend to only be prescribed them for the minimum period of time. It is widely accepted that the minimum period that they should be prescribed for is six months after all symptoms have disappeared. This figure comes from studies which found that in patients who had responded to antidepressant therapy, those who were switched to placebo were more than twice as likely to relapse in the following six months when compared to those who remained on antidepressant therapy. Allowing for between two and three months for all symptoms to respond to therapy means that most patients will need to take an antidepressant for around nine months for any single episode of depression. Individuals who have experienced one episode of depression are at an increased risk of further episodes. For those patients who have had two or more episodes of depression, 75% will remain well for five years if they continue to take their medication, whereas only 10% of those who stop their medication will remain well for the same period. Patients who have had multiple episodes of depression therefore may benefit from long-term therapy with an antidepressant.

Outline a pharmaceutical care plan for Miss CT.

A6 **The pharmaceutical care plan for Miss CT should include the following:**

(a)   Ensure the antidepressant and benzodiazepine are restarted at a dose appropriate for the presenting symptoms.
(b)   Ensure that the benzodiazepine is prescribed for as long as anxiety remains a problem, but it is stopped before addiction occurs.
(c)   Counsel Miss CT about the potential side-effects of both agents and also how they will be of benefit.
(d)   Explain how long it will take before any antidepressant response is seen.
(e)   Reassure Miss CT that antidepressants are not addictive.
(f)   Monitor her for signs of side-effects.

What treatment options are available to the GP now?

A7 **Change to a different antidepressant. Other options could include non-drug strategies or ECT.**

If the first-line antidepressant fails to produce a therapeutic response despite being prescribed for an adequate length of time at an adequate dose then an alternative antidepressant will need to be considered. An adequate length of time is usually defined as being at least four weeks, but if some response is seen then there is benefit in continuing with the antidepressant for longer. Defining what constitutes an adequate dose can be more difficult. Most SSRIs are effective at their initial starting dose, although there is some debate as to whether sertraline is effective at

50 mg daily so doses of at least 100 mg/day are sometimes preferred. For TCAs doses need to be at least 100 mg/day. Studies have shown that 70 or 75 mg doses fail to produce a consistent response. One way of considering whether an appropriate dose has been used is to ensure that the maximum tolerated dose has been given. If patients are unable to tolerate a TCA dose greater than 50 or 70 mg/day then there is little point trying to force the dose any higher. It would then make more sense to consider switching to an alternative antidepressant.

The choice of alternative antidepressant will again depend upon the potential side-effects that may be seen, as well as on which antidepressant was initially used. Although an individual's response to different drugs in the same class should be different, in practice the response seen differs only minimally. This is particularly true with SSRIs as they share a common mechanism of action. With TCAs there is some individual difference to response as they have slightly different receptor affinities. However, it is usual to select a second choice antidepressant that is from a different class to the first.

Other treatment options at this point may include non-drug therapies, although if the depression is severe then this may impair the patient's ability to engage with such therapies. If the symptoms are particularly severe then ECT may be indicated, although as Miss CT is remaining under the care of her GP it is unlikely that her depression is severe enough to warrant ECT.

In summary, Miss CT has failed to respond adequately to the first antidepressant that was prescribed. She should be switched to another agent from a different class. This could be either a TCA or one of the newer agents, e.g. venlafaxine or mirtazapine. There is no evidence to suggest one would be more effective than another so the choice would be based upon likely side-effect profiles and overall tolerability.

Was the starting dose of venlafaxine appropriate?

A8 **It is recommended that therapy with venlafaxine be initiated at 75 mg/day. As venlafaxine has a wide dose range Miss CT will gain more benefit from a higher dose, especially as the drugs noradrenergic effect is only seen at higher doses.**

The major benefit of choosing venlafaxine for Miss CT is it has a different mechanism of action to the SSRIs. In addition to blocking the reuptake of serotonin by presynaptic neurones venlafaxine also blocks the reuptake of noradrenaline. This dual effect may be advantageous as Miss CT failed to respond to an SSRI. As many of its side-effects are dose related, especially nausea, sedation and postural hypotension, a low starting dose is used; however, at these low doses venlafaxine predominantly has an effect on serotonin pathways, so has a mechanism of action similar to an SSRI. It is only after the dose is increased beyond 112.5 mg/day that any activity on noradrenaline reuptake is seen. In order to gain maximum benefit from prescribing venlafaxine the dose will therefore need to be increased to 150 mg/day after a couple of weeks.

How should venlafaxine therapy be monitored?

A9 **Response to therapy can be monitored subjectively or objectively using an appropriate rating scale. Particular side-effects that need to be monitored for are sedation, nausea and (possibly) changes in blood pressure.**

Therapeutic response can be measured subjectively by assessing the patient and seeing if key depressive symptoms are resolved. For Miss CT this will be assessing to see if mood improves, if she takes more of a pride in her appearance and if any weight is gained. If necessary, objective assessment of her mental state can be made by using a standard depression rating scale.

Venlafaxine causes a considerable number of side-effects, including constipation, nausea, dizziness, headache or dry mouth. Dose-related hypertension is seen with venlafaxine and in patients with existing hypertension close monitoring of blood pressure may be necessary if the dose is increased above 150 mg/day. Venlafaxine can also cause increases in serum cholesterol, particularly following prolonged use. Again, in susceptible patients routine monitoring may be advisable.

What options are there to improve Miss CT's mood further?

A10 **If only a partial response is seen then the dose of antidepressant can be increased further, a new antidepressant can be prescribed or an augmenting strategy can be considered.**

Miss CT is already at the maximum dose of venlafaxine that she can tolerate so the option of a further increase in dose would seem inappropriate. Using a sustained-release formulation of venlafaxine can help reduce the incidence of nausea but the maximum licensed dose for this formulation is 225 mg/day. If another antidepressant was to be considered then either a TCA, mirtazepine or possibly even a MAOI might be appropriate. MAOIs are infrequently used in clinical practice due to their adverse effects, and their interactions with other medicines and foods. However, they are still indicated for atypical depression, where symptoms include pronounced phobic anxiety. Moclobemide differs from other MAOIs in that it reversibly inhibits monoamine oxidase type A enzyme. This allows an antidepressant effect without any interaction with foodstuffs plus a quicker offset of action.

The main disadvantage of switching antidepressant therapy at this stage would be the time that a switch would take. In order to minimise any withdrawal symptoms it would be necessary to gradually reduce the dose of venlafaxine over two weeks; however, a specific washout period would not be required if either a TCA or mirtazapine were prescribed.

As there has been some response to venlafaxine then it may be possible to augment its effect by adding another agent to the regimen. Several agents have been suggested as possible augmentation agents including: levothyroxine, liothyronine, tryptophan, anticonvulsants or lithium. Another means of augmenting antidepressant therapy might be to add a second antidepressant into the regimen. Generally this approach is only recommended as a last resort and should be undertaken by somebody experienced in using antidepressant combinations due to the potential that many antidepressants have for interacting with other antidepressants.

Is augmentation with lithium appropriate?

A11 **Lithium is a recognised augmentation option for patients who fail to respond or only partially respond to antidepressant therapy.**

Several studies have shown that the addition of lithium to antidepressant therapy is beneficial in reducing depressive symptoms in patients who are not suffering from a bipolar illness. Antidepressants studied in combination with lithium include lofepramine, fluoxetine, sertraline, citalopram and venlafaxine. When using lithium as an augmentation agent the same plasma level should be aimed for as when lithium is used to treat bipolar disorder, i.e. at least 0.4 mmol/L.

What baseline checks need to be performed before lithium is started and how frequently should lithium levels be monitored?

A12 **Before lithium therapy is commenced the following baseline checks are needed: renal function, thyroid function and general health, including cardiac function. Once an appropriate plasma level has been reached lithium levels should be checked monthly for the first three months, then every three to six months thereafter.**

It is essential to check renal function before commencing lithium therapy as lithium is excreted predominantly unchanged by the kidneys. If renal function is reduced, especially if glomerular filtration rate is less than 50 mL/min, then lithium clearance will be correspondingly reduced and a lower starting dose may be required.

An assessment of thyroid function is necessary because lithium therapy can cause changes in thyroid function in 5–20% of patients. Lithium-induced hypothyroidism can be managed by administering replacement levothyroxine and is reversible when lithium therapy is withdrawn.

There is some debate about the clinical significance of the electro-cardiogram (ECG) changes which lithium therapy can produce. They are largely thought to be benign but initial assessment can be useful in determining if any subsequent ECG abnormalities are due to lithium treatment.

Lithium therapy should be started at a dose of 400 mg lithium carbonate each night (200 mg in the elderly or those who are physically frail). Four to five days after the first dose, a lithium level should be taken 12 h after the last dose and the dose adjusted to the range of 0.4–1.0 mmol/L. Once a stable plasma level has been reached, the level should be rechecked every month for the first three months, then every three to six months after that.

What points should be covered when counselling Miss CT about her lithium therapy?

A13 **Before lithium is started Miss CT needs to be told that lithium will be a long-term treatment; that regular blood tests will be required and why; what the side-effects of lithium are; how to recognise toxicity; the dangers of dehydration or low-salt diets, and which over-the-counter medicines should be avoided.**

The common side-effects of lithium include fine tremor, polyuria (passing a lot of urine), polydipsia (increased thirst), nausea or diarrhoea.

These are usually mild and transient. Other side-effects can also be a sign of lithium toxicity. These include blurred vision, confusion, drowsiness or palpitations and if any of these are experienced then the patient needs to have an urgent lithium level taken.

As the body handles lithium in the same way as sodium ions, so altered sodium levels in the body can affect lithium levels. Thus if sodium levels fall, either due to dehydration or reduced dietary intake, the body will in compensation reduce the amount of sodium excreted by the kidneys and, as a consequence, will also reduce lithium excretion. This in turn will lead to lithium toxicity. Patients taking lithium need to know how dangerous dehydration or low-salt (sodium) diets can be.

Several medicines can potentially interact with lithium, including angiotensin-converting enzyme inhibitors, diuretics and non-steroidal anti-inflammatory drugs. Patients need to be warned about avoiding aspirin or aspirin-like painkillers if they self-medicate, and they need to tell any doctor who prescribes medicines for them that they are taking lithium.

How long should treatment with lithium and venlafaxine be continued?

A14   **If a response is seen with this combination then therapy may need to be continued for a considerable length of time, well beyond the six months of therapy recommended for uncomplicated cases of depression.**

The prognosis for Miss CT is not good as her depressive episode failed to respond to the first two antidepressants prescribed. This may mean that therapy should be continued for longer than the six months after the resolution of symptoms recommended in straightforward cases. Anti-depressant therapy for up to five years, and possibly longer, will continue to prevent the return of symptoms. If there was a desire to withdraw therapy, then each agent should be gradually withdrawn one after the other, starting with lithium first. It should be remembered that even if gradually withdrawn, the risk of relapse would be high.

What other treatment options could be considered if Miss CT fails to respond to this therapy?

A15   **Other treatment options might be augmentation with a different agent, prescribing two antidepressants together or ECT.**

Alternatives to lithium augmentation might include sodium valproate, tryptophan or a thyroid hormone. The use of tryptophan or a thyroid hormone to treat depression requires specialist knowledge and experience, and would best be undertaken by a consultant psychiatrist. Tryptophan, an amino acid precursor of the neurotransmitter serotonin, is sometimes used to treat resistant depression. Due to an association with eosinophilia myalgia syndrome (EMS), it can only be prescribed on a named patient basis by hospital specialists. Patients receiving tryptophan require routine blood monitoring to prevent the development of EMS.

ECT would be indicated for Miss CT if she continued to lose weight or started to refuse fluids. Miss CT's care would need to be referred to a consultant psychiatrist in order for ECT to be used.

Further reading

Anderson I, Nutt D, Deakin J. Evidence-based guidelines for treating depressive disorders with antidepressants: a revision of the 1993 British Association for Psychopharmacology guidelines. *J Psychopharmacol* 2000; **14**: 3–20.

Bollini P, Pampallona S, Tibaldi G. Effectiveness of antidepressants: meta-analysis of dose-effect relationships in randomised clinical trials. *Br J Psychiatry* 1999; **174**: 297–303.

Cookson J. Lithium: balancing risks and benefits. *Br J Psychiatry* 1997; **171**: 120–124.

Davidson J, Meltzer-Brody S. The underrecognition and undertreatment of depression: what is the breadth and depth of the problem? *J Clin Psychiatry* 1999; **60**(suppl. 7): 4–9.

Edwards J. Long term pharmacotherapy of depression. *Br Med J* 1998; **316**: 1180–1181.

Furukawa T, Streiner D, Young L. Antidepressant plus benzodiazepine for major depression (Cochrane Review). In: *The Cochrane Library 2*. Update Software, Oxford, 2003.

Gelder M, Gath D, Mayou R. *Oxford Textbook of Psychiatry.* Oxford University Press, Oxford, 1998.

Gilbody S, House A, Sheldon T. Routinely administered questionnaires for depression and anxiety: systematic review. *Br Med J* 2001; **322**: 406–409.

Peveler R, Carson A, Rodin G. ABC of psychological medicine: depression in medical patients. *Br Med J* 2002; **325**: 149–152.

Reimherr FW, Amsterdam JD, Quitkin F *et al.* Optimal length of continuation therapy in depression: a prospective assessment during long-term fluoxetine treatment. *Am J Psychiatry* 1998; **155**: 1247–1253.

Williams JW, Mulrow CD, Chiquette E *et al.* A systematic review of newer pharmacotherapies for depression in adults: evidence report summary: clinical guideline, part 2. *Ann Intern Med* 2000; **132**: 743–756.

19

Dementia

Denise Taylor

Day 1 Mr LD, a 76-year-old retired sales manager, attended a memory clinic at his local district general hospital with his wife. He had a two-year history of aphasia, mild memory difficulties and problems with activities of daily living. His wife reported that he needed help in dressing appropriately, often putting on pyjamas or suits at the wrong time of day unless she laid out his outfits each morning and evening. She said that he also used to be the one who looked after all the household bills but now he just ignored his bank statements and has also misplaced his chequebook.

The Mini Mental State Examination (MMSE Folstein) score was 25/30 and the Activities of Daily Living (ADL) score was 16/20. He exhibited no extrapyramidal signs, had no medical history of note and scored 12 on the Hamilton Depression (HAMD) rating scale. His blood pressure was 145/85 mmHg, pulse 75 beats per minute, capillary blood sugar 4.6, and his urea and electrolyte levels were all within normal range. Tests for folate, B_{12}, haemoglobin, thyroid and liver function were also all within normal range.

Q1 Briefly describe the purpose and function of the MMSE, ADL and HAMD rating scores.
Q2 What is the purpose of the other baseline measures assessed for Mr LD?

Mr LD agreed to start an antidepressant and attend the memory clinic once a month for review. He was given information on methods to improve his memory and a prescription for fluoxetine 20 mg each morning.

Q3 What is the purpose of trying to improve Mr LD's memory?
Q4 Was fluoxetine therapy appropriate for Mr LD?

Month 3   Mr LD arrived for the day dressed in his pyjama bottoms, and a shirt and tie. He was adamant that he had been brought against his will and that there was nothing wrong with him, and he accused the ambulance driver of stealing his wallet. He became very agitated and displayed mild symptoms of aggression (shouting and pacing up and down) until one of the nurses distracted him with a photo-album depicting London in wartime. Eventually he agreed to see the doctor. His MMSE score was now 21/30, the HAMD score 4, ADL rated 12/20 and his ADAS-cog score was 22.

A computed tomography (CT) scan showed enlarged lateral ventricles, widening of the sulci and atrophy of the medial structures in keeping with a neurodegenerative disorder. No space occupying lesions or cerebral ischaemia was seen.

Q5   What is an 'ADAS-cog' score, how is it calculated and what is the relevance of the final score?

Q6   What is the relevance of the CT results?

Q7   What is the probable diagnosis for Mr LD and how can it be confirmed?

Mr LD's wife was contacted and asked if she could accompany her husband to his next memory clinic appointment. At this appointment, they were informed that Mr LD probably had Alzheimer's disease (AD).

Q8   Why is an early diagnosis of AD better for the patient and their family?

Q9   What are the pharmacological treatment options for Mr LD?

Q10   What therapy would you recommend? Outline a dosing and monitoring schedule.

Q11   Outline a pharmaceutical care plan for Mr LD.

Month 7   Mr LD had his three-monthly assessment after starting rivastigmine. Mr LD had complained of feeling nauseous and dizzy when the rivastigmine was initially started, but he had eventually tolerated the dose increases until the last increase to 4.5 mg twice daily, when he had begun to vomit and feel unwell in himself. On observation he was lethargic and pale, and reluctant to speak. He refused to complete any of the assessment scales because he was feeling so poorly.

Q12   What is the possible cause of these side-effects and how might they be treated?

Mrs LD asked whether her husband should take any herbal remedies as she had heard at the Alzheimer's support group that they could help.

Q13 What is the role of ginkgo biloba and other dietary supplements in the symptomatic treatment of AD?

Month 8   Mr LD was looking much brighter and was telling the nursing staff about his day out to the zoo with his great-grandchildren at the weekend. His MMSE score was now 24/30, ADL rated 16/20 and the ADAS-cog score was 18. His wife thought that he 'was doing brilliantly', and that he seemed much happier and contented in himself.

Month 12   Mr LD was admitted to a general medical ward with deteriorating cognitive function and increasing confusion. That morning Mrs LD had woken up to find her husband was missing from their bedroom. She could not find him downstairs, then had heard 'banging noises' coming from the upstairs bedroom. She found Mr LD in the front bedroom wardrobe 'hiding from the b....... Germans'. Mr LD's GP arranged his admission to hospital for further investigation.

On examination Mr LD was increasingly confused and would not settle for a full physical examination. Observations noted were: a temperature of 39°C, an empty bladder and no signs of constipation. He had an increased respiratory rate, with a 'chesty' cough and crepitations at the left base.

He then became extremely anxious and 'escaped' from behind the curtains to the safety of the corridor near the nurses' station. He now believed that he was back in the army and had to 'take control of the lake' to protect everybody. He would not allow anyone to come near him and was having conversations with an imaginary person he referred to as 'Captain.'

Q14 What is the likely diagnosis for Mr LD?
Q15 Would you recommend antipsychotic therapy for Mr LD at this point?

Two days later   Mr LD's cognitive symptoms had resolved and his temperature was now normal. Antibiotics had controlled his chest infection and he now wanted to go home to be with his wife. He complained that the ward was 'full of old people.'

Month 24   Mr LD's dose of rivastigmine had been increased three months previously to the maximum licensed dose of 6 mg twice daily. This was in response to a fall in his MMSE, ADAS-cog and ADL scores. Since then, there had been no improvement in the scores (MMSE 14/30, ADAS-cog 38 and ADL 8/20), but no further fall in scores. His wife was distressed because Mr LD was now very agitated and shouted at her for bringing 'strangers into the house'. (The strangers were his grandchild and great-grandchildren). He had started to wander aimlessly from room to room and seemed unable to settle. He had also been having increasingly frequent episodes of urinary incontinence and Mrs LD was feeling 'at the end of my tether'.

Q16 What are the next therapeutic options?

Q17 What care issues are necessary for Mrs LD?

Month 40   Mr LD was now very frail (he had lost 8 kg since the first diagnosis of probable AD). He had been admitted to a nursing home three months earlier when Mrs LD no longer felt able to cope. Although his medication of memantine 10 mg twice daily had been continued after admission, he now no longer seemed to be aware of his surroundings. He no longer recognised his wife or any of his family. Increasingly he had been calling for his mother, getting very agitated in the evenings and had difficulty in sleeping. He was often observed 'talking' to an imaginary person who sat at the end of his bed. His speech was rambling and confused, and mainly incoherent. He was also now doubly incontinent and unable to feed himself successfully.

Q18 How might Mr LD's increasing agitation and hallucinations be controlled?

Q19 Outline a pharmaceutical care plan for the treatment of double incontinence.

Q20 When might pharmacological treatment for Mr LD be withdrawn?

Briefly describe the purpose and function of the MMSE, ADL and HAMD rating scores.

A1 **These provide a baseline measurement of a patient's cognitive function, their ability to carry out activities of daily living and to ascertain if a clinical depression is present.**

(a) MMSE.

The Folstein MMSE tests eight domains of cognitive function including: orientation, memory, recall, language and attention. It takes 10–15 minutes to complete. It is scored from 0 (lowest) to 30. A score of 27–30 = normal cognitive function, 25–26 = possible dementia, 10–24 = mild to moderate dementia, 6–9 = moderate to severe dementia and below 6 = severe dementia. The MMSE score is used as an indicator as to when to start a patient on an acetylcholinesterase inhibitor (AchEI) if appropriate, and when to withdraw.

The Abbreviated Mental Test Score (AMTS), e.g. Hodkin's, which takes less than four minutes to complete, is scored from 0 (lowest) to 10, with 7 or less indicating cognitive impairment.

The results of these tests help to establish the level of a person's cognitive impairment. Where a shortfall in performance is seen within a particular domain, the effect on day-to-day activities such as following commands, orientation to time, person and place or the ability to remember new concepts can be determined.

These tests are not without drawbacks. For example, English needs to be the patient's first language. Also, if the patient being tested has learning difficulties or a poor educational background, they may have never have known the answers to some of the questions. The tests are also relatively insensitive to change. However, there is proven sensitivity to the effects of AchEI when compared to placebo in mild to moderate AD. There is also a proven statistically significant inverse correlation between the MMSE score and the ADAS-cog score (see Answer 5). This means that as the MMSE score decreases (reflecting increasing severity of cognitive impairment and/or dementia), there is an increase in the ADAS-cog score (reflecting an increasing severity in the AD).

(b) ADL.

In a clinical setting, the Barthel Assessment scale rates the patient's ability to complete basic ADLs. These include: dressing; continence, grooming, eating, bathing and walking. It is scored out of a total of 20 (best outcome). A score of less than 16 is associated with the need for care services or carer support. It must remembered that as cognitive function declines, the ability of the patient to perform physical tasks will also decline because the memory is no longer present for that particular task.

Complicated ADLs can also be rated and these include: shopping, cooking, finances and keeping appointments.

(c) HAMD.

Severe depression may present with the same symptomatology as a dementia (e.g. slowing down, memory loss, social withdrawal, low mood or personality change. These symptoms may also be reflected in low MMSE and/or ADL scores). When depression presents in this fashion it is often termed a 'pseudo-dementia'. However, because depression is eminently treatable, and effective treatment reduces the associated morbidity and mortality, every patient suspected of having cognitive dysfunction, including dementia, should be assessed for depression. The HAMD scale rates a series of 17 domains ranging from mood to insomnia to anxiety and to somatic symptoms. These are then attributed a score. A score of 0–7 = absence of depression, 8–17 = mild depression, 18–25 = moderate depression and above 26 is associated with a severe depressive episode.

What is the purpose of the other baseline measures assessed for Mr LD?

A2   These results (if normal) rule out the presence of a treatable cause for the cognitive disturbance.

Cardiovascular assessment should include: blood pressure monitoring, heart rate (undiagnosed arrhythmia), heart failure (possible hypoxia) and history of stroke or ischaemic disease (cause of cerebral ischaemic lesions).

Biochemical monitoring should include: blood glucose (to detect hypoglycaemia or untreated diabetes), serum urea and creatinine (renal failure is a rare cause of cognitive decline), serum electrolytes (hyponatraemia and hypercalcaemia are a common cause of cognitive dysfunction, including delirium in the elderly and are often medicine related), haematological indices such as haemoglobin, and folate and B_{12} levels (severe anaemias of any type may produce cognitive impairment in the elderly and these should be treated if detected. Thyroid function should also be assessed as hypo- and hyperthyroidism can be associated with cognitive abnormalities. Liver function tests are generally done to complete the work-up and to establish baseline levels when starting certain pharmacological treatments.

A full medical examination is also necessary as making a diagnosis of probable AD is one of exclusion. All other possible causes for the symptoms observed should be eliminated. Common causes of cognitive dysfunction (especially delirium) in the elderly include infection (urinary, chest or skin, while less common causes are HIV or syphilis) and concomitant medication.

What is the purpose of trying to improve Mr LD's memory?

A3 **Memory dysfunction is a common complaint in ageing. This dysfunction may be not be related to a neurodegenerative processes.**

Often older people complain about changes in their memory. This may or may not be associated with changes after formal cognitive assessment. If minor changes are found but nothing else of note, the person is said to have age-related cognitive decline (ARCD). If slightly more abnormalities are found but insufficient to make a diagnosis of probable dementia, then the person is said to have mild cognitive impairment (MCI). It is thought that about 15% of people presenting with MCI will go on to develop dementia at a later stage.

Giving people with ARCD or MCI hints on how to remember things and/or improve memory allows the person to have some control over the complaints, but also these skills may often normalise the initial symptoms.

Such hints include:

(a)   The use of diaries or notebooks to act as memory aids.
(b)   Repeatedly practising a task.
(c)   Using alarm clocks to remember appointments (with a note by the clock of the reason for its alarming).
(d)   Using strategies such as mnemonics to remember an action plan (sometimes only the mnemonic can be remembered and not the reason why it is remembered).
(e)   When being introduced to new people, to repeat their name immediately once or twice to ensure that it enters the memory.
(f)   To concentrate on things that are important to remember and ignore the less important, e.g. keep telephone numbers in a telephone book for referral.

(g) Establish routines for placing frequently 'lost' items, e.g. always place car keys in a specific place. Carry spectacles on a neck-chain so they cannot be lost.

(h) To admit to others that there is a problem with short-term memory and ask for assistance and prompting.

Was fluoxetine therapy appropriate for Mr LD?

A4 **Yes. Mr LD had a HAMD score which indicated mild depression. The choice of an antidepressant in an elderly patient is dependent on co-morbidity and concomitant medication. In patients with cognitive impairment it is best to select an agent with fewer anticholinergic side-effects, as these side-effects may enhance the impairment. Fluoxetine is thus an appropriate choice.**

Mr LD's HAMD score of 12 indicates a mild depression, therefore it would be reasonable to initiate effective treatment to achieve resolution of his depressive symptoms.

There is little therapeutic difference in terms of efficacy between any group of antidepressants, especially between the tricyclic antidepressants (TCAs) and selective serotonin reuptake inhibitors (SSRIs).

Treatment decisions are dependent on patient acceptability, tolerability, toxicity, suicide risk and cost. Due to age-related changes in pharmacokinetic and pharmacodynamic parameters, the elderly are most susceptible to the adverse effects of any medication. These adverse effects may also be exacerbated by concomitant medication and/or pathology.

In the elderly, pharmacokinetic changes markedly reduce clearance and the elimination half-life of TCAs. These changes can lead to increased plasma concentrations and increased risk of dose-related toxicity. Pharmacodynamic changes in the elderly mean that organ sensitivity is increased to the adverse effects that are associated with these pharmacokinetic changes. The adverse effects of TCAs are well known and the cognitive impairment resulting from their anticholinergic activity precludes their use in patients with dementia.

Due to the heterogeneity of the elderly and often the concurrent pathology and associated polypharmacy, it is appropriate to use an SSRI first-line, with the particular choice of agent governed by patient factors, such as anticipated pharmacokinetic changes and tolerability. Mr LD has no cardiovascular disease (citalopram is more cardiotoxic in overdose), no history of movement disorders (which may preclude treatment with fluoxetine or paroxetine), and his renal and hepatic function (reduced clearance with citalopram, paroxetine and fluoxetine) is unremarkable. Mr LD is not on any other medication which might lead to drug–drug interactions, seen with many of the SSRIs.

Therefore, fluoxetine is a reasonable choice; however, the time to therapeutic effect may be delayed because of the long half-life of fluoxetine and its active metabolite norfluoxetine in the elderly. Therefore the full therapeutic effect may not be attained for one to three months.

What is an 'ADAS-cog' score, how is it calculated and what is the relevance of the final score?

A5 **ADAS-cog (The Alzheimer's Disease Assessment Scale-cognitive subscale) is a tool designed for research and clinical purposes to monitor the progression of disease, and also response to pharmacological treatment.**

The ADAS-cog (there is also a non-cognitive subscale, which is used less frequently) was developed to measure all the major symptoms of AD, and the severity and progression of the symptoms in a variety of settings and languages. It is a performance-based test, which assesses 11 domains of cognitive function, including: word recall, naming, orientation, commands, praxis, word recognition, spoken language and comprehension, word-finding, and recall. It takes about one hour to complete and is scored from 0 (no errors) to 70 (profoundly demented). Patients with moderate dementia (untreated) show an annual rate of change of about 13 points (in comparison with those that are mildly or severely affected who have a point change of about 6 and 7, respectively.

What is the relevance of the CT results?

A6 **A CT scan is used to eliminate reversible causes of dementia and to act as a baseline measurement for disease progression.**

The first purpose of an MRI or CT scan in AD is to rule out reversible causes such as tumours, strokes, haemorrhages, hydrocephalus, ischaemia and other lesions. The findings on CT of enlargement of lateral ventricles and sulci, and the appearance of cerebral atrophy are only supportive diagnostic indicators of dementia. In normal ageing, brain volume reduction is estimated at 5–10% at 80 years, with enlargement of the lateral and third ventricles and cortical cerebral sulci. False positives (apparent cerebral atrophy in normal subjects) and false negatives (appearances within the normal range in definite dementia) are frequently made. The use of follow-up rescanning and identification of progressive changes makes for a more accurate diagnostic test.

What is the probable diagnosis for Mr LD and how can it be confirmed?

A7 **The diagnosis is probable Alzheimer's disease. Confirmation is only possible via post-mortem necropsy.**

Dementia has been defined as a syndrome consisting of progressive impairment in two or more areas of cognition (memory, language, visuospatial and perceptual ability, thinking and problem-solving, and personality), which is sufficient to interfere with work, social function or relationships and represents a significant change from the previous level of function. It generally occurs in the absence of delirium or major non-organic psychiatric disorders such as depression or schizophrenia, or impaired consciousness.

The Diagnostic and Statistical Manual of Mental Disorders (DSM)-IV diagnostic criteria should be referred to before a diagnosis of probable dementia is made.

The histopathological indicators of AD found at necropsy include neurofibrillary tangles, amyloid plaques and, in some cases, the presence of Lewy bodies. These cannot presently be detected via any visualisation techniques whilst the patient is still alive. Research is currently underway to determine a less-invasive screening tool, such as urinary analysis. However, the specificity of such tests remains as yet unproven.

Why is an early diagnosis of AD better for the patient and their family?

A8 **It allows the patient and their family the opportunity to arrange things such as wills, power of attorney and long-term care arrangements, whilst the patient has insight and can make informed choices in these areas.**

An early definitive diagnosis is becoming more important, both for the patient, their carers and loved ones, as well as the patient's physician and multidisciplinary team.

Other benefits of early diagnosis are:

(a)   Reversible conditions can be excluded.

(b)   It allows early access by the patient and their family to support groups (Alzheimer's Disease Association) for further information and planning purposes.
(c)   It helps to determine the prevalence of the disease.
(d)   It permits future research into treatments that may slow or halt the progression of the disease to be more effectively targeted to the right stage of the disease.
(e)   It enables the appropriate medical treatment to be started at the most beneficial time for the patient.

What are the pharmacological treatment options for Mr LD?

A9   **There are currently three licensed AchEIs for the symptomatic treatment of mild to moderate AD in the UK.**

AchEIs increase the bioavailability of acetylcholine (a neurotransmitter which is depleted in AD) by decreasing its hydrolysis. All have shown statistically significant improvement in randomised controlled trials against placebo in patients with mild to moderate AD. However, not all patients will show a response to treatment and some will only have a partial response. It is estimated that approximately 25% of patients show a definite response and that 40–50% of all patients are likely to show some benefit. The reason for these findings is unclear, but perhaps due to the heterogeneity of the dementias as a disease. Patients with the apolipo-protein allele-4 (a genetic risk factor for AD) seem to have a different response rate than those patients without. However, this result is inconsistent in many studies.

The numbers needed to treat (NNT) with reference to a significant improvement in cognition, ADL or global functioning are relatively low (ranging from three to seven for a low dose of any AchEI), indicating this therapy is a clinically significant treatment. A higher NNT would also be acceptable in view of the chronic nature of the disorder.

Each of the agents available has a different side-effect profile, and different cautions and contra-indications to use. Therefore, the choice of the pharmacological agent chosen is dependent on the patient's concomitant pathology and medication.

Other agents have also been investigated. Long-term studies of patients taking NSAIDs or oestrogen (hormone replacement therapy) have shown a reduced incidence of dementia when compared with normal population groups; however, there is currently no evidence for their use in established dementia.

What therapy would you recommend? Outline a dosing and monitoring schedule.

A10 An AchEI is justified. The choice and dose regimen is dependent on patient co-morbidity and local prescribing guidelines. For Mr ID, rivastigmine is an appropriate choice.

Mr LD is suitable for treatment with an AchEI because he had been diagnosed as having probable mild to moderate AD by a specialist physician. The choice of AchEI is dependent on patient concomitant disease factors. The presence of severe hepatic or renal disease precludes the use of galantamine; and the presence of respiratory and cardiovascular disease is a caution for use of AchEIs in general.

Rivastigmine is a reasonable choice. It is generally well tolerated, with the most common side-effects being drowsiness, nausea, vomiting and diarrhoea, which occur most commonly with upward dose titration.

Rivastigmine has a short half-life of about two hours, but a prolonged action, as AchE is inhibited for up to 10 hours after the parent drug has been eliminated from the plasma. Excretion of inactive metabolites is via the kidney. There is no hepatic metabolism and little protein binding.

The starting dose is generally 1.5 mg twice daily increasing slowly by steps of 1.5 mg twice daily at fortnightly intervals to a maximum of 6 mg twice daily. This is in an attempt to increase the tolerability to rivastigmine and to determine the most effective response to a particular dosage. Rivastigmine is marketed in 1.5, 3, 4.5 and 6 mg strengths to aid flexibility in titration. Some patients may need a longer titration interval, e.g. by increments of 1.5 mg daily at fortnightly intervals.

The monitoring requirements of the cholinesterase inhibitor selected will be guided by local policy, but will generally include a barrage of cognitive, physical and psychological assessments. It has been suggested that prior to initiation of therapy, a mutually agreeable end point for withdrawal of therapy is agreed with the patient and their carer. Therapy is usually reassessed during titration of dosing and then every two to four months after a maintenance dose is achieved. Often it takes longer than three months to achieve a therapeutically effective maintenance dose due to a patient's inability to tolerate dose increments. Once reached, assessment can be made every six months and the agent continued if the MMSE remains above 12. However, overall benefit is still judged in terms of patient behaviour, sleep disturbance and ADLs in patients with MMSE scores of less than 12.

Guidance on when to withdraw treatment in those patients that have previously demonstrated a therapeutic response, but have since not shown any improvement, is not currently available. One could argue that if the disease progression itself is being held in a static position and no deterioration is shown, then the treatment should continue.

In those patients who demonstrate no therapeutic response to a first-line agent, there is anecdotal evidence to suggest that they may respond to an alternative AchEI.

Outline a pharmaceutical care plan for Mr LD.

A11 **The pharmaceutical care plan for Mr LD should include the following:**

(a) The patient's (and carer's) understanding of the illness and its treatment should be fully assessed with reference to local support services.

(b) All members of the health care team providing care to the patient should be involved with the pharmaceutical care plan.

(c) Pharmaceutical needs may include: need for concomitant medication, advice and treatment about adverse effects, titration schedule, medicine reminder devices, patient education information, patient and carer agreement with the treatment plan, and monitoring of efficacy.

(d) At each titration of dose, a medicine review may aid the early detection of intolerable adverse effects.

(e) Identification of main carer and relevant carer needs.

What is the possible cause of these side-effects and how might they be treated?

A12 **They are probably due to the cholinergic side-effects of the increasing rivastigmine dose.**

Susceptible patients may find it increasingly difficult to tolerate dose increases due to increased vomiting and nausea. This may be so severe that the patient loses a clinically significant amount of weight. If there is no evidence of a movement disorder such as Parkinson's disease or Lewy body dementia, then prescribing a long-acting form of metoclopramide for two days prior to the dose increase and the first week of the increased dose may help. Also staggering the upward titration over a greater period of time may help (e.g. 4.5 mg each morning and 6 mg each evening for two weeks prior to a final increase to 6 mg twice daily). In those patients with movement disorders then domperidone 10 mg four times daily as a regular medication, again starting two days prior to dose increases and continuing until tolerance is achieved, may help.

What is the role of ginkgo biloba and other herbal agents in the symptomatic treatment of AD?

A13 **There is some evidence to support their efficacy but few robust data are available.**

(a) Ginkgo biloba.

The *Ginkgo* (sometimes spelled *Gingko*) *biloba*, or maidenhair tree, dates back some 200 million years. Its leaves have been used in the treatment of asthma and as a memory enhancer for perhaps 5000 years in Chinese medicine. It has been licensed in Germany for the symptomatic treatment of cognitive disorders, intermittent claudication and vertigo of vascular origin. It is becoming increasingly popular in the US and UK as a dietary supplement taken to enhance memory.

The active ingredients are unknown and may include one or all of the following: flavonoids, terpenoids or organic acids. This means there is no product standardisation and different formulations have different ingredients and dosage specifications.

Ginkgo biloba is thought to produce a vaso-regulatory effect on arteries, capillaries and veins, which improves blood flow, and to antagonise platelet-activating factor. There is a theoretical increased risk of adverse bleeding events if it is taken by patients on either aspirin or warfarin. However there are only isolated case reports in the literature.

A randomised, double-blind, placebo-controlled trial with 309 patients with either vascular dementia or AD of mild to moderate classification over 52 weeks showed improved cognitive function in 50% of those patients receiving active compound compared to 29% of those receiving placebo. A Cochrane Review updated in August 2002 suggests that there is promising evidence of improved cognition, function (as measured by ADL scores), and mood and emotional function associated with ginkgo biloba. There is as yet no data available on the effects on quality of life measures of depression or dependency.

(b) Dehydroepiandrosterone (DHEA) supplementation.

Results of DHEA in a one-year trial in AD are awaited, as are results of long-term trials in normal older men and women. Previous studies have been for two weeks or three months and have shown inconsistent results, with women reporting improvement in immediate and delayed recall, but no benefit reported for men. Recommended doses are 50 mg for men and 25 mg for women, but there is no evidence to support this difference in dose or indeed efficacy at the recommended dose.

(c)   Vitamin E supplementation.

Vitamin E supplementation has been demonstrated to slow decline in cognitive function associated with age and in patients with dementia. However, dose recommendations are unclear and the one high quality study showed a reduction in numbers of patients reaching an endpoint of severe dementia in the active supplementation arm, but also an increased number of falls in this active group of the study. This finding requires further evaluation.

(d)   Lecithin supplementation.

A Cochrane Review found no evidence to support the use of lecithin in the treatment of patients with dementia.

What is the differential diagnosis for Mr LD?

A14 **Infection-induced delirium superimposed on a background of dementia. Supporting factors include: signs of infection, sudden onset, and both visual and auditory hallucinations.**

Delirium is extremely common in this age group, affecting as many as 24% of all hospital admissions. There are many triggers for delirium and the reader is referred to the DSM-IV criteria, which aids in the final diagnosis by outlining the exclusions and investigations that need to be made. The most common triggers for delirium are:

(a) Infection, especially of the urinary or lower respiratory tract (the elderly have a delayed immune response to infection and can become systemically very unwell before changes in x-rays, temperature or blood cultures are seen), but also skin infections and more rarely neurosyphilis or HIV.

(b) Metabolic and endocrine disorders, especially thyroid disorders and electrolyte disturbances.

(c) Neurological disorders, especially stroke and transient ischaemic attacks.

(d) Cardiovascular disease, especially heart failure (poor cerebral perfusion) and arrhythmias.

(e)   Medication toxicity, including intoxication, withdrawal effects and side-effects of certain pharmacological classes.
(f)   Other medical conditions such as chronic constipation, chronic pain or urinary retention.

Impairment of consciousness is defined in DSM-IV terminology as 'reduced awareness of the environment'. In delirium this fluctuates throughout the day, with the intensity of the impairment generally greater at night. This can often present as a disturbance in the sleep–wake cycle, where the patient experiences daytime sleepiness and night-time agitation. Sometimes complete reversal of the sleep–wake cycle can occur. The patient's behaviour and thought process is often slow and muddled, visual perception is distorted, and hallucinations frequently present. The patient can present with mood changes, disorientation for time and place and memory disturbance.

Emotional disturbances such as anxiety, fear, depression, irritability, anger, euphoria and apathy may also be demonstrated, with a rapid and unpredictable shift from one emotional state to another. Fear may distress the patient to such an extent that they try to climb out of the bed while still attached to medical equipment such as intravenous lines and urinary catheter bags. They may also attack those people that are falsely perceived to be threatening, e.g. the nurse trying to get them back into bed.

Would you recommend antipsychotic therapy for Mr LD at this point?

A15   No. Antipsychotic therapy is only indicated if Mr LD's behaviour puts either himself or others at risk of physical harm.

The underlying principle for the successful treatment of a delirium is to treat the physical condition or the underlying cause. During the acute phases of cognitive impairment it is important to relieve the distress of the patient and to prevent behaviour that may result in an injury to themselves or others.

Where possible, non-pharmacological methods should be employed to treat behavioural disturbances in this age group. Patients who have poor concentration are often easily distracted and behavioural intervention methods are recommended. These include:

(a)   Creating an environment which is calming.
(b)   Providing activities to reduce boredom and loneliness.

(c)   Providing a regular routine.
(d)   Providing pro-active non-confrontational patient care.
(e)   Ensuring the physical environment is optimum, i.e. temperature control, space to walk.

Other psychological strategies include the ABC analysis. The patient is carefully observed over a two-week period for:

(a)   Antecedents (television programme, meal times, nurse of the opposite sex involved in bathing routine).
(b)   Behaviour (clear description of behaviour exhibited).
(c)   Consequences (if the consequence is unimportant, does the behaviour require treatment?).
(d)   The next step is to record what stops the behaviour (so that it can be employed again if necessary).

Recent research has demonstrated a statistically significant association between the rate of cognitive decline and the prescribing of antipsychotics. Current advice is not to use antipsychotic medication unless the behavioural symptom places the patient and/or others at risk of personal injury.

The Omnibus Budget Reconciliation Act (OBRA) legislated in the US in 1998 recommends that behaviour is observed for up to one month in patients with neurodegenerative disease before any pharmacological treatment is initiated. This is to ensure that the behaviour is not just a short-term manifestation of disease progression. Unnecessary medication puts the elderly patient at risk of increased morbidity and mortality by possible precipitation of iatrogenic illness.

Behavioural problems can include: restlessness, irritability, nocturnal wakening, aggressive behaviour and resistive behaviour. The first course of action is to attempt to identify any underlying treatable cause. The following questions should be considered:

(a)   Is the patient in pain? (Remember, these patients have reduced visuospatial awareness and are often confused and therefore at greater risk of falls or walking into things.)
(b)   Is there an underlying depression causing the apathy and lethargy?
(c)   Is there a superimposed delirium due to infection or some other cause?
(d)   Is the patient's communication hampered by visual or hearing or speech difficulties? (Always remember to check for glasses, hearing-aids or false teeth when communicating with an elderly patient.)

(e)   Has the patient recently moved from another care environment? (Changes in environment can greatly distress patients with dementia as they no longer have familiar items by which to reorient themselves by.)

(f)   Does the patient becomes more distressed in certain situations (e.g. when being bathed by a member of the opposite sex, mealtimes, etc.)? In which case, try to establish the causative factor.

Each problem should be analysed to identify causality if possible, and specific procedures for assessment and treatment should be agreed so that all members of the multidisciplinary team and any visitors can handle the behaviour problem in the same manner.

In 1998, *The Expert Consensus Guidelines for the Treatment of Agitation in Older Persons with Dementia* were published. They give guidance on two treatment strategies: environmental intervention and the use of medication. The guidelines describe mild agitation as being behaviour which is somewhat disruptive, but non-aggressive, such as moaning, pacing, crying or arguing. They describe severe agitation as behaviour that is aggressive or endangers others (or themselves) to possible physical harm, e.g. screaming, kicking, throwing objects, scratching others or self-injury. Their first recommendation is that the family and/or care-giver(s) are educated about dementia and agitation, and are encouraged to join a support group. The most important aim is to identify the trigger for any problem behaviour.

Efforts should be made to decrease disorientation, e.g. at night-time try using low lights so that the patient can orientate to place, and to avoid over and under sensory stimulation. It may be easier to care for restless agitated patients in a side room where there is less disturbance from noise and other patients.

What are the next therapeutic options?

A16   **Memantine, a novel *N*-methyl-D-aspartate (NMDA) antagonist, is licensed for the symptomatic treatment of moderate to moderately severe AD.**

Transfer to an alternative AchEI may be tried at this point, but it would seem more logical to initiate (or co-prescribe, depending on local policy) the non-competitive NMDA receptor antagonist, memantine. Memantine was licensed in the UK in late 2002 for the symptomatic treatment of moderately severe to severe AD. When a patient is classified as having moderate to moderately severe dementia it is often difficult to assess their cognitive function. Therefore the burden on the care-giver is measured in relation to assisting the patient with ADL.

Placebo-controlled double-blind studies have demonstrated significant improvement in cognitive impairment, lack of drive, motor dysfunction, ADL and elevation of mood (with decreased lability of affect also reported). In two double-blind placebo-controlled randomised trials, memantine demonstrated statistically significant improvement in the following domains of activities of daily living as measured by the Global Deterioration Scale: overall behaviour, ability to move, to wash and to dress.

Memantine targets excitatory amino acids such as glutamate. A chronically released high level of glutamate is associated with the pathomechanism of neurodegenerative dementia. An excess of glutamate causes over-stimulation of NMDA receptors, which allows the free flow of calcium into the cell. Sustained elevation of glutamate leads to a chronic overexposure to calcium, which in turn leads to cell degeneration and ultimately neuronal cell death. Memantine is thought to bind to NMDA receptor sites, thereby reducing this overexposure to calcium. However, although memantine blocks the glutamate-gated receptor channels allowing the physiological activation of the receptors (involved in memory formation), it blocks the pathological activation.

Due to the pharmacological effects and mechanism of action of memantine, there are several medicine–medicine interactions and the reader is advised to refer to the agent's latest 'Summary of Product Characteristics' for further information.

The initial dose is 5 mg once daily, increasing to twice daily, then 10 mg each morning and 5 mg in the evening, eventually leading to the maximum dose of 10 mg twice daily. Dose increments should be made at weekly intervals. Memantine is available as 5 mg tablets or a solution to aid dosing regimens). This slow, upward titration is to reduce the incidence of side-effects, the most common being hallucinations, confusion, dizziness, headache and tiredness. Uncommon adverse reactions include anxiety, hypertonia (increased muscle tone), vomiting, cystitis and increased libido.

What care issues are necessary for Mrs LD?

A17 **Mrs LD requires a personal care plan agreement for her own emotional, physical and psychological needs to be met.**

Carers of people with AD need a great deal of support to ensure that their own physical, mental and social care needs are optimum. The institutionalisation of patients with AD is generally dependent on when the carer feels unable to cope with the demands of a 24-hour, seven-day week regimen of caring. Early intervention for carer needs is vital as many will suffer from depression, and many will be frail and elderly themselves, with concomitant health care needs.

It is advised that each carer has a care plan agreement which outlines respite care needs, additional service needs, community psychiatric nurse monitoring, psychiatric care support programme, carer and patient counselling/support/stimulation activities, and local day hospital services. There should also be a social worker assessment.

How might Mr LD's increasing agitation and hallucinations be controlled?

A18 **The treatment of agitation and hallucinations should be by non-pharmacological methods if possible. However, if these fail, an atypical antipsychotic may be warranted.**

Patients with AD often have associated psychotic presentations such as persecutory delusions and hallucinations. Historically these symptoms were often treated first-line by the use of antipsychotic medication. Recent research has demonstrated a statistically significant association between the rate of cognitive decline and the prescribing of an antipsychotic.

However, if all measures in Answer 15 have been followed and the behavioural presentations justify pharmacological treatment, then the following may be used as guidance.

Increasingly studies involving the treatment of behavioural problems associated with AD are showing a statistically significant reduction in problems as a response to treatment with an AchEI. There is some evidence to show that the effects may differ between the three agents.

Pharmacokinetic changes in the elderly, which lead to higher plasma concentrations at low doses of antipsychotics, increase susceptibility to side-effects which will occur at much lower doses than in younger patients.

If absolutely necessary, risperidone starting at a dose of 500 micrograms at night (and increasing in 500-microgram increments using a twice daily dosing regimen) can lead to symptom control. Increasing side-effects (extrapyramidal effects and postural hypotension) are seen at doses above 2 mg daily. Risperidone does not reduce the seizure threshold, block histamine receptors and has no anticholinergic side-effects.

Quetiapine is well tolerated in the elderly, has a low incidence of seizures, no anticholinergic activity and sedative effects similar to chlorpromazine; however, postural hypotension can be a problem if titration is too rapid. Clearance rates are reduced (30–50%) in the elderly and therefore it is recommended that dosing is started at 25 mg once daily, increasing by 25 mg increments every one to three days until a therapeutic effect is reached.

Olanzapine has been used extensively for the treatment of psychoses in the elderly. In comparison with risperidone, less extra-pyramidal side-effects (EPSEs) have been reported, but there is a 10% incidence of drowsiness, anticholinergic effects and weight gain. Therefore, it is less useful in elderly patients with worsening cognitive dysfunction.

The efficacy of clozapine is well documented in this age group, but its use is associated with many side-effects, including sedation, hypersalivation, tachycardia, hypotension, hypertension, constipation and urinary incontinence. Its propensity to cause fever and agranulocytosis also necessitates mandatory monitoring of blood cell counts on a regular basis. It also has high anticholinergic activity and therefore will adversely affect cognitive function.

Use of the typical antipsychotics in the elderly is associated with increased sensitivity to the histaminergic, adrenergic, muscarinic, cardiovascular and extrapyramidal side-effects. Age-related changes affect the pharmacokinetics and pharmacodynamics of the typical antipsychotics. The elderly have reduced lean body mass, with a corresponding increased lipophilic store and decreased serum albumin, all of which affect the distribution and transportation of a pharmacological agent. For example, the larger lipophilic stores in the elderly lead to a correspondingly greater volume of distribution for lipid-soluble agents (e.g. benzodiazepines and phenothiazines). Clinically this means that when dosing with a lipophilic agent it may seem to take an unexpectedly long period of time before therapeutic effect is reached. Ageing also results in decreased renal and hepatic mass (indeed all organ mass is reduced), which affects the body's ability to metabolise and then excrete medicines. A corresponding reduction in hepatic and renal blood flow also exacerbates this delay in clearance.

Whatever agent is chosen, if an antipsychotic is being prescribed, the dose, frequency and continued use of the medication should be reviewed on a daily basis. As the patient responds to the treatment of the behavioural disturbance, antipsychotic therapy should be decreased and withdrawn as soon as possible. It is also prudent to remember that the neurodegenerative process will be ongoing and that as this progresses, the observed behaviour will change in response.

Outline a pharmaceutical care plan for the treatment of double incontinence.

A19 **Double incontinence puts the patient at risk of infection and skin problems. It is often a leading reason for institutionalisation of the patient by carers.**

As social awareness declines and the patient no longer remembers that they actually physically need to go to the toilet or they cannot find the toilet in the first place, alternative measures are needed. Behavioural treatment suggests a toilet-training regimen, e.g. taking the patient to the toilet at regular intervals during the day, such as on wakening, after breakfast, lunch and dinner, and then again before going to bed. The co-prescription of agents such as oxybutynin is not to be recommended as they have anticholinergic side-effects and may exacerbate confusion. Continence pads are also an option. Catheterisation is generally not an accepted option (due to problems with bladder infections and the distress associated with changing the catheter) unless the patient is bed-bound and has no bladder control.

If the patient is doubly incontinent, the use of a 'constipating and laxative' regimen is often employed. This is where the patient is kept deliberately constipated using codeine or loperamide and then has a stimulant laxative or enema once or twice weekly so that the bowel actions can be controlled. Toilet-training options involve less drug taking, and less distress and discomfort for the patient. Dietary interventions are often less effective due to the reduced appetite in the patient.

It is also important to be aware of the risk of the skin breaking down and leading to chafing or pressure areas. The use of a good barrier cream, such as Drapolene or Morhulin ointment, will help to protect vulnerable areas.

When might pharmacological treatment for Mr LD be withdrawn?

A20 **When there is no halt in progression of baseline disease monitoring scales for at least three months.**

There is no current guidance available for the withdrawal of memantine from patients with end-stage AD. However, it would seem circumspect that if there is no halt in the progression of the disease and if the patient is requiring full nursing care that pharmacological agents for the treatment of AD be withdrawn. Death is commonly due to bronchopneumonia or embolism (as a result of reduced mobility). Also, loss of awareness of hunger and thirst often results in profound weight loss and/or dehydration. The principles of palliative medicine apply to the care of patients in the end stages of AD.

Further reading

Alexopoulos GS, Silver JM, Kahn DA *et al*. eds. *The Expert Consensus Guideline Series: Agitation in Older Persons with Dementia. A Postgraduate Medicine Special Report*. McGraw-Hill, New York, 1998. Also available on-line as 'Treatment of Agitation in Older Persons with Dementia' at: www.psychguides.com/gagl.html (carer and health care professional guidance).

Ballard C, O'Brien J. Treating behavioural and psychological signs in Alzheimer's disease. *Br Med J* 1999; **319**: 138–139.

Birks J, Flicker L. Selegiline for Alzheimer's disease (Cochrane Review). In: *The Cochrane Library 2*. Update Software, Oxford, 2003.

Birks J, Grimley Evans J *et al*. Rivastigmine for Alzheimer's disease (Cochrane Review). In: *The Cochrane Library 2*. Update Software, Oxford, 2003.

Birks JS, Melzer D, Beppu H. Donepezil for mild to moderate Alzheimer's disease (Cochrane Review). In: *The Cochrane Library 2*. Update Software, Oxford, 2003.

Clegg A, Bryant J, Nicholson T *et al*. Clinical and cost-effectiveness of donepezil, rivastigmine and galantamine for Alzheimer's disease: a rapid and systematic review. *Health Technol Assess* 2001; **5**: 1.

DeVane CL, Pollock BG. Pharmacokinetic considerations of anti-depressant use in the elderly. *J Clin Psychiatry* 1999; **60**(suppl. 20): 38–44.

Higgins JPT, Flicker L. Lecithin for dementia and cognitive impairment (Cochrane Review). In: *The Cochrane Library 2*. Update Software, Oxford, 2003.

Hughes CM, Lapane KL, Mor V. Impact of legislation on nursing home care in the Unites States: lessons for the United Kingdom. *Br Med J* 1999; **319**: 1060–1063.

Huppert FA, Van Niekerk JK. Dehydroepiandrosterone (DHEA) supplementation for cognitive function (Cochrane Review). In: *The Cochrane Library 2*. Update Software, Oxford, 2003.

Jones R. *Drug Treatment in Dementia*. Blackwell Sciences, Oxford, 2000.

Krall WJ, Sramek JJ, Cutler NR. Cholinesterase Inhibitors: a therapeutic strategy for Alzheimer's disease. *Ann Pharmacother* 1999; **33**: 441–450.

Kumar V, Brecher M. Psychopharmacology of atypical anti-psychotics and clinical outcomes in elderly patients. *J Clin Psychiatry* 1999; **60**(suppl. 13): 5–9.

Mayeux JJ, Wood MD. Treatment of Alzheimer's disease. *N Engl J Med* 1999; **341**: 1670–1679.

Masand PS. Side-effects of anti-psychotics in elderly. *J Clin Psychiatry* 2000; **61**(suppl 8): 43–49.

McShane R, Keene J, Gedling K *et al.* Do neuroleptic drugs hasten cognitive decline in dementia? Prospective study with necropsy follow up. *Br Med J* 1997; **314**: 288.

Mittman N, Herrmann N, Einarson TR *et al.* The efficacy, safety and tolerability of anti-depressants in late life depression: a meta-analysis. *J Affect Disord* 1997; **46**: 191–217.

Newhouse PA. Use of serotonin selective reuptake inhibitors in geriatric depression. *J Clin Psychiatry* 1996; **57**(suppl 5): 12–22.

Scottish Intercollegiate Guidelines Network. *Interventions in the Management of Behavioural and Psychological Aspects of Dementia*. SIGN, Edinburgh, 1998.

Small GW. What we need to know about age related memory loss. *Br Med J* 2002; **324**: 1502–1505.

Tabet N, Birks J, Grimley Evans J *et al.* Vitamin E for Alzheimer's disease (Cochrane Review). In: *The Cochrane Library 2*. Update Software, Oxford, 2003.

20

Infection in the immunocompromised patient

Maxwell Summerhayes

Day 1 Fifty-five-year-old Mr CR was admitted from his local hospital, where he had been receiving supportive care during R-CHOP chemotherapy for stage IVB, diffuse large B-cell non-Hodgkin's lymphoma (DLBCL).

For the last 30 years, CHOP has been the 'gold-standard' treatment for this type of lymphoma and, like the majority of current chemotherapy regimens, it incorporates a number of antineoplastic agents from different therapeutic classes (the alkylating agent, cyclophosphamide; the cytotoxic antibiotic, doxorubicin; the antimitotic agent, vincristine; and the steroid, prednisolone). Combination treatments are designed to maximise the chances of including drugs to which the patient's disease is sensitive, to prevent the emergence of drug-resistant tumour cell populations and to enable lower, less-toxic doses of individual agents to be used than would be the case during monotherapy.

In CHOP, drugs are administered once every 28 days. The aim is to repeat the cycle six to eight times with curative intent. The limiting toxicity of the regimen is usually bone marrow suppression due, primarily, to cyclophosphamide and doxorubicin.

Over the last three decades many unsuccessful attempts have been made to improve on CHOP. The rationale behind these has, generally, been the exposure of the lymphoma to a greater number of conventional cytotoxic drugs than are contained in CHOP. These more complex regimens have not resulted in better outcomes than CHOP, possibly because the addition of extra drugs has required reductions in the doses of those components of the regimen with the highest activity against lymphoma. However, evidence has recently emerged that the addition of the monoclonal antibody rituximab to CHOP (the R-CHOP regimen) results in significantly improved survival compared with CHOP alone. Rituximab is a chimeric antibody which recognises the CD20 antigen found on the surface of almost all B-cell non-Hodgkin's lymphomas (NHLs) as well as normal B lymphocytes, but not the progenitor cells from which they are derived. Rituximab is given as a short intravenous infusion, over about four hours, with each cycle of CHOP. It is believed to kill lymphoma cells by a variety of mechanisms, including recruitment of cell-mediated and cell-independent host immune processes and enhancement of cytotoxic drug-induced apoptosis.

Mr CR had attended his local hospital 10 days earlier for a nadir blood count after his seventh course of R-CHOP. This had revealed a very low neutrophil count of 0.2×10^9/L (reference range $2.2–7.0 \times 10^9$). As Mr CR also exhibited clinical evidence of a chest infection, he was admitted for antibiotic treatment. He remained pyrexial after three days on ceftazidime 2 g intravenously three times daily and erythromycin 1 g intravenously twice daily, but his temperature had settled after the following antituberculants were added: Rifinah 300 (rifampicin 300 mg, isoniazid 150 mg) two each morning, ethambutol 600 mg each morning. However, he had continued to feel very unwell, had little appetite for food (his weight had declined by 10 kg to 68 kg in 11 weeks) and he was anxious to return to this hospital for further treatment.

On admission Mr CR was afebrile, but very short of breath at rest. He had a cough productive of white sputum. Examination revealed abnormal breath sounds suggestive of a left-sided chest infection. The hepatomegaly noted at previous out-patient appointments could not be felt.

In addition to the antibiotics and antituberculants, Mr CR was taking the following therapy:

- Nystatin mouthwash, 2 mL orally four times daily
- Bendroflumethiazide 5 mg orally each morning
- Propranolol 20 mg orally twice daily
- Naproxen 500 mg orally when required for an arthritic big toe

Mr CR stated that he had given up smoking 30 years earlier and rarely consumed alcohol. His serum biochemistry and haematology results were:

- White blood cells (WBC) 9.1×10^9/L (reference range $4–11 \times 10^9$)
- Neutrophils 7.55×10^9/L ($2.2–7.0 \times 10^9$)
- Sodium 134 mmol/L (134–148)
- Potassium 3.9 mmol/L (3.4–5.0)
- Urea 6.4 mmol/L (2.5–7.5)

- Creatinine 104 micromol/L (50–130)
- Phosphate 1.23 mmol/L (0.8–1.5)

- Liver function tests: within normal limits

His antibiotic and antituberculant therapies were stopped and a bronchoscopy was arranged for the next day, with washings and biopsy samples to be sent for bacteriology and cytology. He was left on his bendroflumethiazide, naproxen and nystatin. A plain x-ray examination of the chest was performed which revealed diffuse left-sided shadowing with a cavitating spherical lesion in the middle of the lung.

Day 2 Mr CR remained apyrexial. Bronchial washings did not stain for acid-fast bacilli or show any abnormality other than an increased number of white cells. Samples were to be cultured overnight. A presumptive diagnosis of systemic mycosis was made. In view of Mr CR's poor condition and his presumptive diagnosis, systemic treatment with liposomal amphotericin 200 mg/day (3 mg/kg/day) and low-dose molgramostim (150 micrograms/day) was started.

Q1 Outline a pharmaceutical care plan for Mr CR.
Q2 Your hospital formulary includes both conventionally formulated (colloidal) and liposomal amphotericin (AmBisome), but dictates that the latter should be reserved for patients with pre-existing renal impairment or intolerant of conventional amphotericin. Mr CR falls into neither category – is it appropriate for him to receive the lipid formulation?
Q3 Other lipid formulations of amphotericin B are available. Would these be equally suitable for Mr CR?
Q4 Are there any alternatives to parenteral amphotericin B for treating Mr CR?
Q5 Is monotherapy with amphotericin B appropriate for Mr CR?
Q6 Why has Mr CR been prescribed molgramostim when he is not neutropenic?
Q7 Does Mr CR still require topical antifungal therapy?
Q8 What parameters would you monitor during Mr CR's antifungal therapy?

Day 4 Although his condition had stabilised, Mr CR was still very unwell and being fed via a nasogastric tube. The materials obtained during bronchoscopy had failed to provide evidence of infection. His neutrophil count was now 25×10^9/L ($2.2–7 \times 10^9$).

Q9 Is it appropriate to continue Mr CR's antifungal and molgramostim therapy?

Day 7   The agency nurse looking after Mr CR reported that for the first time he had had a serious reaction to his amphotericin infusion, with severe rigors and chills. She had taken the infusion bag down and kept it: the 500 mL bag of 5% glucose solution was about one-third full of a clear, golden-yellow liquid.

Q10 What has happened?
Q11 What are the likely consequences?
Q12 What course of action would you recommend?

Day 10   Mr CR was now feeling much better and was not requiring the use of oxygen. His chest x-ray was also much improved, with the diffuse changes almost resolved.

Serum biochemistry results were:

- Sodium 136 mmol/L (134–148)
- Potassium 3.0 mmol/L (3.4–5.0)
- Urea 21.7 mmol/L (2.5–7.5)
- Creatinine 315 micromol/L (50–130)

- Calcium 1.92 mmol/L (2.1–2.6)
- Phosphate 1.93 mmol/L (0.8–1.5)

Q13 What do these laboratory results indicate?
Q14 Is any modification needed to Mr CR's current treatment?

Day 17   Mr CR was discharged. He was feeling much better, eating normally, breathing easily and with an almost normal and still improving chest x-ray. His renal function had improved, but was still impaired with a creatinine clearance of 30 mL/min, calculated from his serum creatinine concentration.

Day 90   Mr CR was readmitted as an emergency. He had received miniBEAM chemotherapy for relapsed lymphoma two weeks earlier. MiniBEAM is an intensive regimen of carmustine, etoposide, cytarabine and melphalan which has the advantage of including drugs from three different groups from those already received by Mr CR. As Mr CR had relapsed so soon after initial therapy, his prognosis was poor. The aim of this treatment was to test the sensitivity of his disease to further chemo- therapy and, provided there was evidence of responsiveness to proceed to high-dose chemotherapy with peripheral blood progenitor cell support (a 'peripheral stem cell transplant').

On admission Mr CR was febrile, anorexic, dehydrated and gen- erally unwell. He weighed 67 kg. Blood samples were taken for culture and it was decided to start Mr CR on piperacillin plus tazobactam

(Tazocin) 4.5 g intravenously four times daily and intravenous gentamicin therapy, pending culture results, as well as giving 3 L sodium chloride 0.9% via his permanently implanted Hickman venous access catheter to rehydrate him.

Serum biochemistry and haematology results were:

- WBC 2.0×10^9/L $(4-11 \times 10^9)$
- Neutrophils 0.6×10^9/L $(2.2-7.0 \times 10^9)$
- Sodium 145 mmol/L (134–148)
- Potassium 4.3 mmol/L (3.4–5.0)
- Urea 9.0 mmol/L (2.5–7.5)
- Creatinine 135 micromol/L (50–130)
- Liver function tests: within normal limits

Q15 Is the antibiotic regimen selected for Mr CR appropriate?

Q16 Suggest an appropriate dosing regimen for Mr CR's gentamicin therapy.

Q17 How would you monitor Mr CR's therapy?

Day 93 Mr CR's blood cultures were all reported to be negative. He was feeling a little better, but still had a fever with a temperature spiking to 39.2°C. While talking to his ward pharmacist, Mr CR complained of a 'prickly heat' rash around his waist and asked if he could have some calamine lotion for it.

Serum biochemistry results were:

- Gentamicin trough off scale (less than 1 mg/L)
- Sodium 139 mmol/L (134–148)
- Potassium 4.0 mmol/L (3.4–5.0)
- Urea 8.5 mmol/L (2.5–7.5)
- Creatinine 120 micromol/L (50–130)

Q18 Should antibiotic treatment be continued in view of the negative blood cultures and Mr CR's failure to respond to broad-spectrum antibiotics?

Q19 Why are the gentamicin levels so high and what should be done about them?

Q20 Are any of Mr CR's other blood parameters a cause for concern?

Q21 Is it appropriate to ask the House Officer looking after Mr CR to prescribe calamine lotion?

Day 94 In view of the possibility that Mr CR had a *Staphylococcus epidermidis* infection, further blood samples were sent to the microbiology department for culture and his gentamicin treatment was replaced by vancomycin at a dose of 250 mg intravenously four times daily. There were no further instructions on the drug chart relating to this antibiotic. Mr CR was also started on aciclovir 800 mg five times daily by mouth.

Q22 Is vancomycin the drug of choice for Mr CR and is the dose appropriate?

Q23 Are the dosage instructions for vancomycin adequate?

Q24 How should Mr CR's vancomycin therapy be monitored?

Q25 Should Mr CR's aciclovir be given intravenously?

Day 95   Mr CR's fever was subsiding and he was feeling much better. His rash was starting to turn crusty but was not getting any bigger.

Serum biochemistry results were:

- Vancomycin peak (three hours after infusion start) 30 mg/L (25–30)
- Vancomycin trough 7 mg/L (5–10)

- Urea 8.7 mmol/L (2.5–7.5)
- Creatinine 135 micromol/L (50–130)

Q26 Would you recommend any modification to Mr CR's vancomycin therapy?

Day 98   Mr CR continued to improve. His laboratory results were substantially unchanged.

Day 100   After five days of vancomycin and aciclovir therapy Mr CR felt much better and both drugs were discontinued. His renal function had not deteriorated further. He still had a low neutrophil count of 1.22×10^9/L ($2.2–7.0 \times 10^9$). He was discharged from hospital, with a view to commencing a programme of stem cell mobilisation on an out-patient basis the following week.

Q27 In view of his persistently low neutrophil count does Mr CR require any prophylactic antimicrobial therapy to take home with him?

Outline a pharmaceutical care plan for Mr CR.

A1 **The pharmaceutical care plan for Mr CR should include the following:**

(a) Advising on the choice and dose of any drug therapy required for Mr CR and ensuring that any therapeutic or prophylactic anti-microbial regimen is selected with regard to his current level of immunocompetence.

(b) Ensure that any drugs needed by Mr CR are made available as quickly as the urgency of the clinical situation dictates.

(c) Ensure, by verbal and written communication with nursing and medical staff, that all prescribed therapy is administered appropriately.

(d) Ensure that all desired therapeutic outcomes are met with the minimum of toxicity by monitoring therapy for efficacy and side-effects and ensuring that any measures necessary for toxicity containment are taken.

(e) Counsel Mr CR on his prescribed medication and on other aspects of his care, as appropriate.

(f) At discharge, ensure that plans for Mr CR's continued drug therapy are clear and that drug-related information is communicated to appropriate carers so that therapy can be continued as intended.

Your hospital formulary includes both conventionally formulated (colloidal) and liposomal amphotericin (AmBisome), but dictates that the latter should be reserved for patients with pre-existing renal impairment or intolerant of conventional amphotericin. As Mr CR falls into neither category – is it appropriate for him to receive the lipid formulation?

A2 **Probably. Mr CR is presumed to have a pulmonary fungal infection which requires urgent and effective treatment, and his serious condition probably justifies the use of the less-toxic liposomal formulation which can be given at full dose from the first day of treatment.**

Mr CR is showing the clinical signs of a pulmonary fungal infection (chest infection which fails to respond to broad-spectrum antibiotics, lack of purulent sputum, cavitating lung lesion). His infection is possibly aspergillosis, which carries a very high risk of mortality, especially in the immunocompromised, and for which there are few treatment options. He requires urgent treatment with an antifungal that has activity against *Aspergillus* spp. Until very recently, the only such agent was parenteral amphotericin B. However, the precise role of the newer amphotericin B formulations such as liposomal amphotericin (AmBisome) remains controversial.

A recent meta-analysis by the Cochrane collaboration looking at the use of lipid-based amphotericin formulations in neutropenic cancer patients concluded that none of these had an impact on mortality superior to that of the, much cheaper, colloidal preparation. This is possibly because most antifungal trials in cancer patients recruit patients on the basis of their failure to respond to broad-spectrum antibiotics rather than because of good evidence of active fungal infection. Under these circumstances, it is likely that many do not have a fungal infection, making it difficult to alter survival in the group as a whole by use of antifungals, especially as mortality from other causes is very high. However, in a large case series of patients with proven aspergillosis, liposomal amphotericin has shown very impressive activity. It is also much less toxic than the original parenteral formulation of the drug, a fact recognised by the Cochrane Review team. This allows the administration of full therapeutic doses from the start of treatment without the need to escalate doses slowly and usually obviates the need for dose reductions resulting from drug toxicity. This is advantageous, because it not only allows extremely ill patients to receive a specific treatment for their disease without delay, but also prevents their condition becoming complicated by the significant toxicities (chills, rigors, anaemia, phlebitis, renal dysfunction) which are almost invariably associated with conventional amphotericin infusion. Renal dysfunction is dose-limiting with conventional amphotericin and, once established, makes therapy with the other nephrotoxic or renally excreted drugs that severely ill patients often require much more difficult. This advantage is lost if the approach recommended by the hospital formulary of withholding liposomal amphotericin until patients develop treatment-induced renal impairment is followed.

For this reason, it has become the practice, in at least one large teaching hospital, to start treatment in severely ill patients with liposomal amphotericin, with a view to switching to lower doses of conventional amphotericin after three days, if the patient's condition has stabilised at a satisfactory level or is improving. This approach is the subject of ongoing research, but is a logical approach to balancing the undoubted benefits of liposomal amphotericin against the cost of a wholesale replacement of the conventional product.

Thus, overall, the use of liposomal amphotericin with its higher cost, but reduced toxicity, seems to be justified in Mr CR's case.

> Other lipid formulations of amphotericin B are available. Would these be equally suitable for Mr CR?

A3 **The products are not identical and the relative value of each remains unclear, but none of the others are likely to offer advantages over liposomal amphotericin.**

There are three novel formulations of parenteral amphotericin available. They are often referred to collectively, and erroneously, as liposomal amphotericin. Only AmBisome is a liposomal formulation; Amphocil is a colloidal dispersion of disc-shaped cholesteryl sulphate–amphotericin B complexes (ABCD) and Abelcet is a suspension of amphotericin B–phospholipid complexes (ABLC). Additionally, there have been reports of conventional amphotericin being administered in lipid emulsions, such as Intralipid, in an attempt to obtain the benefits of lipid-based formulations at low cost. This approach is to be deprecated. Although a recent meta-analysis found no difference in fungal outcomes between amphotericin administered in glucose or Intralipid, and administration in lipid was less nephrotoxic, this approach has not been the subject of large trials, there is uncertainty about the stability of amphotericin given in this way and there are concerns that it may exacerbate non-renal toxicity.

There is no single trial comparing the efficacy and safety of liposomal amphotericin, ABLC and ABCD.

Under these circumstances, and since all three have been shown to be less nephrotoxic than conventional amphotericin in randomised clinical trials, choice is often based on local acquisition costs. Although this seems logical when the most commonly cited reason for their use is avoidance of renal damage, it should not be allowed to obscure the differences between the products.

In terms of efficacy, only liposomal amphotericin has been shown (at a dose of 3 mg/kg) to outperform conventional amphotericin (at a dose of 1 mg/kg) in a randomised trial, in this case conducted in neutropenic patients with pyrexia resistant to broad-spectrum antibiotic treatment. As far as toxicity is concerned, liposomal amphotericin appears to have distinct advantages. Indirect comparison of clinical trial data suggests that it has the lowest potential of all for nephrotoxicity and it almost certainly has the least propensity for producing infusion reactions. In a randomised trial it was better in this respect than ABLC, whereas ABCD appeared to be worse than conventional amphotericin. Although infusion reactions (fever, chills and rigors) are seldom life-threatening they are very unpleasant. They complicate the care of patients who are already extremely unwell and are, in reality, often the spur for clinicians to move from conventional amphotericin to an alternative formulation.

Are there alternatives to parenteral amphotericin B for treating Mr CR?

A4 Yes.

Until very recently the answer to this question would have been no, but two new antifungals with good activity against *Aspergillus* spp. have recently received regulatory approval.

Caspofungin is the first of an entirely new class of antifungal agents, the echinocandins. It appears to offer a good balance of efficacy and acceptable toxicity but, at present, is only recommended for patients with invasive aspergillosis which is refractory to, or intolerant of, other antifungals.

The other novel agent is voriconazole, a triazole antifungal. Unlike other triazoles which have negligible (fluconazole, ketoconazole) or modest (itraconazole) activity against *Aspergillus* spp., voriconazole has a very broad spectrum of action which includes good activity against this organism. It is unique in having demonstrated superior efficacy to amphotericin B (response rates and 12-week survival) in a large randomised trial in patients with invasive aspergillosis. It also exhibits much better tolerability than conventional amphotericin B.

Since voriconazole is well absorbed orally, it offers the option of prolonged therapy without the need for hospital attendance in those patients who require such treatment but who are well enough to be discharged.

No study has yet compared voriconazole with lipid-based formulations of amphotericin B. However, since it is unproven that lipid amphotericins offer survival benefits over conventional formulations, it seems possible that voriconazole may become the new benchmark in the treatment of invasive aspergillosis.

Is monotherapy with amphotericin B appropriate for Mr CR?

A5   **Yes.**

Conventional amphotericin B has, in the past, often been used in combination with flucytosine, with which it has a synergistic action, for the following reasons:

(a)   To produce greater antifungal activity.
(b)   To reduce drug toxicity by allowing lower doses of both agents to be used.
(c)   To achieve better penetration of areas like the cerebrospinal fluid (CSF) which are poorly penetrated by amphotericin (the level of amphotericin in the CSF is 3% of the serum concentration).

Although Mr CR was very unwell at the start of his systemic antifungal treatment, the (possibly unnecessary) addition of a drug to which resistance is common seems unwise for three reasons:

(a)   Liposomal amphotericin is so much less toxic than the original formulation, there is little restraint on administering an effective dose.
(b)   Flucytosine has significant bone marrow toxicity, to which Mr CR might be expected to be particularly vulnerable having just recovered from his fifth course of cytotoxic therapy.
(c)   The combination of flucytosine and liposomal amphotericin has not been studied.

There is no evidence to support the use of other antifungals in combination with amphotericin. There is also a theoretical constraint on the combination of triazoles and amphotericin: the former decrease the production of the ergosterol component of the fungal cell wall, to which the latter binds, thus possibly reducing its efficacy.

Why has Mr CR been prescribed molgramostim when he is not neutropenic?

A6   **It has been prescribed with the intention of enhancing his own macrophage defences to fungal infection.**

Macrophages are known to play a key role in combating fungal infection and molgramostim (granulocyte macrophage colony-stimulating factor) increases both the number of circulating macrophages and their functional capacity to deal with invading organisms, suggesting a useful role in the treatment of serious fungal infections. Although there are case reports of molgramostim being used successfully as part of antifungal regimens, trials are lacking and molgramostim should probably only be used in this way either when a haematopoietic growth factor is to be used anyway, because of low neutrophil counts, or when better, proven therapies have been tried and failed. Its use in Mr CR's case is difficult to justify.

Does Mr CR still require topical antifungal therapy?

A7   No.

Mr CR was started on prophylactic treatment with the non-absorbable polyene antifungal nystatin when he was profoundly neutropenic after chemotherapy. However, recent meta-analysis of 1464 patients entered into eight trials has shown that topical nystatin is no better than placebo when administered prophylactically or therapeutically to severely immunocompromised patients. Therefore, if prophylaxis was necessary, a systemic option would be required. Since Mr CR is currently receiving a full therapeutic dose of amphotericin additional measures of this type are not required.

What parameters would you monitor during Mr CR's antifungal therapy?

A8   Red blood cell count, renal function (serum creatinine, urea) and white blood cell count.

Although liposomal amphotericin is substantially less toxic than conventional formulations it is not without side-effects and it is still prudent to monitor the first two parameters for evidence of anaemia and amphotericin-induced renal toxicity, although probably no more closely than they would be for any patient who is as ill as Mr CR is at present. Mr CR's white blood cell count also needs to be monitored because of the risk of molgramostim-induced leucophilia.

Is it appropriate to continue Mr CR's antifungal and molgramostim therapy?

A9   Liposomal amphotericin therapy should be continued but molgramostim administration should be suspended.

It is unsurprising that bronchoscopy has failed to confirm the clinical diagnosis. Unequivocal diagnosis of systemic fungal infections, especially aspergillosis, is very difficult and the majority of patients treated with systemic antifungals receive them on the basis of clinical symptoms rather than a pathologically confirmed diagnosis. In Mr CR's case, fungal infection remains the most likely cause of his lung problems and his condition has stabilised on antifungal treatment, although molgramostim has caused a profound neutrophilia. Therefore, liposomal amphotericin should be continued, but molgramostim should be suspended, at least until his neutrophil count has returned to normal.

What has happened?

A10 **Mr CR has been given conventional amphotericin B in place of the liposomal product.**

Liposomal amphotericin infusions are cloudy and opalescent (like banana milk-shake), whereas conventional amphotericin forms a clear, golden-yellow liquid when diluted ready for use. When questioned, the nurse admitted that she did not know that there was a difference between liposomal and conventional amphotericin B, and had prepared Mr CR's infusion with some vials of conventional amphotericin which were in the ward refrigerator.

What are the likely consequences?

A11 **Apart from the acute toxicity already experienced, there is a danger of significant renal damage.**

The maximum dose of conventional amphotericin is 1.5 mg/kg/day. However, not all patients will tolerate this dose and a starting dose of 0.25 mg/kg/day should be used. This should be increased to 1–1.5 mg/kg/day over a few days. Additionally, doses should be infused over six hours to minimise side-effects, and consideration should be given to pre-medicating the patient with paracetamol, hydrocortisone and chlorphenamine to reduce acute toxicity.

Mr CR has received the majority of a 3 mg/kg dose of conventional amphotericin infused in less than one hour as a first dose and with no premedication. There is a significant risk that this will result in renal impairment developing over the next few days.

What course of action would you recommend?

A12 **The error must be documented, the patient monitored carefully and an attempt made to prevent recurrence of the error. Additionally, the nature of the error and its consequences should be fully explained to Mr CR.**

An incident of this kind has obvious medico-legal implications and the error needs to be fully documented, both in the patient's notes and according to any local procedure for reporting drug errors. The doctors caring for Mr CR must also be informed promptly.

There are no accepted procedures which will minimise the risk of Mr CR developing amphotericin-induced renal damage. His renal function must be carefully monitored and his drug therapy kept under review to ensure that as far as possible other nephrotoxic drugs are not prescribed until the effects of this incident on his renal function are known.

Preventing a recurrence of an error such as this is difficult. In the short-term, stocks of conventional amphotericin injection could be removed from the ward if not required for other patients. In the longer-term, a nurse education programme may be necessary, although this would not necessarily have prevented the current incident which resulted from the actions of an agency nurse. Additionally, consideration should be given to the centralised preparation of all intravenous amphotericin doses. This would not only avoid problems like that experienced by Mr CR, but would also ensure that the precise requirements for preparing stable and safe infusions of conventional amphotericin are met: i.e. dilution only with 5% glucose of pH greater than 4.2 (buffered by the addition of phosphate buffer if necessary) to a concentration of less than 0.1 mg/mL plus the provision of protection from light and an in-line filter with a mean pore diameter greater than 1 micrometre between the infusion and the patient.

What do these laboratory results indicate?

A13 **That Mr CR is suffering from very significant amphotericin-induced renal damage.**

This is indicated by his low potassium and calcium levels, and by his raised urea, creatinine and phosphate concentrations. Using the Cockcroft and Gault equation, where:

$$\text{Creatinine clearance (CrCl) (in males)} = \frac{1.2\ (140 - \text{age}) \times \text{body weight (kg)}}{\text{serum creatinine concentration (micromol/L)}}$$

it can be calculated that Mr CR's creatinine clearance has fallen to around 20 from 87 mL/min when he was admitted to hospital (reference range 50–130).

It should be noted that the Cockcroft and Gault equation is only reliable when applied to patients whose renal function is at steady state. It should not be used for patients whose serum creatinine levels are fluctuating by more than about 40 micromol/L/day. Mr CR's renal function has deteriorated fairly rapidly since he was inadvertently overdosed with amphotericin and any estimation of renal function based on serum creatinine concentration should be viewed with caution.

Is any modification needed to Mr CR's current treatment?

A14 **No.**

Mr CR is responding to treatment and the cause of his impaired renal function is almost certainly the single, excessive, dose of conventional amphotericin B he received three days earlier, rather than his current therapy. However, a close watch should be kept on his renal function with a view to stopping treatment if further deterioration occurs, especially as Mr CR has now received a cumulative amphotericin B dose of almost 2 g, which may be sufficient to deal with his presumed fungal infection.

Is the antibiotic regimen selected for Mr CR appropriate?

A15 **Not entirely.**

Blind treatment of presumed infection in neutropenic patients requires a broad-spectrum regimen that will be active against the most likely sources of infection, such as coliforms and skin commensals. Most oncology units have a preferred regimen for this purpose which takes into account local resistance problems. Regimens generally fall into one of two groups: monotherapy with one of the newer, extended-spectrum, beta-lactam antibiotics or a combination of one of these with an aminoglycoside. The theoretical benefits of adding an aminoglycoside include extended spectrum of antibiotic cover, especially against *Pseudomonas* spp., synergy between the two agents and reduced risk of selecting out resistant organisms. On the other hand, there is more risk of bacterial strains with dual resistance emerging and patients are exposed to an increased risk of treatment side-effects. Toxicity is a particular issue with aminoglycosides like gentamicin, which have significant potential for nephro- and ototoxicity.

A recent meta-analysis concluded that combination therapy with a beta-lactam and aminoglycoside offers no advantage over treatment with a newer beta-lactam alone. Therefore, Mr CR would be better off with tazobactam plus piperacillin alone, especially in view of the fact that his kidneys are still recovering from the insult provided by an inappropriate dose of amphotericin B.

Suggest an appropriate dosing regimen for Mr CR's gentamicin therapy.

A16 **A dose of 320 mg infused over 30 minutes and repeated every 24 hours provided that the trough serum concentration is below 1 mg/L.**

Although Mr CR's serum creatinine concentration is just above the upper limit of the normal range, it is only slightly elevated and so he can be dosed using the approach now used for the majority of patients with normal renal function of once-daily dosing. This results in very high peak gentamicin levels ensuring that the minimum inhibitory concentration of even relatively resistant organisms is exceeded. The long dose interval also allows for the period of reversible refractoriness that appears to follow a dose of gentamicin to expire before the next dose is given, so that patients are not treated with the antibiotic at a time when their infection would be expected to be resistant to it. Additionally, once daily gentamicin regimens appear to have reduced potential for nephro-toxicity, possibly because gentamicin uptake into the renal cortex is a saturable process, so that dosing schedules with very high peak levels result in less renal drug exposure than regimens employing more frequent lower doses.

There are many once-daily dosing schedules in use. It is difficult to define an optimal one because of uncertainty around desirable peak and trough serum concentrations. The best known and largest study of once-daily gentamicin dosing, carried out at the Hartford Hospital (Massachusetts, USA) used a dose of 7 mg/kg with the dose interval adjusted according to a random level drawn 6–14 hours post-dose. In practice, many hospitals use a lower dose, typically 4–5 mg/kg with the dose interval extended if the serum trough level exceeds 1 mg/L, 24 hours after dosing. Many hospitals have local policies on gentamicin dosing and monitoring which should be followed.

In Mr CR's case a dose of 5 mg/kg was used. Mr CR is not obese so his dose should be calculated on the basis of his actual body weight. If he were obese, ideal body weight should be used. Therefore, his calculated dose is 67 × 5 mg once daily. Rounding down to 320 mg (to make the dose a convenient, whole number, of 40 mg vials) would be appropriate.

How would you monitor Mr CR's therapy?

A17 **Blood biochemistry should be scrutinised for signs of worsening renal function resulting from gentamicin toxicity and regular gentamicin assays are essential.**

Gentamicin monitoring should start 24 hours after the first gentamicin dose. The next dose should not be given until the blood level from the previous dose is below 1 mg/L. In most patients this will be within 24 hours of drug administration. If it is not, the next dose should be withheld until the blood concentration has decayed to a satisfactory level. A reduced dose should then be administered or the planned dose interval extended. If after three days of treatment at the same dose trough levels are consistently satisfactory and the patient's renal function is stable, the frequency of gentamicin assays can be reduced to every third day.

Should antibiotic treatment be continued in view of the negative blood cultures and Mr CR's failure to respond to broad-spectrum antibiotics?

A18 **Yes.**

It is too early to conclude that Mr CR's febrile episode is not infective in nature. Negative blood cultures are of little significance in febrile neutropenia, where a causative organism is often never isolated during episodes of clinical sepsis. However, the fact that Mr CR's fever is not settling suggests that the organism causing his condition may be resistant to the antibiotics in use. A frequent cause of infection in neutropenic patients with in-dwelling venous catheters is *Staphylococcus epidermidis*, a skin commensal. It is often resistant to first-line antibiotics and, unless especially asked for, is often not reported by hospital bacteriology laboratories (as it is considered to be a sampling contaminant with only 6% of blood cultures containing this organism representing true staphylococcal bacteraemias). At this point it would be reasonable to carry out repeat blood cultures and start empirical treatment with vancomycin or teicoplanin for *S. epidermidis*.

Why are the gentamicin levels so high and what should be done about them?

A19 **They are probably incorrect and the tests should be repeated.**

The most likely explanation is that an inexperienced phlebotomist has withdrawn blood samples for assay through a lumen of Mr CR's Hickman line which was still heavily contaminated from its use during drug administration. Repeat sampling is necessary using blood from a peripheral vein. However, treatment should be withheld until the blood level of gentamicin is clear.

Are any of Mr CR's other blood parameters a cause for concern?

A20 **No.**

The fall in concentration of his blood electrolytes, urea and creatinine probably represents increased dilution as dehydration is reversed.

Is it appropriate to ask the House Officer looking after Mr CR to prescribe calamine lotion?

A21 **No. Mr CR's self-diagnosis of prickly heat is almost certainly incorrect.**

What Mr CR is describing (a small group of tense vesicles, clustered *unilaterally* around his waist and whose appearance was preceded by a stabbing irritation) sounds more like the beginning of a local herpes zoster infection (shingles), triggered by his immunosuppression. In contrast, prickly heat typically presents as a large area of *itchy* red papules distributed *bilaterally* and not associated with paraesthesias which precede the appearance of the rash. In an immunosuppressed patient, shingles may lead to a life-threatening generalised infection. Thus, the doctor looking after Mr CR must be informed promptly of his symptoms so that antiviral therapy can be started, if appropriate.

Is vancomycin the drug of choice for Mr CR and is the dose appropriate?

A22　No. Vancomycin may not be the best choice of antibiotic but, if it is used, a dose of 300 mg intravenously twice daily is appropriate for Mr CR.

A glycopeptide antibiotic (vancomycin or teicoplanin) is certainly appropriate for Mr CR given the presumed diagnosis of *S. epidermidis* which is often multiresistant, but usually still sensitive to glycopeptides.

Choice of glycopeptide may well be governed by local resistance patterns and antibiotic policies designed to restrict the use of antimicrobials in order to conserve their utility. However, aside from these constraints, teicoplanin might be a better choice for Mr CR – it is less nephrotoxic and monitoring of blood levels is not required. It also only requires once-daily administration. As well as reducing nursing workload, simplifying intravenous treatment regimens can be important for patients like Mr CR who are receiving several drugs by this route and may run out of 'line time'. (i.e. the total administration time for all of the intravenous drugs exceeds 24 hours x the number of intravenous lines available).

If vancomycin is selected, Mr CR's renal impairment requires that the dose of this nephrotoxic and renally excreted drug be reduced from the normal adult dose of 2 g daily. Recalculating from the patient's current blood chemistry shows him to have a creatinine clearance of 39 mL/min. Using the dosage nomogram supplied by the drug's manufacturers it can be calculated that Mr CR should be receiving a vancomycin dose of 630 mg/day. This could be administered as 150 mg four times daily; however, a dose of 300 mg twice daily reduces the risk of drug accumulation. It is also more convenient and should be recommended.

Are the dosage instructions for vancomycin adequate?

A23　No. Vancomycin should never be given by rapid intravenous injection, as this can lead to the 'red man syndrome' which is caused by widespread release of histamine within the body.

The syndrome is characterised by sudden and severe hypotension, flushing and/or rash on the face, neck, chest and upper extremities. Occasionally death can occur as a result of cardiac arrest or seizures. Administering vancomycin over at least one hour, as an infusion in saline or glucose, usually prevents this problem. Restricting the infusion volume to 250 mL should avoid fluid-overloading Mr CR. This is always a possibility in patients with impaired renal function.

How should Mr CR's vancomycin therapy be monitored?

A24 **Regular assays of Mr CR's serum vancomycin levels should be performed.**

Although the relationship between plasma concentration and toxicity is less clear for vancomycin than for the aminoglycosides, peak levels should be between 25 and 30 mg/L and trough levels in the range 5–10 mg/L.

Should Mr CR's aciclovir be given intravenously?

A25 **Not initially.**

At the time of starting aciclovir therapy Mr CR's lesions are well localised and he is no longer profoundly neutropenic. If oral treatment is successful in preventing the appearance of new lesions, then intravenous treatment is not indicated. However, if oral treatment does not halt the spread of Mr CR's skin lesions, then intravenous treatment should be started without delay.

Would you recommend any modification to Mr CR's vancomycin therapy?

A26 **No.**

Mr CR's vancomycin levels are in the therapeutic range and he is responding to treatment. However, there has been a modest elevation in his serum creatinine and urea levels since he started his vancomycin treatment. This may well be due to day-to-day variation in the patient or in laboratory assay procedures. Alternatively, it may indicate that Mr CR is suffering some renal toxicity from his vancomycin treatment. At present, this is not a cause for concern when set against the risks of inadequate treatment. Treatment should be continued and a close watch kept on his vancomycin levels and renal function.

In view of his persistently low neutrophil count does Mr CR require any prophylactic antimicrobial therapy to take home with him?

A27 **Probably.**

Mr CR's neutrophil count is still below the 1.5 x 10^9/L level at which the risk of bacterial infection rises sharply and his count is rising only slowly. He must also be considered at high risk of recrudescence of his presumed aspergillosis, since this condition is very difficult to eradicate completely. In view of this it would be sensible to prescribe prophylactic antibiotics and antifungals for him. However he is very anxious to have a few days taking the minimum of medications. Under these circumstances, it is reasonable to try and reach a compromise with Mr CR. He should stay on antifungal prophylaxis, since a recurrence of his aspergillosis not only presents a very immediate high risk it will also be difficult to treat, and will also compromise further treatment. He can stop antibacterial prophylaxis as long as he understands that he must contact the hospital promptly if he develops a sore throat, fever or signs of a chest infection. Provided it is dealt with swiftly and correctly, a bacterial infection is unlikely to have long-term consequences for Mr CR.

Acknowledgement

The author would like to thank Dr Steven Schey for his helpful comments on earlier versions of this chapter.

Further reading

American Society of Clinical Oncology. 2000 update of recommendations for the use of hematopoietic colony-stimulating factors: evidence-based, clinical practice guidelines. *J Clin Oncol* 2000; **18**: 3558–3585.

Blum RA, Rodvold KA. Recognition and importance of *Staphylococcus epidermidis* infections. *Clin Pharm* 1987; **6**: 464–475.

Bodey GP, Anaissie EJ, Gutterman J et al. Role of granulocyte macrophage colony-stimulating factor as adjuvant treatment in neutropenic patients with bacterial and fungal infection. *Eur J Clin Microbiol Infect Dis* 1994; **13**(suppl. 2): 18–22.

Bodey GP, Buckley M, Sathe YS et al. Quantitative relationships between circulating leukocytes and infection in patients with acute leukemia. *Ann Intern Med* 1966; **64**: 328–340.

Coiffier B, Lepage E, Briere J et al. CHOP chemotherapy plus rituximab compared with CHOP alone in elderly patients with diffuse large-B-cell lymphoma. *N Engl J Med* 2002; **346**: 235–242.

Cockcroft DW, Gault MH. Prediction of creatinine clearance from serum creatinine. *Nephron* 1976; **15**: 31–41.

Denning DW, Stephens DA. Antifungal and surgical treatment of invasive aspergillosis: review of 2121 published cases. *Rev Infect Dis* 1990; **12**: 1147–1201.

Dranitsaris G. Clinical and economic considerations of empirical antibacterial therapy of febrile neutropenia in cancer. *Pharmacoeconomics* 1999; **16**: 343–353.

Evans WE, Schentag JJ, Jusko WJ, eds. *Applied Pharmacokinetics: Principles of Therapeutic Drug Monitoring*, 3rd edn. Applied Therapeutics, Virginia, WA, 1992.

Farmaki E, Roilides E. Immunotherapy in patients with systemic mycoses: a promising adjunct. *BioDrugs* 2001; **15**: 207–214.

Fisher RI, Gaynor ER, Dahlberg S *et al.* Comparison of a standard regimen (CHOP) with three intensive chemotherapy regimens for advanced non-Hodgkin's lymphoma. *N Engl J Med* 1993; **328**: 1002–1006.

Fleming RV, Kantarjian HM, Husni R *et al.* Comparison of Amphotericin B Lipid Complex (ABLC) vs. AmBisome in the treatment of suspected or documented fungal infections in patients with leukemia. *Leuk Lymphoma* 2001; **40**: 511–520.

Gilbert DN. Meta-analyses are no longer required for determining the efficacy of single daily dosing of aminoglycosides. *Clin Infect Dis* 1997; **24**: 816–819.

Gotzsche PC, Johansen HK. Routine versus selective antifungal administration for control of fungal infection in patients with cancer (Cochrane Review). In: *The Cochrane Library 2*. Update Software, Oxford, 2003.

Hagemeister FB. Treatment of relapsed aggressive lymphomas: regimens with and without high-dose therapy and stem cell rescue. *Cancer Chemother Pharmacol* 2002; **49**(suppl. 1): S13–20.

Hatala R, Dinh TT, Cook DJ. Single daily dosing of aminoglycosides in immunocompromised adults: a systematic review. *Clin Infect Dis* 1997; **24**: 810–815.

Herbrecht R, Denning DW, Patterson TF *et al.* Voriconazole versus amphotericin B for primary therapy of invasive aspergillosis. *N Engl J Med* 2002; **347**: 408–415.

Johansen HK, Gotzsche PC. Amphotericin B lipid soluble formulations versus amphotericin B in cancer patients with neutropenia (Cochrane Review). In: *The Cochrane Library 2*. Update Software, Oxford, 2003.

Klastersky J. Science and pragmatism in the treatment and prevention of neutropenic infection. *J Antimicrob Agents Chemother* 1998; **41**(suppl. D): 13–24.

Marcus RE, Goldman JM. Management of infection in the neutropenic patient. *Br Med J.* 1986; **293**: 406–408.

Mills W, Chopra R, Linch DC *et al.* Liposomal amphotericin B in the treatment of fungal infections in neutropenic patients: a single centre experience of 133 episodes in 116 patients. *Br J Haematol* 1994; **86**: 754–760.

Nicolau DP, Freeman CD, Belliveau PP *et al*. Experience with a once-daily aminoglycoside program administered to 2184 adult patients. *Antimicrob Agents Chemother* 1995; **39**: 650–655.

Nikkels AF, Pierard GE. Recognition and treatment of shingles. *Drugs* 1994; **48**: 528–548.

Paul M, Soares-Weiser K, Grozinsky S *et al*. Beta-lactam versus beta-lactam-aminoglcoside combination therapy in cancer patients with neutropenia (Cochrane Review). In: *The Cochrane Library 2*. Update Software, Oxford, 2003.

Perry CM, Markham A. Piperacillin/tazobactam: an updated review of its use in the treatment of bacterial infections. *Drugs* 1999; **57**: 805–843.

Pizzo PA. Fever in immunocompromised patients. *N Engl J Med* 1999; **341**: 893–900.

Prentice HG, Hann IM, Herbrecht R *et al*. A randomised comparison of liposomal versus conventional amphotericin B for the treatment of pyrexia of unknown origin in neutropenic patients. *Br J Haematol* 1997; **98**: 711–718.

Rolston KV, Rubinstein EB, eds. *Textbook of Febrile Neutropenia*, 1st edn. Martin Dunitz, London, 2001.

Souhami R, Tobias J. Non-Hodgkin's lymphomas. In: *Cancer and Its Management*, 4th edn. Blackwell Science, Oxford, 2003: 401–425.

Summerhayes M. Myeloid haemopoietic growth factors in clinical practice. A comparative review. Part 1. *Eur J Hosp Pharm* 1995; **1**: 30–36.

Summerhayes M. Myeloid haemopoietic growth factors in clinical practice. A comparative review. Part 2. *Eur J Hosp Pharm* 1995; **1**: 67–74.

Timmers GJ, Zweegman S, Simoons-Smith AM *et al*. Amphotericin B colloidal dispersion (Amphocil) vs fluconazole for the prevention of fungal infections in neutropenic patients: data of a prematurely stopped clinical trial. *Bone Marrow Transplant* 2000; **25**: 879–884.

Tiphine M, Letscher-Bru V, Herbrecht R. Amphotericin B and its new formulations: pharmacologic characteristics, clinical efficacy, and tolerability. *Transplant Infect Dis* 1999; **1**: 273–283.

Wagstaff AJ, Faulds D, Goa KL. Aciclovir. A reappraisal of its antiviral activity, pharmacokinetic properties and therapeutic efficacy. *Drugs* 1994; **47**: 153–205.

White MH, Anaissie EJ, Kusne S *et al*. Amphotericin B colloidal dispersion vs amphotericin B as therapy for invasive aspergilosis. *Clin Infect Dis* 1997; **24**: 635–642.

Wingard JR, White MH, Anaissie E *et al*. A randomised, double-blind comparative trial evaluating the safety of liposomal amphotericin B versus amphotericin B lipid complex in the empirical treatment of febrile neutropenia. *Clin Infect Dis* 2000; **31**: 1155–1163.

21

Peripheral blood progenitor cell transplantation (PBPCT)

Maxwell Summerhayes

Case study and questions

Day 1 Fifty-six-year-old Mr CR was admitted to hospital in order to start the programme of cytotoxic and growth factor treatment necessary to increase the numbers of progenitor cells in his peripheral blood prior to harvesting for a peripheral stem cell transplant. He had received R-CHOP immunochemotherapy for non-Hodgkin's lymphoma (described in the previous chapter) but had relapsed soon after achieving a complete remission of his disease. His disease was then tested for chemosensitivity with a course of miniBEAM (carmustine, etoposide, cytarabine, melphalan). This produced significant tumour shrinkage indicating that it was worthwhile to attempt to cure with high-dose chemotherapy followed by reinfusion of autologous peripheral blood progenitor cells (PBPC) in order to reconstitute his haematopoietic system which will be seriously damaged by the high-dose chemotherapy.

On examination Mr CR was found to be fit and well. He was five feet eight inches in height and weighed 67 kg. The only medication he was taking was his antihypertensive, which had recently been changed to enalapril 10 mg each morning, following a change of GP.

The haematology registrar looking after Mr CR prescribed the following regimen:

- 0.9% sodium chloride 1 L by intravenous infusion over two hours immediately before:
- Mesna 1.5 g/m^2 = 2.8 g by intravenous injection immediately before:
- Cyclophosphamide 4 g/m^2 = 7 g by intravenous infusion over one hour in 500 mL 0.9% sodium chloride, immediately before:

- Mesna 1.5 g/m² = 2.8 g by intravenous infusion over four hours in 1 L 0.9% sodium chloride for two doses
- Furosemide 40 mg orally every 12 hours for three doses starting at the same time as the intravenous fluid therapy
- Granulocyte colony-stimulating factor (G-CSF) 670 micrograms once daily for 10 days by subcutaneous injection

Appropriate anti-emetics had also been prescribed.

Q1 Is the cytotoxic regimen prescribed for Mr CR appropriate for mobilising PBPCs?

Q2 Mr CR wants to know why he has to have more chemotherapy and growth factor treatment to mobilise his PBPCs for harvest. Could they have been collected during recovery from his G-CSF-supported miniBEAM treatment?

Q3 Is 'G-CSF' a suitable abbreviation for the growth factor prescribed for Mr CR?

Q4 Is the dose of G-CSF prescribed for Mr CR appropriate?

Q5 Could granulocyte macrophage colony-stimulating factor (GM-CSF; molgramostim) be used instead of G-CSF?

Q6 It is unclear from the prescription when Mr CR should start using G-CSF. When should treatment commence?

Q7 Why has Mr CR been prescribed furosemide?

Day 2 Mr CR had tolerated his cyclophosphamide treatment very well. This was given, following the pharmacist's intervention, according to the hospital's current regimen of cyclophosphamide 1.5 g/m² given as a one-hour intravenous infusion, preceded by an intravenous injection of 300 mg/m² mesna, and followed by two doses of 600 mg/m² mesna given as tablets two and four hours after starting the cyclophosphamide infusion. Mr CR was trained to self-administer his filgrastim with the aid of an instructional video and was ready to go home.

Q8 Apart from his filgrastim and the remainder of his anti-emetics, what other medications should Mr CR be given to take home?

Days 9–12 Mr CR received three consecutive daily apheresis procedures during which his blood was passed via an extracorporeal circuit through a cell-separator which collected his nucleated cells (including the PBPCs required for transplantation) before returning the remainder to his circulation. A very disappointing harvest of only 0.2×10^8 nucleated cells/kg body weight were obtained. This was considerably less than the 1×10^8/kg body weight required for a transplant at this hospital.

Q9   Suggest reasons for this poor harvest. Are any of these avoidable?

Mr CR was rather dispirited at this point and while talking to the ward pharmacist asked if he could just have some of his bone marrow removed and preserved for use after chemotherapy. He had heard of this being done and thought that it would solve his current problems.

Q10   What is the answer to Mr CR's question?

Day 21   Mr CR commenced a second course of mobilisation identical to the first. This time an adequate harvest was obtained, the cells were cryopreserved and a date arranged for Mr CR to be admitted to the transplant unit for high-dose chemotherapy and PBPCT.

Day 40   Mr CR was admitted to start six days of high-dose conditioning chemotherapy using BEAM200 (carmustine, etoposide, cytarabine, melphalan).

Q11   Why is this combination of drugs used?

According to the transplant unit policy, Mr CR was prescribed prophylaxis against bacterial, viral and fungal agents at the time of starting chemotherapy as follows:

- Ciprofloxacin 500 mg orally twice daily
- Aciclovir 200 mg orally four times a day
- Itraconazole 200 mg orally twice daily
- Amphotericin B 10 mg by nebuliser twice daily

The first three agents were prescribed according to transplant unit prescribing policies; however, amphotericin B was an unusual addition.

Q12   What are the objectives and limitations of antimicrobial prophylaxis in Mr CR's case?

Q13   What other measures can be taken to minimise Mr CR's risk of infection?

Q14   Would the newer antiviral agents valaciclovir or famciclovir offer advantages over aciclovir in this situation?

Q15   Suggest a reason for the deviation from transplant unit policy in the choice of Mr CR's antifungal prophylaxis. (His relevant medical history is outlined in the previous chapter.)

Q16   Why is itraconazole the prophylactic triazole of choice when fluconazole generally has better gastrointestinal tolerability?

Q17 Are there any problems associated with combining amphotericin and itraconazole treatment?

Day 42 Mr CR was on the second day of his BEAM200 chemotherapy and was due to receive cytarabine and etoposide. A nurse looking after Mr CR asked whether he should be receiving steroid eye-drops, as she had seen other haematology patients receiving these whilst on high-dose chemotherapy.

Q18 Should Mr CR be prescribed steroid eye-drops?

Day 47 Mr CR had completed his high-dose chemotherapy. He had tolerated this well except for moderate nausea and vomiting which had blunted his appetite for food. On this day he received his cryopreserved PBPCs via his permanently implanted Hickman (venous access) catheter.

Q19 Should Mr CR be prescribed haematopoietic growth factors to stimulate recovery of haematopoietic function?

Day 51 Mr CR's blood count was:

- White blood cells (WBC) 0.5×10^9/L (reference range $4–11 \times 10^9$)
- Neutrophils 0.3×10^9/L $(2.2–7.0 \times 10^9)$
- Platelets 113×10^9/L $(150–400 \times 10^9)$
- Haemoglobin 9.6 g/dL (13.5–17.5)

Mr CR was now pancytopenic and his white cell count had fallen by about 70% since the previous day. Because he would soon be profoundly neutropenic he was put into protective isolation. He was suffering from severe and painful buccal ulceration which was starting to interfere with his food intake.

Q20 Could Mr CR's mucositis have been prevented?
Q21 How can it be alleviated?
Q22 Should you recommend total parenteral nutrition for Mr CR?

Day 58 Mr CR's neutrophil count had recovered to 0.5×10^9/L from undetectable levels three days earlier. His mucositis was improving rapidly and his appetite was returning. He had been apyrexial for 24 hours but remained on broad-spectrum antibiotics (ceftazidime 2 g intravenously three times daily plus teicoplanin 400 mg intravenously once a day) started for a febrile episode five days earlier. The decision was made to allow Mr CR out of isolation and to stop his intravenous antibiotics after another 24 hours if his neutrophil count stayed above $0.5 \times 10^9/L$ and he remained apyrexial.

Day 61 Mr CR had been off antibiotics for 24 hours. His neutrophil count was $0.9 \times 10^9/L$. He remained on prophylactic antivirals and antifungals and was anxious to leave hospital. His consultant told him that he could leave as soon as he wished, although he would have to return to the day-case unit in two days time to have his blood count checked and receive a platelet transfusion if necessary.

Q23 What prophylactic antimicrobials should Mr CR take home with him?

Is the cytotoxic regimen prescribed for Mr CR appropriate for mobilising PBPCs?

A1 Not really.

Although this dose of cyclophosphamide, given in conjunction with G-CSF, will result in PBPC mobilisation and has been widely used for this indication in the past, in most centres it has been abandoned in favour of regimens incorporating lower doses of cyclophosphamide.

The ideal mobilisation regimen would be highly efficient in mobilizing PBPCs with minimal toxicity. It should also do this in a predictable fashion, so that the optimum time for harvesting can be accurately forecast without the need to monitor the number of PBPCs in the blood. Doses of cyclophosphamide as high as that prescribed for Mr CR fall short of this ideal in two ways. First, they are likely to produce excessive toxicity: they require intensive intravenous hydration to prevent urothelial damage and are likely to result in severe nausea and vomiting and prolonged neutropenia. Secondly, they produce an unpredictable pattern of myelosuppression and recovery, making it difficult to estimate in advance the best days for PBPC collection, which are the days immediately after the nadir white blood cell count when haematopoietic regeneration is occurring.

As experience of PBPC mobilisation has grown, most transplant centres have reduced the dose of cyclophosphamide used. Many centres now use a dose of 1.5 g/m^2. Given in conjunction with a suitable course of haematopoietic growth factor treatment this results in little toxicity and the reliable mobilisation of PBPCs on the 10th day after chemotherapy. For some patients, a single apheresis procedure on this day will yield sufficient PBPCs for transplantation, whereas for the majority the pooled product from consecutive aphereses carried out on days 10 and 11 will be adequate.

Mr CR wants to know why he has to have more chemotherapy and growth factor treatment to mobilise his PBPCs for harvest. Could they have been collected during recovery from his G-CSF-supported miniBEAM treatment?

A2 Theoretically, yes.

Many cytotoxic regimens have been used with haematopoietic growth factors to mobilize PBPCs and the rise in PBPCs during recovery from chemotherapy is probably a universal phenomenon. However, there are three reasons why no attempt was made to harvest PBPCs after Mr CR's miniBEAM chemotherapy. First, the kinetics of PBPC release after different chemotherapy regimens are variable, making it difficult to predict the best time for harvesting unless a regimen is used for this purpose on a regular basis. In the absence of good predictive data, multiple, poor-yield aphereses may have to be performed in an attempt to obtain an adequate harvest. This is inconvenient for patients and takes up valuable staff time, equipment time and expensive disposables. Secondly, any attempt to harvest PBPCs after miniBEAM would have required Mr CR to receive larger doses of G-CSF than he had been getting for support during chemotherapy. This would have been an expensive gamble given the uncertainty of obtaining a good harvest. Thirdly, a decision had been made that Mr CR would only be transplanted if his disease remitted with miniBEAM. Therefore, the expense of harvesting his PBPCs would have been unjustified until now.

Is 'G-CSF' a suitable abbreviation for the growth factor prescribed for Mr CR?

A3   **No. There are two G-CSFs commercially available in the UK.**

Both of these agents share the same peptide backbone, but one has apparently human-identical glycosylation of this backbone (lenograstim), and the other is non-glycosylated and has an extra terminal methionine residue (filgrastim). The recommended doses of the two are different and it is clear from the dose that the prescriber intends Mr CR to receive filgrastim, which is licensed for the mobilisation of PBPCs at a dose of 10 micrograms/kg/day.

Is the dose of G-CSF prescribed for Mr CR appropriate?

A4   **Yes and no!**

The prescriber has calculated that, based on his body weight, Mr CR should receive 67 x 10 = 670 micrograms filgrastim daily. Whilst this is correct, it is not a convenient dose given that the product is available in 300- and 480-microgram vials. Generally, it is much easier, and less wasteful of this costly agent, to teach patients to inject an appropriate number of whole vials of filgrastim each day. In Mr CR's case it would be reasonable to round-off the dose to 600 micrograms daily.

Could GM-CSF (molgramostim) be used instead of G-CSF?

A5   Yes, but it has disadvantages.

GM-CSF shares with G-CSF the ability to mobilise PBPCs, although the relative efficacy of the two agents in this situation has not been well characterised. However, the greater toxicity of GM-CSF, the use of which is associated with a high incidence of fluid retention and febrile and injection site reactions, plus its lack of a UK product licence for this application, make its routine use for PBPC mobilisation inappropriate.

It is unclear from the prescription when Mr CR should start using G-CSF. When should treatment commence?

A6   Twenty-four hours after chemotherapy.

Haematopoietic growth factors should not be administered within 24 hours of cytotoxic chemotherapy of any sort. If administered earlier than this, there is a danger that they will stimulate haematopoietic progenitor cells into active growth rendering them more vulnerable to residual cytotoxic drug and thus exacerbating rather than ameliorating the mye-lotoxicity of chemotherapy. However, when counselling Mr CR, it is appropriate to explain that the timing of growth factor administration is not too critical, so that he can start treatment at any convenient time *approximately* 24 hours after finishing his cyclophosphamide. In some centres it is the practice to delay the start of growth factor treatment for three to five days after chemotherapy. This seems to work and significantly reduces the cost of mobilisation.

Why has Mr CR been prescribed furosemide?

A7   Because of the possible antidiuretic effect of cyclophosphamide.

Mr CR was originally prescribed 3.5 L of fluids intravenously with a view to stimulating the production of copious urine to dilute out and encourage voiding of the acrolein metabolites of cyclophosphamide which are responsible for its urothelial toxicity. Cyclophosphamide, particularly at high doses, is capable of exerting an antidiuretic action which will counteract the effects of hyperhydration. The furosemide is intended to ensure that this does not happen. However, it is doubtful whether diuretics are needed with the lower doses of cyclophosphamide now routinely used, and ultimately administered to Mr CR for PBPC mobilisation.

Apart from his filgrastim and the remainder of his anti-emetics, what other medications should Mr CR be given to take home?

A8 **A suitable analgesic, allopurinol and a prophylactic antibiotic.**

The only adverse effect likely to be experienced by Mr CR as a result of his filgrastim treatment is bone pain. This is a toxicity common to all those haematopoietic growth factors currently marketed for increasing neutrophil production and it may be inseparable from the therapeutic response. It can be quite severe at the doses used for PBPC mobilisation and so a suitable analgesic, such as co-proxamol, should be given to Mr CR to take, as required, if symptoms develop.

Although Mr CR does not have a large tumour burden, the administration of a high-dose of cyclophosphamide would be expected to cause the death of a substantial number of cells, both malignant and normal, with the release of nucleic acid components which can be converted into uric acid by xanthine oxidase. The prophylactic administration of the xanthine oxidase inhibitor allopurinol will prevent the formation of large quantities of this poorly soluble compound which can precipitate in the kidneys causing urate nephropathy (tumour lysis syndrome). Mr CR should receive allopurinol 300 mg orally once daily for seven days, starting on the day of cyclophosphamide treatment.

The cyclophosphamide dose given to Mr CR will cause significant myelosuppression, with a white cell nadir occurring between days 6 and 8. Although recovery from this period of myelosuppression is normally uneventful, prophylactic treatment with a broad-spectrum antibiotic (e.g. ciprofloxacin 500 mg orally twice daily for five days, starting on the fourth day after cyclophosphamide administration) is probably a wise precaution, especially as any infective episode experienced by the patient will interfere with the harvesting process. An aborted harvest makes planning patient treatments difficult and is very wasteful of resources.

Suggest reasons for this poor harvest. Are any of these avoidable?

A9 **The factors which determine whether a good harvest of PBPCs can be obtained from an individual are poorly understood, although extensive prior chemotherapy seems to damage the bone marrow in a way which makes PBPC mobilisation more difficult.**

In Mr CR's case the reason was more prosaic. When he attended the hospital for harvesting he returned 10 unused filgrastim vials. When he was questioned about this, he said that he had injected the contents of one vial of filgrastim each day instead of two, because that was what was shown on the patient education video he had seen. This demonstrates the importance of absolute clarity in any educational material supplied to patients, particularly those receiving complex and novel therapies.

What is the answer to Mr CR's question?

A10 **Yes, but it would not be the best solution.**

Although autologous bone marrow transplantation (BMT) is an option for patients such as Mr CR it has been almost completely replaced by PBPCT for several reasons. First, collection of PBPCs is generally preferable to bone marrow harvesting as it does not require the patient to receive a general anaesthetic. More importantly, PBPCT is associated with significantly shorter periods of profound neutropenia and thrombocytopenia than is BMT. Most PBPCT patients recover a neutrophil count of $0.5 \times 10^9/L$ about 10 days after PBPC reinfusion and a platelet count of $50 \times 10^9/L$ about 14 days after progenitor cell return, compared with about 14 and 30–40 days, respectively, after BMT supported by haemopoietic growth factors after reinfusion. This dramatic reduction in the period of transplant-associated pancytopenia makes PBPCT much less hazardous and unpleasant for patients than BMT.

Why is this combination of drugs used?

A11 **BEAM200 was chosen for Mr CR because it contains four drugs with high activity against non-Hodgkin's lymphoma, only one of which he received during his initial treatment. This minimises the risk of Mr CR's disease being resistant to the combination. Additionally, the sensitivity of his disease to this combination of drugs has been tested with the course of miniBEAM that he has already received. MiniBEAM comprises the same drugs as BEAM200, but at non-myeloablative doses.**

There are many combinations of high-dose chemotherapy which are used either alone or in conjunction with total body irradiation as conditioning treatment prior to transplantation. Each of these has characteristics which makes it particularly suitable for a given patient group.

Conditioning regimens generally contain drugs with a high level of activity against the disease being treated and with myelosuppression as their dose-limiting toxicity. Because PBPCT and BMT will only ameliorate the myelotoxicity of chemotherapy, they do not facilitate significant dose-escalation of drugs such as the anthracyclines which have substantial toxicity against other organ systems.

Regimens containing high doses of cyclophosphamide and total body irradiation are profoundly immunosuppressive and their use is generally confined to patients receiving transplantation with donor bone marrow, for whom immunosuppression is essential to prevent graft-versus-host disease.

BEAM200 is a widely used conditioning regimen for patient's with non-Hodgkin's lymphoma and is one of the few drug combinations to have been assessed in a randomised trial comparing high-dose chemotherapy plus BMT with the same combination of cytotoxics given at non-myeloablative doses. In a British National Lymphoma Investigation trial, patients were found to benefit from high-dose treatment.

What are the objectives and limitations of antimicrobial prophylaxis in Mr CR's case?

A12   **The main aim of antimicrobial prophylaxis is the suppression of those potentially pathogenic endogenous organisms which present most risk to Mr CR. The efficacy of prophylaxis is limited by the impossibility of sterilizing the skin and gut, and the resistance of certain common organisms with pathogenic potential to those antibiotics suitable for prophylactic use.**

While he is profoundly neutropenic Mr CR will be nursed in isolation, in a clean room with filtered air. His diet will be controlled to ensure that he does not become infected with food-borne microorganisms and people with infectious diseases will be kept away from him. In such circumstances, Mr CR's most likely source of infection is his own microbial flora, particularly those organisms which colonize the gut and skin surface.

However, it is generally recognised that attempting to sterilize the gut is counterproductive, as the process creates an ideal environment for the overgrowth of pathogens. Instead, the concept of selective bacterial decontamination with quinolone antibiotics has become popular. These are effective in suppressing the most common potential pathogens, but leave the (generally harmless) anaerobic flora untouched.

What other measures can be taken to minimise Mr CR's risk of infection?

A13 **Other prophylactic measures can be divided into environmental controls and personal hygiene measures.**

Mr CR should be nursed in isolation, preferably in a purpose-built room designed to prevent the accumulation of dirt and dust. It should have non-porous surfaces and sealed joints between walls and other structural elements, and a HEPA-filtered air supply. The last measure is particularly useful for removing spores of *Aspergillus niger*, a mould which causes life-threatening and difficult-to-treat infections in the profoundly immuno-suppressed. The room should be thoroughly disinfected before Mr CR moves in.

While he is neutropenic, Mr CR's diet should be controlled to eliminate those items such as uncooked and reheated food which can carry a particularly high bacterial burden.

Personal hygiene measures which should be adopted to suppress Mr CR's endogenous microbial flora include daily skin cleansing with washes containing chlorhexidine or povidone iodine.

Good oral hygiene is also important because the mucositis which usually follows high-dose chemotherapy allows easy access of oral micro-organisms to the systemic circulation. A regimen of regular mouthwash-ing with an antimicrobial such as chlorhexidine gluconate should be instituted once treatment begins. However, toothbrushing should only be carried out with a very soft brush and only then if it can be done without causing trauma which will encourage microbial entry into the blood-stream: it is probably best avoided altogether once mucositis has developed. Additionally, before admission to hospital Mr CR should have received a thorough dental examination with any necessary dental work being completed prior to high-dose therapy.

The exit site of any permanently implanted venous access device is a major site of bacterial ingress in neutropenic patients and any unhealed scar should be cleaned each day with povidone-iodine or chlorhexidine. However, in Mr CR's case the exit site had completely healed and no special treatment was required.

Would the newer antiviral agents valaciclovir or famciclovir offer advantages over aciclovir in this situation?

A14 **Theoretically yes, but there are few clinical data to support their use in this situation.**

Aciclovir is not well absorbed from the gastrointestinal tract and this problem is exacerbated in patients who have had high-dose chemotherapy.

Both the aciclovir prodrug valaciclovir and famciclovir are better absorbed in immunocompetent patients. Unfortunately, there are no published data on their absorption after high-dose chemotherapy and no randomised trials of their use as prophylactic agents in this situation.

Of the two agents the evidence for valaciclovir is the strongest. In a comparison with placebo it significantly reduced the incidence of cytomegalovirus (CMV) disease in patients immunosuppressed after *renal* transplantation. The reduction in clinical infection was similar to that previously reported with aciclovir. Additionally, in a series of patients treated with valaciclovir as prophylaxis after progenitor cell transplantation and compared with historical controls, herpes simplex reactivation rates were similar to those seen in patients receiving intravenous aciclovir and much lower than those receiving no prophylaxis. Overall, it is unlikely that valaciclovir will provide worse protection than aciclovir, but there is no convincing evidence that its use would add additional benefits.

Suggest a reason for the deviation from transplant unit policy in the choice of Mr CR's antifungal prophylaxis. (His relevant medical history is outlined in the previous chapter.)

A15   **Mr CR has already experienced an episode of presumed respiratory infection with *A.niger* (see Chapter 20).**

It is therefore reasonable to suppose that he may still be carrying the organism, leaving him at risk of recrudescence once he becomes immunocompromised. Nebulised amphotericin B is an attempt to deliver high concentrations of amphotericin to the point of possible latent infection, whilst avoiding the toxicity of systemic administration of amphotericin B which remains the gold-standard antifungal. Unfortunately this approach has not been adequately tested in large-scale clinical trials. In fact, because the risk of aspergillosis must be considered very high in Mr CR's case and because this will pose such a grave risk to him if it does develop, prophylaxis with systemic amphotericin B should be considered. In a recent Cochrane meta-analysis, although fluconazole, itraconazole and amphotericin B all reduced the incidence of invasive fungal infections, only amphotericin B showed a clear trend towards reducing mortality when administered as a prophylactic measure to neutropenic cancer patients. The apparently greater utility of amphotericin B as a *prophylactic* agent should, however, be viewed with caution. In the studies used in the meta-analysis amphotericin B was more likely to be used for pre-emptive treatment of individuals with fever resistant to antibacterials and the triazoles were more likely to be used as true prophylactic agents. Thus the amphotericin B studies were more likely to have enrolled patients with significant fungal infections whose course could be altered by intervention.

The drawback of using systemic amphotericin B as a prophylactic agent is its toxicity, especially its nephrotoxicity. This can be circumvented by the use of lipid formulations of amphotericin B (see Chapter 20), though these are, generally, too costly to use prophylactically, except in the highest risk patients.

It seems likely that in the future newer antifungal agents with a better balance of toxicity and efficacy will be used for prophylaxis in high-risk patients like Mr CR. For example, the recently marketed triazole, voriconazole, has a broad spectrum of antifungal activity with good activity against *Aspergillus* spp. It is orally active and has an acceptable toxicity profile. However, it is expensive and has not yet been the subject of published prophylactic trials and cannot be considered a prophylactic agent suitable for routine use. In a patient such as Mr CR, where treatment can be considered more as pre-emptive therapy than prophylaxis, voriconazole treatment might, possibly, be justified during this very immunosuppressive procedure.

Why is itraconazole the prophylactic triazole of choice when fluconazole generally has better gastrointestinal tolerability?

A16 **Because it has greater activity against *Aspergillus* spp.**

Mortality rates of up to 90% have been reported with proven *A. niger* infection. Therefore, preventing infection with this common environmental contaminant is a high priority when selecting a prophylactic agent. Additionally, there appear to be more problems with *Candida* spp. resistant to fluconazole than itraconazole. Some patients appear to tolerate itraconazole capsules better than the oral liquid formulation; however, the liquid formulation should be used where possible since it is better absorbed than the encapsulated drug. Poor absorption appears to be a particular problem in patients who have received high-dose chemotherapy and/or total body irradiation.

As indicated in the answer to the previous question, newer, more potent triazoles may, in due course, replace fluconazole and itraconazole as prophylactic agents in immunosuppressed patients, though there is as yet insufficient evidence to support their routine use in this situation.

Are there any problems with combining amphotericin and itraconazole treatment?

A17 **Theoretically. Itraconazole could reduce the efficacy of amphotericin.**

Itraconazole reduces the synthesis of fungal cell membrane ergosterols and it is to these that amphotericin binds to exert its effect. The clinical significance of this interaction is unclear and it seems best to avoid giving the two agents together systemically. However, in Mr CR's case, where very high local concentrations of amphotericin will be achieved in the lungs, it seems unlikely that reduced ergosterol binding will prevent its action and the risk of interaction is probably offset by the benefit of co-administering a non-toxic, but hopefully effective, systemic antifungal.

Should Mr CR be prescribed steroid eye-drops?

A18 **Possibly.**

Cytarabine is excreted in tear fluid and, when given in high doses, can cause a severe and painful chemical conjunctivitis. This can be prevented by the use of steroid eye-drops (usually prednisolone 0.5% two drops four times a day). Steroid prophylaxis is definitely required at doses of cytarabine above 1 g/m²/day. At the doses of 100–200 mg/m² used in many leukaemia regimens it is not routinely required. With BEAM200 Mr CR receives 400 mg/m²/day and he may suffer ocular irritation but is unlikely to develop severe conjunctivitis. Overall, it is reasonable to provide steroid prophylaxis, on the basis that a short course of steroid eye-drops is unlikely to be harmful and conjunctivitis is a problem best avoided if possible.

Should Mr CR be prescribed haematopoietic growth factors to stimulate recovery of haematopoietic function?

A19 **No.**

In contrast to their use after BMT, there is no convincing evidence that currently licensed growth factors will significantly accelerate haemato-poietic recovery when administered after PBPCT. This may be because PBPCs are more mature than the cells used in BMT and less susceptible to the effects of growth factors.

Could Mr CR's mucositis have been prevented?

A20 **No.**

One of the problems with PBPCT is that although, as with BMT, it offers a satisfactory way of circumventing the dose-limiting myelotoxicity of chemotherapy, dose escalation results in the unmasking of other toxicities. Mucositis, which results from damage to the rapidly dividing and therefore highly chemosensitive cells of the buccal mucosa, is a common problem after high-dose chemotherapy and will be experienced by almost all transplant patients.

How can it be alleviated?

A21 **Numerous treatments have been suggested to alleviate the pain and discomfort of mucositis. Few of these have been evaluated in high quality clinical trials. Amongst the most popular are benzydamine and carbenoxolone mouthwashes, sucralfate suspension used as a mouthwash, lidocaine gel and cocaine mouthwash.**

Lidocaine gel must be used with caution for two reasons. First, because there may be significant systemic absorption when it is applied to a large area of ulcerated mucosa. Secondly, and probably more importantly, because, as it finds its way to the throat, it can interfere with the gag reflex.

Extemporaneously prepared cocaine mouthwash, which seems to be popular in some hospitals, is best avoided. Apart from the problems inherent in local anaesthetic preparations, which it shares with lidocaine, cocaine has other undesirable properties. Systemic absorption of cocaine from a 5 or 10% solution is likely to be significant through the ulcerated and denuded mucosal surface. This could lead to systemic cardiac toxicity as well as undesirable central nervous system effects. A review article recently criticised the continued use of cocaine during ear, nose and throat procedures on these grounds. There is even less reason to use cocaine in mucositis where its sympathomimetic action is of no value.

Although the use of topical agents along with non-drug measures such as the introduction of a bland, liquidised diet and the substitution of mouthwashing for toothbrushing may all help, they are often inadequate to control the pain of severe mucositis and the use of strong opiates to control the pain should not be considered excessive.

Should you recommend total parenteral nutrition for Mr CR?

A22 **Not at this stage.**

Mr CR is still taking some solid food and his oral intake can be enhanced by the use of a bland, liquidised diet and high-calorie dietary supplements. It is also reasonably certain that the mucositis which underlies Mr CR's eating problem will start to resolve in the next five to seven days. Premature introduction of parenteral nutrition for Mr CR will not only add to the cost of his treatment but will also complicate his regimen of intravenous drug treatment unnecessarily. This is an important consideration given that most PBPCT patients will, during the course of their treatment, need to receive large numbers of intravenous anti-infectives, along with other drugs and blood products, via the limited access provided by a single, double or triple lumen central venous catheter. Finding sufficient 'line time' to administer them all can become a problem.

What prophylactic antimicrobials should Mr CR take home with him?

A23 **Ciprofloxacin, aciclovir and itraconazole liquid would be a reasonable combination.**

Although Mr CR's neutrophil count is rising rapidly and he clearly has a functioning graft, he is still neutropenic and it would probably be prudent to continue prophylaxis until his neutrophil count enters the normal range. Mr CR is tolerating these agents well and so there is no reason to deviate from the transplant unit policy. Of the three agents required itraconzole is the one most likely to cause problems since it causes an unpleasant sensation of nausea in a significant proportion of patients. For patients in whom this is likely to cause non-compliance, a change to encapsulated drug (less reliably absorbed, but generally better tolerated) or to fluconazole may be considered. As has already been explained, fluconazole has a reduced antifungal spectrum, but this is probably acceptable in the majority of patients during this phase of recovering immunocompetence. A patient who complies with a less effective therapy is better protected than one who fails to take a more active one. However, Mr CR must still be considered, on the basis of his previous history, to be at significant risk of recurrent aspergillosis and he should be strongly encouraged to continue with itraconazole for the time being, even if he finds it unpalatable.

Acknowledgement

The author would like to thank Dr Steven Schey for his helpful comments on an earlier version of this chapter.

Further reading

American Society of Clinical Oncology. 2000 update of recommendations for the use of hematopoietic colony-stimulating factors: evidence-based, clinical practice guidelines. *J Clin Oncol* 2000; **18**: 3558–3585.

Boogaerts M, Winston DJ, Bow EJ *et al.* Intravenous and oral itraconazole versus intravenous amphotericin B deoxycholate as empirical anti-fungal therapy for persistent fever in neutropenic patients with cancer who are receiving broad-spectrum antibacterial therapy: A randomised, controlled trial. *Ann Intern Med* 2001; **135**: 412–422.

Conneally E, Cafferkey MT, Daly PA *et al.* Nebulised amphotericin B as prophylaxis against invasive aspergillosis in granulocytopenic patients. *Bone Marrow Transplant* 1990; **5**: 403–406.

Craddock C Haematopoietic stem-cell transplantation: recent progress and further promise. *Lancet Oncol* 2000; **1**: 227–234.

Cruciani M. Antibacterial prophylaxis. *Int J Antimicrob Agents* 2000; **16**: 123–125.

Dignani MC, Mykietiuk A, Michelet M *et al.* Valacyclovir prophylaxis for the prevention of Herpes simplex virus reactivation in recipients of progenitor cells transplantation. *Bone Marrow Transplant* 2002; **29**: 263–267.

Ford CD, Reilly W, Wood J *et al.* Oral antimicrobial prophylaxis in bone marrow transplant recipients: randomised trial of ciprofloxacin versus ciprofloxacin-vancomycin. *Antimicrobial Agents Chemother* 1998; **42**: 1402–1405.

Gazitt Y. Comparison between granulocyte colony-stimulating factor and granulocyte-macrophage colony-stimulating factor in the mobilization of peripheral blood stem cells. *Curr Opin Hematol* 2002; **9**: 190–198.

Gluckman E, Lotzberg J, Devergie A *et al.* Prophylaxis of herpes infections after bone marrow transplantation by oral acyclovir. *Lancet* 1983; **2**: 706–708.

Hagemeister FB. Treatment of relapsed aggressive lymphomas: regimens with and without high-dose therapy and stem cell rescue. *Cancer Chemother Pharmacol* 2002; **49**(suppl. 1): S13–20.

Karthaus M, Rosenthal C, Ganser A. Prophylaxis and treatment of chemo- and radiotherapy-induced oral mucositis – are there new strategies? *Bone Marrow Transplant* 1999; **24**: 1095–1098.

Ketterer N, Salles G, Moullet I *et al.* Factors associated with successful mobilisation of peripheral blood progenitor cells in 200 patients with lymphoid malignancies. *Br J Haematol.* 1998; **103**: 235–242.

Lastorre F, Klimek L. Does cocaine still have a role in nasal surgery. *Drug Safety* 1999; **20**: 9–13.

Ljungman P. Prophylaxis against Herpesvirus infections in transplant recipients. *Drugs* 2001; **61**: 187–196.

Marr KA. Antifungal prophylaxis in hematopoietic stem cell recipients. *Curr Opinion Infect Dis* 2001; **14**; 423–426.

Morgenstern GR, Prentice AG, Prentice HG *et al*. A randomised controlled trial of iraconazole versus fluconazole for the prevention of fungal infections in patients with haematological malignancies. *Br J Haematol.* 1999; **105**: 901–911.

Rolston KV, Rubinstein EB, eds. *Textbook of Febrile Neutropenia*, 1st edn. Martin Dunitz, London, 2001.

Russell JA, Chaudhry A, Booth K *et al*. Early outcomes after allogeneic stem cell transplantation for leukemia and myelodysplasia without protective isolation: a 10–year experience. *Biol Blood Marrow Transplant* 2000; **6**: 109–114.

Souhami R, Tobias J. Non-Hodgkin's lymphoma. In: *Cancer and its Management*. 4th edn. Blackwell Science, Oxford, 2003: 401–425.

Summerhayes M. Myeloid haemopoietic growth factors in clinical practice. A comparative review. Part 1. *Eur J Hosp Pharm* 1995; **1**: 30–36.

Summerhayes M. Myeloid haemopoietic growth factors in clinical practice. A comparative review. Part 2. *Eur J Hosp Pharm* 1995; **1**: 67–74.

Thomas ED, Blume KG, Forman SJ, eds. *Hematopoietic Cell Transplantation*, 2nd edn. Blackwell, Oxford, 1999.

Wagstaff AJ, Faulds D, Goa KL. Aciclovir. A reappraisal of its antiviral activity, pharmacokinetic properties and therapeutic efficacy. *Drugs* 1995; **47**: 153–205.

Worthington HV, Clarkson JE, Eden OB. Interventions for treating oral mucositis for patients with cancer receiving treatment (Cochrane Review). In: *The Cochrane Library 2*. Update Software. Oxford, 2003.

22

Symptom control in palliative care

Colin Hardman

Day 1 Mrs PF, an 80-year-old lady, was admitted to hospital after a visit at home by her consultant surgeon. She had a six-month history of weight loss, altered bowel habits, rectal bleeding and abdominal pain. Investigations had revealed a carcinoma in her colon, but she had declined treatment. She had thus been referred to her GP for palliative care and had initially been prescribed co-proxamol and temazepam.

She lived with her 85-year-old husband in their own house and they had no children. She did not smoke and drank only very rarely. She had no other medical problems and did not take any regular medication other than that provided by her GP. She rarely bought medicines and in general did not like taking them. She looked after her husband who had had a myocardial infarction some years ago and now had angina pectoris that limited his activities.

Recently, her pain had become more frequent and more severe. She had experienced nausea and vomiting, and had little appetite. She had not slept well for some time. Her GP had given her metoclopramide 10 mg orally every six hours, with little effect, and Diconal to be taken every six hours when needed for severe pain, but she has been reluctant to take them. She was now in constant pain, bed-bound and was experiencing frequent bouts of vomiting. She reluctantly agreed to let her consultant admit her to hospital for control of her symptoms.

On the ward she was noted to be drowsy, but responded appropriately when asked questions. She was dehydrated. White plaques were seen in her mouth, and areas of her tongue were red and sore. Masses were palpable in her abdomen. She described her pain as constant, but said it varied in intensity. The pain was largely confined to her abdomen. A rectal examination was not carried out because Mrs PF would not agree to it. The clinical impression was that Mrs PF had partial bowel obstruction from her tumour and constipation.

Her serum biochemical results were as follows:

- Glucose 4.1 mmol/L (reference range 3.3–11)
- Sodium 131 mmol/L (136–148)
- Potassium 3.0 mmol/L (3.6–5.0)
- Calcium (corrected for albumin) 2.31 mmol/L (2.1–2.6)

- Urea 10.1 mmol/L (2.5–10)
- Creatinine 125 micromol/L (55–120)

She was initially prescribed intravenous fluids and the following oral drugs:

- Morphine sulphate 10 mg (as solution) every four hours
- Prochlorperazine 12.5 mg every six hours by intramuscular injection

- Co-danthramer liquid 25/200 10 mL at night
- Temazepam 10 mg orally at night

Q1 Outline a pharmaceutical care plan for Mrs PF.

Q2 What factors are likely to be contributing to Mrs PF's drowsiness?

Q3 Why is Mrs PF vomiting so frequently?

Q4 Do you agree with the choice of anti-emetic therapy?

Q5 What might be the cause of Mrs PF's oral problems and what action would you recommend?

Q6 Was morphine sulphate solution the most appropriate analgesic for Mrs PF's initial pain control? Is the starting dose appropriate?

Q7 What should be considered when starting a patient on opiate therapy?

Q8 What might be the cause of Mrs PF's abdominal masses?

Q9 Was co-danthramer liquid the best choice of laxative?

Day 2 She was still in pain so her morphine dose was increased to 20 mg every four hours. She was less nauseated but still vomited once or twice a day. The consultant noted that she had a palpable liver edge.

Q10 What is the significance of Mrs PF's palpable liver?

Day 3 Mrs PF still complained of some abdominal pain. She added that it was different to her original pain, but difficult to describe. Dexamethasone 16 mg daily by mouth was prescribed and the dose of co-danthramer was increased to 10 mL twice daily.

Q11 Why has dexamethasone been prescribed for Mrs PF and is the dose appropriate for this indication?

Q12 How should the dexamethasone therapy be monitored?

Q13 Should an H$_2$-receptor antagonist be co-prescribed?

Q14 Would Mrs PF benefit from the addition of a non-steroidal anti-inflammatory drug (NSAID) to her therapy?

Q15 Is doubling the dose of co-danthramer the best way of managing Mrs PF's continuing constipation?

Day 4 She passed some soft stools.

Day 6 Mrs PF reported that her pain was better. Intravenous access had been removed and she was drinking but not eating much. She still vomited, but rarely, and had little nausea.

Q16 Would you recommend any changes to Mrs PF's morphine therapy?

Q17 What other analgesics could be considered if Mrs PF develops pain unresponsive to her current therapy?

Day 12 She was not sleeping well and complained of pain at night. Additional doses of morphine were given as required, with occasional benefit.

Q18 What other factors may affect Mrs PF's pain control and how should they be addressed?

Day 14 Mrs PF was feeling better but a little drowsy. She complained of a headache and was given paracetamol with good effect.

Q19 Why does paracetamol work in the presence of morphine?

Day 17 Transfer was arranged to a local hospice for continuing care. Her medication regimen at transfer was:

- Slow-release morphine 80 mg orally twice daily
- Haloperidol 0.5 mg orally at night
- Co-danthramer liquid 25/200 10 mL orally twice daily
- Temazepam 10 mg orally at night
- Diazepam 2 mg orally twice daily
- Morphine sulphate 10 mg/5 mL liquid for breakthrough pain

Q20 What factors may affect Mrs PF's compliance with this regimen?

Q21 If Mrs PF becomes unable to tolerate her therapy orally, what options could be considered?

Outline a pharmaceutical care plan for Mrs PF.

A1 **The pharmaceutical care plan for Mrs PF should include the following:**

(a) Ensure that all her symptoms are defined and managed optimally by considering all sources of the symptoms and choosing drugs appropriate to those sources.

(b) Define possible adverse drug reactions or interactions and plan a monitoring system.

(c) Ensure that Mrs PF can manage the regimen prescribed in her current state of health. Be certain that the dose forms are appropriate and that she can physically and mentally comply with the regimen.

(d) Counsel Mrs PF (and/or her carer) on her regimen and be able to answer any anxieties she may have about the drugs prescribed confidently and honestly.

(e) Monitor any relevant laboratory tests which may be available.

(f) As her regimen evolves, ensure that the drugs prescribed are easily available in the community.

(g) Review her regimen regularly to ensure that all drugs and doses are relevant to her current problems.

(h) Recognise that many uses of medicines in palliative care are unlicensed and consider who will need to be aware of such uses.

What factors are likely to be contributing to Mrs PF's drowsiness?

A2 **Several factors may be contributing. These include her advancing disease, divergence from normal sleep patterns as a result of pain and constipation, and her drug therapy. Prolonged nausea and vomiting prior to admission have probably also made her very tired. Uraemia and hypercalcaemia can also cause drowsiness, but these are not contributory factors in Mrs PF's case.**

It is important to consider all possible causes of symptoms in a patient such as Mrs PF who has terminal malignant disease, as each symptom may have a variety of causes, only some of which may be drug-related. In Mrs PF's case there are two possible iatrogenic causes of her drowsiness:

co-proxamol contains dextropropoxyphene and Diconal contains dipipanone, an opioid, and cyclizine, an antihistamine. Older people are more prone to central nervous system side-effects from drugs and this tendency could have been increased in Mrs PF's case by her underlying malignancy.

Why is Mrs PF vomiting so frequently?

A3 **Intestinal obstruction from her advancing disease, constipation, anxiety and her drug therapy are all possible contributory factors.**

Her original disease has not been actively treated and has continued to grow, and possibly to metastasise, and her bowel may be partially or completely obstructed. There is a well-recognised association between obstruction and nausea and vomiting. In addition to this, she is dehydrated, has been bed-bound for some time and has been taking opiates, which are all contributory causes to constipation. Constipation in advanced cancer can cause nausea with or without vomiting. However, Mrs PF does not have significant hypokalaemia or hypercalcaemia, which are also possible contributory factors to the pathogenesis of vomiting.

Anxiety is a factor which can create or exaggerate many symptoms and if Mrs PF is concerned about her disease, symptoms or her invalid husband then this could be a source of her increasing symptoms. In addition, she has not been sleeping well and insomnia adds to the overall perception of many symptoms.

Furthermore, since her admission to hospital she has been prescribed oral morphine regularly in place of irregular doses of a combined opiate plus anti-emetic (Diconal). The introduction of opiates, or a dose increase, is a common cause of vomiting and may lead to an increase in her symptoms if inadequately treated.

Do you agree with the choice of anti-emetic therapy?

A4 **No. Oral haloperidol 1.5 mg at night, plus oral cyclizine 50 mg as required would be a better choice. The prescription should also allow each drug to be given by an appropriate alternative route if Mrs PF is vomiting.**

It is important to determine the source(s) of vomiting (Answer 3) because this facilitates the selection of the most appropriate treatment.

Drug-induced vomiting, such as that associated with opiates, is mediated through the chemoreceptor trigger zone, which in turn is linked to the vomiting centre. Both sites lie in the floor of the fourth ventricle. Opiate-induced vomiting is not inevitable and is normally short-lived (remitting within a period of three to four days), but when it occurs, or has been known to occur in the past, then haloperidol is often effective in a starting dose of 1.5 mg at night. This dose could be increased if necessary, but with care because of Mrs PF's age (extra-pyramidal side-effects should be monitored for).

Mrs PF's bowel obstruction is another probable cause of her vomiting so an anti-emetic such as cyclizine, which has a direct effect on the vomiting centre, should also be considered. As pro-kinetic anti-emetics such as domperidone or metoclopramide may cause colic in patients with obstruction, these should be avoided. Levomepromazine in a dose of 12.5–25 mg daily is an alternative if the above do not produce an adequate response.

If Mrs PF continues to vomit then the absorption of drugs from the gastrointestinal tract must be considered to be unreliable and alternative routes should be used until such time as her vomiting is adequately controlled. For many patients with intestinal obstruction a realistic goal is to eliminate nausea, but to be prepared for the patient to vomit occasionally. It should also be remembered that many anti-emetics can cause constipation and this must be considered as a cause of prolonged nausea and vomiting.

Finally, if anxiety is an important component of Mrs PF's vomiting and if this cannot be resolved by non-drug means, then a low dose of a benzodiazepine such as diazepam might be effective. Although cumulative drowsiness caused by haloperidol, cyclizine and diazepam may be a problem, it can be controlled by dosage adjustment. Regular review of laboratory tests which give an indication of renal and hepatic function can provide a guide to dosage and help to minimise the risk of adverse reactions.

What might be the cause of Mrs PF's problems and what action would you recommend?

A5 **The most likely cause is a *Candida albicans* infection which should be treated by fluconazole 50 mg daily (as syrup) plus regular mouthcare.**

Oropharyngeal and oesophageal candidiasis are a common consequence of chronic illness which can be made worse by factors such as immunosuppressive drugs, a dry mouth caused by antimuscarinic drugs or dehydration and poor oral hygiene. The soreness and discomfort produced by the infection may further reduce the intake of food and liquid, thus compounding the patient's problems. Treatment with drugs such as nystatin, amphotericin or fluconazole will normally be effective: fluconazole syrup has the added advantage of providing a topical and systemic therapeutic effect.

Additional symptomatic support such as artificial saliva solutions for a dry mouth may be useful, while sucking small pieces of ice or pineapple can help to relieve discomfort by stimulating saliva production. Good oral hygiene will help to maintain improvement. Careful attention should also be paid to factors such as adequate cleaning of dentures or they may become a source of continuing infection.

Was morphine sulphate solution the most appropriate choice for Mrs PF's initial pain control? Is the starting dose appropriate?

A6   **Yes. Her pain was not controlled by co-proxamol (an analgesic for mild to moderate pain), but is at least partially opiate-responsive. The starting dose is appropriate but an 'as required' dose of 10 mg for breakthrough pain could have been added.**

Three-quarters of patients with advanced cancer experience pain and of those one-fifth have one pain, four-fifths have two or more pains and one-third have four or more pains. It is important to establish the sources of a patient's pain in order to choose drugs with the greatest chance of achieving analgesia.

Not all pains are reliably relieved by opiates and neither do all pains require strong opiates immediately – it is often worth trying simple or intermediate analgesics before progressing to morphine. In this case oral morphine is appropriate, but it is important to choose an initial dose carefully. As Mrs PF has only used weak opioids regularly before admission (her Diconal use was intermittent), then 10 mg morphine sulphate (as solution) every four hours is appropriate. Morphine and diamorphine have a duration of analgesia of four hours and it is important to adhere to this regimen wherever possible. Morphine is available in a variety of presentations which allows greater individualisation of drug regimens to improve compliance and so maintain analgesia. Diamorphine is usually reserved for injection, where its greater solubility allows a wide range of doses to be administered in small injection volumes – it is particularly useful for continuous subcutaneous infusions.

When oral morphine is introduced it is important to increase the daily dose regularly until pain relief is obtained or side-effects are encountered. Morphine solution should be administered every four hours regularly and the same dose prescribed 'as required' for breakthrough pain. After one or two days the total daily dose of morphine needed to control the pain should be calculated, and from this the new four-hourly dose and breakthrough dose can be created. If it becomes apparent that morphine is not treating the pain adequately then the prescription should be reviewed.

Continual review of a patient's response to analgesia is essential because pains may increase or diminish, and new or different pains may arise which require separate consideration. When monitoring pain control it is important to always remember that pain is what the patient says hurts.

What should be considered when starting a patient on opiate therapy?

 A7   (a)   **That predictable side-effects should be managed appropriately by prophylactic therapy.**

(b)   **Less predictable side-effects should be monitored for and action taken as appropriate.**

(c)   **The opiate dose should be optimised according to response.**

(d)   **Any concerns expressed by the patient or a carer about taking regular opiate therapy must be addressed.**

The predictable side-effects associated with opiate therapy are drowsiness, nausea, vomiting and constipation, and have already been discussed. Appropriate advice and treatment should be provided and monitored. Although patients may become tolerant to the drowsiness, nausea and vomiting, they will not become tolerant to the constipation and regular laxative therapy will be essential.

The dose of morphine can be titrated according to response by increasing the dose by 25–50% overall in regular increments every 24 hours, with any extra doses that have been necessary on an 'as required' basis during the previous 24-hour period being added into the next day's regimen. About two-thirds of patients never need more than 30 mg morphine every four hours, although much higher doses are sometimes necessary.

Morphine does not cause respiratory depression in patients who have chronic pain, nor does dependence become a problem. Doses of morphine can be reduced if other analgesic procedures such as radiotherapy or nerve blocks prove effective, and can sometimes be stopped altogether and be replaced by simple analgesics. Alternative oral opiates include hydromorphone and oxycodone. These may be considered when side-effects from morphine become intolerable but morphine remains the oral opiate of choice. Hydromorphone and oxycodone each have their own range of adverse effects and the prescriber should be familiar with them before changing a prescription.

What might be the cause of Mrs PF's abdominal masses?

A8   The most likely causes are tumour or constipation.

Colonic tumours tend to spread locally, but unrelieved constipation should also be considered as this may also be a source of her symptoms on presentation.

Was co-danthramer liquid the best choice of laxative?

A9   Mrs PF has a combination of constipation and partial obstruction and co-danthramer may exacerbate some of her symptoms. However, overall, laxative therapy is necessary for her and a small dose of co-danthramer is probably the best choice under the circumstances.

Mrs PF has constipation arising from a number of causes which include dehydration (which is being corrected with intravenous fluid replacement), poor diet and her drug therapy. Mrs PF may also have a history of constipation and she should be asked what her normal bowel habits were prior to her current illness. She had taken co-proxamol before being admitted to hospital and she is now taking regular morphine, which carries an almost inevitable risk of causing constipation. It is also important to appreciate that elderly patients are more prone to opioid side-effects. As Mrs PF has elected not to have her tumour treated and is being treated symptomatically, it is important that she is prescribed laxative therapy.

Laxatives can be broadly divided into bulk-forming agents, stool softeners, stimulants and osmotic laxatives. Where constipation is an established problem, then bulk-forming agents may add to the stool mass and should be avoided. Where stools are capable of being moved, then simple measures such as glycerine suppositories may help, along with simple stimulants such as senna or bisacodyl although if there is proven or suspected obstruction from tumour then stimulant drugs should ideally be avoided. Very often stools need softening before they will move and drugs such as docusate alone (as a softening agent), co-danthramer or co-danthrusate (which contain both stool softeners and stimulants) are appropriate. The latter are particularly useful in opiate-induced constipation. Where stimulant laxatives cause pain and discomfort, then lactulose may be preferable.

Mrs PF did not allow a rectal examination on admission so it was not possible to say whether or not her rectum was loaded with faeces. Had this been the case, or if it was suspected, then a glycerine suppository should have been used. In the event of continuing constipation not responding to changes of laxative or an increase in laxative dose, then a phosphate enema could be suggested to her.

What is the significance of Mrs PF's palpable liver?

A10 **That she may have secondary disease in the liver. Colonic tumours tend to expand locally and to metastasise to the liver.**

Liver capsule pain is often opiate-responsive, but dexamethasone therapy may also be helpful.

Why has the dexamethasone been prescribed for Mrs PF and is the dose appropriate for this indication?

A11 **The dexamethasone has been prescribed primarily to relieve her probable bowel obstruction. The dose is appropriate for this indication.**

Dexamethasone is a corticosteroid which is seven times more potent than prednisolone and this means that a dose of 16 mg dexamethasone is approximately equivalent to 112 mg prednisolone. Corticosteroids are powerful anti-inflammatory drugs and are prescribed to reduce inflammation and oedema around the site of the tumour, which in turn may reduce local pressure and thus pain.

Corticosteroids are also used for the symptomatic relief of a range of other problems, including nerve pains, spinal cord compression, dyspnoea, superior vena cava obstruction, liver capsule stretch and other symptoms with an inflammatory component. The use of dexamethasone as a co-analgesic may help to improve effective analgesia and in doing so reduce opiate requirements. In addition, steroid therapy may improve appetite and general well-being. Several studies have demonstrated a noticeable, if short-lived, improvement in appetite which in turn may help to reduce nausea, pain perception and analgesic consumption. Patients report an improvement in quality of life during dexamethasone treatment, but the use of corticosteroids for prolonged periods must be balanced against the risk of side-effects.

The use of dexamethasone in bowel obstruction is controversial and some authorities believe that its value in these circumstances is unproved. Doses of 16–24 mg/day for five days have been advocated although other centres have used 4 mg twice daily for five days with a maintenance dose of 5 mg daily if improvement is noted. High initial doses of dexamethasone are sometimes required in order to achieve a response. The dose is then gradually reduced to one which maintains symptom control. Dexamethasone is often given in divided doses, although some authorities prefer a single daily dose. Where divided doses are used, then the last dose should be given no later than 6 p.m. to avoid insomnia.

How should the dexamethasone therapy be monitored?

A12 Dexamethasone therapy should be monitored clinically and biochemically.

Regular monitoring of urine (for the presence of glucose), blood pressure (for signs of hypertension) and for signs of oedema is necessary.

Mrs PF should be asked regularly about her mouth as corticosteroids may cause candidiasis. Mental disturbances may also occur. These include euphoria or more florid symptoms such as psychosis and are especially associated with high doses or prolonged treatment. Signs and symptoms of Cushing's syndrome may occur with high doses while corticosteroids have a weak association with peptic ulceration.

Should an H$_2$-receptor antagonist be co-prescribed?

A13 Mrs PF does not need an H$_2$-receptor antagonist at this stage.

The causes of gastrointestinal problems in a patient with terminal cancer can be very varied and range from features of the cancer itself to drugs and other unrelated causes. Mrs PF does not have a history of peptic ulceration and she does not complain of symptoms such as heartburn. Although drug-induced causes of gastrointestinal symptoms are common in advanced cancer where polypharmacy increases the number of potential causative agents, Mrs PF is not taking an NSAID as well as dexamethasone. She is thus in a low risk category and prophylaxis is unnecessary.

Would Mrs PF benefit from the addition of an NSAID to her therapy?

A14 **No, as she has no evidence of bone metastases.**

NSAIDs are widely used for the relief of pain associated with bone metastases and the effectiveness of this group of drugs is believed to derive from their action on blocking prostaglandin synthesis although the evidence for their efficacy is limited. Any potential benefits must also be balanced against the potentially serious side-effects that they can produce. Mrs PF does not have signs or symptoms of metastatic bone pain and colonic cancers do not normally metastasise to bone. NSAID therapy is thus not justified.

Is doubling the dose of co-danthramer the best way of managing Mrs PF's constipation?

A15 **Yes, as an initial step.**

Mrs PF has not opened her bowels since her admission and her constipation is probably contributing significantly to her symptoms. It is essential to review the extent and causes of her constipation regularly, to ensure that therapy is as effective as possible.

Mrs PF is now taking oral opiates regularly and the need for protection against worsening constipation is very important. She has been taking dexamethasone for her presumed obstruction and as she has not experienced colic with her previous dose of co-danthramer, then a cautious increase in dose is appropriate. If she eventually passes hard, dry stools, then consideration should be given to prescribing extra stool softeners, such as docusate.

Would you recommend any changes to Mrs PF's morphine therapy?

A16 **A change to twice-daily slow-release morphine tablets is now appropriate.**

Her pain control has reached a level that provides acceptable analgesia so the opiate component may be changed to slow-release morphine as a more convenient but equally reliable method of opiate administration.

To do this the total daily intake of morphine is calculated and converted to two equal doses of a slow-release preparation. A small extra increase in dose is often included.

Mrs PF has been taking 20 mg of oral morphine every four hours which makes a total of 120 mg/day. She has also taken an extra 20 mg daily on an 'as required' basis to give a daily total of 140 mg. This can be rounded up to 160 mg to give a little extra analgesia and to give a convenient dose of 80 mg twice each day of slow-release morphine tablets. Mrs PF can be reassured that this change in treatment will not affect her pain control and she can also be told that the dose can be increased when necessary. Modified-release dose forms of hydromorphone and oxycodone could be considered as alternatives.

What other analgesics could be considered if Mrs PF develops pain unresponsive to her current therapy?

A17   **A number of agents have value as adjuvant treatments for a variety of pains.**

When a patient continues to experience pain while taking opiates then the causes of pain should be reviewed again. There are some pains that are less responsive to opiates and adjuvant treatment may help to bring such pains under control. A common example would be bone pain, which may respond to NSAIDs although radiotherapy is often preferred.

Pains from nerve-related sources are frequently encountered and patients will often describe them as shooting, stabbing or burning types of pain. Antidepressants, anticonvulsants and corticosteroids can be prescribed in these situations and have varying degrees of success. Gabapentin is licensed for the treatment of neuropathic pain. Flecainide and mexiletine have also been used for some neuropathic pains, while colic may be relieved by hyoscine.

What other factors may affect Mrs PF's pain control and how should they be addressed?

A18   **Fear and anxiety or depression may be affecting her pain control.**

Factors such as fear, anxiety, uncertainty about the future and spiritual crises can all have a profound effect on an individual's perception of pain and on their response to treatment. Mrs PF may be worried about her husband and what will happen to him if she dies. In this situation appropriate professionals simply listening to her anxieties may help to improve the situation, while it may also be possible to suggest some practical solutions.

Where necessary, severe anxiety may be helped by low doses of an anxiolytic such as diazepam and this may be appropriate for Mrs PF. Taking into account her age and concurrent therapy a modest dose of diazepam (e.g. 2 mg twice daily) could be initiated. Alternatively, if depression is diagnosed then active treatment for that should be considered, with the choice of drug and dose being individualised as necessary.

Why does paracetamol work in the presence of morphine?

A19 **Simple analgesia often works for simple symptoms.**

Patients with advanced cancer are as likely to experience minor problems as the rest of the population and symptoms from simple causes, such as an occasional headache, frequently respond to simple therapy.

What factors may affect Mrs PF's compliance with this regimen?

A20 **The main factors are the number of drugs that are frequently required for effective palliative care, together with the physical problems that accompany a terminal illness.**

Good palliative care regimens may eventually require a large number of drugs to treat all of the patient's symptoms. The potential complexity of the treatment may lead to problems in timing for the patient, and confusion about uses and doses. In addition, drug-induced symptoms such as a dry mouth or oral candidiasis can make swallowing solid dose forms difficult. The pharmacist can help by providing detailed counselling, and by helping to simplify and manipulate the regimen to provide the best symptom control. Liquid preparations may help to ease swallowing difficulties, and the use of appropriate compliance aids may help to resolve the organisation of drug administration. Mrs PF was reluctant to take medication before her admission and counselling should focus on helping her to understand the importance of the regular use of her slow-release morphine to maintain her analgesia, and the purpose and value of the other components of her regimen.

If Mrs PF becomes unable to tolerate her therapy orally, what options could be considered?

A21 **Her treatment may be provided rectally, transdermally, by the buccal route or via a syringe pump.**

Some drugs are available for administration by a variety of routes. Although alternative routes of administration may be suitable in some situations, there are also some potential disadvantages. For example, someone with a dry mouth may not be able to absorb a drug effectively by the buccal or sublingual route, while rectal administration may not be practical in someone with rectal disease or diarrhoea.

A continuous subcutaneous syringe driver is a convenient and practical method for administering a range of drugs, including analgesics and anti-emetics. Diamorphine is the analgesic of choice for subcutaneous administration by virtue of its greater solubility and has been subjected to laboratory studies to define its stability in solution, both alone and with a variety of other drugs. When a patient is changed from oral morphine to subcutaneous diamorphine appropriate dosage adjustment is required – guidance on this can be found in the current edition of the *British National Formulary*.

Octreotide is a somatostatin analogue that has been used in palliative care for the relief of diarrhoea and large-volume vomiting. Intestinal obstruction has also been treated with octreotide but its value for this indication is uncertain. It can be administered by subcutaneous infusion or as bolus subcutaneous injections. Octreotide should be used on the advice of a palliative care specialist.

Fentanyl transdermal patches are an alternative method of opiate administration. The patches are changed every 72 hours. The choice of starting dose with transdermal fentanyl depends on whether or not the patient has previously received opioids – when a change is made from oral morphine to fentanyl patches an appropriate dose can be calculated from information provided with the patches. Transdermal fentanyl should not be used for the treatment of acute pain because of the nature of its formulation, and if fentanyl patches are withdrawn for any reason, then the transfer to another form of analgesia must take into account the gradual fall in fentanyl serum concentration.

Further reading

Dickman A, Littlewood C, Varga J. *The Syringe Driver – Continuous Subcutaneous Infusions in Palliative Care*. Oxford University Press, Oxford, 2002.

Doyle D, Hanks GWC, Macdonald N. *Oxford Textbook of Palliative Medicine*, 3rd edn. Oxford University Press, Oxford, 2003.

Twycross RG. *Introducing Palliative Care*, 4th edn. Radcliffe Medical Press, Oxford, 2002.

Twycross RG, Wilcock A. *Symptom Management in Advanced Cancer*, 3rd edn. Radcliffe Medical Press, Oxford, 2001.

Twycross RG, Wilcock A, Charlesworth S *et al. Palliative Care Formulary*, 2nd edn. Radcliffe Medical Press, Oxford, 2002.

23

Human immunodeficiency virus (HIV) disease: opportunistic infections and antiretroviral therapy

Elizabeth Davies

Day 1 Mr IH, a 34-year-old homosexual male, presented to A & E with a 10-day history of increasing shortness of breath. He also complained of a non-productive cough, with fevers and night sweats, but he had had no haemoptysis. His appetite had decreased over the last few days and his weight had fallen from 73 to 64 kg during the last month.

On examination he was pyrexial with a temperature of 39.5°C and tachycardic with a pulse of 125 beats per minute. He was also tachypnoeic with a respiratory rate of 30 breaths per minute. He had poor lung expansion on both sides; however, his breath sounds were clear with no bronchial breathing or crepitations. His blood pressure was 120/80 mmHg. He had white plaques with surrounding areas of inflammation on his tongue suggestive of *Candida albicans* infection. The rest of his examination was unremarkable.

A chest x-ray was requested which showed diffuse bilateral shadowing with no signs of consolidation. Pulse oximetry without supplementary oxygen showed an oxygen saturation (O_2 sat) of 82% at rest.

His arterial blood gases on admission (on 40% oxygen) were:

- PaO_2 7.2 kPa (reference range 11.9–13.2)
- $PaCO_2$ 4.1 kPa (4.8–6.3)
- HCO_3 21 mmol/L (22–30)
- pH 7.42 (7.35–7.45)

From his presentation, a clinical diagnosis of either *Pneumocystis carinii* pneumonia (PCP) or another atypical pneumonia was made. Mr IH was admitted to hospital and nursed in a negative-pressure isolation room until a diagnosis of tuberculosis could be excluded.

Mr IH's serum biochemistry and haematology on admission were:

- Sodium 138 mmol/L (135–144)
- Potassium 3.9 mmol/L (3.1–4.4)
- Calcium 2.2 mmol/L (2.15–2.55)
- Albumin 35 g/L (30–42)
- Urea 4.9 mmol/L (2.2–7.4)
- Creatinine 91 micromol/L (60–115)

His liver function tests were within normal ranges.

- White blood cells (WBC) 2.3 × 10^9/L (4–11 × 10^9)
- Neutrophils 1.5 × 10^9/L (2.0–7.5 × 10^9)
- Lymphocytes 0.7 × 10^9/L (1.5–4.0 × 10^9)
- Monocytes 0.1 × 10^9/L (0.2–0.8 × 10^9)
- Haemoglobin 11 g/dL (13–18)
- Mean cell volume 108 femtolitres (85–95)
- Platelets 238 × 10^9/L (150–400 × 10^9)

Q1 How should Mr IH be treated to cover for PCP and atypical pneumonias?

Q2 Would you recommend the use of steroids to help manage Mr IH's hypoxia?

Day 2 An induced sputum was performed for further respiratory microbiological examination. His arterial blood gases (on 60% oxygen) were:

- PaO$_2$ 11.6 kPa (11.9–13.2)
- PaCO$_2$ 3.28 kPa (4.8–6.3)
- HCO$_3$ 30.3 mmol/L (22–30)
- pH 7.46 (7.35–7.45)
- O$_2$ sat 90% at rest

Mr IH had been started on high-dose intravenous co-trimoxazole and intravenous steroid therapy the previous evening. His current drug therapy was:

- Co-trimoxazole 3840 mg (40 mL) intravenously twice daily
- Methylprednisolone 40 mg intravenously four times daily
- Metoclopramide 10 mg intravenously three times daily (for prevention of co-trimoxazole-induced nausea)
- Fluconazole 100 mg orally once daily
- Erythromycin 500 mg orally four times daily

HIV testing was discussed and after Mr IH had consented, pre-test counselling was arranged with a health advisor. Mr IH was subsequently found to be positive for HIV antibody. A CD4 lymphocyte count was found to be low, at 33/mm^3.

Q3 Is a systemic agent appropriate for treating Mr IH's oral *Candida* infection?

Day 4 Results of the induced sputum confirmed the diagnosis of PCP. Mr IH was now apyrexial with a temperature of 37°C and was feeling better, although he was still short of breath and tired. His nausea was controlled with regular metoclopramide.

Day 7 As Mr IH had improved it was decided on the ward round to change his co-trimoxazole therapy from intravenous to oral administration. His intravenous steroids were changed to oral prednisolone. A dose of 40 mg prednisolone twice daily was prescribed with a reducing regimen to follow, which reduced the dose to zero over the next 10 days.

Q4 What oral dose of co-trimoxazole would you recommend?

Day 9 Mr IH's respiratory symptoms were improving. However, he complained of painless blurred vision, which had worsened over the last few days. Examination revealed retinal haemorrhage with exudates in the right eye characteristic of cytomegalovirus (CMV) retinitis.

Q5 What agents are available for the treatment of CMV infection? What are their advantages and disadvantages?

His haematology, urea and electrolytes were all within normal range. It was decided to commence treatment with intravenous ganciclovir at a dose of 5 mg/kg twice daily.

Q6 What monitoring is necessary throughout treatment with intravenous ganciclovir?

Q7 Would you now consider any adjustment to his PCP treatment, in view of the need to commence ganciclovir?

Day 14 Mr IH was feeling much better. The PCP treatment course was due to be completed and the CMV retinitis was being treated. Mr IH's drug therapy was as follows:

- Clindamycin 600 mg orally four times daily
- Primaquine 30 mg orally once daily

- Prednisolone 40 mg orally once daily
- Metoclopramide 10 mg orally three times daily
- Fluconazole 50 mg orally once daily
- Ganciclovir 320 mg intravenously twice daily

Q8   What PCP prophylaxis would you recommend for Mr IH?

Mr IH was to complete a three-week induction course as treatment of his CMV retinitis, at which point he would then continue on maintenance therapy with oral valganciclovir 900 mg once daily.

In view of his low CD4 count and diagnosis of PCP and CMV retinitis, it was decided that Mr IH ought to commence antiretroviral therapy.

Q9   When should antiretroviral therapy be commenced?
Q10 What antiretroviral options are available for Mr IH? What factors ought to be considered when choosing a regimen?
Q11 Is any other drug therapy required in view of his low CD4 cell count?

Day 23   Mr IH was discharged from hospital following completion of his PCP and CMV treatment.

Q12 Outline a pharmaceutical care plan for Mr IH.

Day 28   Mr IH returned to the out-patient clinic for follow-up and to discuss antiretroviral therapy. He was taking the following medication:

- Co-trimoxazole 960 mg once daily
- Valganciclovir 900 mg once daily
- Azithromycin 1250 mg once weekly

Following discussion Mr IH felt that he required a simple regimen, which he could take once daily if possible.

Q13 Which antiretroviral regimen would you recommend?

It was agreed that Mr IH would commence lamivudine, didanosine and efavirenz taken as a once-daily regimen.

Q14 Which classes of pharmacological agents would you advise Mr IH to avoid whilst on his chosen antiretroviral regimen?

Month 6   Mr IH was now taking the following medication:

- Co-trimoxazole 960 mg once daily
- Valganciclovir 900 mg once daily

- Azithromycin 1250 mg once weekly
- Didanosine 400 mg once daily
- Lamivudine 300 mg once daily
- Efavirenz 600 mg once daily

His CD4 lymphocyte count was 280 cells/mm^3 and his viral load was undetectable (below 50 copies/ml).

Q15 Is it safe for Mr IH to discontinue his prophylactic medication for PCP, CMV and *Mycobacterium avium* complex (MAC)?

How should Mr IH be treated to cover for PCP and atypical
pneumonias?

A1 **Co-trimoxazole at a dose of 120 mg/kg/day intravenously in
two divided doses (usual dose 3840 mg intravenously twice
daily unless under 60 kg) plus a macrolide antibiotic.**

Co-trimoxazole is highly effective for the treatment of HIV-associated
PCP. Treatment should be continued for 14–21 days depending on the
severity of infection. As Mr IH has presented with severe disease, a three-
week course is indicated. Although co-trimoxazole is well absorbed from
the gastrointestinal tract, in severe disease it should initially be administered intravenously, switching to oral therapy as the patient improves.
Local practice often deviates from the administration guidelines recommended by the manufacturers. Practice also varies between hospitals,
although a common regimen is to infuse intravenous co-trimoxazole
3840 mg in 500 mL 5% glucose over a two-hour period. Higher concentrations have been used, e.g. in patients in whom fluid restriction is
necessary. In practice, if large doses are given quickly the patient is at
greater risk of developing nausea and vomiting. Patients receiving high-
dose co-trimoxazole should always be co-prescribed an anti-emetic. An
appropriate choice is intravenous metoclopramide, which is effective at
controlling drug-induced nausea and vomiting through its action on D_2
receptors in the chemoreceptor trigger zone area of the brain. At higher
doses metoclopramide also acts as a 5-hydroxytryptamine $(5\text{-}HT)_3$ receptor antagonist. However, HIV-positive patients appear to be more susceptible to extrapyramidal side-effects of metoclopramide at high doses. If
these occur, domperidone is a suitable alternative, although there is no
intravenous preparation. As Mr IH's HIV status on admission is unknown
it is important to consider other possible causes of his chest infection
such as *Legionella* or *Mycoplasma*. Co-trimoxazole is a suitable choice of
antibiotic for most bacterial chest infections, but the addition of an oral
macrolide antibiotic will cover atypical pneumonias. Once a diagnosis of
PCP is confirmed this can be discontinued. While Mr IH is on high-dose
co-trimoxazole his renal, liver function and full blood count should be
monitored twice each week.

Would you recommend the use of steroids to help manage Mr IH's hypoxia?

A2   **Yes. In patients with moderate to severe PCP and hypoxia there is evidence that by reducing inflammation in the alveoli, gaseous exchange is improved, hypoxia is reduced and the need for mechanical ventilation is prevented.**

Current local practice recommends that patients presenting with a PaO_2 less than 8 kPa should be prescribed steroids, but many centres use a lower PaO_2 threshold. Various regimens have been described (different regimens are used in different treatment centres). One suggested regimen is 40 mg intravenous methylprednisolone four times daily until the PaO_2 is above 10 and there is clinical improvement. This should be followed by a switch to a reducing dose of oral prednisolone starting with 40 mg twice daily for five days then once daily for five days.

There are risks associated with prescribing steroids in patients with HIV infection, particularly if establishing a definitive diagnosis of PCP is difficult. Patients with tuberculosis or disseminated fungal infections may present with clinical and radiological features similar to PCP. For this reason steroids should be tailed off at the earliest opportunity. In addition, a long-term complication of receiving steroids in HIV infection is osteonecrosis. Finally, it should always be ensured that the steroid courses are completed prior to the patient completing the treatment course of co-trimoxazole.

Is a systemic agent appropriate for treating Mr IH's oral *Candida* infection?

A3   **Yes. Patients with early HIV infection can often be managed with topical agents such as nystatin suspension and amphotericin lozenges. However, as they become more immunosuppressed it becomes necessary to use systemic therapy. As Mr IH is acutely unwell and receiving large doses of antibiotics and steroids, it is unlikely that topical treatment will clear his oral *Candida* infection.**

There are three oral azole antifungal agents that can be used for the treatment of oral *Candida*: ketoconazole, fluconazole and itraconazole. Treatment choices will vary between centres. Ketoconazole is currently used to a lesser extent because it is metabolised in the liver via the cytochrome P450 microsomal enzyme system, and therefore has the potential to interact with drugs metabolised via the same route, of which there are many used in HIV infection. Fluconazole is predominantly excreted unchanged in the urine so drug interactions are less common. Itraconazole is another option and is often used in its liquid formulation for oesophageal involvement, although, some centres prefer to reserve the use of itraconazole to treat conditions such as aspergillosis or dermatophyte infections. For uncomplicated oral *Candida* a suitable choice is a single dose of fluconazole 400 mg orally. Therapy should be confined to single doses where possible, and treatment courses should be reserved for more severe infections, to minimise the risk of resistance. Mr IH is on steroids and so the *Candida* infection is likely to persist. For this reason it is reasonable to prescribe fluconazole as a course until the oral steroids have been discontinued. A suitable dose would be 50–100 mg daily.

As all three agents have been associated with hepatotoxicity, baseline and then regular liver function tests should be carried out on patients prescribed azole antifungals.

What oral dose of co-trimoxazole would you recommend?

A4 **Dosage adjustment is not required when changing from intravenous to oral co-trimoxazole. Mr IH's intravenous dose of 3840 mg twice daily can be converted to 4 × 960 mg tablets twice daily or more commonly 2 × 960 mg tablets four times each day.**

Co-trimoxazole is rapidly and well absorbed from the gastrointestinal tract. Patients should be counselled to take the tablets after meals to decrease the probability of gastrointestinal side-effects.

What agents are available for the treatment of CMV infection? What are their advantages and disadvantages?

A5 **There are four agents available for the treatment of CMV retinitis: intravenous ganciclovir, foscarnet, cidofovir and the oral preparation valganciclovir.**

Ganciclovir is a nucleoside analogue closely related in structure and mode of action to aciclovir, but with activity against additional members of the herpes group of viruses, including CMV. The treatment dose is 5 mg/kg intravenously twice daily for three weeks. Its main disadvantage is bone marrow suppression. Foscarnet is a pyrophosphate analogue which inhibits the replication of herpes viruses and some retroviruses, including HIV. The treatment dose is 90 mg/kg intravenously twice daily for three weeks. Its main disadvantages are nephrotoxicity, electrolyte disturbances and the fact that there is no oral preparation available. Cidofovir is a nucleotide analogue which is administered once weekly for two weeks during induction therapy and then once every two weeks as maintenance therapy, each dose being 5 mg/kg. The main advantage of treatment with cidofovir is the convenient dosing schedule. The main drawback is its renal toxicity. Patients must receive concomitant intravenous hydration and oral probenecid, which protects the kidneys by blocking secretion of the drug into the renal tubules. Co-administration of other nephrotoxic drugs is absolutely contra-indicated, which can often lead to treatment problems.

Most centres will use ganciclovir as first choice treatment, reserving cidofovir and foscarnet for patients with bone marrow suppression or those who have relapsed on ganciclovir treatment.

Valganciclovir is an oral prodrug of ganciclovir. It is administered at a dose of 900 mg twice daily as induction treatment and 900 mg once daily as maintenance therapy thereafter. Its main advantage is that is allows treatment as an out-patient, but many ophthalmologists may be hesitant about using this for sight-threatening CMV retinitis as treatment success relies upon patient adherence to therapy. Its main disadvantage is its high cost and it shares all the same toxicities as ganciclovir.

Local therapy is also available in the form of a ganciclovir ocular implant and some patients receive direct intraocular injections of ganciclovir or foscarnet. These options are usually given as adjuvant therapy, as they do not offer any systemic protection if used alone.

Mr IH has no specific contra-indications to any of the above treatment options. Although his WBC count and haemoglobin levels seem low, these are relatively normal for someone with advanced HIV disease and do not contra-indicate the use of ganciclovir/valganciclovir.

What monitoring is necessary throughout treatment with intravenous ganciclovir?

A6 **All patients should have a full blood count and urea and electrolyte monitoring performed twice weekly during induction therapy.**

The major side-effect of ganciclovir is bone marrow suppression. If neutropenia occurs patients may require treatment with colony-stimulating factor, or a switch to alternative therapy. Ganciclovir is excreted renally, and dose adjustment is required with declining renal function. Electrolyte results should be monitored twice weekly and the patient's calculated creatinine clearance should be checked to ensure the dose prescribed is still appropriate.

Would you now consider any adjustment to his PCP treatment in view of the need to commence ganciclovir?

A7   **One option is to switch to clindamycin and primaquine as alternative treatment for his PCP.**

As previously discussed the major toxicity of ganciclovir is bone marrow suppression. Co-trimoxazole can also cause haematological changes, mainly leucopenia, neutropenia, thrombocytopenia and to a lesser extent agranulocytosis. There is a high risk of neutropenia if the two drugs are co-prescribed. Different treatment centres will have different protocols for treatment, but one option is to consider an alternate form of PCP treatment, particularly now that clinical improvement has been made. Second-line treatment for PCP is clindamycin 600 mg orally or intravenously four times daily in combination with primaquine 30 mg orally once daily. The other option is to continue with the co-trimoxazole and monitor for haematological toxicity, and use colony-stimulating factors when necessary.

What PCP prophylaxis would you recommend for Mr IH?

A8   **Oral co-trimoxazole 960 mg once daily or three times each week.**

HIV-positive patients are at risk of PCP infection once their CD4 lymphocyte count falls below 200 cells/mm^3. It is recommended practice to prescribe primary prophylaxis for all patients with CD4 counts below 200 cells/mm^3. Secondary prophylaxis should be given to all patients following an acute episode of PCP. Mr IH should continue with PCP prophylaxis until such time as his immune system function has been restored sufficiently by the use of antiretroviral medication. Co-trimoxazole has been shown in large clinical trials to be the most effective agent for both primary and secondary PCP prophylaxis. A thrice-weekly dosage of 960 mg, usually taken on Monday, Wednesday and Friday, appears to be as effective as 960 mg daily and is accompanied by a lower incidence of side-effects. In addition, co-trimoxazole will offer patients some protection against infection with *Toxoplasma gondii*, a protozoan affecting the brain, as well as some other bacterial infections.

Other agents that can be used for PCP prophylaxis in the presence of co-trimoxazole allergy include dapsone (100 mg daily), nebulised pentamidine isetionate (300 mg every two to four weeks) or atovoquone (750 mg twice daily). Up to 20% of patients develop a skin rash whilst taking co-trimoxazole. These patients can be changed to one of the alternative agents described above or a desensitisation regimen can be tried. This involves minute doses being given initially, increasing gradually over a ten-day period to the therapeutic dose of 960 mg. There is an increased risk of a rash in patients treated with dapsone who have previously had a co-trimoxazole-associated rash.

When should antiretroviral therapy be commenced?

A9 **Antiretrovial therapy should be commenced in all patients with late disease/symptomatic HIV infection who have a CD4 lymphocyte count below 200 cells/mm^3 and in ALL patients who have had an AIDS-defining illness such as PCP. In asymptomatic disease, the decision of when to start treatment is dependent on the CD4 count.**

In symptomatic disease this is because of the high risk of further opportunistic infections, which although treatable may cause irreversible damage or be life-threatening.

In asymptomatic patients the decision of when to start treatment is driven by the CD4 count. A value of 200 cells/mm^3 represents the minimum level at which treatment should be advised. Treatment should be initiated when the CD4 cell count is between 200 and 350 cells/mm^3 and the exact timing should depend upon individual factors such as symptoms, patient preference, likely adherence and potential toxicity. In this range the rate of CD4 decline, viral load and age provide additional information to the CD4 count on the short-term risk of progression.

Mr IH has a diagnosis of PCP and CMV retinitis – both are classified as AIDS-defining diagnoses. He should therefore commence antiretroviral therapy. A decision has to be made as to whether treatment is urgent, in which case it should be instituted as soon as possible, or whether it is better to wait until the acute infections have been treated. Mr IH is severely immunocompromised and therefore there is some urgency to start therapy. It is not known whether the institution of highly active antiretroviral therapy (HAART) during treatment for PCP improves the clinical outcome. However, due to the possible theoretical benefits and the known rapid reductions in viral load and restoration of the immune system that can occur with HAART during the first few weeks of therapy, early initiation of HAART has been attempted. However, there are reports of acute respiratory failure following initiation of HAART soon after treatment for PCP. This is thought to be a manifestation of immune restoration disorder where the immune system reacts in an exaggerated fashion to microbial antigens.

Consideration also needs to be given to the need for adherence to antiretroviral therapy. Adherence is vital for treatment success, therefore it may be more appropriate to allow patients time to recover from their acute episode and adjust to their new HIV diagnosis before treatment is initiated. It also provides time for the pharmacist/doctor/nurse specialist to educate the patient about the medication, side-effects and the importance of complete adherence.

What antiretroviral options are available for Mr IH? What factors ought to be considered when choosing a regimen?

A10 **There are now a range of antiretroviral agents available to choose from. Mr IH needs to commence a combination of three drugs (triple therapy). Factors such as number of tablets, side-effects, resistance patterns, etc., need to be considered before deciding on a regimen.**

HAART is now the standard of care for HIV infected individuals who require treatment in the developed world. HAART is a combination of at least three active drugs.

Currently, recommended standard first-line treatment is two nucleoside reverse transcriptase inhibitors (NRTIs) plus a non-nucleoside reverse transcriptase inhibitor (NNRTI).

Combinations which include a protease inhibitor may also be considered as first-line therapy, although they are used less frequently in this scenario nowadays due to the large pill burden, toxicity and drug–drug interactions.

For patients with very high viral loads there is some evidence that more than three active drugs may result in a more rapid decline in viral load. Studies are in progress to determine whether this will lead to better long-term outcomes than the standard three drug HAART.

The following parameters should be considered for each patient when choosing a regimen, and therapy individualised accordingly:

(a) Potency.
(b) Likelihood of adherence.
(c) Potential toxicity.
(d) Resistance.

(e)   Scope for salvageability (the likelihood that other drugs will remain active following failure of the current drug – many drugs exhibit cross-resistance).

(f)   Co-infection with hepatitis B.

(g)   Drug–drug interactions.

Some patients acquire a drug-resistant virus, so therapy should always be guided by resistance testing.

Is any other drug therapy required in view of his low CD4 cell count?

A11 **Mr IH should be commenced on azithromycin 1250 mg once a week as prophylaxis against MAC.**

Mr IH has a CD4 lymphocyte count of only 33 cells/mm^3. The Centres for Disease Control (CDC) and other guidelines indicate that patients with CD4 cell counts below 50 cells/mm^3 should receive prophylaxis for MAC. Clarithromycin or azithromycin are the preferred prophylactic agents for MAC but if they cannot be tolerated rifabutin is an alternative, although rifabutin-associated drug interactions can make this agent difficult to use. A suitable prophylactic regimen for Mr IH would be azithromycin 1250 mg orally once weekly.

Outline a pharmaceutical care plan for Mr IH

A12 **The pharmaceutical care plan for Mr IH should include the following:**

(a)   Ensure PCP prophylaxis is prescribed in the form of co-trimoxazole 960 mg once daily or three times each week.

(b)   Ensure that the steroid course is reduced to zero prior to discharge, as remaining on steroids after completion of the PCP treatment course is not recommended.

(c)   Ensure the patient is prescribed the correct dose of oral valganciclovir as maintenance treatment for his CMV retinitis following completion of the three weeks treatment with intravenous ganciclovir.

(d)   Ensure that arrangements have been made for the patient to have blood monitoring performed at least every two weeks while he is taking valganciclovir.

(e)   Counsel Mr IH on his discharge medication.

(f)   Issue the patient with some written information regarding antiretroviral therapy, to read prior to returning to the out-patient clinic to commence his HAART regimen.

Which antiretroviral regimen would you recommend?

A13   **Standard first-line treatment in the UK at present is to prescribe two NRTIs plus an NNRTI, e.g. Combivir plus nevirapine or efavirenz. However, Mr IH has expressed a wish for a simple regimen which he can take once daily if at all possible. A combination of didanosine, lamivudine and efavirenz may be taken as a once-daily regimen.**

Didanosine, lamivudine, tenofovir and efavirenz are available as once-daily preparations.

Other drugs are occasionally prescribed once daily outside their product licence when adherence is likely to be an issue and their pharmacokinetics support once-daily dosing.

Since there is concern over the effectiveness of using three NRTIs alone, a suitable regimen would be one which included the NNRTI efavirenz used in combination with two drugs chosen from either didanosine, lamivudine or tenofovir. Current opinion would be to opt for didanosine and lamivudine, as tenofovir is often reserved for treating patients already exposed to several antiretrovirals.

Which classes of pharmacological agents would you advise the patient to avoid whilst on his chosen antiretroviral regimen?

A14   **Mr IH should be advised to avoid medicines capable of inducing liver enzymes, e.g. phenytoin, carbamazepine and St John's Wort, and also the antihistamine terfenadine, due to the risk of cardiac arrhythmias when this is co-prescribed with enzyme inhibitors.**

Efavirenz is primarily metabolised in the liver via the cytochrome P450 microsomal enzyme system. The primary enzyme responsible for its metabolism is CYP4503A4. This enzyme is responsible for the metabolism of many other drugs, and is also subject to potential enzyme induction or inhibition. Enzyme induction would lead to a reduction in plasma efavirenz drug levels, thereby increasing the development of drug resistance and virological failure. Mr IH should be advised to consult a specialist HIV Pharmacist or HIV Physician prior to receiving any prescribed medicines from a GP. Rifampicin is another enzyme inducer which interacts with efavirenz; however, this may be prescribed with careful dose adjustment by a physician specialising in both HIV and tuberculosis.

Efavirenz itself acts as a mixed enzyme inducer/inhibitor. It has been shown to lower plasma methadone levels and induce withdrawal in patients stabilised on methadone maintenance. An increase in the patient's methadone maintenance dose may sometimes be required.

Lamivudine and didanosine are renally excreted and therefore do not exhibit metabolic drug–drug interactions.

Is it safe for Mr IH to discontinue his prophylactic medication for PCP, CMV and MAC?

A15 **It is safe for him to stop his PCP prophylaxis and MAC prophylaxis. His CMV retinitis maintenance therapy may be stopped providing his CMV infection is quiescent.**

PCP prophylaxis may be safely discontinued if the CD4 count is maintained above 200 cells/mm^3 for 3 months. If the CD4 count falls below 200 cells/mm^3, prophylaxis should be recommenced.

The CDC guidelines indicate that patients with CD4 lymphocyte counts less than 50 cells/mm^3 should receive prophylaxis for MAC. Primary prophylaxis can be discontinued with minimal risk of developing MAC in patients who have responded to HAART, with an increase in the CD4 count to greater than 100 cells/mm^3 for at least 3 months. Secondary prophylaxis or maintenance therapy is life-long unless immune reconstitution occurs as a consequence of HAART. There are few firm recommendations on when to discontinue secondary prophylaxis, but patients appear to have a low risk of recurrence if they have completed a course of at least 12 months of MAC treatment, are clinically well and have a sustained increase over three to six months in their CD4 count to more than 100 cells/mm^3 with HAART. Prophylaxis should be reintroduced if the CD4 count decreases to below 100 cells/mm^3 – (although some physicians use a lower cut off of 50 cells/mm^3 for primary prophylaxis).

In CMV retinitis infection a maintenance regimen must be chosen for the patient in order to prevent reactivation of disease and risk of blindness. The maintenance phase for CMV retinitis is indefinite or until an adequate CD4 count rise has been achieved with HAART. Maintenance treatment can often be safely discontinued once the CD4 count has risen above 100 cells/mm^3. As some patients will not receive specific CMV immunity despite an increase in CD4 lymphocyte cells, these patients require regular ophthalmological follow-up. In addition the CD4 count needs to be monitored as patients may relapse if it falls below 50 cells/mm^3. There are no definitive guidelines for when to stop CMV maintenance therapy but local practice is to treat the patient until the CD4 count rises to above 100 cells/mm^3. Therapy is then continued for three months, at which point therapy may be stopped if the CMV is inactive, the CD4 remains above 100 cells/mm^3 and the patient's HIV RNA viral load is undetectable.

Acknowledgements

I would like to acknowledge the help of colleagues at Chelsea & Westminster Hospital, Dr John Morlese MBBS, Dr Mark Nelson MA MBBS FRCP and Barry Jubraj MRPharmS. I would also like to thank Claire Richardson, the previous author of this chapter.

Further reading

BHIVA Writing Committee on behalf of the BHIVA Executive Committee. British HIV Association (BHIVA) Guidelines for the treatment of HIV-infected adults with antiretroviral therapy. *HIV Med* Autumn 2003; also available at www.bhiva.org.

Bartlett J, Gallant J. *2001–2002 Medical Management of HIV Infection.* Johns Hopkins University School of Medicine, Baltimore, MD, 2002.

Currier JS, Williams PL, Koletar SL *et al.* Discontinuation of *mycobacterium avium* complex prophylaxis in patients with antiretroviral induced increases in CD4 cell count: a randomised double blind placebo controlled trial. AIDS Clinical trial group 362 study team. *Ann Intern Med* 2000; **133**: 493–503.

Furrer H. Opportunistic infections: an update. *J HIV Therapy* 2002; **7**: 2–7.

Gazzard B, ed. *AIDS Care Handbook*. Mediscript, London, 2002.

Jabs DA. Discontinuing anticytomegalovirus therapy in patients with cytomegalovirus retinitis and AIDS (Editorial). *Br J Ophthalmol* 2001; **85**: 381–382.

Lopez Bernaldo de Quiros JC, Miro JM, Pena JM *et al.* A randomized trial of the discontinuation of primary and secondary prophylaxis against PCP after highly active antiretroviral therapy in patients with HIV infection. *N Engl J Med* 2001; **344**: 159–167.

24

Type 1 diabetes in childhood

Stephen Tomlin

Case study and questions

Day 1 Miss VT, a six-year-old girl, who lived with her mother and two younger sisters was brought into the A & E by her mum. She weighed 22 kg and had always been a healthy active child. The whole family had had colds and fevers over the last few weeks, but Miss VT was still suffering from flu-like symptoms as well as having some nausea, vomiting and a recurrent stomach ache. Miss VT's mum was concerned because her symptoms were not improving and she appeared to have lost weight over the last few weeks.

On questioning, it became apparent that Miss VT had been drinking large quantities of water and juice over the last couple of months. She had also been wetting the bed on a number of occasions, which her mum had put down to Miss VT not getting on well at school.

Laboratory values for blood taken in A & E were:

- Glucose 22 mmol/L (3.5–10)
- Bicarbonate 11 mmol/L (22–29)
- Blood pH 6.7 (7.35–7.45)
- Ketones 5.5 mmol/L

Her urine also tested positive for ketones (normally 0).

A diagnosis of mild ketosis was made presenting secondary to newly diagnosed Type 1 diabetes.

Q1 Describe the presenting symptoms that lead to a diagnosis of Type 1 diabetes.
Q2 How do these symptoms compare to a classic presentation of the disease? Could there have been a misdiagnosis?
Q3 What are the aims of treatment for Miss VT?
Q4 What initial treatment would you recommend for Miss VT?
Q5 What long-term therapy would you recommend and why?

Miss VT was managed as an in-patient over the next few days and was then started on Humulin M3 insulin (7 units in the morning and 4 units before her evening meal). She was monitored carefully and given a lot of information from members of the multidisciplinary team. After five days she was discharged home, but had daily home visits from the diabetic nurse for the following four days.

Q6   Outline a pharmaceutical care plan for Miss VT.
Q7   How should Miss VT's therapy be monitored at home after discharge?

Week 5   Miss VT was taken to a GP while on holiday complaining of headaches and nightmares. The mother admitted that they had not been checking the blood sugars as often as they were recommended since they had been on holiday and that they had also missed the last hospital appointment. On top of this, Miss VT had probably been running around more than usual on the beach. Her insulin regimen had not altered much over the first few weeks and from her last consultation was still 7 units in the morning and 4 units in the evening of Humulin M3. The mother also had concerns that Miss VT's eating habits had become more erratic, even before the holiday, and was not sure of the consequences of this.

Q8   What do the presenting symptoms tell us about Miss VT's condition?
Q9   Why is it so important to keep a close eye on blood sugar levels in the first few months after starting treatment?
Q10   What treatment changes would you recommend for Miss VT?
Q11   What are the possible options for treating Type 1 diabetes in children with erratic eating habits?

Miss VT was discharged after another long consultation with the consultant paediatrician and diabetic nurse. Her insulin type had not been changed, but the dose had been reduced to 4 units in the morning and 3 units at night.

Over the next few months Miss VT was not a regular attender at clinic and her blood sugar diary was not well filled in; however, she did remain fairly well.

Month 6, day 1   Miss VT was once again brought back to A & E by her mother. She was looking very pale and lethargic. She had been unwell for a few days with diarrhoea and vomiting following a friend's birthday party. Her mother said they had omitted the last couple of doses of insulin as Miss VT had not been eating, but that she had carried on going downhill.

On examination Miss VT was very lethargic, but just about responding. Her eyes looked sunken and her mouth was very dry. There was a distinctive fruity odour on her breath. Her abdomen was very tender and her pulse rate high at 125 beats per minute. She was breathing deeply.

Laboratory results:

- Blood glucose 25 mmol/L (3.5–10)
- Sodium 150 mmol/L (135–147)
- Potassium 5.6 mmol/L (3.5–5.0)
- Chloride 110 mmol/L (95–105)
- Bicarbonate 5mmol/L (22–29)

- Creatinine 180 micromol/L (80–120)
- Urine 2% glucose and ketones (normal for both is 0)
- Weight 20 kg (last recorded weight was 23 kg a month ago)

Miss VT's therapy had not varied greatly over the last few months, and her last regimen had still been using Humulin M3 at a dose of 4 units in the morning and 3 units at night.

Q12 What is the clinical diagnosis for Miss VT?
Q13 Why might this have occurred?
Q14 What are the aims of treatment now?
Q15 What treatment would you recommend for Miss VT?

Day 2   After 36 hours Miss VT was able to tolerate oral feeds.

Day 3   Her fluid balance and electrolytes were finally completely corrected. She was given the first dose of her usual subcutaneous insulin just before her insulin infusion was turned off.

Because of the recent problems and a real loss of confidence in the treatment regimen on the part of Miss VT and her mother, a thorough review was conducted by the consultant and specialist nurse. The options were discussed with Miss VT and her mother, including the use of insulin glargine, lispro and insulin pumps. However, it was decided that Miss VT would be better off at this time carrying on with the twice-daily biphasic insulin with regular support from the diabetic nurse.

Q16 Discuss the advantages and disadvantages associated with the alternative methods and types of insulin. Why it is likely that the current regimen was finally decided upon?
Q17 How should Miss VT's mother be advised to manage minor illness in the future?
Q18 How should Miss VT's specialist consultant and GP monitor her long-term therapy?

Describe the presenting symptoms that lead to a diagnosis of Type 1 diabetes.

A1 **Abdominal pain, weight loss, enuresis, thirst, elevated blood glucose, and ketones and glucose in the urine.**

The onset of Type 1 diabetes is often preceded by an acute viral illness which can cause an autoimmune destructive response in the pancreas leading to impaired insulin production.

Abdominal symptoms are often seen as the presenting symptoms of diabetic ketoacidosis, which is still fairly mild in Miss VT's case. The ketoacidosis is due to an excessive mobilisation of free fatty acids to the liver where they are metabolised to ketones. This process is activated by low insulin levels.

The weight loss will be the product of several of the presenting symptoms. When glucose levels reach the renal threshold, glucose spills into the urine taking water with it by the process of osmotic diuresis. The loss of calories in water in this way leads to polyuria, enuresis, thirst, weight loss and fatigue. In addition, there will also be weight loss due to the ongoing viral illness decreasing Miss VT's wish to eat.

How do these symptoms compare to a classic presentation of the disease. Could there have been a misdiagnosis?

A2 **Miss VT's symptoms are classic, but in children such symptoms may initially be associated with urinary tract infection, failure to thrive, gastroenteritis or psychological problems.**

Miss VT's symptoms are typical of Type 1 diabetes, with a relatively acute onset of symptoms at a young age following a traumatic life event (e.g. viral illness). Unlike Type 2 diabetes, there is rarely an association with a family history of diabetes and the patient is rarely obese.

It is uncommon for infants (under one year of age) to get diabetes, but the incidence increases with age with particular peaks between four and six years, and the largest peak in early adolescence.

Polyuria and bed wetting in children are often linked to urinary tract infection and this diagnosis is further supported by the presence of abdominal pain. Because of the gastrointestinal upset caused by the presenting ketoacidosis there is often weight loss due to lack of eating, vomiting and also the higher urine output. This in turn leads to fatigue and irritability. Consequently there are often problems at school which may be picked up by the parents or teachers; but these problems at school are then often blamed for the bed-wetting and emotional instability, thus leading to an initial misdiagnosis.

Miss VT's height and weight have been normal for her age and the sequence of events alongside the laboratory results have led to the correct diagnosis.

What are the aims of treatment for Miss VT?

A3   **To obtain optimal glucose control, prevent diabetic complications (chronic and acute), and to achieve normal growth and development.**

Miss VT had normal growth velocity before the onset of illness; however, any acute or chronic illness in a child can have a dramatic long-term influence on height and weight. They can thus be used as markers for the overall well-being of Miss VT as she grows up. The weight loss that Miss VT has already experienced should be corrected easily and quickly now that the diagnosis has been made. Her height and weight should be plotted at regular clinic appointments on a standard growth chart, so that progress can be monitored.

The Diabetes Control and Complications Trial Group demonstrated that tight blood glucose control decreased the incidence of complications, both in terms of microvascular (retinopathy and renal failure) and macrovascular (stroke, angina, myocardial infarction) complications. In older children and adults it is recommended that intensive control of blood sugar is adhered to, in order to reduce the long-term sequelae of diabetes. The same principal applies to younger children, but greater care must be taken in the implementation of this. Over-zealous control could lead to hypoglycaemias and these must be avoided in children under the age of eight years as brain development may be impaired.

Glucose control can be assessed by measuring glycated haemoglobin. The HbA_{1c} fraction is commonly measured. It comprises the majority of glycated haemoglobin and is the least affected by recent fluctuations in sugar levels. It measures the percentage of haemoglobin A that has been irreversibly glycated and its value is determined by the plasma glucose levels and the life span of a red blood cell (about 120 days). It can thus be said that HbA_{1c} is an indicator of glycaemic control over the preceding two to three months.

Glycated haemoglobin is thus normally monitored on a 3-monthly basis to give a longer-term view of blood sugar control. It is carried out on a finger-prick of blood. It has been shown that lowering the HbA_{1c} can delay or stop the development of long-term complications. A normal HbA_{1c} is 4–6.5%; levels greater than 8.5% are seriously elevated. The target HbA_{1c} for a child such as Miss VT would be 4–7.5% but children will often have an HbA_{1c} of 8–10%. Children's blood sugars are notoriously hard to control due to their varied life styles and lack of compliance. It is important to encourage tight glucose control and praise when progress is being made rather than condemn for being outside a specified range.

What initial treatment would you recommend for Miss VT?

A4   **As Miss VT has significant signs of ketoacidosis she should probably be started on a sliding-scale insulin regimen for about 24 hours, in order to get her condition under control.**

The sliding-scale insulin method is probably still the most common initial treatment of newly diagnosed patients. The amount of insulin given over the first 24 hours is no longer used as a predictor of the insulin requirements of the patient; however, it is a safe way to gain initial control of hyperglycaemic symptoms.

A sliding scale works as follows. An intravenous infusion is set up of soluble insulin (Human Actrapid) 50 units made up to 50 mL with sodium chloride 0.9% in a syringe pump (i.e. 1 mL = 1 unit insulin). The giving-set is flushed with insulin solution before it is connected to the child, in order to saturate the plastic's absorption of insulin.

The blood glucose level should be measured as soon as the insulin is started and the infusion rate adjusted according to the table below in order to keep the blood glucose between 4 and 11 mmol/L. Blood glucose levels should be measured every hour for the first four hours and then reduced to every two hours until stable. Once Miss VT is stable, her ongoing insulin needs must be met.

Blood Glucose (mmol/L)	Insulin Infusion (units/kg/h)
0–5	0
6–10	0.05
11–15	0.1
16–20	0.15
>20	0.2

What long-term therapy would you recommend and why?

A5 **She should start on a twice-daily subcutaneous insulin regimen using a biphasic insulin mix via a pre-loaded pen. The dose should be based on 0.5 units/kg/day, with two-thirds given in the morning before breakfast and one-third given before the evening meal.**

Severe insulin deficiency in combination with the physical and psychological changes that accompany normal development through childhood make the management of Type 1 diabetes particularly difficult.

Since it is more important to prevent hypoglycaemia (which is potentially life-threatening) than hyperglycaemia, initial treatment should be cautious.

Initial insulin dosing in this age group will usually start at 0.25 units/kg/day but will be higher if there are signs that ketoacidosis has been present for a while. Dosing of greater than 0.9 units/kg of insulin per day are rarely required in pre-pubertal children, but the dose may increase up to 1.8 units/kg/day during puberty due to the increased growth hormone release at this time leading to decreased insulin sensitivity.

As Miss VT has shown signs of ketosis for some days she should be started on a dose of 0.5 units/kg/day with two-thirds of the dose being given in the morning before breakfast and one-third before the evening meal. A variety of insulins are available for long-term treatment and their characteristics are summarised on page 470.

The mixed preparations of insulin (biphasic) give a high initial peak and then a sustained level throughout the day when used twice daily. This is a good combination for children of school age as they have limited support during lunchtime. These combinations have the advantage of providing peaks of insulin around main meal times (breakfast and evening meal), as well as continual lower levels throughout the day without the user having to draw up two different insulins. It is normal to start with the 70:30 ratio, e.g. Humulin M3 (70% isophane and 30% regular) and to make any necessary changes thereafter.

Miss VT could start by using a pen device giving 7 units in the morning and 4 units each evening (0.5 units/kg/day). These mixes may cause hypoglycaemic times in young children due to the short-acting insulin peaks, so one or both of the doses may have to be swapped for an intermediate-acting insulin on its own, or to a different ratio of biphasic insulin. If Miss VT shows signs of hypoglycaemia after a meal, the proportion of short-acting insulin is obviously too large and a different ratio biphasic could be tried, such as 80:20 (e.g. Humulin M2).

Insulin type	Example brand name	Properties
Ultra short-acting	Humalog, NovoRapid	Lasts 2–5 h; acts fast enough to be given immediately prior to meals
Short-acting (soluble)	Humulin S, Actrapid	Peak action 2–6 h post-injection so dose needed 30 min prior to food; lasts up to 8 h
Intermediate-acting	Humulin I, Humulin Lente, Humulin Zn, Monotard, Insulatard, Ultratard	Peak action 4–12 h; lasts 8–14 h
Long-acting	Lantus	Lasts for 24 h
Biphasic	Humulin M2, M3, M5; Humalog Mix25, Mix50; Mixtard 10,20,30,40,50	Combinations of short- and intermediate-acting insulin; number represents the short-acting component; Humalog uses the insulin short-acting lispro

Once children have lost their baby fat, subcutaneous injections are not as easy to give and care must be taken when choosing an injection site. During this period the abdomen may be a difficult site to use, so injections should be rotated between the thighs and upper buttock area. Insulin pens have different size needles so that the insulin is delivered directly into the subcutaneous tissue. The specialist nurse will assess a patient for the correct needle size.

Outline a pharmaceutical care plan for Miss VT.

A6   The pharmacist should contribute to the overall care and management of Miss VT by providing information to her and to her family specifically about storage, administration and monitoring of insulin therapy. It is also essential that the pharmacist reinforce information on all relevant aspects of diabetic care given by other health care professionals.

The care plan for an individual with Type 1 diabetes must be individualised as the treatment will affect their whole life plan. The key players will be the consultant who will perform the formal clinical assessments of the child, initially on a monthly basis; the specialist nurse who will have regular contact with the family; and the dietitian, who will be involved initially to advise on diet and then intermittently, depending on Miss VT's progress.

The key information Miss VT and her carers need include:

(a) Education on how to use an insulin pen device (the easiest initial method of administration). This includes checking the insulin expiry date; using a different needle each time; how to insert, hold and then remove the needle. It is also important that the family know how to use a syringe in case the pen is lost or damaged.

(b) The need to rotate injection sites (usually the abdomen, buttocks and thighs) as injecting into the same site can cause lumps to form which will affect insulin uptake in the long-term. Rotation guides are available if these are deemed necessary.

(c) How to dispose of needles safely.

(d) The need to keep spare insulin cartridges in the fridge. Opened insulin can be stored for one month out of the fridge.

(e) How to take blood glucose levels and, hopefully, keep them at 4–8 mmol/L. A single blood drop from the side of a finger (not thumb) is usually put onto a test strip. It is important that blood level diaries are kept so that trends can be seen.

(f) How to assess for hyper- and hypoglycaemia and to treat them. It is essential that this aspect of care is understood by all carers of the child, e.g. teachers. If a child has symptoms of hypoglycaemia they should take some sugar or a sugary drink straightaway followed by a sandwich or biscuit. If they are unable to swallow, Hypostop can be used (a sugary gel that can be rubbed into the lips or gums). If these measures do not work, glucagon injections may be given by the carer if they are deemed to have a good level of understanding of their use. Otherwise the patient and carer should be advised to go to a doctor. It is important that Miss VT and her family always carry sugar or sweet food with them.

(g) Normal dietary advice includes:

   (i)   Avoiding fatty foods.
   (ii) Eating mainly vegetables, fruit, cereal, rice and pasta.
   (iii) Eating only small amounts of refined sugar (jam, sweets etc.).
   (iv) Eating at regular intervals.
   (v)   Carrying glucose tablets or sweets in case of hypoglycaemia.

(h) Information on what to do when the child is ill.

(i) Useful contact numbers.

How should Miss VT's therapy be monitored at home after discharge?

A7 **Initial monitoring should involve blood glucose monitoring before each meal and at bedtime. This level of monitoring can usually be reduced over time.**

Immediately following diagnosis, monitoring is essential before each meal along with a final daily check prior to going to bed. Once glycaemic control is stable and appropriate then monitoring can drop to two to three times a week, with three or four tests on each of those days prior to meals, or to twice daily each day to help compliance. Monitoring should be increased during acute illness and at times of changed life style.

Blood samples are usually taken from finger-pricks, although in younger children heel-pricks and earlobes may provide an alternative site.

Blood glucose monitoring must be tailored to an individual's life circumstances and this is particularly important with children going to school. Enforcing a regimen that is not what the child wants when they are at school (this will vary with age) is likely to produce a child who carries out no monitoring at all. Ideally, blood glucose levels should be maintained at 4–8 mmol/L

Parents should be taught to monitor as often as possible and to respond to altering glucose concentrations. If glucose levels are high, they may be taught to give additional insulin on top of the normal requirements. This will normally involve doses of short-acting insulin in doses of about 0.1 units/kg. These doses should not be given more frequently than four-hourly to avoid hypoglycaemia. If this additional requirement is recurrent, then changes in dose will be recommended. In reality most additional insulin dose adjustments are made by the diabetic nurse and not taken on fully by the carer. Dose adjustments of the biphasic insulin, whether up or down, are usually made in increments of 10–20% of the original dose.

Children are usually monitored, either within a clinic or at home through visits by a specialist diabetic nurse on a regular basis, varying initially from daily to weekly. They will be given dietary advice on avoiding high glucose-containing foods and drinks. They are encouraged to fill in glucose diaries so that trends can be seen in blood glucose patterns.

What do the presenting symptoms tell us about Miss VT's condition?

A8 **That Miss VT is being over-treated with insulin and is suffering from hypoglycaemia.**

Nightmares, as in the case of Miss VT, poor sleep and crying are all potential signs of hypoglycaemia. Hypoglycaemia is a very serious and life-threatening consequence of diabetic treatment. It is particularly hard to spot in children and is more likely to occur due to their very varied activity levels throughout a day. Nocturnal hypoglycaemia has also been observed more frequently in children than adults and, perhaps more worrying, it is often asymptomatic.

> Why is it so important to keep a close eye on blood sugar levels in the first few months after starting treatment?

A9 **A lot of patients have a 'honeymoon' period for the first few months after starting treatment, with their insulin requirements dropping off dramatically.**

Apart from the lack of sugar monitoring that Miss VT has been receiving and the increased exercise burning off more sugar, she is at increased risk in the first few months post-diagnosis of having lower insulin requirements.

Around a quarter of all patients who get Type 1 diabetes develop what is known as a 'honeymoon' period within days or weeks of the onset of treatment. It is as if the patient has gone into remission and it can be confusing for the patient/carer as it would appear that the condition has corrected itself. Some patients actually require no insulin during this phase and this may last for weeks or months. It is usually best to keep treating with insulin even if the requirements are negligible, to avoid possible insulin allergy upon re-exposure and also to maintain a treatment regimen and not give false hope to the patient.

> What treatment changes would you recommend for Miss VT?

A10 **Miss VT now needs increased monitoring and probably a reduction in insulin dose, especially in the evening.**

The nightmares indicate that the hypoglycaemia is occurring at night, but increased daily monitoring should be encouraged to rule out an overall 'honeymoon' period. Both bedtime and early morning blood glucose monitoring should be carried out. It is important to have a good picture of what is happening to ensure the best changes to treatment. If a biphasic insulin is being given before the evening meal the overall dose may be too large, or perhaps the soluble insulin component needs altering. The most common treatment change to avoid nocturnal hypo-glycaemia is to use a different ratio of biphasic insulin, such as 80:20 (e.g. Humulin M2) thus decreasing the amount of fast-acting insulin. The use of biphasic insulin containing a very fast-acting phase such as Humalog

Mix25 could also be considered, as the action of the lispro insulin is short-lived. Alternatively, control may be almost correct and the only intervention needed is to give a small snack just prior to going to bed to keep the blood sugar up.

What are the possible options for treating Type 1 diabetes in children with erratic eating habits?

A11 **The answer to this is very patient-specific, but may involve giving short-acting insulin more frequently (three times daily) and an intermediate-acting insulin before bed.**

Set regimen and combination (biphasic) insulins are the most convenient form of insulin to administer providing that the person's life style and eating habits do not fluctuate greatly. Children are renowned for eating erratically, and for the quantity and content of what they eat having little to do with their daily routine (or lack of it).

Using the same total daily insulin dose, the soluble insulin may be given before the three main meals of the day (breakfast, lunch and dinner), then a fourth dose of intermediate insulin is given prior to going to bed.

Another option could be to use insulin lispro as the short-acting insulin in the regimen above. It is a fast-acting insulin (onset in about 15 minutes, peaking at one hour) with short duration (about five hours). It can solve some of these problems as it can be used when necessary and will even be effective if it is given directly after a meal, instead of before.

In reality, erratic eating habits often go hand in hand with poor compliance and education is the main support of treatment (see Answer 15).

What is the clinical diagnosis for Miss VT?

A12 **Miss VT has acute, life-threatening diabetic ketoacidosis**

As in the initial diagnosis, Miss VT has signs of ketoacidosis. However, this time the signs and symptoms, as well as the laboratory results, show that it is serious and potentially life-threatening.

Miss VT has presented with a high blood glucose level, which in turn has led to an increase in plasma osmolarity. Osmotic diuresis has then set in with loss of fluid and electrolytes. Dehydration can be rapid, causing changes in skin texture, sunken eyeballs and eventually loss of consciousness. Excessive ketone production causes a distinctive fruity odour on the breath. High levels of ketones also cause a fall in pH since they are organic acids. Hypercapnia then results, due to the respiratory rate increasing to try to compensate for the metabolic acidosis.

Why might this have occurred?

A13 **Misinterpretation of her symptoms, leading to non-administration of insulin.**

Miss VT was vomiting after the party. It could be assumed that she had gastroenteritis, and thus was not eating and therefore would not be needing any insulin. In reality, the nausea and vomiting were probably the first signs of ketoacidosis due to a large glucose intake at the party. Non-administration of the insulin doses has only made the situation worse, and has caused a critical ketoacidosis to develop.

What are the aims of treatment now?

A14 **The main aims of treatment for Miss VT are to correct her dehydration and the hyperglycaemia.**

What treatment would you recommend for Miss VT?

A15 **Fluid correction is vital and must be initiated immediately. This must be done cautiously, while bringing the blood sugars back under control.**

Children who are greater than 5% dehydrated and/or drowsy will almost certainly require urgent intravenous fluids with electrolyte correction; however this must be done with caution to avoid cerebral oedema and hypokalaemia, which are the leading causes of death in such cases.

Miss VT is 3 kg lighter than she was a month ago and has therefore lost greater than 10% of her body weight through dehydration (weight loss should be based, as near as possible, on her current weight against her weight before dehydration started). This is severe dehydration with 1 kg of weight loss equating to 1 L of fluid loss. Treatment will be as if the dehydration is 10%, as using figures greater than this can lead to more complications and assessment can never be regarded as totally accurate. In cases of greater than 10% dehydration with shock, or in the young, it would be normal practice to treat the patient on a paediatric intensive care unit.

Children who are in shock due to the severity of the ketoacidosis (tachycardia, poor capillary refill time and hypotension) should initially be given 10 mL/kg of sodium chloride 0.9%. Miss VT has some of these symptoms and this should be the first treatment that she receives.

After this initial fluid a continuous rehydration infusion should be set up alongside an insulin infusion.

The rehydration regimen should be calculated as follows:

24 h correction = maintenance fluid + deficit + any continuing
losses (vomiting)

Maintenance = 0–2 years   80 mL/kg/24 h
          3–5 years   70 mL/kg/24 h
          6–9 years   60 mL/kg/24 h
          10–14 years   50 mL/kg/24 h
          >15 years   35 mL/kg/24 h

Deficit (ml) = % dehydration × body weight (kg) × 1000

For Miss VT:

Maintenance = 60 mL × 23 kg = 1380 mL
Deficit = 10/100 × 23 × 1000 = 2300 mL

Thus, 24 hour correction for Miss VT = 1380 mL + 2300 mL = 3680 mL, i.e. 3680 mL needs to be run over the next 24 hours. Providing she is not anuric (which she is not), this fluid should be sodium chloride 0.9% with 20 mmol of potassium in each 500 mL bag.

An electrocardiogram monitor should be set up and her potassium levels should be checked every two to four hours throughout the first 24 hours. Levels should be corrected to keep them between 4 and 5 mmol/L.

The insulin regimen should be as follows. A continuous infusion of soluble insulin (Actrapid) should be set up. The insulin should be diluted to 1 unit/mL in a syringe using sodium chloride 0.9%. The infusion should be started at 0.1 units/kg/h. If the rate of fall of glucose level is greater than 5 mmol/h, then the rate of the infusion should be halved. Rates of fall greater than 5 mmol/h can lead to large osmolarity changes and this can in turn lead to cerebral oedema. When the blood glucose is 12 mmol/L the insulin infusion should be reduced and the fluid changed to glucose 5% + sodium chloride 0.45% with or without potassium, still running at the same rate.

Blood glucose levels should be held between 10 and 11 mmol/L. If levels start to dip below 7 mmol/L the glucose input should be increased. The insulin should not be stopped as insulin is required to switch off ketone production.

Acidosis is usually self-limiting; however, profound acidosis with a pH below 7 with shock and circulatory failure will require sodium bicarbonate infusion to reverse the acidosis slowly. This should be a very rare requirement if rehydration has been managed appropriately.

> Discuss the advantages and disadvantages associated with the alternative methods and types of insulin. Why it is likely that the current regimen was finally decided upon?

A16 **The use of alternative methods do have their advantages, but they are generally felt to be best suited to patients with a thorough understanding of their disease state and high level of motivation. This is not the case for Miss VT and her family, so continuing with the current regimen is the best option for her.**

Insulin glargine is a new long-acting insulin analogue. It is designed to have a flat release profile to mimic natural insulin release and has a longer duration of action than isophane insulin. A lower incidence of nocturnal hypoglycaemia has been demonstrated in some trials, although early morning hypoglycaemia may occur. There are some data in paediatrics, but at the time of writing there is no paediatric UK licence. Short-acting insulins still need to be administered before meal times, and thus the number of injections daily is likely to be four or five, making it less convenient for patients with poor compliance.

Insulin pumps are available and being reviewed for their place in therapy. They provide an alternative to multiple injections. The insulin pump is a battery-operated pump with a computer that programs the pump to deliver predetermined amounts of soluble insulin from a chamber into a subcutaneously implanted catheter. They can deliver constant flow as well as be activated for boluses by the operator 30 minutes before meals. Lispro insulin is also now being combined with the pumps so that shots of insulin can be given whenever a meal is eaten rather than the user having to pre-plan and inject 30 minutes before meals. This type of device is likely to increase in favour as it can mimic normal insulin flow reasonably well; however, users must be highly motivated to use the device efficiently and not all children take kindly to having a pump attached to them. This may well be a suitable device in the future for Miss VT.

Miss VT and her family are typical in terms of concordance with treatment of Type 1 diabetes. The best way to improve treatment is to encourage compliance continuously and get concordance with their treatment and social setting.

How should Miss VT's mother be advised to manage minor illness in the future?

A17   **Miss VT's mother should be advised never to stop giving insulin to her daughter even if she is unwell and not eating.**

Even when she is unwell and not eating, Miss VT's body is still producing glucose from its stores. If the insulin is stopped, then Miss VT could become hyperglycaemic and seriously ill. The dose of insulin may need to be adjusted during periods of illness and thus careful monitoring of the patient is essential. Blood sugars usually rise during illness, especially if fever is involved and thus increases in insulin may be necessary. This increase in insulin requirements is usually short-lived and decreases will need to be made as soon as levels start dropping again. Increased requirements are usually only in the region of 10–20% of the original dose.

Hyperglycaemia is more common if dehydration occurs and this is common during episodes of fever. Therefore good fluid intake should be encouraged throughout the day.

If solid foods are not being taken then alternatives such as milk, fruit juice, soup, ice cream and fizzy drinks will help maintain the carbohydrate allowance thus avoiding hypoglycaemia.

During illness her urine should be monitored for sugar and ketones. The presence of both of these substances in the urine will indicate a lack of insulin. If there is no sugar and only ketones then there is an indication of a lack of food intake, especially carbohydrates.

Miss VT's mother should be advised to contact the health care team for advice during periods of illness.

How should Miss VT's specialist consultant and GP monitor her long-term therapy?

A18   **Alongside the blood glucose and HbA$_{1c}$ monitoring there are a number of other parameters which should be monitored regularly. These include growth and development, injection-site checks, and retinal field checks.**

Growth and development must be plotted regularly at this age on a standard growth chart.

It is important that the injection sites are checked to ensure that the sites are being rotated. If sites are used over and over again they may become red and lumpy, a condition called lipodystrophy. Insulin injected into these sites may not work properly, due to poor absorption.

Due to the long-term risk of retinal damage, eye checks should be performed not only at initial diagnosis, but also on a yearly basis thereafter. This practice usually only starts once the child is 12 years old, but many clinicians will do random eye checks before this time, especially if diagnosis is at a very early age.

Further reading

Anon. When and how should patients with diabetes test blood glucose? *MeReC Bull* 2002; **13**(1).

Diabetes Control and Complications Trial Research Group. The effect of intensive diabetes treatment on the development and progression of long-term complications in adolescents with insulin-dependent diabetes mellitus. *J Pediatr* 1994; **125**: 177–188.

Koda-Kimble MA, Young LY, Kradjan WA *et al.*, eds. *Applied Therapeutics: The Clinical Use of Drugs*, 7th edn. Lippincott Williams & Wilkins, Philadelphia, PA, 2001.

Rudolph CD, Rudolph AM, eds. *Rudolph's Pediatrics*, 21st edn. McGraw-Hill, New York, 2001.

Schober E, Schoente E, Van Dyk J *et al.* Comparative trial between insulin glargine and NPH insulin in children and adolescents with type 1 diabetes mellitus. *Pediatr Endocrinol Metab* 2002; **15**: 369–376.

Scottish Study Group for the Care of the Young Diabetic. Factors influencing glycaemic control in young people with Type 1 diabetes in Scotland. *Diabetes Care* 2001; **24**: 239–244.

Sperling MA. Continuous subcutaneous insulin infusion and continuous subcutaneous glucose monitoring in children with Type 1 diabetes mellitus: boon or bane? *Paediatr Diabetes* 2001; **2**: 49–50.

Tamborlane WV, Bonfig W, Bowland E. Recent advances in treatment of youth with Type 1 diabetes: better care through technology. *Diabetic Med* 2001; **18**: 864–870.

Thompson R, Hindmarsh P. Management of Type 1 diabetes in children. *Prescriber* 2002; 19 April: 77–85.

Tupola S, Komulainen J, Jääskeläinen J *et al.* Post-prandial insulin vs. human regular insulin in prepubertal children with Type 1 diabetes mellitus. *Diabetic Med* 2001; **18**: 654–658.

25

Type 2 diabetes mellitus

Judith A Cantrill and Jayne Wood

Case study and questions

Day 1 Mrs PK, a 68-year-old housewife, was seen in the chiropody department. She had had a poorly healing ulcer on the plantar aspect of her left foot for three weeks. This had been cleaned and dressed daily by the district nurse. On examination, the area around the ulcer was found to be red, inflamed and tender. The foot was swollen. She had been feeling generally unwell and lethargic for several months, but worse in the last week. The lesion on her left foot had been painful for some time. She described the pain as 'burning'.

Mrs PK had been diagnosed as having Type 2 diabetes three years earlier. At the time of diagnosis she was found to be hypertensive. Her only other complaints were of occasional ankle swelling and shortness of breath on exertion.

Her current drug therapy was:

- Gliclazide 80 mg orally twice a day
- Bendroflumethiazide 2.5 mg orally in the morning
- Atenolol 50 mg orally in the morning
- Co-proxamol one or two orally as required

She lived with her husband, smoked 20 cigarettes a day and drank approximately 15 units of alcohol a week.

The chiropodist asked for the opinion of the diabetologist, who arranged for her admission the following day.

Day 2 Mrs PK was admitted to hospital. On examination she was found to be pyrexial (temperature 38°C) and unwell. Her blood pressure was elevated (180/100 mmHg) and she was obese (weight 92 kg).

Her left foot was extremely swollen and very tender. The ulcer was approximately 3 cm wide and 1.5 cm deep and filled with pus. She had no pinprick sensation over either foot, and absent reflexes at both knees and ankles. She had background retinopathy and microaneurysms in her right eye. She was also noted to have mild ankle oedema and some basal crepitations in both lungs.

Blood cultures and swabs of the ulcer site were sent to the micro-biology department for culture and sensitivity, and an x-ray of her left foot was requested.

Her serum biochemistry and haematology results were:

- Sodium 135 mmol/L (reference range 135–145)
- Potassium 4.2 mmol/L (3.5–5.0)
- Urea 22.7 mmol/L (2.5–7.5)
- Creatinine 180 micromol/L (60–120)
- Random blood glucose 22 mmol/L (3.5–10.0)
- White blood cells (WBC) 15.6×10^9/L (4–11×10^9)
- Total serum cholesterol 5.5 mmol/L (below 5 mmol/L)

Urine testing on the ward showed moderate amounts of protein and glucose, but no ketones.

Q1   What are the overall therapeutic aims for Mrs PK?

Q2   What would be an appropriate choice of antibiotic(s) for Mrs PK and by what route should it (they) be administered?

Q3   What factors might have contributed to the development of Mrs PK's ulcer?

Q4   How should Mrs PK's ulcer be cleansed and dressed?

Q5   What other therapy may aid wound healing?

Q6   Why is insulin therapy indicated for Mrs PK?

Q7   How should the insulin be administered and monitored?

Q8   How should her neuropathic pain be managed?

Day 5   Mrs PK was apyrexial, and her foot was much less swollen and inflamed. Her blood glucose was well controlled on insulin and ketones were absent from her urine. The x-ray of her foot showed no evidence of osteomyelitis.

On the ward round she was asked how she monitored her diabetes prior to coming into hospital. She replied that she used to test her urine occasionally, but did not record her results. On questioning about dietary habits she admitted to eating biscuits and sweets. A request was made for the dietitian to see her. Mrs PK was changed to oral antibiotics.

Serum biochemistry results were:

- Sodium 137 mmol/L (135–145)
- Potassium 4.5 mmol/L (3.5–5.0)
- Urea 15 mmol/L (2.5–7.5)
- Creatinine 180 micromol/L (60–120)
- Glycated haemoglobin (HbA_{1c}) 11.4% (5.5–8.5)

Her urinary protein excretion was found to be 2.3 g in 24 hours and her blood pressure was 175/105 mmHg.

Q9 What is the significance of Mrs PK's elevated HbA_{1c}?

Q10 What is a likely explanation for Mrs PK's elevated urinary protein excretion?

Q11 Was the combination of atenolol and bendroflumethiazide appropriate antihypertensive therapy for Mrs PK?

Q12 How should Mrs PK's hypertension be managed in the future?

Day 14 Mrs PK was now apyrexial and her left foot appeared normal in size and was not tender. The ulcer, although improving, was approximately the same size as on admission and was still producing a moderate exudate. It was decided to continue Mrs PK's antibiotics, mobilise her slowly and observe her wound closely.

Mrs PK's blood sugar was well controlled on her current insulin regimen. She had been seen by the dietitian, who reported that Mrs PK had previously received very little dietary advice. The dietitian had recommended a calorie-restricted diet and given general advice about healthy eating and reducing her sugar intake.

It was decided to plan for discharge the following week and to put Mrs PK back on to oral antidiabetic therapy.

Q13 What oral antidiabetic regimen would you recommend for Mrs PK and why?

Q14 What other drug therapy should Mrs PK receive?

Q15 How should Mrs PK monitor her diabetes after discharge?

Q16 How should Mrs PK's ulcer be managed?

Day 20 Mrs PK was discharged and given appointments with the chiropodist in two weeks and the diabetic clinic in six weeks' time.

Her discharge medication was:

- Gliclazide 80 mg orally twice daily
- Ramipril 5 mg orally twice daily
- Furosemide 40 mg orally in the morning

- Simvastatin 10 mg orally at night
- Aspirin 75 mg orally daily

Her oral antibiotics also continued and were to be reviewed in two weeks.

She was also given a box of blood glucose testing strips and a demonstration of how to use them.

Q17 What should be included in the pharmaceutical care plan for Mrs PK at discharge?

Q18 What foot-care advice would be appropriate for Mrs PK?

Week 9   The ulcer was now fairly clean but had not healed as well as expected. Mrs PK felt generally a little unwell and lethargic.

Her HbA_{1c} was 10.3% (5.5–8.5). Her blood pressure was well controlled (140/75 mmHg) and her weight was 91 kg.

Q19 How should Mrs PK's diabetes be managed now?

What are the overall therapeutic aims for Mrs PK?

A1 **The aims of treatment for Mrs PK are to:**

   (a)   Keep her symptom-free.

   (b)   Treat her hypertension optimally.

   (b)   Improve and maintain her well-being.

   (c)   Prevent serious hypoglycaemia.

   (d)   Heal her foot ulcer.

   (e)   Prevent the progression and further development of complications.

Historically, Type 2 diabetes was termed 'mild diabetes' and little thought was given to the aims of treatment in these patients. However, the age- and sex-related mortality rates for patients with Type 2 diabetes are twice those of their non-diabetic counterparts. Thus, more attention is now being focused on this group, who represent approximately 80% of the total diabetic population.

   All adults with diabetes need high quality care, including optimisation of blood glucose, blood pressure control and management of other risk factors for developing the complications of diabetes. The UK Prospective Diabetes Study Group clearly showed that optimisation of blood glucose alone is insufficient to prevent the development of complications in Type 2 diabetes. Standard 4 of the National Service Framework (NSF) for Diabetes provides guidance on the clinical care of adults with diabetes. The key recommendations underpinning the NSF can be summarised as follows:

(a)   Improve blood glucose control.
(b)   Control hypertension.
(c)   Reduce raised cholesterol levels.
(d)   Encourage smoking cessation.

These strategies will reduce the risk of microvascular (retinopathy, nephropathy) and macrovascular (cardiovascular) complications of diabetes.

What would be an appropriate choice of antibiotic(s) for Mrs PK and by what route should it (they) be administered?

A2 **Appropriate antibiotic therapy would be: amoxicillin 500 mg intravenously every eight hours, flucloxacillin 500 mg intravenously every six hours and metronidazole 1 g rectally every eight hours.**

Seemingly benign, superficial ulcers can progress to extensive cellulitis, osteomyelitis and systemic toxicity. It is therefore imperative that infection is treated aggressively in the management of a diabetic foot. Even in moderately infected ulcers, therapy with a single antibiotic seldom provides adequate cover. Bacteriological cultures usually reveal two or three isolates from a single site. Aerobic Gram-positive organisms are the most prevalent, being present in 85% of cultures. These organisms are most commonly *Staphylococcus aureus, S. epidermidis* and *Streptococcus* spp. Gram-negative aerobes are present in about half the cases, most commonly *Proteus* spp. Anaerobic cultures are positive in about one-third of patients. A fetid odour emanating from the ulcer is particularly characteristic of the presence of anaerobic organisms.

Broad-spectrum intravenous antibiotic therapy should be commenced initially, but not before appropriate swabs have been sent for culture and sensitivity. Superficial swabs are not ideal for culturing, as both colonising and infecting organisms are recovered. More reliable specimens are obtained from the base of the ulcer after debridement. A combination of amoxicillin, flucloxacillin and metronidazole usually provides appropriate initial therapy; in a patient such as Mrs PK, who is pyrexial and in whom bacteraemia is suspected, the parenteral route should be used. A wide variety of other antibiotic regimens have been suggested. However, it is not possible to state the optimum regimen because objective data are lacking. Other proposed regimens include: ciprofloxacin monotherapy, ceftriaxone monotherapy, imipenem/cilastatin monotherapy, meropenem monotherapy, vancomycin, metronidazole and aztreonam, and co-amoxiclav with an aminoglycoside.

Therapy can be changed to the oral route once there is an adequate clinical response, usually after five to seven days. Initially, metronidazole can be administered rectally rather than parenterally, as there is near-complete absorption by this route, thus ensuring adequate blood concentrations. If an extended course of intravenous antimicrobial therapy is indicated, home administration can be considered.

What factors might have contributed to the development of Mrs PK's ulcer?

A3 **Neuropathy and lack of education.**

Absence of sensation may cause a patient with neuropathy to ignore the development of calluses (a sign of excessive pressure) or to be unaware of injury to the foot.

Mrs PK has signs of neuropathy (absent pinprick sensation). She also has neuropathic pain (burning). She will require advice about the prevention of future foot problems.

How should Mrs PK's ulcer be cleansed and dressed?

A4 **Sugar paste dressings are one suitable form of treatment. The wound should be cleansed with sterile, isotonic saline between dressings.**

Sugar paste dressings exert an antimicrobial effect, principally through an osmotic action. Controlled trials of ulcer dressings are very difficult to perform, but there are several reports of success with these preparations. Following application, the paste is held in place with an absorbent pad. With all formulations, twice-daily application is desirable. The pastes rapidly absorb wound exudate, liquefy and then flow away from the ulcer, which acts to clean the wound. The use of sugar paste has not been shown to have a detrimental effect on glycaemic control. There are a number of different formulations of sugar paste: one commonly used is in polyethylene glycol. Other alternatives for autolytic wound debridement include Debrisan, Sterigel, GranuGel and Intrasite Gel.

In almost all situations, the most appropriate method of gentle cleansing when the dressing is changed is the use of a sterile solution of isotonic saline.

Cetrimide and chlorhexidine are both active against Gram-positive and, to a lesser extent, Gram-negative organisms. However, there are few clinical data to confirm their benefit in either preventing or treating infection. Cetrimide also has potentially useful surfactant properties, but it has been shown to have a markedly toxic effect upon fibroblasts and can cause skin irritation and occasionally sensitisation. Hydrogen peroxide 10 volume (3%) is an antiseptic that is used for its oxidising effect, which destroys anaerobic bacteria. Unfortunately, it loses this effect when it comes into contact with organic material such as pus or gauze. Hydrogen peroxide assists in rapid removal of slough, but if it is used on granulating tissue, air blisters form which burst and lead to wound breakdown. Hydrogen peroxide interacts chemically with other agents and irrigation under pressure or into enclosed body cavities may have serious consequences, such as oxygen emboli. Hydrogen peroxide may also be caustic to skin surrounding the wound.

What other therapy may aid wound healing?

A5 **Limb elevation and optimal control of blood glucose concentrations.**

Limb elevation is essential in the management of an infected foot ulcer. This promotes drainage, alleviates the swelling and removes pressure from the foot. The heels should be protected, e.g. with a sheepskin dressing.

Why is insulin therapy indicated for Mrs PK?

A6 **Because Mrs PK is hyperglycaemic and has a febrile illness.**

Insulin therapy is indicated for all diabetic patients with hyperglycaemia and a febrile illness. In this situation, insulin is the only means by which optimum control of blood glucose can be obtained. If the blood glucose level remains even mildly elevated, infection is more likely to persist as a result of impaired leucocyte function.

How should the insulin be administered and monitored?

A7 **Administration should be by subcutaneous injection of insulin. Blood glucose should be monitored regularly.**

In patients who require insulin during intercurrent illness but who are not normally treated with insulin, a neutral preparation such as Humulin S or Actrapid can be given three times daily with a small dose of isophane insulin at bedtime to control blood glucose quickly and eliminate symptoms. The most commonly quoted regimen is 6 units of neutral insulin before each meal and 6 units of isophane insulin at bedtime. The dose is adjusted according to four times daily blood glucose measurements. The aim should be to maintain Mrs PK's blood glucose concentration between 4.5 and 11 mmol/L.

How should her neuropathic pain be managed?

A8   **Co-proxamol is unlikely to control neuropathic pain. A low dose of a tricyclic antidepressant (TCA) is more likely to be effective.**

Diabetic neuropathy is characterised by burning, aching (dysaesthesia) or sharp stabbing pain which does not respond to conventional analgesia. TCAs are the agents of choice for symptomatic relief of painful diabetic neuropathy. The majority of evidence is with amitriptyline, although imipramine is a popular alternative. Amitriptyline is usually started at a dose of 10–25 mg at night and increased gradually (depending on how the patient tolerates treatment) to 150–200 mg if necessary. However, the majority of patients will get at least 50% pain relief with the median preferred dose of 75 mg at night within two to eight days of reaching this dose. Gabapentin would be a suitable alternative as it is licensed for the treatment of neuropathic pain. It is usually started at a dose of 300 mg daily and the dose is then increased in steps of 300 mg daily to a maximum of 1.8 g daily.

What is the significance of Mrs PK's elevated HbA_{1c}?

A9   **The HbA_{1c} measurement provides objective evidence that Mrs PK has had poor glycaemic control over the previous six to eight weeks.**

HbA_{1c} is the name given to a subfraction of haemoglobin to which glucose binds. If the blood glucose level is persistently high, the percentage that binds to haemoglobin is increased. This is an irreversible process and persists throughout the lifespan of the red blood cell. The measurement of HbA_{1c} thus provides a means of assessing overall blood glucose control over the preceding six to eight weeks. High levels are indicative of poor diabetic control, but HbA_{1c} measurement provides no evidence of the fluctuations between high and low levels of blood glucose, and thus cannot be used for making day-to-day adjustments in treatment. In the out-patient and GP settings, it has largely replaced the measurement of random blood glucose concentrations. Mrs PK had an elevated blood glucose level on admission to hospital, but this could have been explained by the presence of infection. However, the subsequent finding of an HbA_{1c} of 11.4% is indicative of chronic, poor diabetic control. Long-term poor control is also supported by the presence of complications including neuropathy and retinopathy. The therapeutic aim should be to obtain an HbA_{1c} below 7%.

What is a likely explanation for Mrs PK's elevated urinary protein excretion?

A10   She has underlying renal disease.

Normal subjects excrete up to 0.08 g protein per day in the urine. Such amounts are undetectable by the usual screening tests. Proteinuria of more than 0.15 g/day is usually indicative of underlying pathology, most commonly renal disease. After 15 years duration of diabetes, up to 33% of patients have persistent proteinuria. Many patients with proteinuria also develop renal insufficiency, as indicated by raised serum urea and creatinine concentrations. Hypertension and retinopathy also co-exist in the majority of diabetic patients with renal insufficiency. Mrs PK has significant proteinuria at this time, but the test should be repeated to see if this is a consistent finding. She is also hypertensive and has a calculated creatinine clearance of approximately 38 mL/min.

Was the combination of atenolol and bendroflumethiazide appropriate antihypertensive therapy for Mrs PK?

A11   No. These agents are not optimal therapy for this patient as an angiotensin-converting enzyme inhibitor (ACEI) should be considered first-line in patients with proteinuria. In addition, Mrs PK has symptoms suggestive of heart failure which would also benefit from treatment with an ACEI.

The interaction between beta-blockers and diabetes is complex. The use of these agents is not absolutely contra-indicated and each patient should be assessed individually, considering the following points:

(a)   Beta-blockade inhibits beta-adrenergic-mediated insulin secretion. In Type 2 diabetes, beta-blockers can potentially impair insulin release and worsen glucose tolerance.

(b)   Beta-blockers mask some of the symptoms of hypoglycaemia (e.g. anxiety, tachycardia, tremor), but not all of them (e.g. sweating). This problem is less likely to occur with cardioselective agents.

(c)   Beta-blockers can elevate total peripheral resistance, causing vasoconstriction and reduced blood flow to most peripheral vascular beds. This may severely impair exercise tolerance and intensify intermittent claudication. Cardioselective agents are less likely than non-selective agents to exacerbate peripheral vascular disease.

(d)   Both cardioselective and non-selective beta-blockers have been shown to elevate very low-density lipoprotein triglycerides and reduce high-density lipoprotein (HDL) cholesterol levels, so should be used cautiously in diabetic patients with hyperlipidaemia.

(e)   Cardiac failure due to coronary heart disease, hypertensive heart disease and cardiomyopathy is frequent in the diabetic population. Beta-blockade may precipitate or exacerbate heart failure.

A beta-blocker was therefore not the optimum choice of antihypertensive therapy for Mrs PK, who has chronic hyperglycaemia and evidence of heart failure.

Diuretic therapy would appear to be a reasonable choice in a patient who has both hypertension and cardiac failure. However, the following points should be considered:

(a)   In Type 2 patients who still depend on some endogenous insulin secretion, diuretic-induced hypokalaemia can impair insulin release and worsen glucose tolerance. This is a dose-dependent phenomenon which can be minimised by using small doses, e.g. bendroflumethiazide 2.5 mg in the morning. Thiazide diuretics may also interfere with insulin action at a cellular level. Loop diuretics are less likely than thiazide diuretics to cause hyperglycaemia.

(b)   Thiazide diuretics are effective when renal function is normal; however, when the serum creatinine level is significantly elevated, loop diuretics should be used.

(c)   Diuretics can also produce a reduction in HDL cholesterol, an increase in low-density lipoprotein (LDL) cholesterol and elevation of triglycerides. These lipid abnormalities are dose-related, usually transient and their long-term significance has yet to be established.

For Mrs PK, use of an ACEI first-line would have been more appropriate due to its additional benefit on renal function.

How should Mrs PK's hypertension be managed in the future?

A12 **With an ACEI inhibitor plus a loop diuretic, together with a weight-reducing diet and advice to stop smoking.**

Thiazides, beta-blockers, ACEI, calcium-channel blockers (CCBs) and alpha-adrenoceptor blockers are all effective in lowering blood pressure and reducing the risk of cardiovascular events. The results of the UK Prospective Diabetes Study indicated that 30–40% of patients with hypertension required three or more agents to achieve adequate control so it is likely that Mrs PK will require more than one agent to achieve her target blood pressure of less than 140/80 mmHg.

Co-existing hypertension and diabetes act as additive risk factors in the acceleration of vascular complications which include cardiovascular disease, nephropathy and retinopathy. It is therefore essential that Mrs PK's hypertension is adequately treated by both pharmacological and non-pharmacological means. She should be strongly advised to lose weight and to stop smoking.

There are several pharmacological agents that can be considered:

(a) Alpha-adrenoceptor blockers. These agents can effectively reduce blood pressure in the diabetic patient without altering metabolic control. However, the side-effect of orthostatic hypotension may be a problem in the diabetic with clinical or subclinical autonomic neuropathy. Alpha-adrenoceptor blockers appear to have a beneficial effect on lipid profiles (an increase in HDL cholesterol and a decrease in triglycerides).

(b) CCBs. Because the process of insulin secretion from the pancreas is dependent on calcium entry into the beta cell, these agents may theoretically inhibit insulin release. However, there are only a few isolated case reports describing reversible deterioration in blood glucose control following the use of these agents. CCBs may also have beneficial vasodilator effects in patients with peripheral vascular disease.

(c) ACEIs. ACEIs confer unique benefits in the management of diabetic nephropathy by reducing both systemic and intraglomerular arterial pressure. These agents can control hypertension and may slow the progression of renal disease, as assessed by a decline in urinary albumin excretion rate and an improvement in the glomerular filtration rate. They should, however, be used with caution in renal insufficiency as they can cause an acute deterioration in renal function, notably in patients with renal artery stenosis. Although Mrs PK has renal impairment this is unlikely to be due to renal artery stenosis, therefore cautious introduction of an ACEI is justified. However, in such patients, close monitoring of renal function and serum electrolytes is required in the early stages of treatment and periodically thereafter.

All three classes of drug are suitable for use in patients with diabetes. However, Mrs PK also has symptoms of congestive cardiac failure and diabetic nephropathy. Ramipril would thus be a suitable agent and may have additional benefits as suggested by the results of the Heart Outcomes Prevention Evaluation study. This showed that ramipril reduced cardiovascular morbidity and mortality. Interestingly, the cardiovascular benefit was greater than that attributable to blood pressure reduction alone. In order to enhance the effect of ramipril and minimise the dose required, furosemide 40 mg in the morning should be added to the regimen. The dose of ramipril should be titrated until the desired hypotensive effect is achieved. A blood pressure of less than 140/80 mmHg would be desirable in Mrs PK.

> What oral antidiabetic regimen would you recommend for Mrs PK and why?

A13 **Commence gliclazide at the same dose as on admission (80 mg orally twice daily).**

The treatment options are as follows:

(a)   Continue with the gliclazide therapy which Mrs PK had been treated with prior to admission to hospital. Although her control was poor on admission, this could have been due to chronic infection. In addition, she has now been given dietary advice including a calorie-restricted diet.

(b)   Change to another sulphonylurea. However, gliclazide is a relatively potent sulphonylurea and it is unlikely that there would be any benefit in changing to another agent.

(c)   Add metformin to her drug regimen. In over 50% of patients, the addition of metformin to maximum doses of sulphonylureas achieves good metabolic control. However, metformin should be used with caution in patients with any disease that allows accumulation of the drug or any disease that predisposes to the accumulation of lactate. Lactic acidosis is a very rare, but potentially life-threatening, complication of metformin therapy. Metformin is eliminated totally by the kidney and should not be used in a patient with renal insufficiency, such as Mrs PK.

(d)   Add acarbose. Acarbose is a reversible, competitive inhibitor of alpha-glucosidase enzymes. The effect is to delay the digestion of starch and sucrose, resulting in a lowering of post-prandial hyperglycaemia and smoothing of daily blood glucose fluctuations. It can be used alone when dietary restriction has failed or in combination with other agents. However, acarbose does not appear to achieve significant improvements in blood glucose profiles in many diabetic patients. This is probably related to the high incidence of side-effects such as flatulence and so acarbose is rarely a realistic option.

(e) Stop gliclazide and start repaglinide. Repaglinide is a post-prandial glucose regulator which has a very rapid onset and short duration of action. However, it cannot be used in combination with a sulphonylurea and is unlikely to significantly improve her glycaemic control.

(f) Add a thiazolidinedione (glitazone), e.g. rosiglitazone or pioglitazone. The glitazones work by enhancing insulin action and thus promoting glucose utilisation in peripheral tissues. They act additively with other oral agents, including sulphonylureas and metformin. They are not licensed at the time of writing for monotherapy or for use in combination with insulin. However, as Mrs PK has symptoms of heart failure, glitazone therapy is contra-indicated as these agents can cause fluid retention.

(g) Change to insulin therapy. The incidence of secondary failure to oral hypoglycaemic agents is 5–6% per year. Secondary failure is defined as a good initial response to oral agents followed by a gradual decrease in effectiveness and eventual failure. Such patients subsequently require treatment with insulin. There is often a great reluctance amongst both doctors and patients to initiate insulin therapy. As a result many patients continue on oral hypoglycaemic agents when the aims of treatment may be better achieved by the use of insulin therapy.

Finally, in addition to pharmacological therapy, it is essential that Mrs PK adheres to the dietary advice and is encouraged to lose weight.

What other drug therapy should Mrs PK receive?

A14 **A statin and low-dose aspirin.**

Both the NSF and the National Institute of Clinical Excellence guidance recommend the use of a statin for primary prevention in patients with Type 2 diabetes and a raised cholesterol. Targets for cholesterol reduction are the same as for patients with cardiovascular disease. Once commenced, the effect of therapy should be assessed within three months and the dose titrated if required. With regard to aspirin, the current Diabetes UK recommendations are that low-dose aspirin should be considered in any patient over the age of 30 with one or more risk factors for cardiovascular disease. Mrs PK has a number of risk factors, including a high cholesterol level, hypertension plus she is a smoker.

How should Mrs PK monitor her diabetes after discharge?

A15   **By home blood glucose monitoring.**

Although urine glucose monitoring is adequate for most patients treated with oral hypoglycaemic agents, those who may be heading for secondary failure should be encouraged to perform home blood glucose monitoring. However, guidance on this subject is variable.

The European consensus guide states that urine testing is useful when blood testing is not possible. The American Diabetic Association position statement adds that although urine testing is low in cost and easy to perform, its limitations (e.g. it does not identify impending hypoglycaemia) make blood testing the preferred method of measuring glycaemic control.

There is no evidence that blood testing is more effective than urine testing at improving blood glucose control in people with Type 2 diabetes. Four trials that compared blood and urine testing found no significant difference between the two techniques. Urine testing can be used by people who find blood testing difficult or for those who do not like it. Blood testing is more expensive than urine testing and meters are not available on NHS prescription although they are often loaned to patients.

Overall, Mrs PK would benefit from monitoring her blood glucose levels. She should be taught how to use the blood glucose test strips, when to do the tests and be provided with a booklet in which to record results.

How should Mrs PK's ulcer be managed?

A16   **Alginate dressings are appropriate for clean wounds with moderate to heavy exudate.**

Mrs PK requires a dressing that she or the district nurse can easily manage at home. Alginate dressings are haemostatic, highly absorbent and biodegradable. The frequency of dressing changes will depend upon the condition of the wound. A clean, granulating ulcer will only require dressing twice weekly. The dressing is easily removed by irrigation with normal saline.

There is also a wide range of foam, gel and hydrogel dressings which may be equally effective. Consideration should be given to their cost and availability on GP prescription.

What should be included in the pharmaceutical care plan for Mrs PK at discharge?

A17 **The pharmaceutical care plan should include:**

(a)   Counselling

    (i)   Prescribed medication, including:

        Medication changes.

        Potential side-effects of new medication, e.g. dry cough with ramipril, diuresis with furosemide.

        Timing of doses, especially gliclazide and furosemide.

        Anticipated duration of antibiotics.

        Availability of items on GP prescription, e.g. finger-pricking devices for blood glucose tests are not available so she will need to obtain replacements from hospital.

        Obtaining further supplies of dressings. Alginate dressings are available in the community but not in all presentations. In addition, they may not be stocked by the community pharmacist.

    (ii)   Over-the-counter medication, including:

        Informing the pharmacist when purchasing over-the-counter medicines that she has hypertension and diabetes, as not all products are suitable.

        Not to self-treat foot problems; she should seek the advice of a state registered chiropodist.

    (iii)   General advice:

        The desirability of stopping smoking and the availability of nicotine substitutes.

(b)   Liaison with community pharmacist

    (i)   Medication changes.

    (ii)   Requirement for dressings.

    (iii)   Support required to encourage Mrs PK to stop smoking, including use of nicotine replacement therapy.

What foot-care advice would be appropriate for Mrs PK?

A18 **Detailed foot-care advice is essential and should include:**

    (a)   Avoid extremes of heat.

    (b)   Avoid walking barefoot.

(c) Examine feet regularly.

(d) Wear well-fitting footwear.

(e) Report problems immediately.

(f) Keep feet dry between the toes (use unscented talcum powder).

(g) Do not let feet get dry and cracked (use moisturising lotion, but not between the toes).

(h) Do not use corn remedies.

(i) See a chiropodist regularly.

How should Mrs PK's diabetes be managed now?

A19 **With insulin therapy.**

Mrs PK's diabetes is poorly controlled: she has a high random blood glucose level and, more importantly, a persistently elevated HbA_{1c}. In addition, she has not achieved any significant weight reduction, the ulcer has failed to heal and she feels generally unwell. All of this is clear evidence that a change in therapy is now required.

Insulin should be started with twice-daily subcutaneous injections. This may be an intermediate-acting insulin alone (e.g. isophane insulin) or a combination of intermediate and neutral insulins. If Mrs PK requires combination therapy but has difficulty mixing the insulins, a fixed mixture preparation could be used. She should be assessed by a diabetes specialist nurse to determine the preferred mode of insulin delivery, i.e. conventional, pre-filled cartridge or disposable syringe. The dose should be calculated from her insulin requirements while in hospital and then decreased a little to compensate for her extra mobility at home.

Further reading

Anon. When and how should patients with diabetes mellitus test blood glucose? *MeReC Bull* 2002; **13**(1).

Backonja M, Beydoun A, Edwards KR *et al*. Gabapentin for the symptomatic treatment of painful neuropathy in patients with diabetes mellitus: a randomised controlled trial. *J Am Med Assoc* 1998; **280**: 1831–1836.

Cantrill JA, Wood J. Diabetes mellitus. In: *Clinical Pharmacy and Therapeutics*. R Walker, C Edwards, eds. Churchill Livingstone, Edinburgh, 2002: 657–677.

Chantelau E, Tanudjaja T, Altenhofer F *et al.* Antibiotic treatment for uncomplicated neuropathic forefoot ulcers in diabetes: a controlled trial. *Diabetic Med* 1996; **13**: 156–159.

Clifford RM, Batty KT, Davis TME *et al.* A randomised controlled trial of a pharmaceutical care programme in high risk diabetic patients in an outpatient clinic. *Int J Pharm Prac* 2002; **10**: 85–90.

Coster S, Gulliford MC, Seed PT *et al.* Monitoring blood glucose control in diabetes mellitus: a systematic review. *Health Technol Assess* 2000; **4**: 1–93.

Day C. Thiazolidinediones: a new class of antidiabetic drugs. *Diabetic Med* 1999; **16**: 179–192.

Department of Health. *National Service Framework for Diabetes*. Department of Health, London, 2001.

Diabetes Control and Complications Trial. The effect of intensive treatment of diabetes on the development and progression of long-term complications in insulin dependent diabetes. *N Engl J Med* 1993; **329**: 977–986.

Diabetes UK. *Care Recommendation – Aspirin Treatment in Diabetes*. Diabetes UK, London, 2001. Available at: diabetes.org.uk/infocentre/carerec/aspirin.htm

European Diabetes Policy Group. A desktop guide to Type 2 diabetes mellitus. *Diabetic Med* 1999; **16**: 716–730.

Hansson L, Zanchetti A, Carruthers SG *et al.* Effects of intensive blood-pressure lowering and low-dose aspirin in patients with hypertension: principal results of the Hypertension Optimal Treatment (HOT) randomised trial. HOT Study Group. *Lancet* 1998; **351**: 1755–1762.

Hutchinson A, McIntosh A, Feder G *et al.* Effects of ramipril on cardiovascular and microvascular outcomes in people with diabetes mellitus: results of the HOPE study and MICRO-HOPE substudy. Heart Outcomes Prevention Evaluation Study Investigators. *Lancet* 2000; **355**: 253–259.

Levin SR, Coburn JW, Abraira C *et al.* Effect of intensive glycaemic control on microalbuminuria in Type 2 diabetes. *Diabetes Care* 2000; **23**: 1478–1485.

Lewis EJ, Hunsicker LG, Bain RP *et al.* The effect of angiotensin-converting-enzyme inhibition on diabetic nephropathy. The Collaborative Study Group. *N Engl J Med* 1993; **329**: 1456–1462.

Macleod AF. Diabetic neuropathy. *Medicine* 1997; **25**: 36–38.

Max MB, Lynch SA, Muir JA *et al.* Effects of desimipramine, amitriptyline and fluoxetine on pain in diabetic peripheral neuropathy. *N Engl J Med* 1992; **326**: 180–186.

McQuay HJ, Tramer M, Nye BA *et al.* A systematic review of antidepressants in neuropathic pain. *Pain* 1996; **68**: 217–227.

Neal B, MacMahon S, Chapman N. Effects of ACE inhibitors, calcium antagonists, and other blood-pressure-lowering drugs: results of prospectively designed overviews of randomised trials. Blood Pressure Lowering Treatment Trialists' Collaboration. *Lancet* 2000; **356**: 1955–1964.

National Institute for Clinical Excellence. *Management of Type 2 Diabetes: Management of Blood Pressure and Blood Lipids*. NICE, London, 2002.

Pahor M, Psaty BM, Alderman MH *et al*. Health outcomes associated with calcium antagonists compared with other first-line antihypertensive therapies: a meta-analysis of randomised controlled trials. *Lancet* 2000; **356**: 1949–1954.

Royal College of General Practitioners. *Clinical Guidelines and Evidence Review Type 2 Diabetes. Prevention and Management of Foot Problems*. Royal College of General Practitioners, London, 2000.

Royal Pharmaceutical Society of Great Britain. *Guidelines for Community Pharmacists on the Care of Patients with Diabetes*. Royal Pharmaceutical Society of Great Britain, London, 2001.

Scheen AJ, Lefèbvre P. Oral antidiabetic agents: a guide to selection. *Drugs* 1998; **55**: 255–236.

Scheen AJ. Drug treatments of non-insulin dependent diabetes mellitus in the 1990s: achievements and future developments. *Drugs* 1997; **54**: 355–368.

Scottish Intercollegiate Guidelines Network. *Lipids and The Primary Prevention of Coronary Heart Disease: A National Clinical Guideline*. SIGN, Edinburgh, 1999.

Scottish Intercollegiate Guidelines Network. *Secondary Prevention of Coronary Heart Disease following Myocardial Infarction: A National Clinical Guideline*. SIGN, Edinburgh, 2000.

UK Prospective Diabetes Study Group. Intensive blood-glucose control with sulphonylureas or insulin compared with conventional treatment and risk of complications in patients with Type 2 diabetes. UKPDS 33. *Lancet* 1998; **352**: 837–853.

UK Prospective Diabetes Study Group. Effect of intensive blood-glucose control with metformin on complications in overweight patients with Type 2 diabetes. UKPDS 34. *Lancet* 1998; **352**: 854–865.

UK Prospective Diabetes Study Group. Tight blood pressure control and risk of macrovascular and microvascular complications in Type 2 diabetes. UKPDS 38. *Br Med J* 1998; **317**: 703–713.

UK Prospective Diabetes Study Group. Efficacy of atenolol and captopril in reducing risk of macrovascular and microvascular complications in Type 2 diabetes. UKPDS 39. *Br Med J* 1998; **317**: 713–720.

Winocour PH. Effective diabetes care: a need for realistic targets. *Br Med J* 2002; **324**: 1577–1580.

Wood DA, Durrington P, Poulter N *et al*. (on behalf of the Societies). Joint British recommendations on prevention of coronary heart disease in clinical practice. *Heart* 1998; **80**(suppl. 2): S1–S29.

Yudkin JS, Blauth C, Drury P *et al*. Prevention and management of cardiovascular disease in patients with diabetes mellitus: an evidence base. *Diabetic Med* 1996; **13**(9 suppl. 4): S101–121.

26

Rheumatoid arthritis

David Bryant and Sue Parkinson

Case study and questions

Day 1 Sixty-nine-year-old Mrs SD was admitted to the ward from the rheumatology out-patient clinic. She was complaining of increasing pain and stiffness in her hands and knees. The pain was bad all day, but worse in the morning.

She had been diagnosed with seropositive rheumatoid arthritis (RA) four years earlier. Her other medical history was unremarkable. She had been treated with sulfasalazine from the date of diagnosis. That had been stopped due to loss of efficacy and subsequently she was initiated on gold therapy that was stopped due to side-effects.

At the time of admission she was taking methotrexate 10 mg orally once a week. The dose of methotrexate had been increased in the past, but was not tolerated at doses higher than 10 mg due to gastrointestinal side-effects. Mrs SD was taking both ibuprofen 200 mg and co-codamol 8/500 when required for pain relief. The only other medication she was taking was calcium and vitamin D as prophylaxis against osteoporosis.

On examination Mrs SD was found to have swelling in the joints of both hands and both her knees were swollen and tender. The swollen joints were warmer than the surrounding areas. Rheumatoid nodules could be felt on her elbows and she was suffering from dry eyes (Sjögren's syndrome). She had the following blood results:

- Haemoglobin 10.6 g/dL (reference range 12–16)
- White blood cells (WBC) 12.1×10^9/L (4–11×10^9)
- Neutrophils 5.2×10^9/L (2–7.5×10^9)
- Platelets 456×10^9/L (150–400×10^9)
- Erythrocyte sedimentation rate (ESR) 69 mm/h (0–20)
- C-reactive protein (CRP) 92 mg/L (<10)
- Plasma viscosity (PV) 2.14 mPa.s (1.5–1.72)
- Urea and electrolyte levels and liver function tests were unremarkable.

A flare of her RA was diagnosed and Mrs SD was admitted. The initial plan was to treat her with drug therapy and physiotherapy.

Q1   Comment on the previous disease-modifying antirheumatic drug (DMARD) treatment that Mrs SD had received.

Q2   What are the usual signs and symptoms of a flare in RA?

Q3   What initial drug therapy would you advise to treat Mrs SD's symptoms (rather than her underlying disease)?

Day 2   She was prescribed the following medication:

- Methotrexate 10 mg orally once a week
- Folic acid 5 mg orally daily except on the day of methotrexate
- Calcium 500 mg plus vitamin D 400 units one tablet twice a day
- Co-codamol 8/500 orally, two when required for pain
- Ibuprofen 200 mg orally one three times a day when required for pain
- Tramadol 50–100 mg orally four times a day when required for pain

Since admission Mrs SD had taken eight tablets of co-codamol 8/500, three doses of ibuprofen 200 mg and no tramadol. She complained that although the affected joints felt better since the initial treatment for her flare she was still in considerable pain. The Senior House Officer asked for advice on her pain management. He was particularly interested to know whether addition of a cyclooxygenase (COX)-2 inhibitor would be of benefit to this patient.

Q4   What advice would you give with respect to the use of non-steroidal anti-inflammatory drugs (NSAIDs)?

Q5   What other advice would you give on her pain medication?

Q6   Outline a pharmaceutical care plan for the initial management of Mrs SD.

Day 4   The long-term management of Mrs SD was discussed on the consultant ward round.

Q7   What future DMARD therapy would you recommend for this patient from the options available?

It was decided to continue the patient on methotrexate but to change the route of administration to subcutaneous. It was planned that the dose would be increased if the patient tolerated it. She was started on sulfasalazine enteric-coated tablets 500 mg in the morning to be increased slowly.

In addition it was planned to initiate hydroxychloroquine in four weeks' time.

Day 12   Mrs SD was considerably better and was not suffering any adverse effects from her therapy. She was discharged home.

Q8   What long-term monitoring is required for the therapy she has been prescribed?

Month 7   Mrs SD attended the out-patient clinic complaining of similar symptoms to her previous flare. She was now on subcutaneous methotrexate 25 mg once a week, sulfasalazine enteric-coated tablets 1000 mg in the morning and 500 mg at night, and hydroxychloroquine 200 mg orally twice a day. She had not had any adverse effects and all of her monitoring parameters had remained within normal limits.

It was decided that the combination therapy was no longer effective and she needed alternative therapy.

Q9   What biologic therapies are available for the treatment of RA?
Q10   What are the doses and methods of delivery for these agents?
Q11   What are the considerations and contra-indications to starting a patient on these agents?
Q12   Does Mrs SD fulfil the commonly used criteria for treatment with these agents?
Q13   Which biologic therapy would you recommend for this patient?

Mrs SD was admitted for treatment of the flare. She received analgesia, steroid injections, physiotherapy and hydrotherapy. The flare settled within two weeks. All of her current DMARD therapy was discontinued during the admission and she was started on subcutaneous etanercept injections after her acute flare had settled, which she self-administered twice weekly on a Monday and a Thursday.

Q14   Mrs SD asked how long she will remain on the etanercept. What is your answer?
Q15   What are the long-term prospects for this patient?

Comment on the previous disease-modifying antirheumatic drug
(DMARD) treatment that Mrs SD had received.

A1 **Sulfasalazine is a common first choice of DMARD in RA. It
has a good efficacy profile and low rate of serious adverse
side-effects. Gold is an effective agent in the treatment of
RA, but its use is limited by its adverse side-effect profile.
Methotrexate is the 'gold standard' choice of DMARD in
rheumatoid arthritis.**

The DMARDs currently used in clinical practice include methotrexate,
sulfasalazine, injectable or oral gold, antimalarials, ciclosporin, penicillamine, azathioprine and leflunomide. DMARDs are used to try and
prevent joint deformation, and hence reduce disability in rheumatoid
patients. The precise mechanism of action of DMARDs is unclear. All
DMARDs inhibit the release of, or reduce the activity of, inflammatory
cytokines. The choice of DMARD by a clinician is dependent upon the
balance between adverse effects and efficacy, and on its suitability for the
patient being treated. All the DMARDs possess a slow onset of action and
complete response to treatment can take up to four to six months.
Sulfasalazine and methotrexate are generally regarded as first-line therapies due to their higher efficacy rate (approximately 40% response rates)
and high continuation rates compared to the other DMARDs.

Sulfasalazine is one of the most commonly prescribed DMARDs. It
has a low incidence of serious adverse effects and has been shown to slow
disease progression. It is often used in mild to moderate disease. The
monitoring requirements are less arduous than for most other DMARDs,
which is a significant benefit for the patients. In order to reduce the
problem of nausea, the dose is usually titrated upwards slowly from
500 mg daily, increasing at weekly intervals up to 1 g twice daily. Only
the enteric-coated tablets are licensed for the treatment of RA.

Methotrexate is seen as the 'gold standard' therapy in most centres.
It is generally used in patients with moderate to severe disease, especially
in those with a poor prognosis. It has a relatively rapid onset of action of
four to six weeks and is easy to administer as a single weekly dose, given
orally or by intramuscular or subcutaneous injection (the latter route
being unlicensed). Nausea and stomatitis are common side-effects but
can be managed by the addition of oral folic acid therapy to the
methotrexate regimen. The optimal dose of folic acid has yet to be
established, but ranges from 5 to 30 mg weekly in divided doses. Most

centres omit the folic acid on the day methotrexate is administered, due to the potential interaction. Bone marrow suppression is also a concern for patients receiving methotrexate therapy and can be related to either too high a maintenance dose or accidental overdose. This has occurred in patients who have inadvertently taken methotrexate daily rather than weekly or due to confusion between the 2.5 and 10 mg strength tablets, and happens more frequently in the elderly population. Patients *must* be carefully counselled on how many tablets to take and to take them only once a week on the same day. Any signs of infection, e.g. unexplained fever or sore throat etc., must be reported to a doctor immediately. Patients should be advised to avoid contact with people who may have chickenpox. Methotrexate can also derange liver function tests and these should be monitored regularly. Methotrexate is largely cleared unchanged from the body by renal excretion. NSAIDs can potentially reduce this excretion due to reductions in renal perfusion caused by NSAID inhibition of prostaglandin synthesis. Co-prescription of these two agents should be undertaken with care in patients with impaired renal function.

Sodium aurothiomalate (gold injection) is a long-established DMARD and is a very effective agent in the treatment of RA, although its use is limited by its side-effect profile. Patients are more likely to stop gold therapy due to toxicity than with any other DMARD. Important adverse events include rashes, stomatitis, proteinuria, leucopenia and thrombo-cytopenia. Despite this, injectable gold can provide benefit to some patients for many years and it may be a useful agent for those with progressive disease failing other therapies.

There has been a major shift in the treatment of RA over the last decade. Traditionally the therapeutic pyramid was employed whereby initial treatment was conservative, with the use of NSAIDs for several years and progression on to DMARDs when disease was not controlled. This approach has been replaced by early treatment with DMARDs, as there is evidence that most patients develop joint destruction within the first two years of their disease. Treatment aims not only to treat the symptoms, but also to slow or prevent the underlying disease process.

What are the usual signs and symptoms of a flare in RA?

A2   Joint pain and loss of function are the most obvious symptoms of RA flare. The peripheral joints of the hands and feet are usually involved first and symmetrically. During a disease flare there is increased pain and swelling at the

affected joints. There is also morning stiffness that can last for several hours after rising. These factors lead to decreased mobility.

There are also non-specific indicators of inflammatory processes. The ESR, CRP and PV may be raised. These inflammatory markers can be used as indicators as to the success of treatment, but it should be remembered that the inflammatory markers are not specific and normal results do not preclude active disease. There is also often a raised WBC count due to the disease processes, but it may be high for another reason such as infection. The WBC count can also be low – an example would be in Felty's syndrome. Rheumatoid factor and antinuclear antibodies (ANA) are often also measured.

What initial drug therapy would you advise to treat Mrs SD's symptoms (rather than her underlying disease)?

A3 **Pain relief in the form of an NSAID plus simple analgesia, with steroid injection into the worst affected joints.**

Pain relief is important in the early stages of a flare to enable the patient to start to mobilise and be able to receive physiotherapy. Choices of pain relief in RA patients are discussed in greater depth in Questions 4 and 5. An NSAID would be beneficial to this patient.

Systemic corticosteroids have long been used in the management of RA and were the first drugs to result in reversibility of the disease, however; their place in long-term therapy is still controversial. Corticosteroids have a potent anti-inflammatory effect and recent studies have suggested their use leads to a slowing of radiological progression. However, side-effects associated with long-term, high-dose therapy (e.g. osteoporosis, diabetes mellitus, hypertension, etc.) have severely limited their long-term use in RA. Corticosteroids would, however, be considered appropriate to control a flare. Steroids administered by the intramuscular route may be useful for patients with an acute flare of disease, while intravenous pulses of methylprednisolone are particularly helpful in controlling rheumatoid vasculitis. Intra-articular steroid administration (e.g. methylprednisolone acetate or triamcinolone acetonide) can effectively relieve pain, increase mobility and reduce deformity in one or more joints. The duration of response to intra-articular steroids is variable. The dose used is dependent upon the joint size, with methylprednisolone acetate 40–80 mg or triamcinolone acetonide 20–40 mg appropriate for large joints such as knees. The frequency at which injections may be given is controversial, but repeated injections are usually given at intervals of one to five weeks or more, depending on the degree of relief obtained from the first injection.

What advice would you give with respect to the use of NSAIDs?

A4 **Due to Mrs SD's age and her concurrent medication, a standard NSAID in combination with a proton pump inhibitor (PPI) or a COX-2 selective agent on its own should be used. Ibuprofen, diclofenac and naproxen (in increasing order of relative risk) have the lowest risk of gastrointestinal toxicity of standard NSAIDs.**

Although the NSAIDs differ in chemical structure, they all have similar pharmacological properties in terms of anti-inflammatory and analgesic action, and have similar drug interactions. Despite numerous clinical trials, differences between NSAIDs in terms of objective measures of efficacy have not emerged. Patient response to NSAIDs is highly variable, with about 60% of patients responding to any one drug, and therapeutic trials with several NSAIDs may be necessary to determine the best agent for an individual. It is recommended that the drug should be changed after one week of non-response if an analgesic effect is the desired outcome or after three weeks if an anti-inflammatory effect is the desired outcome. Approximately 10% of patients will not find any NSAID beneficial.

Gastrointestinal adverse reactions range from superficial damage with minor symptoms (dyspepsia, abdominal pain and diarrhoea) through to duodenal and gastric ulceration and potentially fatal complications. Patients generally complain of nausea and indigestion, but some of those presenting with bleeding or perforation will have no history of dyspepsia. The prevalence of symptomatic ulcers has been reported to be between 14 and 31%, with gastric ulcers most prevalent. The options for reducing gastric side-effects due to NSAIDs are: to avoid the use of NSAIDs and use simple analgesia; to use an NSAID with the lowest associated gastrointestinal side-effects and use it at the lowest possible dose; to prescribe a gastro-protective agent; or to prescribe a selective COX-2 inhibitor. From studies it would appear that proton pump inhibitors are most effective, for the prevention of gastrointestinal complications associated with NSAID use. Renal function should also be regularly monitored for patients on the combination of methotrexate and an NSAID.

The main mechanism of action of NSAIDs is believed to be the inhibition of the enzyme COX. COX converts the fatty acid arachadonic acid into endoperoxidases, prostaglandins and thromboxanes in a cell-specific manner. It has been shown that there are two isoforms of COX: COX-1 and COX-2. COX-1 is thought to function mainly as a physiologic enzyme producing the prostaglandins critical for maintaining normal renal function, gastric mucosal integrity and haemostasis. COX-2 is virtually undetectable in most tissues under physiologic conditions but is induced by certain inflammatory stimuli.

NSAIDs act by direct inhibition of COX-1 and COX-2, via blockade of the COX enzyme site. The subsequent inhibition of prostaglandin production reduces inflammation but also results in additional activities on platelet aggregation, renal homeostasis and gastric mucosal integrity. In an effort to reduce the side-effects of NSAIDs, and particularly the gastrointestinal side-effects, agents were developed that selectively block COX-2 and have minimal effect on COX-1.

COX-2 selective agents are recommended for use in patients who are at high risk of developing gastrointestinal side-effects but they are not recommended for routine use. Patients that are at 'high risk' are defined as: those over 65 years of age; those using concomitant medications known to increase the likelihood of upper gastrointestinal side-effects such as steroids and anticoagulants; those with serious co-morbidity such as cardiovascular disease, renal or hepatic impairment, diabetes or hypertension; and those requiring prolonged treatment with high doses of NSAID. It is important to consult the product information when starting a COX-2 selective agent, as many of the contra-indications and side-effects of traditional NSAIDs remain.

Due to Mrs SD's age and her concurrent medication it would be reasonable to assume that she will need some sort of protection from gastric ulceration. The options for this would be to use a standard NSAID in combination with a PPI or to use a COX-2 selective agent. The dose of ibuprofen prescribed is too low and an 'as required' prescription is inappropriate at this stage of her disease. A higher regular dose of ibuprofen such as 400 mg three times a day or diclofenac 50 mg three times a day would be more appropriate, with co-prescription of a PPI. These drugs have been shown to be efficacious, whilst having a lesser gastrointestinal side-effect profile than some of the more potent NSAIDs.

What other advice would you give on her pain medication?

A5 **Paracetamol, paracetamol combinations and dihydrocodeine are all useful for simple pain relief. Although they have no anti-inflammatory properties and do not affect the disease**

process, they do have a place in both early and late stages of the disease. The World Health Organization's analgesic ladder is a good starting point for any decision on analgesia.

Regular prescription of paracetamol 1 g four times a day with a weak opioid analgesic either regularly or when required would be a good initial prescription for Mrs SD. There is a need for regular reassessment dependent on her pain scores. It is important to avoid co-prescription of analgesia that works on the same receptors. The point of the World Health Organization analgesic ladder is to move up the ladder, not across it. The prescription of co-codamol and tramadol on a 'when required' basis is an example of this, and should thus be reviewed.

Outline a pharmaceutical care plan for the initial management of this patient.

A6   The pharmaceutical care plan for Mrs SD should include the following:

(a)   Obtain a detailed drug history. Patients often omit to inform medical staff of any eye-drops, inhalers or medicines they may buy from their chemist. The pharmacist is in the best possible position to elicit the greatest information.
(b)   Contribute to optimising her future treatment according to defined outcomes.
(c)   Counsel on all aspects of her treatment.
(d)   Monitor all treatment for efficacy and side-effects.
(e)   Ensure all treatment initiated during her hospital stay can be continued and monitored successfully following discharge.
(f)   Ensure that she has any aids she might need to manage her medication (e.g. non-child resistant containers).

What future DMARD therapy would you recommend for this patient from the options available?

A7   A number of options can be considered for Mrs SD. The best option would be for her to commence on triple therapy with oral sulfasalazine, subcutaneous methotrexate and oral hydroxychloroquine.

One option is for Mrs SD to be started on one of the other DMARDs currently used in clinical practice. These include penicillamine, antimalarials, azathioprine, ciclosporin, cyclophosphamide or leflunomide.

The precise mechanism of action of DMARDs is unclear. All the DMARDs inhibit the release of, or reduce the activity of, inflammatory cytokines. Activated T lymphocytes appear to be particularly important in this process and it is known that methotrexate, leflunomide and ciclosporin all inhibit T cells. Cytokines, which appear to be important in the inflammatory cascade, include tumour necrosis factor (TNF), interleukin (IL)-1, IL-2 and IL-6. There is good evidence that DMARDs inhibit these cytokines *in vitro* and *in vivo*.

Penicillamine is seldom now used due to problems with toxicity and poor long-term efficacy. There is no evidence that penicillamine reduces joint erosions. Ciclosporin is an immunosuppressive agent recently licensed for use in RA. It has proven efficacy in early and late disease, but long-term data on reducing joint destruction is lacking. The lack of data and its potential toxicity means that it is often reserved for patients who have failed conventional therapies. The antimalarial agents (mainly hydroxychloroquine) are the least toxic of all the DMARDs. Unfortunately they are also the least effective and so are reserved for less severe forms of the disease, or are used in combination regimes.

Azathioprine is often used when treating RA that is refractory to other agents; it may have a steroid-sparing effect. Cyclophosphamide given either orally or as intravenous pulse therapy is mainly reserved for treatment of rheumatoid vasculitis. Both azathioprine and cyclophosphamide have the potential to cause infertility and the development of malignancies. As a result, their use should only be considered when the risks have been balanced against the intended clinical improvement.

Leflunomide is a relatively new DMARD that has both anti-inflammatory and immunomodulatory properties. It acts by inhibiting the synthesis of pyrimidine nucleotides in immune response cells, particularly T cells and it reduces the pro-inflammatory cytokines TNF and IL-1. It is at least as effective as sulfasalazine and methotrexate, and there is some evidence that quality of life measures may be superior with leflunomide. It has a rapid onset of action (four weeks) and is well tolerated. Leflunomide is licensed to be given as a loading dose of 100 mg daily for three days followed by 10–20 mg daily, although there may be local variations to this loading regimen. Some centres feel that although loading a patient will induce a faster response, patients may stop taking therapy due to diarrhoea. As a result some centres choose not to use the loading regimen and commence therapy on 10 or 20 mg daily from day 1. The most common side-effects are gastrointestinal disturbances, reversible alopecia, rash and hypertension. There have also been reports of serious liver reactions after treatment with leflunomide. Liver function tests (LFTs) should thus be checked at initiation of treatment and at monthly intervals for the first six months of treatment, and then every eight weeks thereafter. If the alanine aminotransferase (ALT) increases to more then twice the normal range then the dose should be reduced to 10 mg daily and the LFTs monitored weekly. If it rises to greater then three times the normal level, then leflunomide should be discontinued.

Methotrexate may be given orally or by subcutaneous (unlicensed) or intramuscular injection. Gastric tolerability is improved when the drug is given parenterally. Subcutaneous therapy has the advantage that, with suitable support, patients can be taught to self-inject and can therefore administer their medication at home. Mrs SD has tolerated methotrexate well except for the gastric side-effects. It would thus be reasonable to try changing her oral methotrexate therapy to subcutaneous, and to titrate the dose up as far as it is tolerated.

There is also evidence that combination therapy with different DMARDs is more likely to achieve clinical improvement of the disease. Combination therapy may offer better symptom control, particularly if combining agents with different modes of action. A triple regimen of hydroxychloroquine, methotrexate and sulfasalazine has shown significant advancements over monotherapy with the individual agents. This combination regimen is also well tolerated. Single therapy is usually tried as a first-line, due to the increased risk of toxicity when using more than one agent, but triple therapy is usually the next stage, especially if a patient has a partial response to any single therapy.

As Mrs SD has tolerated both methotrexate and sulfasalazine in the past a suitable option for her would be to try this combination approach. Methotrexate should be switched to the parenteral route. Sulfasalazine should then be started in the usual way. If this is tolerated, then oral hydroxychloroquine may also be added.

What long-term monitoring is required for the therapy she is prescribed?

A8 **Methotrexate and sulfasalazine therapy require baseline LFTs and full blood count (FBC), repeated two-weekly for two months, then monthly for four months, then three-monthly thereafter. If doses change then monitoring should restart from two-weekly. Some centres would remain on monthly monitoring after the four-month period due to the fact she would be on combination therapy.**

Methotrexate requires baseline measurement of FBC, urea and electrolytes and LFTs. FBC and LFTs should be repeated two weekly for two months, then monthly for four months and then at least 3-monthly thereafter. If the WBC count falls to below 4.0, neutrophils below 2.0, platelets below 150, or if aspartate aminotransferase (AST) or ALT levels increase to greater than three times the normal range, then therapy should be reviewed. Mrs SD should be counselled to report any oral ulceration, unusual bruising, rash, fever, cough, shortness of breath, nausea or alopecia, as methotrexate can cause stomatitis, hepatic fibrosis and liver toxicity, severe alveolitis, pneumonitis, and bone marrow suppression.

Sulfasalazine treatment requires baseline assessment of FBC and LFTs. These should be repeated in the same two-weekly, monthly, three-monthly pattern as methotrexate. Sulfasalazine can cause nausea, reversible male infertility, rashes, marrow suppressions and hepatitis.

Hydroxychloroquine generally requires little monitoring. Gastro-intestinal toxicity is its main adverse effect, while some patients may experience tinnitus. Retinopathy has been associated with hydroxy-chloroquine, although the need to perform eye tests and the frequency of such tests is still open to debate. Mrs SD should be counselled to report any visual acuity changes or blurred vision.

Patient information sheets and individual DMARD booklets are recommended for patients taking DMARDs. Counselling should reinforce the need to comply with monitoring requirements, the expected onset of action, potential toxicity and action to take in the event of adverse effects. There have recently been moves towards a shared care approach to managing patients receiving DMARDs. Medication may be supplied by a GP, but overall responsibility for monitoring and dosing will remain with the hospital consultant. The aim of such schemes is to ensure all patients receive adequate monitoring and specialist input without the inconvenience of frequent hospital visits.

What biologic therapies are available for the treatment of RA?

A9 **Infliximab, etanercept, anakinra and adalimumab are biologic therapies which can be used in the treatment of RA.**

The currently available therapies act either on TNF-alpha or IL-1 receptors, both of which are thought to be pivotal pro-inflammatory cytokines. Whilst TNF-alpha is thought to mediate inflammation, IL-1 is thought to mediate bone and cartilage destruction. TNF is a pro-inflammatory mediator found in high concentrations in joints affected by RA. Research has demonstrated its contribution to the pathogenesis of synovitis and joint destruction in RA. Biological therapies that act on TNF-alpha include etanercept, infliximab and adalimumab. Anakinra is the only currently available agent that acts on IL-1 receptors.

Infliximab is a chimeric human-murine monoclonal antibody that binds with high affinity to both soluble and transmembrane forms of TNF-alpha, and hence blocks the functional activity of TNF-alpha.

Etanercept is a recombinant human soluble TNF receptor. The mechanism of action of etanercept is competitive inhibition of TNF. It binds to cell surface or soluble TNF and prevents TNF-mediated cellular responses.

Adalimumab is a recombinant human immunoglobulin (IgG1) monoclonal antibody containing only human peptide sequences. It binds with high affinity and specificity to soluble TNF-alpha. As the first fully humanised monoclonal antibody against TNF-alpha, it is less likely to engender an immune response in the recipient than agents that contain non-human or artificial sequences.

Anakinra is a recombinant form of human IL-1 receptor antagonist (IL-1Ra). Within the IL-1 family there is IL-1-alpha, IL-1-beta and IL-1Ra. IL-1Ra partially blocks the biological activity of IL-1-alpha and IL-1-beta by competitively inhibiting their binding to IL-1 receptors. Because IL-1Ra has this action, the effects of IL-1 on inflammation and bone erosions will be reduced. Anakinra, as a recombinant form of IL-1Ra, also has this effect and so is of benefit in RA.

What are the doses and methods of delivery for these agents?

A10 **Infliximab is given by intravenous infusion at a dose of 3 mg/kg at weeks 0, 2 and 6, and then eight-weekly thereafter. Etanercept is given at a dose of 25 mg by subcutaneous injection twice a week. Adalimumab is given by subcutaneous injection at a dose of 40 mg every other week. Anakinra is given at a dose of 100 mg by subcutaneous injection daily.**

What are the considerations and contra-indications to starting a patient on these agents?

A11 **TNF blockade has significant advantages over the existing DMARD treatments. The efficacy of infliximab and etanercept is very similar with response rates in the region of 60–70% compared with 40% for existing DMARD therapies. Both agents have been shown to reduce disease activity significantly and to improve quality of life. There is also radiological evidence that infliximab halts disease progress.**

Etanercept is generally well tolerated with the commonest adverse event being the development of injection site reactions (approximately 40%

incidence). These are generally mild, transient, and resolve with time and do not usually necessitate stopping treatment. Upper respiratory tract infections (rhinitis, sinusitis, etc.) have also been reported. These are generally mild and transient. There have also been reports of demyelination and other neurological problems in patients treated with etanercept. There is currently no evidence of increased risk of malignancy in patients taking etanercept.

Infliximab must be given with oral methotrexate to prevent the development of murine antibodies; therefore it is not suitable for patients who cannot tolerate methotrexate. It is generally well tolerated with infusion-related events such as headache, diarrhoea, rash, fever, chills, urticaria and dyspnoea being the most common side-effects. These are most likely to occur within the first four infusions. Delayed infusion reactions have also been reported, with symptoms such as fever, rash and arthralgia occurring up to two weeks post-infusion. This is thought to be due to immune complex formation and complement activation. Malignancies, such as lymphomas, breast carcinoma, skin tumours and rectal cancers have developed in a small number of patients. Additionally, pancytopenia has also been described. However because of the low incidence of such events and the concurrent use of DMARDs in many cases, infliximab is not thought to cause cancer or bone marrow suppression. Extra vigilance is advised and a complete medical history is warranted before infliximab initiation. There are reports which show patients on infliximab therapy have an increased risk of upper respiratory tract infection. In addition, reports have implicated a relationship between infliximab and tuberculosis (TB). The precise link is unknown, but it is felt to be a reactivation of latent disease. However as TNF-alpha is known to have a function in regulating the immune response, the possibility of primary TB infection cannot be ignored. Worsening of heart failure has also occurred in New York Heart Association (NYHA) class III and IV congestive heart failure patients taking infliximab. Avoidance of treatment in this patient group is advised. Neurological events such as demyelination have also been reported in relation to infliximab treatment. Whether this is an exacerbation of an underlying disease state or a new presentation is not yet known.

Adalimumab is generally well tolerated. Injection site reactions, headaches and rashes are among the most commonly reported adverse effects. There have been no reported cases of TB to date. In clinical trials there have been no significant differences in rates of infection between adalimumab and placebo groups. As the newest agent there is a need for close post-marketing surveillance to detect any increased rates of adverse events such as TB or demyelination.

Some centres would advise extreme caution in using any of the TNF blocking agents in patients with a history of TB, neurological problems or NYHA stage III or IV heart failure. A careful medical history is required when commencing a patient on any biological therapy. Many of the reports of adverse effects could have been avoided if a complete medical history had been taken. Any decision to initiate therapy in patients with a history of TB, neurological problems or heart failure is at the discretion of the lead clinician.

The most commonly seen side-effect with anakinra is injection site reactions, including pain, erythema, pruritus and rash. More serious reactions include bruising and bleeding. Most commonly reported infections have been upper respiratory tract infections and sinusitis. At the time of writing there are no reports of TB or opportunistic infections. Neutropenia has been reported in patients receiving anakinra, and it has usually resolved upon cessation of the drug. Anakinra should be used with caution in patients with severe or prolonged neutropenia. Various forms of malignancy have been diagnosed in a small number of patients receiving anakinra, but in all cases the tumour was not thought to be secondary to the biological agent.

None of the four agents should be used in patients with active infection. In the UK all patients on biological therapy are registered nationally to monitor any increased incidence of serious adverse events. The outcomes of this register will be keenly awaited.

Finally there are several general considerations involved in choosing a particular agent. Rheumatoid patients may often lack the dexterity to manipulate the syringes required for subcutaneous injection. Without a trained carer, patients who are unable to self-administer may be limited to therapy which is given in a day-unit setting. Smaller hospitals may not have the facilities required for administration of infusions in a day-unit setting. Patients may not have adequate storage facilities for the subcutaneous syringes; or a patient may simply not have a fridge. Although these observations may appear obvious, they should not be overlooked.

> Does this patient fulfil the commonly used criteria for treatment with these agents?

A12 **Yes.**

Current best practice recommends the use of an anti-TNF alpha agent for treatment in adults who have continuing clinically active rheumatoid arthritis that has not responded adequately to at least two DMARDs, including methotrexate unless contra-indicated. The agents should be prescribed in accordance with current guidelines, which set out criteria for eligibility, definitions of failure of standard therapy, exclusion criteria and criteria for withdrawal of therapy. Prescription of these agents and follow-up of treatment should be undertaken only by a consultant rheumatologist specialising in their use. Maintenance therapy in those who respond should be at the lowest licensed dose compatible with a continued clinical response. All patients receiving treatment with a biologic agent should, with their consent, be registered with the Biologics Registry of the British Society for Rheumatology.

Which biologic therapy would you recommend for this patient?

A13 **Treatment of this patient should be with an agent that acts on TNF-alpha.**

At the time of writing, there have been no head-to-head trials between these agents. The agents which act on TNF-alpha generally result in a better clinical response compared to the IL-1Ra, anakinra, as they reduce inflammation acutely. Anakinra has been to shown to reduce bone erosions, but it is not as effective in the acute inflammatory phase. Until comparative data are produced, the anti-TNF therapies will tend to be used first-line, with anakinra reserved as a second-line choice.

The choice of anti-TNF therapy is currently governed by many factors. These include: clinician experience; patient suitability and wishes with respect to the route of administration (e.g. can the patient manipulate a syringe); whether the patient can tolerate methotrexate or not; the facilities in the hospital (whether beds are available for day case administration of infliximab); disease profile (if there is systemic lupus erythematous overlap infliximab may be avoided). Taking all these factors into account, etanercept is a suitable option for Mrs SD, but any anti-TNF could have been prescribed.

The patient asks you how long she will remain on the etanercept. What is your answer?

A14 **Unless they suffer from side-effects that necessitate withdrawal of therapy, patients will normally remain on anti-TNF therapy until their disease becomes uncontrolled by the agent. In this event an alternative will be tried.**

There is some evidence to show that stopping long-term therapy may precipitate a flare. Some clinicians are examining dose escalation when loss of efficacy occurs. In this situation higher, unlicensed doses are used.

This may be necessary due to 'bulk' of disease (an increase in synovitis) or formation of human chimeric antibodies. This elevation in dose would only occur on an individual patient basis.

What are the long-term prospects for this patient?

A15 **Unfortunately, patients with advanced disease will normally continue to progress and symptoms will continue to get worse. There are new therapies continually being trialled, so it is possible that a patient will respond to one of these.**

Mrs SD has not yet been treated with anakinra and so this would be an option for her, although there are limited data to support its use in patients previously treated with anti-TNF agents. Further trials are needed to establish the place of anakinra in therapy. She could also be treated with other available anti-TNF therapies. Although this approach is used in practice, more research needs to be done into whether there is a place for switching to an alternative anti-TNF agent.

Acknowledgement

The authors would like to thank Dr Gaye Cunnane (formerly Senior Lecturer and Consultant in Rheumatology, Leeds General Infirmary), Dr Maya Buch (Specialist Registrar in Rheumatology, Leeds General Infirmary) and Dr Sarah Bingham (Specialist Registrar in Rheumatology, Leeds General Infirmary) for reviewing and commenting on this chapter.

Further reading

Bathron JM, Martin RW, Fleischmann RM *et al.* A comparison of etanercept and methotrexate in patients with early rheumatoid arthritis. *N Engl J Med* 2000; **343**: 1586–1593.

Bombardier C, Laine L, Reicin A *et al.* Comparison of upper gastrointestinal toxicity of rofecoxib and naproxen in patients with rheumatoid arthritis. VIGOR Study Group. *N Engl J Med* 2000; **343**: 1520–1528.

Buch M, Emery P. The aetiology and pathogenesis of rheumatoid arthritis. *Hosp Pharmacist* 2002; **9**: 5–10.

Cunnane G, Doran M, Bresnihan B. Infections and biological therapy in rheumatoid arthritis. *Best Pract Res Clin Rheumatol* 2003; **17**: 345–363.

Cohen S, Hurd E, Cush J *et al.* Treatment of rheumatoid arthritis with anakinra, a recombinant human interleukin-1 receptor antagonist, in combination with methotrexate: results of a twenty-four week, multi-center, randomised, double-blind, placebo-controlled trial. *Arthritis Rheum* 2002; **46**: 614–624.

Furst DE, Fleischmann R, Bibara C *et al.* Efficacy of adalimumab (D2E7), the first fully human anti-TNF alpha monoclonal antibody, administered to rheumatoid arthritis patients in combination with other anti-rheumatic therapy in the STAR trial. *Ann Rheum Dis* 2002; **61**(suppl. S1): 174.

Green C. New drugs in the treatment of rheumatoid arthritis. *Hosp Pharmacist* 2002; **9**: 16–19.

Kavanaugh A, Weinblatt M, Keystone E *et al.* The ARMADA trial: 12 month efficacy and safety of combination therapy with adalimumab (D2E7), the first fully human anti TNF alpha monoclonal antibody and methotrexate in patients with active rheumatoid arthritis. *Ann Rheum Dis* 2002; **61**(suppl. 1): 168.

Kumar P, Clark M. *Clinical Medicine*, 5th edn. Saunders, Philadelphia, PA, 2002.

Maini R, St Clair EW, Breedveld F. Infliximab (chimeric anti-tumour necrosis factor alpha monoclonal antibody) versus placebo in rheumatoid arthritis patients receiving concomitant methotrexate: a randomised phase III trial. ATTRACT Study Group. *Lancet* 1999; **354**: 1932–1939.

Moreland LW, Baumgartner SW, Schiff MH *et al.* Treatment of rheumatoid arthritis with recombinant human tumor necrosis factor receptor (p75)–Fc fusion protein. *N Engl J Med* 1997; **337**: 141–147.

National Institute for Clinical Excellence. *Guidance on the Use of Cyclooxygenase (Cox) II Selective Inhibitors, Celecoxib, Rofecoxib, Meloxicam and Etodolac for Osteoarthritis And Rheumatoid Arthritis*. NICE, London, 2001.

National Institute for Clinical Excellence. *Guidance on the Use of Etanercept and Infliximab for the Treatment of Rheumatoid Arthritis*. NICE, London, 2002.

Parkinson S, Alldred A. Drug regimens for rheumatoid arthritis. *Hosp Pharmacist* 2002; **9**: 11–15.

Rheumatology (various authors). *Medicine* 2002; **8/9**: 1–86.

Royal College of Physicians. *Working Party Report on Osteoporosis – Clinical Guidelines for Prevention and Treatment*. Royal College of Physicians, London, 1999 and update 2003.

Schiff M, Furst DE, Strand V *et al.* A randomised controlled safety trial of adalimumab (D2E7), a fully human anti-TNF alpha monoclonal antibody, given to RA patients in combination with standard rheumatological care: STAR (Safety Trial of adalimumab in rheumatoid arthritis) Trial. *Ann Rheum Dis* 2002; **61**(suppl. 1): 169.

Weinblatt ME, Kremer JM, Bankhurst AD *et al.* A trial of etanercept, a recombinant tumor necrosis factor receptor:Fc fusion protein, in patients with rheumatoid arthritis receiving methotrexate. *N Engl J Med* 1999; **340**: 253–259.

27

Osteoporosis

Jonathan Mason

Day 1 76-year-old Mrs MG attended A & E following a fall at her residential home, where she had been living for the past two years. She had a five-year history of becoming increasingly dependent on others to assist with activities of daily living and had shown signs of developing dementia, with increasing memory loss and wandering, for which her GP had prescribed haloperidol 500 micrograms twice daily. Three years earlier, Mrs MG had been diagnosed as suffering from polymyalgia rheumatica for which she had been initially prescribed prednisolone orally 10 mg daily. This had been reduced to 5 mg daily after one year. She had now been taking this dose for two years. She had been a heavy smoker, smoking some 20–30 cigarettes per day, but had stopped completely nearly 10 years earlier. She only drank alcohol socially.

Her drug history on admission was as follows:

- Prednisolone 5 mg orally daily
- Nitrazepam 5 mg orally every night
- Haloperidol 500 micrograms orally twice daily

Q1 What is the appropriate dose of prednisolone for the treatment of polymyalgia rheumatica?

On examination, Mrs MG was found to be a small-framed lady, 1.62 m tall and weighing 49 kg. Blood biochemistry showed that her urea and electrolyte levels were normal. X-ray revealed a fracture to the right radius (Colle's fracture). She was discharged with a plaster cast and a prescription for co-codamol 30/500 capsules one or two to be taken every four to six hours. She was referred to the multidisciplinary falls clinic.

Q2 What factors might have contributed to her fall?
Q3 Do you agree with the prescribing of co-codamol 30/500 capsules for analgesia?

Q4   What risk factors does Mrs MG have for osteoporosis?
Q5   How could the diagnosis of osteoporosis be confirmed?

Day 5   Mrs MG attended the multidisciplinary falls clinic at the local hospital out-patient department for a full assessment, which included a review of her medication by a pharmacist. An x-ray was taken of her lower spine, which revealed that she had previously suffered three crush fractures of lumbar vertebrae.

Q6   What is the purpose of a falls clinic?
Q7   Outline the key points of a pharmaceutical care plan for Mrs MG.
Q8   What changes would you make to her existing therapy?
Q9   What drug treatment options can be considered for her osteoporosis?
Q10 Which would you recommend for this patient and why?
Q11 What non-pharmaceutical interventions should be recommended for Mrs MG?

Mrs MG was started on alendronate 10 mg tablets and Adcal-D3 (calcium and vitamin D tablets). The falls clinic pharmacist stopped the haloperidol and switched the co-codamol to separate paracetamol and codeine tablets. It was agreed that she would be seen at a pharmacist-run sleep clinic in her local surgery. A letter on her proposed management plan was sent to her GP.

   Her medication at this time was:

- Prednisolone enteric-coated tablets 5 mg daily
- Nitrazepam tablets 5 mg every night
- Paracetamol tablets 500 mg one or two every four to six hours (up to eight tablets in 24 h)
- Codeine tablets 30 mg one every four hours if required
- Alendronate tablets 10 mg daily
- Adcal-D3 tablets two daily

Q12 What key points should Mrs MG and her carers be counselled on with regard to her osteoporosis?

Day 14   Mrs MG attended the sleep clinic. The pharmacist stopped the nitrazepam, and provided her carers with advice about sleep hygiene and how to manage her wandering if it became a problem.

   A prescription was issued for:

- Temazepam tablets 10 mg one every night if required

Month 3   Mrs MG was seen again in the falls clinic. Her carers reported that she was sleeping well and her wandering was manageable during the day, but that she was experiencing problems swallowing both the alendronate and the calcium tablets.

Q13 What changes would you recommend to her therapy?
Q14 How long should treatment for osteoporosis be continued?
Q15 How effective is treatment with a bisphosphonate and/or calcium and vitamin D at reducing the risk of fractures?

What is the appropriate dose of prednisolone for treatment of polymyalgia rheumatica?

A1 **Prednisolone should be started at a dose of 15 mg daily, which should then be gradually reduced to the minimum dose that controls symptoms.**

Polymyalgia rheumatica (PMR) is a chronic inflammatory soft-tissue condition, which is characterised by persistent pain and stiffness of the neck, shoulders and pelvis. It is frequently accompanied by systemic features and inflammatory markers [erythrocyte sedimentation rate (ESR), C-reactive protein (CRP) and plasma viscosity] are typically elevated. PMR is rare under the age of 60 (mean age of onset is 70 years) and the condition is three times more common in women than in men.

Corticosteroid therapy is indicated in all cases and should be started as soon as the diagnosis of PMR is suspected. A dramatic symptomatic response to prednisolone 15 mg daily would be expected, usually within two to four days, whilst inflammatory markers generally normalise over two weeks. No advantage has been shown for using starting doses of prednisolone greater than 15 mg daily and higher doses significantly increase adverse effects.

Corticosteroid doses should then be reduced gradually, taking into account clinical symptoms and inflammatory markers. The patient's symptoms are often a more reliable guide to disease activity than ESR, since it may be normal when the disease is active, and raised when the disease is quiescent.

The median duration of treatment is approximately two years, but may be much longer, with up to 40% of patients still requiring corticosteroid treatment at four years. Neither severity of symptoms nor elevation of inflammatory markers at onset can predict the duration of treatment required. Relapse is common after stopping or reducing the dose of prednisolone, occurring in up to 60% of people, but the relapse usually responds rapidly to an increase in corticosteroid dose. Relapse is most likely in the first 18 months of treatment and within a year of stopping treatment.

What factors might have contributed to her fall?

A2 **A host of factors might have contributed to Mrs MG's fall including psychoactive drug therapy (nitrazepam and haloperidol), confusion, problems with balance and environmental factors within the home.**

There are a number of risk factors for falls in older people. These include:

(a)   Underlying medical conditions, e.g. transient ischaemic attacks or stroke, heart disease, dementia.
(b)   Physical inactivity, which leads to weak muscles and poor balance.
(c)   Poor nutritional status.
(d)   Medication, e.g. antidepressants, hypnotics, sedatives, diuretics, laxatives.
(e)   Sensory disturbance, particularly problems with vision or hearing.
(f)   Environmental hazards such as loose carpets, poor lighting, unsafe stairways, rugs on polished floors, ill-fitting shoes or slippers.

Do you agree with the prescribing of co-codamol 30/500 capsules for analgesia?

A3   **No. Fixed combination analgesics are not recommended since they do not provide flexibility in dosage and can lead to opioid overdose, particularly in older people like Mrs MG who generally require lower doses of opioids.**

Compound analgesic preparations containing a simple analgesic, such as paracetamol, and an opioid, such as codeine, are not generally recommended since there is reduced scope for titration of the individual components to manage pain of varying intensity effectively.

Co-codamol 30/500 is preferable to co-codamol 8/500, since the higher codeine preparation does at least provide a full dose of the opioid; however, older people are particularly susceptible to opioid side-effects. Using co-codamol 30/500 in an older person may result in the patient receiving either too high a dose of codeine, leading to opioid side-effects, particularly constipation, or too low a dose of paracetamol to provide effective analgesia.

What risk factors does Mrs MG have for osteoporosis?

A4   **Mrs MG has a number of risk factors for osteoporosis, including:**

   (a)   Chronic steroid use.

   (b)   Female sex.

   (c)   Increased age.

   (d)   White race.

(e) **Low weight and body mass index (BMI).**

(f) **Decreased mobility.**

(g) **Oestrogen deficiency.**

(h) **Smoking history.**

(i) **Being housebound, with a consequent vitamin D deficiency.**

Long-term corticosteroid therapy, defined as prednisolone 7.5 mg or more daily for longer than 3 months, increases the risk of osteoporosis through a variety of mechanisms:

(a) Decreased gastrointestinal absorption of calcium and increased urinary calcium excretion.

(b) Effects on sex hormones, including decreased adrenal androgens, decreased oestrogen and decreased testosterone, leading to increased osteoclast activity and bone resorption.

(c) Decreased osteoblast activity, leading to decreased bone formation.

(d) Decreased muscle mass.

(e) Effects on growth hormones and growth factors.

Most guidelines recommend prophylaxis for osteoporosis for anyone taking, or planned to be taking, more than 7.5 mg prednisolone (or equivalent) daily for longer than 3 months.

Patient demographics such as female sex, increased age (leading to age-related reduction in vitamin D levels), white race, low weight and low BMI (Mrs MG's BMI is less than 19 kg/m^2) and decreased mobility (on feet for less than four hours per day) are all predictors of low bone mass and consequently increase the risk of osteoporosis. Other risk factors include a strong family history of osteoporosis (particularly maternal hip fracture), personal history of low impact fractures and height loss as a result of crush fractures of the vertebrae, which may lead to kyphosis (hunched back).

A number of diseases also predispose to low bone mass, either as a result of increased bone turnover or as a result of reduced absorption of calcium and/or vitamin D. These include liver disease, thyroid disease, rheumatoid arthritis and diseases leading to malabsorption.

In women, oestrogen deficiency following the menopause results in the net rate of bone resorption exceeding the net rate of bone formation, which in turn leads to a decrease in bone mass. This effect is heightened in women who have an early (defined as aged under 45) natural or surgical menopause, women with pre-menopausal amenorrhoea for more than six months which is not due to pregnancy and women who have had a hysterectomy under the age of 45 with at least one ovary conserved, since this may affect ovarian function.

Smoking is associated with low bone mass and evidence suggests that patients who smoke have at least double the risk of hip fracture, particularly if a post-menopausal woman. Smoking may increase the risk for hip fracture through decreased weight, impaired health status and decreased neuromuscular function. It may take up to 10 years after cessation of smoking before the excess risks disappear.

Other lifestyle/dietary factors such as alcohol and caffeine intake are inconsistently associated with low bone mass.

Vitamin D and its major biologically active metabolite, 1,25-dihydroxyvitamin D, play a central role in maintaining calcium and phosphate homeostasis. Vitamin D is thus essential for skeletal health. Severe deficiency is associated with defective mineralisation resulting in rickets in children or osteomalacia in adults. Less severe deficiency leads to secondary hyperparathyroidism and increased bone turnover. These effects play an important role in age-related bone loss and osteoporotic fractures. Housebound and institutionalised people are at increased risk of vitamin D insufficiency. Natural dietary sources of vitamin D are limited and their contribution to vitamin D status assumes importance in individuals with reduced exposure to sunlight. At-risk populations include older people, housebound and institutionalised people, those who avoid exposure to sunlight and patients with intestinal, liver, renal or cardiopulmonary disease.

How could the diagnosis of osteoporosis be confirmed?

A5 **Osteoporosis is diagnosed in terms of bone mineral density (BMD). Dual x-ray absorptiometry (DXA) scanning of the hip and/or lumbar spine is the gold standard tool for BMD measurement.**

The diagnosis of osteoporosis is confirmed by DXA demonstrating low BMD. Results of DXA scans are reported as T and Z scores, which indicate the BMD as the number of standard deviations (SD) from the mean BMD for young adults and the patient's age group respectively. The T score relates to absolute fracture risk, whilst the Z score relates to the individual's risk for their age.

The World Health Organization defines osteoporosis as a BMD of 2.5 SD or more below the young adult mean value, i.e. a T score of less than, or equal to, −2.5. For every SD below the mean, the risk of fracture is approximately doubled. A score between −1.5 and −2.5 SD is indicative of osteopenia, i.e. low BMD, which is suggestive of osteoporosis, but is not diagnostic. DXA scanning of the hip is generally preferred to the spine, particularly in older people, because it is thought to give more information about cortical and trabecular bone, and is predictive for fracture risk. DXA scanning of the spine, whilst easier to perform and probably faster than for the hip, is not suitable for diagnosis in older people because of the high prevalence of arthrosis and arthritis. However, the spine is the preferred scanning site for assessment of response to treatment.

The use of BMD assessment alone has high specificity but low sensitivity. The low sensitivity means that half of all osteoporotic fractures will occur in women said not to have osteoporosis. Screening of individuals without risk factors for osteoporosis is therefore not recommended. Many guidelines have defined who should be referred for DXA scanning. It is usually recommended that mobile older patients with risk factors for osteoporosis or who have suffered a fragility fracture or one vertebral crush factor should be referred for a lateral thoraco-lumbar spinal x-ray. However, if the patient has suffered two or more vertebral crush fractures this is highly suggestive of osteoporosis and treatment for osteoporosis should be initiated, without referring for DXA scanning.

In Mrs MG's case, because she has so many risk factors and has already suffered vertebral crush fractures and a low impact fracture, DXA scanning is unnecessary and treatment for osteoporosis should be initiated.

What is the purpose of a falls clinic?

A6 **Falls clinics are designed to conduct a comprehensive review of patients with multiple needs who have had a fall and require multifactorial interventions to reduce their risk of further falls.**

Multidisciplinary falls clinics are designed to assess the needs of 'fallers', i.e. older people who have had a number of falls (usually three or more). Patients are referred following an initial assessment to determine whether the faller has single or multiple needs. If a faller has single needs then these are more appropriately addressed by the most relevant service, e.g. occupational therapy, district nurses, social services. Fallers with multiple needs are referred to a falls clinic. The multidisciplinary falls team reviews all aspects of the patient's situation, including medication, vision and hearing, nutrition, walking/gait/balance, environmental hazards, etc.

Outline the key points of a pharmaceutical care plan for Mrs MG.

A7 **The pharmaceutical care plan for Mrs MG should identify and address each of her problems. It should indicate what monitoring is necessary to ensure the desired therapeutic outcomes are achieved with the minimum of adverse effects.**

(a)   Identified problems

    (i)   Cause of fall.
    (ii)   Pain due to Colle's fracture.
    (iii)   PMR.
    (iv)   Osteoporosis and risk of further fractures.

(b)   Care plan

    (i) Review her current drug therapy to ensure that any drugs contributing to her risk of falling are discontinued or changed to drugs that reduce the risks. Other non-pharmaceutical interventions should also be implemented to reduce her risk of further falls.
    (ii) Ensure that appropriate analgesia is provided using paracetamol with or without codeine.
    (iii) Review the need for the continuing use of prednisolone.
    (iv) Prescribe appropriate therapy for her osteoporosis.
    (v) Counsel Mrs MG and her carers on all aspects of her drug therapy, including reasons for changes.
    (vi) Monitoring (for efficacy and side-effects).
    (vii) Monitor for insomnia and behavioural problems.
    (viii) Pain relief. Ensure that paracetamol and codeine provide sufficient analgesia. If necessary increase the dose of codeine or switch to a different opioid. Monitor side-effects of codeine, particularly constipation.
    (ix) Monitor symptoms of PMR and inflammatory markers (ESR, CRP and plasma viscosity).
    (x) Monitor plasma calcium before treatment and at regular intervals thereafter, and whenever nausea or vomiting occurs.
    (xi) Ensure she is referred for DXA scanning of the spine every two years.

What changes would you make to her existing therapy?

A8 **The following changes should be made to Mrs MG's medication:**

   (a) Switch night sedation from nitrazepam to temazepam.

   (b) Stop haloperidol therapy.

   (c) Switch co-codamol 30/500 to separate paracetamol 500 mg and codeine 30 mg formulations.

   (d) Review the use of prednisolone as Mrs MG is now three years post-diagnosis of PMR.

(a) Night Sedation. Benzodiazepines increase the risk of falls, particularly in older people and even more so when used in combination with other psychotropic agents. Benzodiazepines with a longer plasma half-life, such as nitrazepam, are more problematic than those with shorter half-lives, such as temazepam. The benzodiazepines with longer half-lives tend to cause a 'hangover' effect, i.e. their sedative effects persist into the following day.

   It is advisable to switch patients from longer-acting benzodiazepines to a shorter-acting alternative. A number of studies have shown that it is relatively easy to switch patients from nitrazepam to temazepam. Some studies have shown that a third of patients taking nitrazepam long-term can just stop taking it, a third can be switched directly to temazepam, whilst the remaining third will need more intensive support.

(b) Haloperidol. Antipsychotics such as haloperidol have frequently been used to control behavioural disturbances in patients with dementia, even though there is little evidence that they work in such patients. Use of antipsychotics in nursing and residential home patients with dementia is frequently inappropriate, since some behavioural disturbances occur more frequently in people taking antipsychotics, and less than 20% of behavioural problems associated with dementia respond to antipsychotics. A number of studies have found an association between the use of psychotropic drugs and falls, restlessness, wandering and urinary incontinence. In addition, the use of antipsychotics in dementia may increase the rate of cognitive decline, reduce inhibitions, and increase wandering.

   In the USA, the *Nursing Home Reform Amendments* – a component of the *Omnibus Budget Reconciliation Act 1987* (OBRA '87) which came into effect in 1990 – were enacted in an attempt to decrease the unnecessary use of antipsychotics in nursing home residents. The OBRA '87 recommendations specify that antipsychotics should only be used where patients exhibit psychotic symptoms and not for indications such as anxiety, wandering and insomnia. The OBRA '87 guidelines require documentary evidence that other, non-pharmacological methods have been tried and have failed to control symptoms, and reasons for exceeding recommended doses. Following the implementation of the OBRA '87 guidelines there has been a reduction in the use of antipsychotics of between a quarter and a third in US nursing homes with no concomitant increase in prescribing of other psychotropic drugs.

In Mrs MG's case it would be appropriate to just stop the haloperidol and then monitor her behaviour. Withdrawal of antipsychotics has been shown to improve mental state and attention span, and is not associated with an increase in problem behaviour. Mrs MG's carers should be given advice on how to cope with problem behaviour. This could include:

(i)   Create a calm, predictable environment.
(ii) Take steps to avoid boredom and loneliness.
(iii) Ensure a regular routine, with no unnecessary rules and restrictions.
(iv) Review physical environment, paying attention to room temperature, background noise, lighting, etc.
(v)   If patients are prone to wandering, ensure they have plenty of opportunity for physical exercise and are encouraged to take walks.
(vi) Warm milky drinks can help induce sleep.

Carers should record details of problem behaviour as follows: date and time of incident; who recorded it; description, including the context of the behaviour; consequences, including how staff responded to the behaviour; and what was thought to trigger the behaviour.

(c)   Analgesia. As discussed in Answer 3, co-codamol 30/500 does not provide flexibility in analgesic dosage and can lead to opioid overdose. Her prescription should be switched to paracetamol 500 mg tablets one or two up to four times a day, plus codeine 30 mg every four hours only if required.

(d)   Steroid. Since Mrs MG has been taking prednisolone for over three years it would be worth considering a reduction in dose with a view to stopping corticosteroid therapy completely.

A suitable dose regimen for Mrs MG would be to reduce her dose to prednisolone 2.5 mg daily and then monitor her condition closely for several months for signs of a flare-up. If she suffers a relapse in symptoms, her dose of prednisolone should be increased again. If she does not, further reduction or withdrawal could be considered; however, it should be recognised that it may not be possible to completely withdraw corticosteroid treatment.

What drug treatment options can be considered for her osteoporosis?

A9   **A number of treatment options are available:**

(a)   **Hormone replacement therapy (HRT) (either unopposed or with progestogen).**

(b)   **Selective oestrogen receptor modulator (SERM).**

(c)   **Bisphosphonates, such as cyclic etidronate, alendronate and risedronate.**

(d)   **Calcitonin.**

(e)   **Vitamin D derivatives (alfacalcidol and calcitriol).**

(f)   **Calcium supplementation.**

(g)   **Calcium and vitamin D supplementation.**

HRT with oestrogen prevents bone loss and may increase BMD in post-menopausal women. HRT has been shown to reduce the risk of vertebral fractures. It may also have some effect at reducing the risk of non-vertebral fractures, e.g. observational data support a protective effect against hip fracture. There is also some evidence that HRT helps prevent corticosteroid-induced osteoporosis. There appears to be no difference in efficacy between the different formulations; however, the bone protective effect is probably dose related. The usual recommended dosages are 0.625 mg oral conjugated oestrogen daily, 2 mg oral estradiol daily or 50 micrograms transdermal estradiol daily. Lower dosages may also pre-serve bone mass and may be an option in women intolerant of higher dosages. There is no clear evidence concerning either the optimal age for initiation or for duration of therapy. However, most evidence suggests that bone-conserving effects are greatest if HRT is initiated at menopause and continued for up to 10 years, but even this may have little residual effect on BMD among women over 75 years of age, who have the highest risk of fracture.

The choice of HRT as the first-line primary preventative strategy for osteoporosis in post-menopausal women needs to be weighed against the potential risks of long-term HRT. The results of several long-term studies into the risks and benefits of HRT indicate that for long-term treatment with oestrogen the risks of adverse outcomes such as breast cancer and stroke probably outweigh the benefits in terms of prevention of bone loss and fractures. These studies suggest that HRT should not be used purely for prevention of osteoporosis.

Whilst HRT may be appropriate in some older women, the monthly withdrawal bleeds and oestrogenic and/or progestogenic adverse effects generally make it difficult to tolerate in women over the age of 75 years.

Tibolone, which has both oestrogenic and progestogenic effects is licensed for prophylaxis of osteoporosis. However, the benefits of tibolone on BMD have not been demonstrated and there is no evidence that it prevents fractures.

Raloxifene is a SERM which acts as an oestrogen agonist in bone and in the cardiovascular system, and an oestrogen antagonist in the endometrium and breast. Raloxifene prevents bone loss in post-menopausal women, and is licensed for the treatment and prevention of post-menopausal osteoporosis. It prevents bone loss in the lumbar spine and proximal femur. However, whilst raloxifene (in combination with calcium and vitamin D) has been shown to reduce the risk of vertebral fracture, it has not been shown to reduce the risk of non-vertebral and hip fractures. Raloxifene could be considered if HRT or a bisphosphonate is inappropriate or not tolerated; however, its place in the treatment of women beyond 10 years of the menopause is uncertain.

The bisphosphonates [etidronate (taken on a cyclical basis), alendronate and risedronate] are all licensed for the prevention and treatment of osteoporosis. In combination with calcium and vitamin D they prevent bone loss and reduce the risk of osteoporotic fractures. However, the evidence for hip protection is strongest for alendronate and risedronate, particularly in people with established osteoporosis (i.e. T score < -2.5 SD), so these drugs are preferred if hip protection is particularly important.

Alendronate is licensed for the prevention of post-menopausal osteoporosis at a dose of 5 mg daily, treatment of osteoporosis in both post-menopausal women and men at a dose of 10 mg daily, and for the prevention and treatment of corticosteroid-induced osteoporosis. For the latter indication, the dose is 5 mg daily for all categories of patients except post-menopausal women not receiving HRT, for whom the dose is 10 mg daily. Risedronate is licensed for the prevention and treatment of post-menopausal osteoporosis, including corticosteroid-induced osteoporosis, at a dose of 5 mg daily. Etidronate is licensed for treatment of osteoporosis, prevention of bone loss in post-menopausal women, and for the prevention and treatment of corticosteroid-induced osteoporosis. It is taken in 90-day cycles as follows, 400 mg etidronate daily for 14 days followed by 1.25 g calcium carbonate (500 mg elemental calcium) daily for 76 days.

Calcitonin (salmon), in both injectable form (for subcutaneous or intramuscular injection) and as nasal spray, is licensed for the treatment of post-menopausal osteoporosis in combination with calcium and vitamin D supplementation. The efficacy of calcitonin for fracture prevention in corticosteroid-induced osteoporosis remains to be established. It appears to preserve bone mass in the first year of corticosteroid therapy at the lumbar spine, but not at the femoral neck. A Cochrane Review suggests that the protective effect on bone mass may be greater for patients who have been taking corticosteroids for more than three months.

Calcitriol (1,25-dihydroxycholecalciferol), the major active metabolite of vitamin D, is also licensed for the treatment of post-menopausal osteoporosis. Studies of calcitriol on bone loss and fractures have produced conflicting results. It seems to protect against vertebral fracture and is effective in reducing the incidence of vertebral deformity, but it is not known whether it protects against hip fracture. Calcitriol may be useful in younger people, especially women of child-bearing age, in whom bisphosphonates should be used with extreme caution, but there is a lack of data in older men and women. Similarly, alfacalcidol (1-alpha-hydroxycholecalciferol) has been shown to prevent corticosteroid-induced bone loss from the lumbar spine, but it is not licensed for this indication.

Calcium supplements alone may reduce the rate of bone loss in post-menopausal women with osteoporosis and reduce the risk of vertebral fracture, and there may be some effect on non-vertebral and hip fracture risk; however, calcium supplementation alone is less effective than other agents, and is not generally recommended. Calcium supplements should usually be used in combination with other bone protective agents.

Historically, calcium and vitamin D supplements have been regarded as adjuncts to treatment. However, recent evidence from large trials indicates that calcium and vitamin D supplements (providing 800 units vitamin D and 1 g elemental calcium) significantly reduce the risk of both hip and non-vertebral fracture, and may even reduce the risk of falling in older people. It is unclear whether the reduction in risk is due to vitamin D, calcium or the combination of both. Calcium and vitamin D supplementation should be considered as first-line monotherapy prophylaxis for frail elderly, older people in nursing and residential homes and those who are housebound. Calcium and vitamin D should also be used as an adjunct to treatment for those with established osteoporosis.

Which would you recommend for this patient and why?

A10 **Mrs MG should be prescribed a bisphosphonate together with calcium and vitamin D supplementation. Mrs MG has already suffered vertebral crush fractures, a low impact non-vertebral fracture and has a number of other factors putting her at high risk of osteoporosis.**

As discussed above, alendronate or risedronate plus calcium and vitamin D have been shown to prevent bone loss and reduce the risk of osteoporotic fractures at all sites in post-menopausal women. This combination offers the best protection for a woman of Mrs MG's age and fracture history.

What non-pharmaceutical interventions should be recommended for Mrs MG?

A11 **A number of non-pharmaceutical interventions should be recommended. These include: the use of external hip protectors, ensuring adequate nutrition (especially with calcium and vitamin D), increased exercise and modifications to the home environment.**

External hip protectors consist of plastic shields or foam pads, which are kept in place by pockets within specifically designed underwear. They are designed to divert a direct impact away from the greater trochanter during a fall from standing height. At impact the protector transfers released energy to soft tissue and muscles anterior and posterior to the femoral bone. Studies into the effect of hip protectors on hip fractures have shown that hip protectors significantly reduce the risk of hip fractures. Indeed, in studies in which there were hip fractures in the hip protector group, none of the people who suffered a hip fracture were wearing their hip protectors at the time. Other benefits to wearing hip protectors include the fact that they reduce the patient's fear of falling and increase their confidence in participating in exercise and completing activities of daily living.

The main problem with hip protectors is that compliance is generally poor. Studies into compliance with use of hip protectors indicate that only about 50% of patients wear them when they are first issued and compliance rates drop to 25–30% within six months. Daytime compliance rates are generally better than night-time rates. By their very nature, hip protectors are bulky and many wearers stop using them because they find them uncomfortable, they restrict mobility or they cause practical problems, such as incontinence. Causes of discomfort include warmth, being too tight fitting and a feeling that the shells are too hard. Compliance can be improved if carers are enthusiastic about the use of hip protectors and problems with incontinence can easily be overcome by the use of incontinence pads.

At present, hip protectors are not available on NHS prescription, but they can be purchased by the patient or their carers, or may be provided by a hospital or falls clinic.

As discussed earlier, bone loss is influenced by a number of modifiable lifestyle factors, including diet, exercise, smoking, and alcohol consumption. Although it is uncertain what benefit people with established osteoporosis gain from lifestyle changes, in Mrs MG's case it would be sensible to encourage an increase in her dietary calcium and vitamin D.

Sources of dietary calcium include: milk (200 mL provides approximately 250 mg elemental calcium) and other dairy products (e.g. 30 g cheddar cheese provides approximately 200 mg calcium); bread; green vegetables, particularly spring greens, broccoli and spinach; nuts, particularly brazil nuts and almonds; and tofu (120 g provides 1776 mg calcium). Dietary sources of vitamin D include margarine, oily fish (herring, sardines), cod liver oil and eggs.

Patients with osteoporosis should also be encouraged to increase their exercise levels. Although exercise has not been consistently shown to improve bone mass, it does improve general well-being, muscle strength and postural stability. Physiotherapists working as part of a multidisciplinary falls team can provide a programme of muscle strengthening and balance retraining exercises. Exercise programmes prescribed for fallers generally include elements designed to reduce the risks of injury. So, whilst such exercises may not prevent the person from falling, the faller knows how to fall more safely.

Finally, Mrs MG's home environment should be assessed to identify potential hazards and to consider measures to reduce the risk of falls. This ideally involves a combined medical and social services assessment. One of the key components of a falls clinic is to assess the patient's home environment focusing on issues such as provision of night-lights in hallways and bathrooms; provision of footwear with non-slip soles; removal of rugs or the placing of non-slip mats under rugs; the need to ensure that bath, shower and toilet areas are equipped with adequate grab bars, and that stairway railings are sturdy.

What key points should Mrs MG and her carers be counselled on with regard to her osteoporosis?

A12 **Mrs MG and her carers should be counselled on:**

(a) **The importance of regular treatment.**

(b) **How to take alendronate.**

(c) **Diet and exercise.**

(d) **The need to reduce her night-time sedation regimen.**

(e) **Coping strategies for wandering.**

(f) **The benefits of hip protectors.**

Because alendronate can cause oesophageal reactions, the tablets should be taken with a full glass of water on an empty stomach, at least 30 minutes before other drinks and/or breakfast (and any other oral medication). Mrs MG should sit upright or stand for at least 30 minutes and should not lie down until after breakfast. The tablets should not be taken at bedtime or before rising.

What changes would you recommend to her therapy?

A13 **Mrs MG's prescription should be switched to the 70 mg once weekly alendronate formulation and a soluble calcium and vitamin D formulation.**

Alendronate may cause oesophageal reactions (oesophagitis, ulceration, strictures or erosions). These problems can be reduced by using the 70 mg once a week formulation, which is licensed for the treatment of post-menopausal osteoporosis and achieves similar increases in bone density to the 10 mg daily formulation. A less frequent dosing schedule will also help Mrs MG cope with her difficulties around taking a tablet formulation.

Effervescent granule formulations of calcium and vitamin D are available which provide calcium and the recommended amount of vitamin D per sachet.

How long should treatment for osteoporosis be continued?

A14 **The optimal duration of bisphosphonate therapy for osteoporosis has not been established. Calcium and vitamin D should be continued long-term.**

The optimal duration of bisphosphonate therapy for osteoporosis has not been established, because most of the trials have been for less than four years. The best approach to long-term management is to perform a DXA scan on Mrs MG every two years. If her *T* score is greater than –2.5 SD (i.e. indicative of osteopenia) it would be reasonable to consider stopping the bisphosphonate therapy, since bisphosphonates are less beneficial in patients with osteopenia. Calcium and vitamin D therapy should, however, be continued.

How effective is treatment with a bisphosphonate and/or calcium and vitamin D at reducing the risk of fractures?

A15 **Both alendronate and risedronate significantly reduce the risk of osteoporotic fractures at all sites in post-menopausal women. The evidence for efficacy of etidronate is less substantial. Calcium and vitamin D significantly reduce the risks of osteoporotic fractures at all sites in older people (over 65 years of age).**

With regard to corticosteroid-induced osteoporosis, the bisphosphonates have been shown to prevent and treat corticosteroid-induced bone loss, while calcium and vitamin D has been shown to prevent bone loss in patients treated with corticosteroids; however, there is a lack of evidence for these agents' efficacy with respect to fracture prevention.

A number of clinical trials have shown that alendronate prevents osteoporotic fractures in post-menopausal women. For non-vertebral fractures, the absolute risk reductions (ARRs) ranged from 1.5 to 6.5%; whilst for vertebral fractures, the ARR ranged from 1.6 to 6.8%.

However, the trials were of different duration (1–4.25 years) and the rate of fractures in the placebo groups varied between trials (from 3.1 to 4.9% for non-vertebral and from 0.8 to 4.8% for vertebral). Thus the standardised numbers needed to treat (NNTs) for three years (adjusted to a baseline risk of 4%) ranged from 17.3 to 75.3 for non-vertebral fractures and from 16.5 to 18.6 for vertebral fractures.

Risedronate has also been shown to prevent osteoporotic fractures in post-menopausal women. For non-vertebral fractures the ARRs ranged from 1.8 to 5.8% whilst for vertebral fractures the ARRs ranged from 3.9 to 8.8%. Again the trials were of different duration (2.3–3 years) and the rate of fractures in the placebo groups varied between trials (from 2.1 to 7.0% for non-vertebral and from 3.8 to 7.3% for vertebral). For rise-dronate, the standardised NNTs for three years (adjusted to a baseline risk of 4%) ranged from 17.7 to 39.9 for non-vertebral fractures and from 20.6 to 24.2 for vertebral fractures.

A recent Cochrane Review of the use of etidronate for treating and preventing post-menopausal osteoporosis concluded that while etidro-nate increases BMD in lumbar spine and femoral neck, and reduces risk of vertebral fractures, its effects on non-vertebral and hip fractures are uncertain. However, a recent large observational study suggested that etidronate reduces the risk of fractures at all sites.

In a large trial in relatively healthy mobile older women (mean age 84) living in nursing homes, treatment with calcium and vitamin D resulted in a 4% absolute reduction in hip fracture and a 7% reduction in any fracture over three years (NNTs of 25 and 14 respectively). In another trial in community-dwelling older people (both men and women aged over 65) treatment with calcium and vitamin D resulted in a significant reduction in non-vertebral fractures (NNT of 14 over three years).

Further reading

Anon. Raloxifene to prevent postmenopausal osteoporosis. *Drug Ther Bull* 1999; **37**, 33–36.

Black DM, Cummings SR, Karpf DB *et al.* Randomised trial of effect of alendronate on risk of fracture in women with existing vertebral frac-tures. Fracture Intervention Trial Research Group. *Lancet* 1996; **348**: 1535–1541.

Black DM, Thompson DE, Bauer DC *et al.* Fracture risk reduction with alendronate in women with osteoporosis: the Fracture Intervention Trial. FIT Research Group. *J Clin Endocrinol Metab* 2000; **85**: 4118–4124.

Chapuy MC, Arlot ME, Delmans PD *et al.* Effect of calcium and cholecalciferol treatment for three years on hip fractures in elderly women. *Br Med J* 1994; **308**: 1081–1082.

Compston, J.E. Vitamin D deficiency: time for action. *Br Med J* 1998; **317**: 1466–1467.

Cranney A, Welch V, Adachi JD *et al*. Calcitonin for preventing and treating corticosteroid-induced osteoporosis (Cochrane Review). In: *The Cochrane Library 2*. Update Software. Oxford, 2003.

Cranney A, Welch V, Adachi JD *et al*. Etidronate for treating and preventing postmenopausal osteoporosis (Cochrane Review). In: *The Cochrane Library 2*. Update Software. Oxford, 2003.

Cryer C, Knox A, Martin D *et al*. Hip protector compliance among older people living in residential care homes. *Injury Prevent* 2002; **8**: 202–206.

Cummings SR, Black DM, Thompson DE *et al*. Effect of alendronate on risk of fracture in women with low bone density but without vertebral fractures: results from the Fracture Intervention Trial. *J Am Med Assoc* 1998; **280**: 2077–2082.

Grady D, Cummings SR. Postmenopausal hormone therapy for prevention of fractures. How good is the evidence? *J Am Med Assoc* 2001; **285**: 2909–2910.

Dawson-Hughes B, Harris SS, Krall EA *et al*. Effect of calcium and vitamin D supplementation on bone density in men and women 65 years of age or older. *N Engl J Med* 1997; **337**: 670–676.

Department of Health. *National Service Framework for Older People*. Department of Health, London, 2000.

Felson DT, Zhang Y, Hannan MT *et al*. The effect of postmenopausal estrogen therapy on bone density in elderly women. *N Engl J Med* 1993; **329**: 1141–1146.

Gillespie WJ, Avenell A, Henry DA *et al*. Vitamin D and vitamin D analogues for preventing fractures associated with involutional and postmenopausal osteoporosis (Cochrane Review). In: *The Cochrane Library 2*. Update Software. Oxford, 2003.

Harris ST, Watts NB, Genant HK *et al*. Effects of risedronate treatment on vertebral and non-vertebral fractures in women with postmenopausal osteoporosis: a randomised controlled trial. Vertebral Efficacy with Risedronate Therapy (VERT) Study Group. *J Am Med Assoc* 1999; **282**: 1344–1352.

Homik J, Cranney A, Shea B *et al*. Bisphosphonates for steroid-induced osteoporosis (Cochrane Review). In: *The Cochrane Library 2*. Update Software. Oxford, 2003.

Homik J, Suarez-Almazor ME, Shea B *et al*. Calcium and vitamin D for corticosteroid-induced osteoporosis (Cochrane Review). In: *The Cochrane Library 2*. Update Software. Oxford, 2003.

McClung MR, Geusens P, Miller PD *et al*. Effect of risedronate on the risk of hip fracture in elderly women. Hip Intervention Programme Study Group. *N Eng J Med* 2001; **344**: 333–340.

NIH Consensus Development Panel on Osteoporosis Prevention, Diagnosis and Therapy. Osteoporosis Prevention, Diagnosis and Therapy. *J Am Med Assoc* 2001; **285**: 785–795.

Pols HA, Felsenberg D, Hanley DA *et al.* Multinational, placebo-controlled, randomised trial of the effects of alendronate on bone density and fracture risk in postmenopausal women with low bone mass: results of the FOSIT study. FOSAMAX International Trial Study Group. *Osteoporosis Int* 1999; **9**: 461–468.

Reginster J, Minne HW, Sorenson OH *et al.* Randomised trial of the effects of risedronate on vertebral fractures in women with established post-menopausal osteoporosis. Vertebral Efficacy with Risedronate Therapy (VERT) Study Group. *Osteoporosis Int* 2000; **11**: 83–91.

Royal College of Physicians. *Osteoporosis: Clinical Guidelines for Prevention and Treatment.* Royal College of Physicians, London, 1999.

Royal College of Physicians. *Osteoporosis: Clinical Guidelines for Prevention and Treatment. Update on Pharmacological Interventions and an Algorithm for Management.* Royal College of Physicians, London, 2000.

Woolf AD, Akesson K. Preventing fractures in elderly people. *Br Med J* 2003; **327**: 89–95.

28

Anticoagulant therapy

Christopher Acomb and Peter A Taylor

Case study and questions

Day 1 Mr WS, a 52-year-old 65 kg overlooker in the local wool mill, was referred into hospital by his GP with a red, swollen left leg. He said that he had not knocked his leg but that 'it had just come up during the night'. He had taken some painkillers before going to his GP.

His past medical history revealed that he had been started on co-amilozide 5/50 tablets (amiloride hydrochloride 5 mg, hydrochloro-thiazide 50 mg) six months earlier for mild breathlessness on exertion. He had been treated for epilepsy in the past, but had not had any fits for over five years and was not currently taking any medication for this. He had been thinking of going back to his GP because he had recently become more breathless, particularly at night.

On examination, Mr WS was found to be short of breath with a regular pulse and had a raised jugular venous pressure. His left calf was inflamed and painful to the touch. When measured, his calf circum-ferences were: left leg 39.5 cm, right leg 38 cm. His left thigh was also swollen. He was diagnosed as having a left deep-vein thrombosis (DVT) and mild left ventricular failure.

Mr WS was prescribed:

- Furosemide 40 mg orally each morning
- Amiloride 5 mg orally each morning
- Warfarin, loading dose to be given over three days
- Tinzaparin 14 000 units sub-cutaneously once a day

Q1 Why does Mr WS need both low-molecular-weight heparin and warfarin therapy?

Q2 What laboratory indexes would you check before starting oral anticoagulant therapy?

Q3 Was the dose of low-molecular-weight heparin prescribed for Mr WS appropriate?

Q4 How is the low-molecular-weight heparin treatment monitored in the laboratory?

Q5 Is there a place for intravenous unfractionated heparin?

Q6 What loading dose of warfarin would you recommend for Mr WS? What factors did you take into account when making this recommendation?

Q7 How is warfarin treatment monitored in the laboratory?

Q8 Why is it important that a complete drug history is taken from Mr WS?

Q9 Outline the key elements of a pharmaceutical care plan for Mr WS.

Day 2 Mr WS was slightly less breathless, although his leg was still swollen and painful. He was prescribed ibuprofen for the pain.

Q10 What changes in drug therapy would you recommend?

Day 4 Mr WS was still a little breathless and had now developed a cough with green sputum. He was diagnosed as having a chest infection and prescribed erythromycin 500 mg orally three times a day.

His prothrombin time [reported as an international normalised ratio (INR)] was 3.5 (target range 2–3) after a loading dose of 7 mg warfarin daily for three days.

His low-molecular-weight heparin was continued at a dose of 11 600 units subcutaneously once a day and a maintenance dose of warfarin was prescribed.

Q11 How long should Mr WS's low-molecular-weight heparin therapy be continued?

Q12 What maintenance dose of warfarin would you recommend? How should his therapy be monitored after the maintenance dose is initiated?

Q13 How long should Mr WS's warfarin therapy be continued?

Day 5 Mr WS's chest infection appeared to be improving and his leg was much better.

Day 6 Mr WS continued to do well. His low-molecular-weight heparin was discontinued, however, his INR was reported as 5.4 (2–3). Adjustment to his treatment for left ventricular failure was also undertaken by reducing his diuretics and adding the angiotensin-converting enzyme inhibitor, ramipril. Blood pressure was carefully monitored during this change.

Q14 What are the possible causes of Mr WS's high INR?

Q15 How should Mr WS's high INR be managed?

Day 8   Mr WS was doing very well, with both his chest and leg much improved. His INR was 2.9 (2–3) and it was decided to discharge him.
His discharge medication comprised:

- Erythromycin 500 mg orally three times a day for one day, then stop

- Furosemide 20 mg orally daily
- Ramipril 1.25 mg orally daily
- Warfarin 1.5 mg orally daily

His GP was asked to increase the dose of ramipril as necessary, in accordance with the BNF, and to monitor urea and electrolytes.

Q16 What points would you cover when giving medication advice to Mr WS about his warfarin therapy?

Day 12   On his visit to the out-patient clinic, Mr WS's INR was found to be 2.6 (2–3) and his warfarin dose was continued at 1.5 mg orally daily for a further week.

Day 19   At Mr WS's out-patient attendance his INR was found to have fallen to 1.8 (2–3).

Q17 What are the possible causes of Mr WS's low INR?

Mr WS was prescribed warfarin 2.5 mg daily.

Day 33   Mr WS was admitted with epistaxis and haematuria. The only change in treatment was a prescription for azapropazone from his GP two days before admission. The azapropazone had been prescribed for gout.

Q18 What are the probable causes of Mr WS's problems? What action would you recommend?

Q19 What other drugs should be avoided or prescribed with caution and careful monitoring while Mr WS continues to take warfarin?

Why does Mr WS need both low-molecular-weight heparin and warfarin therapy?

A1 **Mr WS requires anticoagulant therapy to prevent the extension of the clot that has formed in his leg. Low-molecular-weight heparin therapy provides an immediate anticoagulant effect until the slower-acting oral warfarin therapy exerts its full anticoagulant activity.**

A low-molecular-weight heparin is now often used alone whilst awaiting a definitive diagnosis by Doppler ultrasound scan. Clinical symptoms and history, along with a positive or equivocal result from either plethysmography (venometry) or D-dimer testing will reduce the likelihood of an incorrect diagnosis, enabling early intervention with a low-molecular-weight heparin and the prevention of a hospital admission. A confirmatory diagnosis can then be made following a planned Doppler ultrasound scan, at which time warfarin can be introduced and the low-molecular-weight heparin stopped once warfarin has achieved therapeutic control. This form of treatment can be easily organised in the community.

Heparin and low-molecular-weight heparin form a complex with antithrombin III which, in therapeutic doses, inhibits the action of thrombin and activated factor X. Warfarin is a vitamin K analogue and prevents the formation of vitamin K-dependent clotting factors II, VII, IX and X.

Low-molecular-weight heparin acts rapidly but it must be given parenterally. The low-molecular-weight heparins have the advantage over unfractionated heparin because (for the treatment of thromboembolism) they can be given as a once-daily subcutaneous injection, whereas unfractionated heparin needs to be given as a continuous intravenous infusion. This simpler administration of low-molecular-weight heparins has led to the development of home/out-patient treatment of deep vein thrombosis and pulmonary embolism. The low-molecular-weight heparin will need to be continued for at least six days and until the warfarin is exerting a full therapeutic effect. Mr WS will be at risk of further thrombosis for a number of weeks after this first incident.

In contrast to heparin, warfarin takes three to four days to exert its full anticoagulant effect and is therefore not effective in limiting the extension of the thrombosis in the early phase. However, being orally active, it is very useful for long-term anticoagulant treatment.

What laboratory indexes would you check before starting oral anticoagulant therapy?

A2 **A pre-treatment clotting screen should be carried out. Although other indexes (such as haemoglobin level, platelet adhesiveness and liver function tests) are indicated in some patients, Mr WS's history does not suggest that these tests are warranted in his case.**

A pre-treatment clotting screen is essential to ensure that a patient has not already been anticoagulated and that organic changes, such as liver disease, have not disrupted his clotting mechanism. Either of these conditions would mean an excessive response to the initial warfarin dose, but not necessarily the heparin dose.

There are other laboratory indexes that will help make anticoagulation safer, but they are not necessary for every patient and they should only be carried out if there is evidence, either from a previous or a current medical history, that they may be abnormal. They include the following:

(a)   A haemoglobin level. A patient with anaemia may have occult bleeding which would be exacerbated by anticoagulation. A baseline haemoglobin level would also be useful to detect bleeding in the future.

(b)   A platelet level. Platelets are involved in the clotting process and thrombocytopenia would make the patient very prone to bleeding. However, platelet counts can be deceptive, as it is the ability to adhere to one another and not just the number of platelets that determines their activity. This adhesiveness is seldom checked routinely, but such a measurement would detect the antiplatelet activity of non-steroidal anti-inflammatory drugs (NSAIDs).

(c)   Liver function tests. The liver is involved in both the production of clotting factors and the metabolism of warfarin. Its normal function is therefore essential for safe anticoagulation.

Mr WS only requires his INR to be measured. Although he may have a history of taking NSAIDs ('painkillers') and there is thus a slight chance he may have had a gastrointestinal bleed, he has given no history of dyspepsia and has no obvious signs of anaemia.

Was the dose of low-molecular-weight heparin prescribed for Mr WS appropriate?

A3 The dose was rather large and should be adjusted.

The low-molecular-weight heparins used to treat thromboembolism are dosed according to body weight. Tinzaparin is dosed at 175 units/kg and so the correct dose for Mr WS is 11 375 units. A dose of 11 000 units (0.55 mL) would be appropriate, being a reasonable volume to be measured. At the time of writing all the low-molecular-weight heparins used for the treatment of thromboembolism come as pre-filled syringes. There are some small differences between the different brands of low-molecular-weight heparins, so the Summary of Product Characteristics should be consulted for specific details on dosing.

How is the low-molecular-weight heparin treatment monitored in the laboratory?

A4 The low-molecular-weight heparins differ from unfractionated heparin in that they do not require therapeutic monitoring. Low-molecular-weight heparins have little effect on APTT (activated partial thromboplastin time, the measure used to monitor unfractionated heparin). Anti-factor Xa has been used in research studies to monitor the effect of low-molecular-weight heparins, but this is not necessary for routine use. The low-molecular-weight heparins are associated with a small incidence of thrombocytopenia and so patients who remain on low-molecular-weight heparin for longer than five days should have a platelet count carried out as part of a full blood count.

Is there a place for intravenous unfractionated heparin?

A5 Dalteparin, enoxaparin and tinzaparin all have an evidence base to support their use in thromboembolism, and are all licensed for DVTs and pulmonary embolism so there is little place for intravenous unfractionated heparin at the start of thromboembolism treatment.

The low-molecular-weight heparins are easier to dose and more consistent in the degree of anticoagulation produced. The main advantage to using intravenous unfractionated heparin is that it is controllable. The relatively short half-life of unfractionated heparin means that stopping an intravenous infusion quickly results in a return to normal clotting status. Furthermore, the effect of unfractionated heparin can be reversed by using protamine. This is in contrast to the low-molecular-weight heparins that once given subcutaneously have an effect for 24 hours and are not fully reversible by protamine. Therefore when it is occasionally necessary to control carefully or stop anticoagulation rapidly, unfractionated heparins still may be used. For example, intravenous unfractionated heparin can be used when therapeutic anticoagulation is required prior to surgery, with the infusion being switched off six to eight hours prior to the procedure.

> What loading dose of warfarin would you recommend for Mr WS? What factors did you take into account when making this recommendation?

A6   **Warfarin 7 mg daily for three days. This loading dose takes into account the fact that Mr WS has left ventricular failure.**

Warfarin is highly protein-bound and has a long half-life. The administration of a loading dose thus reduces the time taken for the drug to achieve steady state.

The standard warfarin loading dose is 10 mg daily for three days. This should be reduced in the presence of conditions which may potentiate the action of warfarin. The following factors should be considered:

(a)   Age. In general, elderly patients are more sensitive to warfarin: it is recommended that a reduced loading dose is given to patients over 60 years of age.

(b)   Body weight. Given that the volume of distribution is at least partially linked to body weight, a reduced loading dose should be given to patients weighing less than 60 kg.

(c)   Plasma protein-binding capacity. This will be reduced in patients with low plasma protein levels or in those already taking drugs that are highly protein-bound. Albumin is the principal plasma protein fraction that binds warfarin.

(d)   Concurrent pathology. Some diseases, such as congestive cardiac failure, reduce the liver's ability to produce clotting factors and to metabolise warfarin effectively.

(e)   Other drugs. Although already mentioned under plasma protein-binding capacity, concurrent drug therapy can also interfere with warfarin activity in many other ways and nearly all types of drug interaction have been reported.

In Mr WS's case his loading dose should be reduced to 7 mg daily for three days on the basis that his left ventricular failure may enhance the activity of warfarin. If he had had two or more of the above factors, then his loading dose should have been reduced to 5 mg daily for three days.

It should be noted that prescribers sometimes reduce the loading dose by giving 10 mg, 5 mg and then 5 mg over the three days. The first dose (10 mg) will often produce an exaggerated response on day 4, which makes calculation of the maintenance dose difficult and can lead to doses being omitted because of the seemingly high INR.

There are a number of nomograms and methods available to initiate warfarin therapy. Certainly we favour lower loading doses, particularly for patients managed on an out-patient basis. Providing patients continue to receive adequate anticoagulation with low-molecular-weight heparin, it is better to be slow and cautious when initiating oral anticoagulation.

How is warfarin treatment monitored in the laboratory?

A7 **Warfarin activity is monitored in the laboratory by measuring the prothrombin time.**

The citrate in the blood sample is neutralised with excess calcium ions and thromboplastin is added. The time taken for the sample to clot is then known as the prothrombin time. Comparing this with a sample containing no anticoagulant will give a prothrombin time ratio.

The thromboplastin used in this test has been standardised so as to allow a patient to be controlled by any laboratory. This standardisation has resulted in the test being named the INR.

INR values in the range of 2.0–4.5 are accepted as being therapeutic, although target INRs within this range are used to cover the various indications for warfarin anticoagulation. In Mr WS's case a target range of 2.0–3.0 would be appropriate to prevent an extension of his DVT.

Why is it important that a complete drug history is taken from Mr WS?

A8 **A drug history is essential prior to starting oral anticoagulant therapy with warfarin or other coumarin derivatives because many drugs can interact with warfarin to a clinically significant extent.**

Two important facts were elicited from Mr WS's medication history. First, it was noted that Mr WS has a history of epilepsy. On questioning, he indicated that he had been taking phenytoin some three months earlier. Phenytoin and other drugs that induce warfarin metabolism may exert their effect for up to six weeks after stopping therapy. This demonstrates that not only current medication, but also any other medication taken over the previous six weeks, should be considered in an effort to reduce potential complications of warfarin treatment.

Secondly, Mr WS had referred to 'painkillers' he had taken at home. When questioned further, he said that he usually took Aspro Clear tablets, but as he had run out he had taken some of his wife's Veganin. Both of these over-the-counter products contain aspirin. This means that he should be counselled regarding their future use, as he will need to avoid aspirin and aspirin-containing products while he is taking warfarin. In addition, attention should be given to the possibility that his recent ingestion of aspirin may cause aspirin-induced low platelet activity, which may lead to bruising or other minor bleeding, despite normal INRs, or that drug-induced gastrointestinal erosions may cause major bleeding complications.

Outline the key elements of a pharmaceutical care plan for Mr WS.

A9   **This is high-risk treatment and a care plan to ensure adequate anticoagulant control is essential.**

All patients starting anticoagulant therapy should have a clear pharmaceutical care plan which ensures, wherever possible, that the patient is protected from the potential risks of treatment.

Warfarin activity monitoring should be planned, with the first significant laboratory result being reported on day 4 after introducing the drug. Thereafter, INRs should be done regularly and with a gradually increasing time interval between tests, as stability is achieved.

The care plan should include discharge arrangements and should allow time for providing medication advice to ensure he has a good understanding of the treatment and its implications, before discharge.

Mr WS will need to be followed up at the anticoagulant clinic after leaving hospital and these arrangements (e.g. when and where) along with communications with the clinic should be included in the care plan. In our own hospital these clinics are run by our pharmacists, making the organisation much simpler. We are also using Intermediate Care Centres (or peripheral clinics) to provide a more local service for patients.

The plan should also consider how to communicate with both the patient's GP and, if possible, their community pharmacist. Good communication is essential in order to reduce the risks to the patient.

What changes in drug therapy would you recommend?

A10 **Consider changing ibuprofen to paracetamol or co-codamol or co-dydramol.**

Although ibuprofen does not usually affect warfarin activity (it does not normally increase INRs), it probably should be stopped because of the small risk of gastrointestinal bleeding associated with NSAIDs. A gastro-intestinal bleed whilst on warfarin can have disastrous consequences. Furthermore, ibuprofen and other NSAIDs could exacerbate Mr WS's heart failure. Paracetamol, co-codamol and co-dydramol should not affect his warfarin activity, unlike co-proxamol, which can enhance warfarin activity.

How long should Mr WS's low-molecular-weight heparin therapy be continued?

A11 **Low-molecular-weight heparin therapy should continue until the desired effect of warfarin has been achieved.**

The INR value on day 4 is the first indication of warfarin activity and is the level from which the maintenance dose of warfarin can be calculated. Mr WS's INR is already in the therapeutic range by day 4; however, we would usually recommend continuing the low-molecular-weight heparin until day 6 as some patients can have high INRs but still have coagulation problems because an imbalance in the clotting process had occurred. This may be seen as a worsening of the DVT. It is usually desirable to overlap the low-molecular-weight heparin with warfarin at therapeutic INRs for at least 24 hours.

What maintenance dose of warfarin would you recommend? How should his therapy be monitored after the maintenance dose is initiated?

A12 **Warfarin 2.5 mg daily. INR monitoring should take place after two to three days then, depending on the results, may be carried out at increased time intervals.**

This dose is calculated using the method of Dobrzanski, which relates the maintenance dose to the cumulative loading dose over three days (in this case 21 mg, rounded down to 20 mg) and the INR achieved on the fourth day. This relationship is shown in the following table. Although many factors can affect this relationship, in general it gives a good conservative estimate of the maintenance dose required.

To use the table, the cumulative loading dose given prior to the time of INR measurement should be calculated.

The horizontal line corresponding to the measured INR should then be followed to the point where it intersects with the vertical column headed by the cumulative loading dose. The value at the point of intersection represents the recommended maintenance dose.

INR	Cumulative warfarin dose (mg)						
	15	20	25	30	35*	40*	45*
2.0	3.5	4	5	5.5	6	7	7.5
2.2	3.5	4	4.5	5	5.5	6	6.5
2.5	3	3.5	4	4	4.5	5	5.5
3.0	2.5	3	3.5	3.5	4	4	4
3.5	–	2.5	3	3	3.5	–	–
4.0	–	–	3	3	3	–	–
4.5	–	–	2.5	3	3	–	–
5.0	–	–	2.5	2.5	3	–	–

* Values of cumulative doses exceeding 30 mg may be found when the INR has not been measured at the correct time. Such values should not normally be used.

Further monitoring should be carried out after two to three days, and then, depending on the results obtained, the interval can be increased, initially to once a week and then to every two, four and even six weeks. If a graph is drawn of INR against time, the slope will indicate the need for more frequent monitoring, e.g. a sharp change in the slope of the graph would indicate the need for more frequent monitoring or intervention to prevent values going outside the agreed limits.

Changes in treatment, or in a patient's pathology, also necessitate more frequent monitoring. The overall aim must always be to ensure that sufficient monitoring is undertaken to enable adverse changes to be detected without inconveniencing the patient excessively.

How long should Mr WS's warfarin therapy be continued?

A13 **For six months, providing there is no recurrence of his DVT.**

A first DVT with no complications is normally treated with warfarin for a period of three months, although some authorities feel that patients who have suffered a thrombotic episode may be predisposed to this condition for much longer. In the case of Mr WS, his mild heart failure could have been a contributing factor: until this is controlled he will continue to be at risk (it was a spontaneous DVT). We would recommend at least six months anticoagulant therapy and, if the DVT should recur, then continuous treatment.

What are the possible causes of Mr WS's high INR?

A14 **There are a number of possible causes of the high INR, including changes in Mr WS's fluid balance (as a result of furosemide therapy), worsening of his heart failure (no clinical signs), drug interactions and failure to take the correct dose. However, the most likely explanation is an interaction between erythromycin and warfarin.**

Erythromycin is known to inhibit the enzyme systems involved in warfarin metabolism (as do trimethoprim and ciprofloxacin) and is best avoided in patients anticoagulated with warfarin. If erythromycin therapy is necessary, a reduction of 50% in the dose of warfarin is required before the antibiotic is started. Weekly monitoring should also be recommended until the effect of the erythromycin is no longer seen, which may be two or three weeks after antibiotic therapy is stopped.

How should Mr WS's high INR be managed?

A15 **Omit one dose then recommence treatment with 1.5 mg warfarin orally daily.**

The *British National Formulary* gives good guidance on the management of excessive anticoagulation. Mr WS has a high INR but no apparent bleeding and the probable cause of the increase in INR is known. He should therefore have one dose of warfarin withheld to reduce quickly the risk of a bleed and he should then continue treatment with a lower dose. Reducing the dose to approximately 50% of that previously suggested would be appropriate. His INR should be monitored after a further two days and the dose readjusted if necessary.

When the erythromycin therapy is stopped, Mr WS's hepatic enzyme systems will return to normal. However, this return will not be as sudden as the inhibition: monitoring should therefore continue at least weekly and his dose of warfarin should be adjusted until he returns to his pre-erythromycin dose.

What points would you cover when giving medication advice to Mr WS about his warfarin therapy?

A16   **It is essential to give medication advice to patients who have been prescribed warfarin for the first time. There is a large amount of information to be conveyed to such patients and it requires a high level of skill and a substantial amount of time. We take the view that it is unethical for a patient on warfarin to be discharged from hospital without being given medication advice.**

The major points to be covered with Mr WS include the following:

(a)   What warfarin is and what it does.

(b)   Why Mr WS is taking warfarin and how its action can help.

(c)   How much to take and how the dose can be described (i.e. the colour or strength of the tablet and how dose changes may involve different combinations of the four strengths of tablet available).

(d)   When to take the dose, what happens if a dose is missed and the importance of regular dosing.

(e)   Factors that affect the action of warfarin. These include food (diets high in vitamin K in particular), social activities (smoking, drinking, travel, exercise), and other medicines, including over-the-counter products and alternative medicines.

(f)   Who Mr WS should tell that he is on anticoagulant therapy (GP, dentist, pharmacist).

(g)   What symptoms to look for which may indicate too much anticoagulant activity (e.g. gum bleeding, bruising, blood in urine), what the significance of each might be and what to do about it.

(h)   Who to contact if there are problems or doubts about treatment.

(i)   What to do about diseases that might occur during treatment (for instance, influenza).

(j)   When to come to clinic and why monitoring is important.

(k)   What the treatment goals are (to help Mr WS visualise his therapy and therefore assist his compliance and cooperation).

The advice and information sessions will also be an opportunity to develop a clinical relationship between Mr WS and the pharmacist which will continue after discharge.

What are the possible causes of Mr WS's low INR?

A17 **His warfarin dose was not increased when his erythromycin therapy was stopped.**

This is the most likely cause of Mr WS's low INR. Assuming non-compliance at this stage would be inappropriate. The effect of hepatic enzyme inhibition may take a week or two to be fully reversed, so monitoring and small dose increases (in this case 0.5-mg aliquots) will be required during this time and until the original activity is resumed. It should be noted that if a patient has very low INRs early on in treatment and is at risk of further thromboembolism, it may be necessary to restart therapeutic doses of low-molecular-weight heparin for a few days until therapeutic INRs are achieved again.

What are the probable causes of Mr WS's problems? What action would you recommend?

A18 **Azapropazone therapy is the most likely cause of his problems. It should be withdrawn and replaced by alternative therapy if needed.**

On admission Mr WS was found to have a very high INR (greater than 7.0), which was most probably caused by the addition of azapropazone to his warfarin therapy.

Most NSAIDs have some antiplatelet activity and, as such, can enhance bleeding, although this does not affect the INR. Similarly, although many NSAIDs are protein-bound, the warfarin that is displaced by their competitive binding is rapidly eliminated by the liver so that, at most, only a small transient rise in INR (usually for no longer that a day or two) may be seen. However, as with the classic reaction between phenylbutazone and warfarin, which is now fortunately rarely seen, azapropazone is not only capable of displacing a significant amount of warfarin from its protein-binding sites, but it can also inhibit hepatic enzyme activity very rapidly. This produces a very profound increase in free warfarin levels and, therefore, in anticoagulant activity.

The use of azapropazone (or phenylbutazone) must be avoided wherever possible in patients already taking warfarin; however, the data sheet for azapropazone gives good guidance on its use if it is deemed necessary.

NSAIDs also affect the gastrointestinal mucosa, causing damage and some blood loss, and this will be enhanced in the presence of warfarin.

Mr WS's acute symptoms of gout may require an NSAID but diclofenac would have been a more appropriate choice, being potent enough to treat the pain while having no effect on warfarin metabolism and only a small effect on the protein-binding of warfarin.

In our experience we have seen problems with high INRs following the use of colchicine for gout. Whether this is a result of an interaction between colchicine and warfarin or a physiological effect of gout on warfarin therapy is unknown. We would welcome other reports of this potential interaction.

The use of allopurinol for long-term prophylaxis of gout may also be considered, provided that increased monitoring of Mr WS's warfarin therapy is undertaken while allopurinol therapy is being introduced, as this drug is also reported to have an effect on anticoagulant therapy. An increase in warfarin activity is likely, although the size of the response varies from patient to patient.

Finally, the diuretics taken by Mr WS should be reviewed to see if improvements in control or choice could be made, as they are the likely cause of his acute episode of gout.

Whichever method is used to control Mr WS's gout, more frequent monitoring of his anticoagulant treatment must be initiated.

What other drugs should be avoided or prescribed with caution and careful monitoring while Mr WS continues to take warfarin?

A19 **Warfarin and related compounds interact with many different drugs. A comprehensive, but not exhaustive, list of compounds involved can be found in the *British National Formulary.***

Patients can vary quite markedly in their response to interactions, sometimes making it difficult to predict the outcome. For this reason it is important to:

(a) Recognise known drug interactions before the interacting medicine is given and initiate treatment changes that will avoid marked disruption of anticoagulant control.

(b) Ensure that the patient (and their GP and community pharmacist) is aware of the problem of drug interactions and that the clinic is informed before any new medication, including alternative and over-the-counter medicines, is started. As more medicines transfer from prescription only to over-the-counter status, e.g. cimetidine, the involvement of the community pharmacist becomes essential. Also, regular reminders should be given to the patient that many health store products taken in large doses can also have a marked effect on anticoagulant control. Ubidecarenone (Coenzyme Q10), vitamin E and fish oils have all been implicated, the latter two probably affecting platelet activity rather than the INR. Patients often do not equate health store products with medical products.

(c)   Remember that changes in the dose of concurrent medication may influence the anticoagulant effect.

(d)   Use the smaller range of medicines known to be safe in the presence of anticoagulants.

(e)   Monitor patients carefully when medication is being changed.

It is very easy to recognize a drug interaction after a marked change in anticoagulant control has occurred. It is more beneficial to the patient if that change is anticipated and prevented.

Further reading

Anon. How to anticoagulate. *Drug Ther Bull* 1992; **30**: 9–12.

Anon. Guidelines on oral anticoagulation: third edition. *Br J Haematol* 1998; **101**: 374–387.

Anon. Low-molecular-weight heparins for venous thromboembolism. *Drug Ther Bull* 1998; **36**: 25–29.

Bourne JG, Pegg M. Pharmacy contribution to out-patient management of oral anticoagulation. *Pharm J* 1987; **238**: 733–755.

Dobrzanski S. Predicting warfarin dosage. *J Clin Hosp Pharm* 1983; **8**: 247–250.

Hirsh J, Poller L, Deykin D *et al*. Optimal therapeutic range for oral anticoagulants. *Chest* 1989; **95**(suppl.): 55–115.

Hirsh J. Lee AY. How we diagnose and treat deep vein thrombosis. *Blood* 2002; **99**: 3102–3110.

Mason PA. Diet and drug interactions. *Pharm J* 1995; **255**: 94–97.

Michiels JJ, Kasbergen H, Oudega R *et al*. Exclusion and diagnosis of deep vein thrombosis in outpatients by sequential noninvasive tools. *Int Angiol* 2002; **21**: 9–19.

Radley AS, Hall J. The establishment and evaluation of a pharmacist-developed anticoagulant clinic. *Pharm J* 1994; **252**: 91–92.

Rivey MP, Peterson JP. Pharmacy-managed, weight-based heparin protocol. *Am J Hosp Pharm* 1993; **50**: 279–284.

Schraibman IG. Milne AA. Royle EM. Home versus in-patient treatment for deep vein thrombosis (Cochrane Review). In: *Cochrane Library 2*. Update Software, Oxford, 2003.

Spigset O. Reduced effect of warfarin caused by ubidecarenone. *Lancet* 1994; **344**: 1372–1373.

Stockley IH. *Drug Interactions*, 5th edn. Pharmaceutical Press, London, 1999.

Taylor P, Acomb C, Simmons AG. *Oral Anti-coagulants – Patient Care and Control*. UK Clinical Pharmacy Association, Leeds University Press, Leeds, 1994.

29

Colorectal surgery

Stan Dobrzanski

Day 1 (pre-operatively) Seventy-four-year old Mr NA, an elective admission to hospital, arrived on a Saturday afternoon to prepare for surgery on Monday morning. He was quite frail and had suffered a change in bowel habit. There had been loss of blood rectally and he had been suffering from tenesmus – a feeling of not having properly evacuated the bowel. He had been using laxatives, but they had proved to be of little use. Mr NA had visited his family doctor. Following a rectal examination that revealed a mass, sigmoidoscopy and biopsy showed a mid-rectal growth.

A magnetic resonance imaging scan had been used to determine the likely resection margins in preparation for surgery. The scan showed no spread to local lymph nodes and so the decision was made that there was no need for pre- or post-operative chemotherapy or radiotherapy. It was arranged that Mr NA would have an anterior resection, where the section of bowel containing the tumour would be cut out and the proximal sigmoid colon joined to the remnants of the lower rectum. It was explained to Mr NA that there might be a possibility that a stoma would have to be created, but if so this might be reversed later on.

Mr NA lived with an extended family. He had been in the UK for some years but originally came from a South Asian background and spoke little English. He confirmed, via his son who acted as an interpreter, that he had no allergies. When the junior doctor asked Mr NA about the tablets that he took, it proved difficult to establish a medication history since he had left his tablets at home. His memory was poor, and while the original referral letter from the family doctor had listed the patient's symptoms and also mentioned that he suffered from polymyalgia rheumatica, it did not list medication taken at home. Eventually, the following details were obtained:

- Ferrograd one daily
- A tablet whose name he could not remember
- A laxative
- Prednisolone enteric-coated (EC) 5 mg daily

The nurses gave him graduated compression stockings to wear and he was prescribed Ferrograd and prednisolone. In addition he was written up for:

- Hydrocortisone 100 mg intravenously four times a day to start immediately before admission to theatre
- Dalteparin 2500 units subcutaneously in the evening
- Temazepam 10 mg at night

The junior doctor wrote 'Little English – Urdu only' in the notes and made a mental note to find out what medication Mr NA actually took at home.

Q1   Why should pharmacists confirm medication histories obtained by doctors?
Q2   What are the advantages of patients bringing into hospital medication prescribed by their GP?
Q3   What steps could the doctor have taken to confirm the medication history?

Day 2 (pre-operatively)   The nurses gave a bowel cleansing solution to Mr NA. He was asked to drink about 4 L of fluid within four to six hours, and a check was made to ensure that the bowel movements he produced were watery and clear. A 'nil orally' notice was placed at the top of his bed. His biochemical results were as follows:

- Sodium 142 mmol/L (reference range 135–145)
- Potassium 4.4 mmol/L (3.5–5.1)
- Haemoglobin 10.9 g/dL (13–18)

Q4   Should the 'nil orally' also apply to Mr NA's medication?
Q5   Was Mr NA at high risk of thromboembolism?
Q6   Why had the doctor prescribed the dalteparin as an evening rather than a morning dose? What are the hazards of administering low-molecular-weight heparin immediately before surgery?

Day 3 (operation day)   An epidural line was inserted by the anaesthetist. Mr NA was given a bolus dose of propofol to make him lose consciousness and the muscle relaxant rocuronium was used to allow intubation and then ventilation. A remifentanil infusion was used for pain control, while anaesthesia was maintained with desflurane administered through a closed low flow 'circle' system.

Q7 Since the patient was unconscious why did the anaesthetist need to infuse a potent analgesic?

Q8 What is a closed low flow 'circle' system?

During the two-hour operation the anaesthetist also administered the following fluids:

- Sodium chloride 0.9%
  3 × 500 mL

- Hartmann's solution 2 × 500 mL

Post-operatively the anaesthetist prescribed:

- Hartmann's Solution, 500 mL over 4 hours
- Glucose 4% sodium chloride 0.18%, 2 L in the following 12 hours
- Cyclizine 50 mg intravenously eight-hourly if required for nausea

- Epidural morphine with bupivacaine to run as an infusion at between 2 and 6 mL/h for pain control

The surgeon performing the operation suggested on the operation record that the patient should receive five days intravenous treatment with cefuroxime 750 mg plus metronidazole 500 mg.

Q9 How could the antibiotic prescribing have been improved?

Q10 When Mr NA returned to the ward, the pharmacist challenged the prescribing of intravenous hydrocortisone 100 mg four times a day. Why?

Q11 Why did the anaesthetist use both Hartmann's solution and sodium chloride 0.9%?

A 25-cm section of rectum and colon had been removed in theatre and sent for histology. A diagnosis was made of Dukes A tumour that had not penetrated deep into the rectal wall and was, therefore, linked with a favourable prognosis for long-term survival. However, because the resulting bowel anastomosis was so near the anal margin, the surgeon was anxious to protect the rectal suture line from any damage caused by the passage of faeces, at least until healing was complete and wound strength was at a maximum. Therefore, a small loop of the patient's ileum had been passed through the abdominal wall and incised so that a loop ileostomy was formed to divert intestinal output into an ileostomy bag. It was planned that the loop ileostomy could later be reversed.

Day 4 During the morning surgical round, the nurses reported that Mr NA had been agitated overnight. His urine output over the past 24 hours had been 940 mL despite an intravenous intake of over 4 L and there was little output in the ileostomy bag. Mr NA had had a nasogastric tube inserted to aspirate his stomach contents as he was suffering from ileus as a result of the major abdominal surgery suppressing gastrointestinal peristalsis. Ileus produces symptoms of abdominal distension, discomfort and nausea as gastric juices build up in the stomach. In addition, Mr NA was mildly pyrexial with a temperature of 37.6°C. The junior doctor prescribed:

- Glucose 4% sodium chloride
  0.18% 1 L intravenously every 8
  hours

Q12 Why was Mr NAs urine output low the first day after surgery?
Q13 What is the likely cause of the mild pyrexia?

The clinical pharmacist checked the drug history listed in the pre-admission clinic notes and then contacted the family doctor to confirm the patient's medication history. He found the following had not been prescribed:

- Levothyroxine 100 micrograms,   - Latanoprost eye-drops, one drop
  one tablet daily   in each eye at night

The clinical pharmacist also spoke to the patient's relatives asking them to bring the patients medication from home. The patient's son complained that his father was experiencing significant pain. As a result the pain management team recommended that the epidural infusion rate was increased to 6 mL/h. In addition he was prescribed:

- Piroxicam (Melt) 20 mg once a
  day

Because of the nature of the operation, use of suppositories was not possible.

Q14 Would the piroxicam help to control the pain?

Day 5   On the surgical ward round it was noted that bowel sounds had returned. Mr NA's urine output had improved to 1754 mL and the ileostomy bag contained about 200 mL of output. Mr NA was started on 15-mL sips of water.

Day 6   Mr NA had experienced a significant diuresis with a urine output of 3456 mL. The patient was now taking 30-mL sips of water and could start taking his normal medication. He was taking regular paracetamol in addition to piroxicam (Melt) for pain control and his epidural pump was discontinued.

His biochemical results were as follows:

- Sodium 133 mmol/L (135–145)   ▪ Potassium 3.5 mmol/L (3.5–5.1)

Q15 Why was Mr NA hyponatraemic?

Day 7 The stoma care nurses visited Mr NA to check that he was learning to deal with his ileostomy. His son brought his medication from home and this included a box of senna tablets. The patient's own medication was locked away in a secure metal drug storage cabinet by the patient's bedside.

Q16 The clinical pharmacist was very concerned that the patient had a supply of laxatives. Why would the use of laxatives be undesirable in a patient with an ileostomy?

Mr NA was very concerned at the dark colour of his stoma output and thought that he could see tablets in it which he claimed could not be working as 'they were passing straight through him'.

Q17 What could explain this observation?

Day 15 Mr NA was thought to be ready for discharge. With the help of his family and interpreters, he had been trained by the stoma nurse to use his ileostomy bag. It was explained he would return to the hospital in a few months time to have the temporary ileostomy reversed. The pharmacist also asked the surgical team to arrange for a bone scan to determine if Mr NA had significant osteoporosis as a result of long-term steroid use.

Q18 How can the pharmacist influence prescribing and minimise delays which might occur at discharge?

Why should pharmacists confirm medication histories obtained by doctors?

A1 **Failure to obtain a complete medication history is the most common of all hospital prescribing errors.**

A hospital survey (Dobrzanski *et al.*, 2002) demonstrated that nearly half of all prescribing errors detected by pharmacists were related to medication history taking. Commonly, the prescribing error was one of omission, where essential medication taken at home, such as anticonvulsants, were simply not prescribed. Perhaps not surprisingly, such prescribing errors were found to be more common in patients with a limited command of English.

It has been claimed that pharmacists are better than doctors at taking medication histories; however, this may not always be the case. Patients are often confused, anxious and disorientated when they arrive in hospital. Medication history taking under such circumstances can thus be difficult for any health care professional. In the case of Mr NA, there was the additional factor that he was admitted at a weekend. The family doctor's surgery from which details of regularly taken medication would usually be obtained was probably closed.

Therefore, omissions, mistakes and misunderstandings are quite likely, whether it is a doctor, nurse or pharmacist who interviews the patient. It is thus likely that medication histories taken by hospital doctors, nurses and pharmacists will complement each other and be more accurate when viewed together than each would separately.

What are the advantages of patients bringing into hospital medication prescribed by their GP?

A2 **It aids the production of an accurate medication history.**

Complete reliance on referral letters provided by GPs for a patient's medication history may not be justified, as they may be incomplete, inaccurate or the medication history may simply not be mentioned. Moreover, in patients who are waiting for surgery where there is a long waiting list, their medication regimen may have altered in the time since referral.

Having the medication brought from home can confirm any information provided by the patient.

This case refers to an elective hospital admission. The problem of poor medication histories in referral letters is also particularly evident in the case of acutely admitted patients, especially where the referral is being made through the deputising doctor service.

What steps could the doctor have taken to confirm the medication history?

A3 **By referring to notes from the pre-admission clinic or by making a formal request for a complete medication history to be obtained by other health care staff.**

Most patients attend pre-admission clinics even for minor surgical procedures. There, a nurse or pharmacist would have taken the drug history since it is important to identify if the patient is taking medication that might need to be discontinued or altered before surgery.

It is very likely that a junior doctor working at a weekend would be 'on call' and likely to go off duty as soon as the surgical team caring for the patient arrive on Monday morning. This scenario carries a risk that any uncertainty that the admitting doctor felt when prescribing for this patient will not be conveyed to his colleagues who take over at the start of the week. A formal 'handover' system where the doctor requests confirmation of medication history from the pharmacist or from nurses could eliminate this risk.

Should the 'nil orally' also apply to Mr NA's medication?

A4 **No.**

Pharmacists should work with pre-admission clinics to produce guidelines about which drugs to stop and which to continue before surgery. Some medicines, such as warfarin or monoamine-oxidase inhibitors are normally stopped before surgery since they may, respectively, cause excessive blood loss and haematoma formation or interact with medication prescribed by the anaesthetist. It is important to establish exactly when such drugs should be discontinued. However, it is also the case that the abrupt withdrawal of medication unrelated to the surgery, and normally taken by the patient, might be undesirable. Omission of anticonvulsants or drugs acting on the cardiovascular system, or the failure to prescribe appropriate peri-operative regimens for diabetics or patients taking large doses of corticosteroids may lead to post-operative complications. Therefore, guidelines also need to be created to help doctors to determine alternative ways of administering drugs when the patient cannot take anything by mouth post-operatively.

These guidelines should be supplemented by formal 'nil orally' guidelines that define the precise meaning of this term. Surgical wards should be clear about when the patient scheduled for surgery should stop the intake of solids, liquids and oral medicaments. A common practice is to allow the patient to take most oral medicaments with a 30-mL sip of water up to one hour before admission to theatre.

Was Mr NA at high risk of thromboembolism?

A5   Yes.

Mr NA is an elderly patient with cancer scheduled for a long operation. The pharmacist should check that each speciality has developed a formal thromboprophylaxis policy so that a formal assessment can be made and documented of the risk of thromboembolism for patients scheduled for surgery, and appropriate prophylaxis ordered.

Why had the doctor prescribed the dalteparin as an evening rather than as a morning dose? What are the hazards of administering low-molecular-weight heparin immediately before surgery?

A6   There might be a theoretical possibility of a vertebral canal haematoma.

In America, the increased likelihood of vertebral canal haematoma formation leading to paralysis has been observed following the placement of epidural catheters immediately following the administration of low-molecular-weight heparin. However, the doses used there were far higher than is usual in the UK. Nevertheless, many anaesthetists prefer that the administration of low-molecular-weight heparin does not immediately precede the insertion of the epidural catheter. Giving the low-molecular-weight heparin the night before means that the peak effects of the drug will have passed by the time the epidural line is being inserted. The same rationale applies to the *removal* of epidural catheters. Preferably removal should be carried out at least 12 hours after the administration of low-molecular-weight heparin.

Since the patient was unconscious why did the anaesthetist need to infuse a potent analgesic?

A7 **The analgesic was part of a balanced anaesthesia regimen.**

Even if the patient is unconscious, surgical incision and manipulation produces pain that can elicit adverse responses such as a steep rise in heart rate. In this case, if the anaesthetist had not used a very powerful analgesic such as remifentanil to prevent the patient reacting as surgery proceeded, there would have been a need to use huge amounts of desflurane so as to induce a very deep anaesthesia to compensate for the patient's increased capacity to sense pain. Use of potent analgesics such as remifentanil means that the patient requires far less volatile or intravenous anaesthetic. Remifentanil is very short-acting and its effects wear off almost as soon as the infusion is stopped.

What is a closed low flow 'circle' system?

A8 **Where the patient rebreathes the volatile anaesthetic that has just been exhaled.**

It is obviously wasteful if, when a patient is being anaesthetised with an expensive volatile anaesthetic such as desflurane, that after breathing in the anaesthetic gas, they exhale it via an 'open' system into the atmosphere. Moreover, high gas flows are needed to provide the anaesthetic and oxygen needed by the patient. A closed low flow 'circle' anaesthetic system means that the patient rebreathes the gases that have been exhaled. However, the exhaled gases are first passed through soda lime to absorb expired carbon dioxide and then supplemented with a 'low flow' small quantity of additional anaesthetic plus top-up quantities of oxygen. Such a system is clearly more economical. Moreover, it reduces the extent of exposure of theatre staff to the gaseous anaesthetics that are exhaled by the patient.

How could the antibiotic prescribing have been improved?

A9 **The patient required a prophylactic dose of antibiotics in theatre.**

Clean surgery, such as a thyroidectomy or a breast biopsy, does not normally require antibiotic prophylaxis. However, where contaminated or dirty surgery is carried out, such as that involving incision of the bowel or the biliary tract, antibiotic prophylaxis helps to prevent post-operative infection. Intravenous broad-spectrum antibiotics such as cefuroxime are commonly used in combination with metronidazole, which has activity against anaerobes. Antibiotic prophylaxis is also used in high risk, albeit clean, surgery where prosthetic materials such as hip or knee replacements or synthetic arterial bypass grafts are implanted, as infection around such prosthetic materials would be disastrous.

To prevent infection, the optimal timing of the prophylactic antibiotic injection is vital. For maximal antibacterial effect, it is important that tissue antibiotic levels are high at the time of surgery. The first intravenous dose of antibiotic is thus usually given by the anaesthetist at around the time of induction of anaesthesia, but in this case there was no mention of any antibiotic being given. If antibiotics are not given at the time of surgery or if their administration is delayed for only a few hours, the 'golden period' during which antibiotic prophylaxis is effective passes and the probability of post-operative wound infection increases.

Antibiotic prophylaxis only applies to elective surgery. For emergency surgical cases such as a burst appendix, perforated duodenal ulcer or ischaemic bowel it is likely that bacterial infection (peritonitis) has taken hold before the patient arrived in hospital. Here, antibiotics are used to treat infection as it is too late to prevent it. The duration of antibiotic use then depends on response to therapy, with cessation of treatment normally being considered when the patient has been apyrexial with a normal white blood cell count for 48 hours.

The surgeon's direction to continue using the antibiotic for five days in this elective surgical case might therefore seem questionable, since one intraoperative dose plus another two more doses at eight-hourly intervals would represent a normal antibiotic prophylaxis regimen. However, a low rectal anastomosis carries a high risk of infection and if this happened, it would be catastrophic. While it would be correct to confirm the duration of antibiotic therapy with the surgeon, it should also to be borne in mind that the surgeon may have experienced technical difficulties in theatre and that this might explain the decision to continue antibiotics for longer than might be expected.

> When Mr NA returned to the ward, the pharmacist challenged the prescribing of intravenous hydrocortisone 100 mg four times a day. Why?

A10   **The dose of hydrocortisone was far in excess of what was required.**

After major surgery cortisol levels rise as part of a natural stress response. This response is impaired in patients who have had long-term steroid therapy and this carries the risk of a hypoadrenal crisis and collapse and shock. Therefore, in these patients there may be a need to give some additional steroids peri-operatively. However, 400 mg of hydrocortisone daily is equivalent to 80 mg of oral prednisolone and represents a huge amount of steroid that will inhibit wound healing. A recent recommendation for major surgery has been to give 25 mg hydrocortisone at induction of anaesthesia, which is then followed by an infusion of 100 mg of hydrocortisone daily for two or three days. This reflects the amount of excess steroid that might be secreted by an individual with a normal hypothalamic–pituitary–adrenocortical axis when undergoing major surgery, and is an amount of steroid much less than originally prescribed for Mr NA.

Why did the anaesthetist use both Hartmann's solution and sodium chloride 0.9%?

A11 **Hartmann's solution resembles blood plasma more closely in terms of electrolyte content.**

Hartmann's is basically 'dirty saline' and includes homeopathic quantities of calcium that increase the possibility of precipitating some medicaments. However, sodium chloride 0.9% does contain more chloride ions (154 mmol/L) than blood plasma, while Hartmann's contains a more physiological quantity of chloride ions (112 mmol/L). When a patient receives only moderate quantities of sodium chloride 0.9%, the chloride excess does not matter. However, large volumes of sodium chloride 0.9% can, in theory, result in the patient having excess chloride ions and this produces hyperchloraemic acidosis. The clinical significance of this is controversial, but it accounts for many anaesthetists choosing to use Hartmann's if large amounts of crystalloid fluid are to be used in theatre.

Why was Mr NA's urine output low the first day after surgery?

A12 **Because surgery increases the secretion of antidiuretic hormone and this reduces urine output.**

The sodium chloride 0.9% and Hartmann's given to Mr NA in theatre were to compensate for blood and body fluid losses, together with insensible loss of water through mechanisms such as sweat. It was also given to compensate for the movement of fluid from the circulation into intercellular and intercavitary spaces as a result of surgical trauma (third space losses). It is preferable to give too much fluid rather than too little. The aim should be to ensure blood pressure and renal perfusion are maintained and there is a urine output of at least 1 L/day.

Post-operatively, the patient retains fluid because surgery stimulates the production of high levels of antidiuretic hormone and because fluid is sequestered at the site of operative trauma. Usually, after about the second or third day, the antidiuretic hormone levels fall and sequestered third space fluids are reabsorbed back into the blood circulation. At this stage a diuresis is usually seen and this was the case here.

What is the likely cause of the mild pyrexia?

A13 **A transient mild post-operative pyrexia of below 38°C is common following elective surgery and may be due to the stress, trauma and inflammation resulting from the surgery itself. It is not caused by infection and is not a reason for prolonging antibiotic use.**

Would the piroxicam help to control the pain?

A14 **The piroxicam would probably have only a limited analgesic effect while the patient had a nasogastric tube in place for nasogastric suction.**

If a patient has post-operative ileus a nasogastric tube is put in place to suck out excess fluid from the stomach until the time peristalsis restarts and the stomach can empty properly again. Piroxicam (Melt) is absorbed intestinally and not buccally. Therefore, the piroxicam (Melt) would be aspirated via the nasogastric tube while ileus persisted. It would only begin to have an effect as normal intestinal motility reappeared.

Why was Mr NA hyponatraemic?

A15 **Because of the continuous administration of a fluid regimen comprising 3 L/day glucose 4% with sodium chloride 0.18% that did not provide sufficient sodium for Mr NA's needs.**

Post-operatively, the aims of prescribing fluids are broadly to maintain a urine output of between 1 and 2 L/day and to assume the need to replace further 'insensible' fluid losses of approximately 1.5 L/day lost through perspiration through the skin and water vapour via the lungs. As an example, an 'average' patient might in 24 hours require: 1 L of sodium chloride 0.9% plus 20 mmol potassium over eight hours and then 2 L glucose 5%, each with 20 mmol potassium over the next 16 hours, by intravenous infusion.

The sodium chloride 0.9% provides 154 mmol of sodium and main-tains extracellular fluid volume. The glucose 5% provides free water which distributes both intra- and extracellularly (adding glucose, to a concentration of 5%, makes the water isotonic and capable of being given intravenously). For a 70 kg patient, the above regimen is very loosely based on giving each day: fluid 40 mL/kg; sodium 2 mmol/kg; potassium 1 mmol/kg.

These are average daily requirements. Other losses from nasogastric aspirate or losses from drains are normally replaced with sodium chloride 0.9% which is given in addition to the regimen above. Maintenance of accurate fluid balance records and monitoring of electrolyte levels is pivotal to the rational prescribing of fluids post-operatively.

Mr NA received only 90 mmol of sodium per day since each bag of 1 L of glucose 4% plus sodium chloride 0.18% only contained 30 mmol of sodium. In addition, the doctor forgot to prescribe potassium. Potas-sium is normally omitted on the day the patient has their operation as surgery causes cellular damage, which results in the release of this ion from intracellular stores. However, it can be restarted on subsequent days and failure to do this resulted in a fall in Mr NA's potassium levels.

The clinical pharmacist was very concerned that the patient had a supply of laxatives. Why would the use of laxatives be undesirable in a patient with an ileostomy?

A16   **Because patients with ileostomies are never constipated.**

Ileostomy output is very liquid. If it is not being produced then the most likely cause is an intestinal obstruction. The patient should then seek medical help and not rely on laxatives. In addition, laxatives can increase the volume of ileostomy output and this may cause dehydration. The colon has a major role in water reabsorption and if it is being bypassed, as in Mr NA's case, then this renders the patient very vulnerable to fluid and electrolyte disturbance.

What could explain his observation?

A17   **Ferrous sulphate in the Ferrograd may darken faecal output. The Ferrograd tablets would not dissolve in the intestine but would appear in the ileostomy bag as spent wax matrix 'ghosts'.**

There are numerous pharmaceuticals which may alter the colour of faecal output and this may be disturbing to the patient looking at their ileostomy bag, so adequate counselling is essential. The effective shortening of the patient's bowel in ileostomy patients means that complete drug absorption is less likely to occur and hence it is preferable that slow release or enteric-coated products are avoided.

How can the pharmacist influence prescribing and minimise any delays that might occur at discharge?

A18   **By acting as a 'discharge medication planner'.**

For most surgical cases the clinical pharmacist can plan discharge medication requirements. Medical prescribing is diagnosis dependent. Surgical prescribing is procedure dependent. Surgery rarely entails substantial alterations to the long-term essential medication prescribed for the patient by their family doctor.

In Mr NA's case the surgical pharmacist would write the pharmaceutical discharge plan on the discharge letter and present it to the surgical ward round. The surgeons would assess the plan and sign the discharge letter that might read:

- Ferrous sulphate 200 mg orally twice a day
- Latanoprost, one drop at night in each eye
- Prednisolone plain, 5 mg orally daily
- Paracetamol 500 mg, one or two tablets orally up to four times a day if required
- Levothyroxine, 100 micrograms orally daily

In view of the ileostomy, the slow-release and enteric-coated tablets that the patient had been taking should be discontinued. The temazepam could also stop. The clinical pharmacist should make the patient aware that laxatives should no longer be used. With the patient's consent, the patient's community pharmacist would be notified about the change in therapy, the need to alter medication because of the temporary ileostomy, and the need to supply stoma care appliances.

Further reading

Anon. Drugs in the peri-operative period. *Drugs Ther Bull* 1998; **37**: 68–70.

Dobrzanski S, Reidy F. The pharmacist as a discharge medication planner in surgical patients. *Pharm J* 1993; **250**(suppl. 1): HS53–HS56.

Dobrzanski S, Jackson MN, Booth CD *et al.* Pharmaceutical protocols of care for surgical patients. *Pharm J* 1994; **252**: 609–610.

Dobrzanski S, Holdsworth H, Khan G *et al.* The nature of hospital prescribing errors. *Br J Clin Gov* 2002; **7**: 187–193.

Kearon C, Hirsh J. Management of anticoagulation before and after elective surgery. *N Engl J Med* 1997; **21**: 1506–1511.

McLatchie RD, Leaper DJ. *Oxford Handbook of Operative Surgery.* Oxford University Press, Oxford, 1996.

Noble DW, Kehlet H. Risks of interrupting drug treatment before surgery. *Br Med J* 2000; **321**: 719–720.

Scottish Intercollegiate Guidelines Network. *Prophylaxis of Venous Thromboembolism. A National Clinical Guideline.* SIGN, Edinburgh, 2002.

Scottish Intercollegiate Guidelines Network. *Antibiotic Prophylaxis in Surgery. A National Clinical Guideline.* SIGN, Edinburgh, 2000.

Schulz NJ. Drug therapy and the ostomy patient. *J Enterostomal Ther* 1986; **13**: 157–161.

Thromboembolic Risk Factors (THRIFT) Consensus Group. Risk of and prophylaxis for venous thromboembolism in hospital patients. *Br Med J* 1992; **305**: 567–574.

Turner DAB. Fluid, electrolyte and acid–base balance. In: *Textbook of Anaesthesia*, 4th edn. AR Aitkenhead, DJ Rowbotham, G Smith, eds. Churchill Livingstone, London, 2001: **489–500**.

Wright J, Prasad N, Dalrymple G. Emergency referral letters from deputising doctors need to be improved. *Br Med J* 1996; **312**: 1304.

30

Cholecystectomy

Sharron Millen and Anne Cole

Day 1 Twenty-one-year-old Miss RW was admitted for an elective chol-ecystectomy. She had first presented to her GP one year earlier complain-ing of pain in the right upper quadrant of her abdomen, which occurred after eating. The pain radiated to the back and usually lasted for about four hours. It was associated with nausea. Her GP made a diagnosis of biliary colic and prescribed paracetamol, diclofenac, dihydrocodeine and metoclopramide. However, the episodes of biliary colic had not resolved and Miss RW had been referred for an ultrasound scan which had revealed a 1.5 cm gallstone in the gallbladder.

Her drug therapy on admission was:

- Paracetamol, one or two tablets orally, up to four times daily, when required
- Diclofenac 50 mg orally, up to three times daily, when required
- Metoclopramide 10 mg orally, up to three times a day when required
- Dihydrocodeine 30 mg orally, four-hourly, to a maximum of 240 mg in 24 hours

Q1 Is metoclopramide a suitable choice of anti-emetic for Miss RW?
Q2 Is diclofenac an appropriate choice of analgesic for biliary colic?

Miss RW had no known allergies. She smoked 20 cigarettes each day and drank occasionally. Her weight on admission was 93 kg and she was noted as being a 'large lady'. She had been taking a combined oral contraceptive pill (ethinylestradiol 30 micrograms and levonorgestrel 150 micrograms) until admission. Her mother had undergone an open cholecystectomy for gallstones several years earlier. Miss RW herself had no other previous medical history of note.

On examination her pulse was 88 beats per minute and regular. Her blood pressure was 140/70 mmHg. Examination of the abdomen revealed no masses, but there was slight tenderness in the right upper quadrant.

A pressure sore assessment risk by the nursing staff gave a score of 5, which indicated that Miss RW was not at risk of pressure sores. A nutritional assessment by the nursing staff triggered a referral to the dietitian.

She was prescribed enoxaparin 20 mg subcutaneously daily at 5pm for prophylaxis against deep-vein thrombosis (DVT) and pulmonary embolism (PE).

Q3 How should her smoking cessation be managed during her admission?

Q4 How should her use of the combined oral contraceptive pill be managed?

Q5 Is thromboembolic prophylaxis important in this case?

Q6 How should enoxaparin be administered?

Q7 Are the nutritional and pressure sore risk assessments important for Miss RW?

Q8 Outline a pharmaceutical care plan for Miss RW.

Day 2 Her serum biochemistry and haematology results were:

- Sodium 137 mmol/L (reference range 135–145)
- Potassium 3.6 mmol/L (3.5–5.0)
- Urea 2.8 mmol/L (3.0–6.5)
- Creatinine 63 micromol/L (60–125)
- Albumin 32 g/L (32–50)
- Liver function tests within normal limits
- White blood cells (WBC) 10.0×10^9/L (4.0–10.0×10^9)
- Haemoglobin 125 g/L (120–160 female)
- International normalised ratio 1.1

A cholecystectomy was planned for the following day. The procedure was outlined to Miss RW and her parents by the surgical house officer, and the associated risks were described. Miss RW agreed that she understood what she had been told and signed a consent form.

The nursing staff measured and fitted Miss RW with graduated below-knee compression stockings, and the importance of her continuing to wear these until discharge was emphasised.

The ward pharmacist spoke to Miss RW about her medication, and it became apparent that she had some ibuprofen tablets in her bedside locker and was continuing to take them because she was in pain. She had not told the doctor about these tablets because she had bought them herself and therefore did not think they were important.

Q9 What should the pharmacist do about this situation?

During the afternoon the anaesthetist visited the ward to review the elective cases for the following day. The anaesthetist spoke to Miss RW about the drugs she would receive peri-operatively and how she would feel during the various stages of the next day. The idea of an epidural or patient-controlled analgesia (PCA) were discussed as suitable means of controlling her post-operative pain and the risk factors were explained. Miss RW consented to have an epidural. Her enoxaparin was prescribed at 5 p.m. so it would be administered at least 12 hours prior to her operation and allow the safe insertion of the epidural catheter.

Q10 What combinations of drugs are used in epidurals?
Q11 How do these agents work?
Q12 What are the side-effects of epidurals and how can they be managed?
Q13 What other methods of opioid analgesic administration could have been used for Miss RW?
Q14 What is meant by 'patient-controlled analgesia' (PCA)?
Q15 When is PCA not a suitable choice of analgesia?
Q16 What counselling points would have needed to be covered if Miss RW had chosen PCA for post-operative analgesia?
Q17 Is there an advantage to using an epidural over PCA for Miss RW?

Day 3   Her serum biochemistry and haematology results were:

- Sodium 136 mmol/L (135–145)
- Potassium 3.7 mmol/L (3.5–5.0)
- Urea 3.2 mmol/L (3.0–6.5)
- Creatinine 65 micromol/L (60–125)

- Albumin 32 g/L (32–50)
- WBC 8.2×10^9/L $(4.0–10.0 \times 10^9)$

The following premedication was administered on the ward at 10 a.m.:

- Temazepam 20 mg orally
- Cyclizine 50 mg intramuscularly

Q18 What is the purpose of 'premedication'?
Q19 Do you agree with the choice of Miss RW's premedication?

Miss RW was drowsy within 30 minutes and was taken down to theatre at 11 a.m. On induction Miss RW received:

- Cefuroxime 750 mg intravenously
- Metronidazole 500 mg intravenously

- Morphine 2 mg intravenously

An intermittent compression device was set up on Miss RW's calves and used for the duration of the procedure. The anaesthetist utilised physiological responses to pain throughout the operation to manage Miss RW's analgesia. Small bolus doses of morphine were administered as needed.

Q20 Why was Miss RW given antibiotics and morphine at induction?

In theatre the surgeon found an inflamed gall bladder containing many large gallstones. The cholecystectomy was performed, a nasogastric tube was inserted and a bile sample was sent for culture and sensitivities.

In recovery, an epidural of bupivacaine 0.15% with fentanyl 2 micrograms/mL was started at 8 mL/h. This was to run via a dedicated, coloured anti-syphon epidural line and the dose titrated accordingly.

Q21 How should patients with epidurals be monitored?
Q22 What methods of thromboembolic prophylaxis are being used for Miss RW?

Miss RW was returned to the ward where she continued to receive the following medication:

- Cefuroxime 750 mg intravenously three times daily
- Metronidazole 500 mg intravenously three times daily
- Enoxaparin 20 mg subcutaneously once daily

- Bupivacaine 0.15% with fentanyl 2 micrograms/mL – 8 mL/h via epidural catheter
- Paracetamol 1 g orally or rectally four times a day

The 'as required' medication was as follows:

- Cyclizine 50 mg intramuscularly up to three times daily
- Diclofenac 100 mg suppositories rectally every 18 hours or 50 mg orally three times a day

Day 3 The epidural was controlling Miss RW's pain well. She was comfortable and apyrexial. During the immediate 24-hour post-operative period Miss RW had received glucose 4% sodium chloride 0.18% plus potassium chloride 0.15% intravenously at 125 mL/h. This was sufficient to replace her losses from the drain at the wound site, losses via the nasogastric tube, urine output, faecal and insensible losses.

Q23 What is meant by 'insensible losses'?
Q24 Is there a rationale for co-prescribing non-steroidal anti-inflammatory drugs (NSAIDs) with opioids post-operatively?

Q25 Should gastrointestinal prophylaxis have been co-prescribed with the NSAID?

Day 4   Her serum biochemistry and haematology results were:

- Sodium 142 mmol/L (reference range 135–145)
- Potassium 4.0. mmol/L (3.5–5.0)
- Urea 3.6 mmol/L (3.0–6.5)
- Creatinine 72 micromol/L (60–125)

- Albumin 28 g/L (32–50)
- WBC 9.8×10^9/L $(4.0–10.0 \times 10^9)$

Bowel sounds had returned and the nasogastric tube and wound drains were removed. Miss RW was commenced on 30-mL sips of water every hour, to increase to 60 mL/h during the afternoon. The epidural was stopped. The bile culture and sensitivity results came back as no growth. Miss RW was apyrexial and her pulse was 50 beats per minute. The intravenous fluid replacement regimen was stopped. Miss RW's medication was now as follows:

- Cefuroxime 750 mg intravenously three times a day
- Metronidazole 500 mg intravenously three times a day

- Enoxaparin 20 mg subcutaneously once a day
- Paracetamol 1 g orally or rectally four times a day

The 'as required' medication was as follows:

- Diclofenac 50 mg tablets orally up to three times daily
- Dihydrocodeine 30 mg four-hourly to a maximum of 240 mg in 24 h

- Morphine 10 mg intramuscularly every two to four hours as required

The pharmacist requested that the surgical house officer discontinued the antibiotics.

Q26 Was the pharmacist right to request this?
Q27 Do you agree with the choice of oral analgesia for Miss RW?
Q28 Should the first dose of morphine be given as the epidural stops?
Q29 How long should her thromboembolic prophylaxis continue?

Day 5   Miss RW was eating a light diet. The dietitian visited her and provided her with some nutritional advice with an aim to achieve a weight loss of no more than 2 kg per week.

Day 6 Miss RW was discharged from hospital, with an out-patient appointment in six weeks. Her discharge medication was as follows:

- Paracetamol 1 g four times a day as required
- Ibuprofen 400 mg three times a day as required

Q30 What advice should Miss RW be given about her medication prior to discharge?

Is metoclopramide a suitable choice of anti-emetic for Miss RW?

A1   **No. Metoclopramide is not a good choice of anti-emetic for children, women, the very old, patients with Parkinson's disease or gastrointestinal obstruction.**

The first-line choice of anti-emetic for Miss RW would be cyclizine, which exerts its effect by an action on histamine and muscarinic receptors in the nucleus tractus solitaris (which stimulates the vomiting centre) and the vestibular nucleus. If additional anti-emetics were needed, domperidone could be considered.

Metoclopramide is a dopamine antagonist which acts centrally by blocking the chemoreceptor trigger zone and peripherally on the gut, to increase lower oesophageal sphincter tone and speed up gastric empty-ing. Phenothiazines, such as prochlorperazine also act centrally as dopa-mine antagonists, but do not have any peripheral action on the gut and they are therefore not as effective as metoclopramide for nausea asso-ciated with gastroduodenal, hepatic or biliary disease. The problem with all centrally-acting dopamine antagonists is that they can sometimes induce acute dystonic reactions such as facial and skeletal muscle spasm and oculogyric crisis. These side-effects are more common in young girls and women and the very old. Cyclizine does not have these side-effects, although occasionally drowsiness can be a problem. If cyclizine failed to be effective on its own then a peripherally-acting dopamine antagonist may be needed. Domperidone is an alternative to metoclopramide which does not readily cross the blood–brain barrier and is therefore less likely to cause dystonic reactions.

Is diclofenac an appropriate choice of analgesic for biliary colic?

A2   **Yes. However, diclofenac is contra-indicated in some situations.**

Diclofenac is a NSAID which may induce or worsen peptic ulcer disease (PUD). If the differential diagnosis of Miss RW's disease had included any possibility of active PUD, dyspepsia or pyloric stenosis, then a NSAID would not have been an appropriate choice of analgesic. NSAIDs must also be avoided in patients with a history of an allergic reaction to NSAIDs and used with caution in patients with a history of PUD, asthma or renal disease. The total daily dose of NSAID can be minimised by the

co-prescribing of additional analgesia. In this case Miss RW was prescribed paracetamol and a weak opioid. Her GP has prescribed dihydrocodeine 30 mg every four hours up to a maximum of 240 mg in 24
hours to minimise the chance of constipation from this agent. If additional analgesia is required then morphine is the opioid analgesic of
choice. Historically pethidine was used in biliary disease because it was
reported to cause less spasm of the sphincter of Oddi (the sphincter at the
base of the gall bladder) than other opioids but this is now disputed. All
opioids can affect smooth muscle tone.

How should Miss RW's smoking cessation during her admission be
managed?

A3 **Unless patients are suffering from severe nicotine
withdrawal, it is not appropriate to initiate nicotine
replacement therapy peri-operatively while patients are out
of their normal environment and usual support network.
However, prior to discharge, Miss RW should be provided
with encouragement and information regarding smoking
cessation, support groups and products available to aid
smoking cessation.**

A good starting point is for Miss RW to make a list of reasons for giving up
smoking and to keep referring back to the list to ensure she maintains her
commitment to stopping. Nicotine replacement therapy has been found
to increase the chance of smoking cessation by about 1.5–2 times. Both
individual counselling and group therapy increase the chance of quitting.
Currently most hospitals have nicotine replacement patches available, but
these are not the only type of smoking cessation aid available. Nicotine
replacement is also available in the form of chewing gum, nasal spray,
inhaler, sublingual tablets and lozenges. There is little direct evidence that
one nicotine replacement product is more effective than another. The
decision about which product to use should be guided by individual preferences. Miss RW should be advised to consult her GP after she has
returned home with a view to attending a specialist smoking clinic.

How should the use of the combined oral contraceptive pill be
managed?

A4 **It is recommended that patients taking a combined oral
contraceptive pill should stop taking it one full cycle prior to
an elective surgical admission in order to prevent this
additional low risk factor for DVT/PE in patients undergoing**

surgery. However, the decision to stop combined oral contraceptives prior to admission should be made on the basis of weighing up additional risk factors for thromboembolism with the risk of pregnancy, if contraception fails.

There is no evidence to suggest that progestogen-only preparations are associated with an increased risk of venous thromboembolism peri-operatively, but compliance is essential because the pill must be taken at exactly the same time each day. Miss RW has not stopped her combined oral contraceptive pill prior to admission so it should be stopped on admission and she should be treated with DVT/PE prophylaxis according to protocol. Miss RW should be counselled to recommence her combined oral contraceptive pill once at home and fully mobile. The course should be recommenced on day 1 of the cycle; if starting on day 4 of cycle or later, additional precautions (barrier methods) are required for the first seven days.

Is thromboembolic prophylaxis important in this case?

A5 **Yes. Miss RW is undergoing abdominal surgery which lasts more than 30 minutes. This carries a significant risk factor on its own for the development of post-operative DVT/PE which may be fatal.**

Miss RW also has other risk factors for the development of post-operative DVT/PE. She is overweight and admits to smoking 20 cigarettes per day. She was taking a combined oral contraceptive pill until admission. Using the Thrift consensus guidelines these factors put her at moderate risk of developing a post-operative DVT/PE and for this reason it is essential that Miss RW receives thromboembolic prophylaxis.

How should enoxaparin be administered?

A6 **Enoxaparin is licensed to be administered into the abdomen by deep subcutaneous injection. The patient should be lying down and the injections should alternate between the left and right sides of the abdominal wall.**

The whole length of the needle should be introduced vertically into a skin fold held between the thumb and index finger. The skin fold should not be released until the injection is complete. The injection site should not be rubbed.

Occasionally patients are too uncomfortable to have an injection into their abdomen or there are too many drains or dressings *in situ*. Enoxaparin can then be administered into the arms or legs by subcutaneous injection, but these are unlicensed sites.

Are the nutritional and pressure sore risk assessments important for Miss RW?

A7 **Yes. Ideally all patients admitted to hospital should have a nutritional and pressure sore risk assessment.**

The reason for performing these assessments when patients are admitted to hospital and during their stay is to identify patients who have deficits in their nutritional status, who may require dietary advice or may be at risk of developing pressure sores. The results of these assessments result in positive action by the nursing staff, which is important from both a quality of care and risk management perspective. Traditionally, nursing staff have underestimated the nutritional risk which patients are under or their risk of tissue breakdown. There is now a wealth of evidence which demonstrates that if nutritional and pressure sore risk assessments are in place, the incidence of post-operative complications and hospital-acquired pressure sores reduces significantly. Regular mattress audits should also be undertaken to ensure worn mattresses are removed from use. During her admission, Miss RW's skin should be examined daily for any sign of tissue breakdown.

Outline a pharmaceutical care plan for this patient.

A8 **The pharmaceutical care plan for Miss RW should consist of a problem list, aims of pharmaceutical treatment, interventions or monitoring required and an evaluation section. The pharmaceutical aspects of Miss RW's care which need to be included in the care plan are:**

(a)   Choice of anti-emetic.
(b)   Choice and method of administration of analgesia.
(c)   Use and duration of prophylactic antibiotics.
(d)   Methods and duration of thromboembolic prophylaxis.
(e)   Discharge medication planning and patient counselling.
(f)   Smoking cessation.

What should the pharmacist do about this situation?

A9 **Discuss the matter with the patient, the nurse in charge of the ward and the patient's surgical house officer.**

The pharmacist should ascertain how long Miss RW has been taking ibuprofen and at what dosage. The pharmacist should then explain the similarity of ibuprofen and diclofenac and the importance of always including over-the-counter medicines when asked about 'current medication'. The pharmacist should not be 'heavy handed' with Miss RW about the situation, but should obtain Miss RW's permission to remove the ibuprofen tablets from her locker. The ibuprofen tablets may be stored either in a locked cupboard on the ward or destroyed with Miss RW's consent. If there is a Patient's Own Drug scheme then it may be beneficial to stop the diclofenac and use Miss RW's ibuprofen, if this provides adequate analgesia.

What combinations of drugs are used in epidurals?

A10 **Epidurals are usually a mixture of a local anaesthetic agent and an opioid. Occasionally local anaesthetic agents are used alone. The most commonly prescribed solution is bupivacaine with fentanyl. The concentrations used in these solutions across the country vary widely. A review of the literature suggests that bupivacaine 0.125–0.15% with fentanyl 2 micrograms/mL results in effective pain relief without increasing the side-effect profile.**

The effectiveness of the analgesia depends on many factors including:

(a)   The drugs chosen.
(b)   The site of the epidural.
(c)   The volume and concentration of the local anaesthetic.

   These all contribute to the degree of sensory and motor block achieved.

How do these agents work?

A11 **These agents have different mechanisms of action and in combination they act synergistically, which reduces the dose of each agent required to produce adequate analgesia. This reduces the incidence of side-effects. Opioids selectively block pain transmission by their action on opioid receptors. Local anaesthetics inhibit nerve transmission.**

(a)   Fentanyl. Opioids diffuse across the dura mater into the cerebrospinal fluid. Here they bind with the opioid receptors in the dorsal horn of the spinal column and modify transmission of pain impulses to the brain. The remainder of the drug is absorbed into the epidural veins and passes into the systemic circulation, which may produce a small degree of systemic analgesia.

(b)   Bupivacaine. Local anaesthetic agents block sodium channels along the nerve fibre, which results in a local block of pain transmission in the spinal canal. The degree of blockade depends on the total amount of drug instilled, which in turn depends upon the solution concentration and the rate of infusion

Small unmyelinated fibres are affected first, large myelinated fibres last. Loss of nerve function occurs in the following order: pain, temperature, touch, deep pressure, skeletal muscle power and finally autonomic blockade.

What are the side-effects of epidurals and how can they be managed?

A12 **Side-effects can include urine retention, hypotension, sensory loss, and (rarely) pruritus, respiratory depression and nausea. Side-effects with epidurals can be minimised by close monitoring of the patient, and adhering to a standardised system and the use of colour-coded, dedicated epidural lines. Serious drug side-effects with epidurals are usually the result of accidental intravenous administration instead of epidural administration. There is also a small risk of paralysis during the insertion of the epidural catheter.**

As a result of media attention about epidurals, patients are often very concerned about having an epidural inserted and this needs to be discussed and informed patient consent obtained. Patients also need to understand that as a result of epidural administration they may become unaware of the need to urinate, as sensory awareness of the bladder can be lost. Depending on local practice, patients will either be routinely catheterised on initiation of therapy or monitored for this adverse event and catheterised if needed.

Specific side-effects are as follows:

(a)   Epidural fentanyl. Side-effects as any opioid.

   (i)   Pruritus is caused by histamine release, although it is not that common with fentanyl. If it occurs it is likely to be on the face, chest and abdomen and within the first few hours of epidural initiation.

(ii) Respiratory depression is uncommon with low-dose infusions because the high solubility of fentanyl confines its effect mainly to the spinal cord. If it is going to occur it is most likely within the first hour of initiating the infusion. It can be reversed with naloxone.

(iii) Nausea is rare with low-dose infusions but is a result of systemic action.

(iv) Urinary retention is a result of the inhibition of the micturition reflex and is not readily reversed.

(v) Slowing of gastrointestinal motility is less likely than with parenteral administration.

(b) Epidural bupivacaine.

(i) Hypotension is the most commonly occurring cardiovascular side-effect, especially if the patient is hypovolaemic. It can result in decreased heart rate and blood pressure. If not a symptom of hypovolaemia then it can be treated with ephedrine, a potent vasoconstrictor (alpha- and beta-agonist), by administering 3–6 mg by slow intravenous injection, repeated every three to four minutes to a maximum dose of 30 mg.

(ii) Sensory loss may include numbness of the legs and tongue and shivering.

(iii) Urinary retention. As a result of the sacral level block there is a reduced ability for the urinary sphincter to relax.

(iv) Neurotoxicity. This is generally only in the case of overdose or accidental systemic administration and includes light-headedness, dizziness, visual/auditory disturbances, e.g. tinnitus and inability to focus. In severe cases twitching, tremors and convulsions may occur.

> What other methods of opioid analgesic administration could have been used for Miss RW?

A13 **The other major methods of administering post-operative opioid analgesia are via fixed regular or 'as required' doses of intramuscular injections, or a PCA system.**

Administering opioid analgesia via fixed regular or 'as required' doses of intramuscular injections is fraught with problems, such as the difficulty in assessing how much opioid will be required and how frequently it should be given for each individual patient. Numerous factors influence the amount and frequency of analgesia required. These include the patient's age, weight, height, sex and type of operation. Many factors also influence the kinetics of an intramuscular dose in a patient after surgery, such as the patient's temperature and circulating blood volume. Therefore, a patient who returns to the ward hypothermic after a lengthy procedure, and hypovolaemic, because of inadequate fluid replacement, will have poor perfusion of skeletal muscle with resultant poor absorption of any opioid analgesia administered. If an increased amount of opioid analgesic is prescribed to overcome this situation and provide an adequate level of pain relief, there is a serious risk that as the contributing factors to the poor skeletal muscle perfusion are corrected, the patient will become 'overdosed' with opioid which may increase the risk of respiratory depression and sedation. Sometimes patients also feel reticent to ask for an injection, either because they do not want to 'bother the nursing staff' or wish to avoid having an injection. This results in inadequate levels of analgesia. Infusion devices, epidurals or PCAs provide much better analgesia and therefore aid recovery.

What is meant by 'patient-controlled analgesia' (PCA)?

A14   **PCA is a method of pain control whereby patients self-administer small doses of an intravenous opioid analgesic using a specially designed pump.**

This method of opioid administration is generally accepted as safe and effective. In contrast to conventional intramuscular opioid analgesia, PCA is associated with fewer adverse effects, better pulmonary recovery after abdominal surgery, decreased nursing time for drug administration, improved individualisation of drug dosages, improved analgesia and reduced length of patient stay in hospital. It also allows patients to take control of their own pain relief.

There are many devices available to administer opioid analgesia via PCA. The electronic infusion pumps used to administer PCA consist of a microprocessor, which is programmed to deliver a set volume of analgesic with a lock-out period, during which time the patient can receive no further doses of analgesic. Some PCA pumps consist of a mini-printer from which a printout of everything which has occurred to the device since it was set up is listed, e.g. the number of times the patient has pressed the demand button, the number of doses received and the volume of analgesic remaining. The disposable devices used to administer PCA are more simple, with a fixed lock-out period and fixed volume delivered by each press of the demand button outside the lock-out period. The various devices used to administer PCA differ enormously and there should be careful multidisciplinary evaluation of the different products available before any choice to purchase is made.

When is PCA not a suitable choice of analgesia?

A15 **Exclusion criteria for the use of PCA would include:**

(a) **Major, complex procedures.**

(b) **Any known allergies to the opioid used for PCA.**

(c) **Pregnancy.**

(d) **Breast-feeding.**

(e) **History of drug abuse.**

(f) **Patients with rheumatoid arthritis or any other disabilities with their fingers which prevent them from operating the device.**

(g) **Patients with pre-existing neurological disease.**

(h) **Patients whose English prevents full understanding of the device, although literature is available for some PCA devices in a number of different languages.**

(i) **Those who do not wish to use PCA.**

(j) **Emergency surgical procedures, when there is insufficient time pre-operatively to explain about PCA and how to use the device or when the patient is too unwell to understand.**

What counselling points would have needed to be covered if Miss RW had chosen PCA for post-operative analgesia?

A16 **If patients are deemed suitable for PCA, it is essential that they receive counselling on its use prior to surgery and also given the opportunity to refuse to use it if they do not wish to take control of their analgesia.**

The nurse, doctor or pharmacist counselling Miss RW prior to surgery would need to explain how PCA works, how to obtain a dose, how hard to press the demand button, the lock-out period, what this means and what to do if she remained in pain. A demonstration PCA kit would have been available for Miss RW, so that she could handle the device and practise pressing the demand button before going to theatre. A patient information booklet about PCA would also have been provided for Miss RW to read through and she would have been encouraged to ask any questions she had about the PCA. There are also videos available to help with patient counselling about PCA. Miss RW would have been made aware that the nursing staff would be assessing her pain score every hour and told how the pain scoring method works. The nursing staff would have regularly monitored the PCA device during use.

Is there an advantage to using an epidural over PCA for Miss RW?

A17   **Yes. Epidurals manage pain more effectively than a PCA.**

A cholecystectomy is a major, abdominal operation. Surgery takes about an hour, and involves abdominal dissection and manipulation to remove the gall bladder. Post-operatively there is likely to be substantial pain and while PCA could be used, an epidural is likely to provide better analgesia.

What is the purpose of 'premedication'?

A18   **The purpose of premedication prior to surgery is to allow patients to go through the pre-operative period free of apprehension and sedated enough to be comfortable, but still rousable and able to cooperate fully in their care.**

Prior to anaesthesia the anaesthetist will explain to Miss RW what is to happen, where she will wake up and that she may feel ill on waking. Pre-medication is best administered one hour prior to surgery.

Do you agree with the choice of Miss RW's premedication?

A19   **Yes. Oral premedication with a short-acting benzodiazepine such as temazepam is common practice, as benzodiazepines meet the criteria outlined in Question 18.**

Anti-emetics are not routinely administered during premedication, but on induction Miss RW will receive an intravenous dose of morphine. As anti-emetics are best administered thirty minutes prior to emetic stimuli, then it is sensible to administer an anti-emetic with the premedication. Also Miss RW is suffering with nausea pre-operatively, therefore it is sensible to treat this prior to induction.

In addition, Miss RW received her last dose of enoxaparin at least 12 hours earlier which will allow an epidural cannula to be inserted without an increased risk of a haematoma.

Why was Miss RW given antibiotics and morphine at induction?

A20 The antibiotics were administered prophylactically and the morphine was administered to supplement the analgesic effects of the anaesthetics.

Antibiotic prophylaxis is defined as 'Administration of an antimicrobial drug in the absence of known infection in order to decrease the likelihood of subsequent infection at a surgical site'. Prophylactic antibiotics are most effective if they are administered during the two-hour period before the surgical incision. This is because high levels of antibiotics are needed in the blood stream and tissues in the minutes after the incision to prevent bacterial seeding of the operative wound.

As Miss RW is to undergo surgery on her biliary tract, the most likely organisms to be encountered are *Enterococci* and *Enterobacteriacae*. The need for metronidazole in this situation is debatable because anaerobes are not usually present in the biliary tract and cefuroxime should provide adequate prophylactic cover for the organisms most likely to be present.

Morphine is administered intraoperatively to supplement the analgesic effects of anaesthetics, which, if used alone, may not provide adequate analgesia for a patient undergoing major surgery. The administration of opioid analgesics, such as morphine, with anaesthetic agents also reduces the total amount of anaesthetic required.

How should patient's with epidurals be monitored?

A21 The detailed monitoring of an epidural will depend on hospital policy. Generally patients with epidurals have blood pressure, heart rate, respiratory rate and level of block monitored every hour. The total amount of drug remaining in the syringe and the total amount infused is also checked hourly to prevent the chance of mechanical error.

Level of block is checked using ethyl chloride spray (because it is cold). This is sprayed over the patient's torso and the patient identifies where they can feel it. If the analgesia is felt to be insufficient then the nurses can increase the epidural rate until the maximum prescribed rate is reached. If the epidural is still not providing adequate relief then an alternative pain system must be used or the epidural re-sited.

What methods of thromboembolic prophylaxis are being used for Miss RW?

A22 **Miss RW is receiving prophylactic subcutaneous enoxaparin injections. She has also been fitted with graduated below-knee compression stockings and an intermittent compression device was used on her calves during surgery.**

A larger reduction in the incidence of post-operative DVT and/or PE is achieved when these three different methods of thromboembolic prophylaxis are used together, rather than in isolation. Enoxaparin is used because it is a once a day injection and it currently costs less than unfractionated heparin. At the time of writing there is no evidence demonstrating that any of the low-molecular-weight heparins available are superior to unfractionated heparin in reducing the incidence of DVT/PE following general surgery. Properly fitted graduated compression stockings increase the velocity of venous return. Below-knee stockings are as effective as above-knee stockings, more comfortable and a fraction of the cost. Intermittent compression devices rhythmically alter the pressure in an envelope around the calves during surgery and reduce the incidence of DVT, especially when continued post-operatively. Early post-operative ambulation may also help to reduce the incidence of DVT, but this is not proven. It has been recommended that individual clinicians, units and hospitals in the UK should develop written policies for prophylaxis, and the use of prophylaxis should be included in clinical audit and care pathways.

What is meant by 'insensible losses'?

A23 **The term 'insensible fluid loss' refers to water loss from the body via evaporation from the skin and water vapour expired from the lungs. It can be estimated at 0.5 mL/kg/h at 37°C.**

Is there a rationale for co-prescribing NSAIDs and paracetamol with opioids post-operatively?

A24 **Yes. Opioid analgesics, paracetamol and NSAIDs have different modes of action and are complementary in their analgesic effects.**

It has been demonstrated that by administering opioids with paracetamol or diclofenac during the post-operative period, opioid requirements can be reduced by one-third. However, NSAIDs should be reserved for patients for whom analgesia cannot be provided by opioids and simple analgesics alone. This is because NSAIDs can have serious side-effects. Also there is a risk that using NSAIDs for post-operative analgesia may lead to wound haematoma, especially if the patient is receiving heparin.

Should gastrointestinal prophylaxis have been co-prescribed with the NSAID?

A25 **No. The National Institute for Clinical Excellence (NICE) have circulated a list of patient risk factors for gastrointestinal ulceration. These should be applied. Miss RW is unlikely to be nil by mouth for very long, she is young, she is not on any other drugs irritant to the gastric mucosa such as prednisolone and she has no history of gastric problems. She does not have predictable risk factors for gastrointestinal ulceration and therefore should just be counselled to take her diclofenac after food, but to stop it immediately if she experiences any symptoms of indigestion.**

Was the pharmacist right to request this?

A26 **Yes. The current local antibiotic prophylaxis guidelines for biliary surgery are for one dose of intravenous cefuroxime and metronidazole on induction and three doses at eight-hourly intervals, post-operatively.**

The answer to this question therefore depends on the surgical antibiotic prophylaxis guidelines in place within the hospital or Trust. Prophylactic antibiotics should not be continued for more than 48 hours, although most of the evidence is for 24 hours only. A limit of 12 hours is desirable for most types of wound and operation, although if spillage of bowel contents occurs during surgery or there is some other form of wound contamination, the surgeon may request that antibiotics are continued for three to five days. This would then be classed as treatment and should be documented as such in the patient's case notes.

Do you agree with the choice of oral analgesia for Miss RW?

A27 **Yes. Once the immediate post-operative requirement for opioid analgesia has passed, a combination of paracetamol with a weak opioid and a NSAID if needed usually provides good analgesia for general surgical patients, providing they**

do not have any contra-indications to receiving NSAIDs. Compound preparations are no better than individual agents and it is more difficult to titrate the dose to achieve the required level of analgesia whilst minimising side-effects.

The nursing staff should be educated that these different forms of analgesia are additive in their effects when given in combination, and they should be encouraged to use them together.

Should the first dose of intramuscular morphine be given as the epidural stops?

A28 **This again would depend on individual hospital guidelines. There is no clinical reason why the first dose of opioid cannot be given immediately the epidural stops but most hospitals have policies which stipulate a gap of about four hours between stopping the epidural and giving the first dose of intramuscular opioid.**

How long should her thromboembolic prophylaxis continue?

A29 **Following general surgical procedures, thromboembolic prophylaxis should continue at least until discharge, rather than for any predetermined time.**

Miss RW is obese, smokes, was taking a combined oral contraceptive pill until admission and has undergone major abdominal surgery. These factors put Miss RW into a moderate risk category for the development of DVT/PE despite the fact she is under 40 years of age and has no history of venous thromboembolism. Prophylaxis with enoxaparin should continue until discharge and consideration should be given to the continued use of graduated compression stockings for four to six weeks post-discharge. Thromboembolism can occur up to six weeks post-operatively and patients should be encouraged to remain mobile following their return home.

Miss RW must not have her epidural cannula removed until at least 12 hours after a dose of enoxaparin to prevent the risk of an epidural haematoma.

What advice should Miss RW be given about her medication prior to discharge?

A30 **There are several important medication counselling points which Miss RW should receive prior to discharge.**

The medication counselling should include the importance of taking the tablets to remain pain free rather than trying just to tolerate the pain. Her own ibuprofen has less gastrointestinal side-effects than diclofenac but is also less potent; however in combination with regular paracetamol this should be adequate. The importance of taking her ibuprofen after food must be stressed to Miss RW, and she should be advised to stop them if she has any signs of dyspepsia and to consult her GP immediately. Prior to admission Miss RW was also taking metoclopramide. Following her surgery, anti-emetics are no longer required and she should be encouraged to return these to her community pharmacist for destruction. If the oral analgesia is ineffective, Miss RW should consult her GP. In this situation an additional prescription for dihydrocodeine would be appropriate. Finally, Miss RW was taking a combined oral contraceptive pill up until admission. This can be recommenced at the first menses occurring at least two weeks after full mobilisation.

Further reading

Anon. Preventing and treating deep vein thrombosis. *Drug Ther Bull* 1992; **30**: 9–12.

Anon. Nicotine replacement therapy. *MeReC Bull* 1999; **10**(3): 9–12.

Badner NH, Komar WE. Low-dose bupivacaine does not improve postoperative analgesia. *Anaesth Anal* 1994; **72**: 337–341.

Benzon HT, Wong CA. The effects of low-dose bupivacaine on post-operative epidural analgesia and thrombelastography. *Anaesth Anal* 1994; **79**: 911–917.

Chan KL, Hung LCT, Suen BY *et al.* Celecoxib versus diclofenac and omeprazole in reducing the risk of recurrent ulcer bleeding in patients with arthritis. *N Engl J Med* 2002; **347**: 2104–2110.

Dollery C, ed. *Therapeutic Drugs*, 2nd edn, Churchill Livingston, Edinburgh, 1998.

Godney JA. Side-effects of epidural infusions of opioid bupivacaine mixtures. *Anaesthiology* 1998; **53**: 1148–1155.

Lancaster T, Stead L, Silagy C *et al.* Effectiveness of interventions to help people stop smoking: findings from the Cochrane Library. *Br Med J* 2000; **321**: 355–358.

McQuay HJ, Moore RA. *An Evidence-based Resource for Pain Relief.* Oxford University Press, Oxford, 1998.

National Institute for Clinical Excellence. *Guidance on the Use of Cyclo-oxygenase (Cox) II Selective Inhibitors, Celecoxib, Rofecoxib, Meloxicam and Etodolac for Osteoarthritis And Rheumatoid Arthritis*. NICE, London, 2001.

Scottish Intercollegiate Guidelines Network. *Guidance on Antibiotic Prophylaxis in the Surgical Patient*, SIGN, Edinburgh, 2000.

Scottish Intercollegiate Guidelines Network. *Guidance on Prophylaxis of Venous Thromboembolism*. SIGN, Edinburgh, 1995.

Thromboembolic Risk Factors (THRIFT) Consensus Group. Risk of and prophylaxis for venous thromboembolism in hospital patients. *Br Med J* 1992; **305**: 567–574.

31

Managing medicine risk

Gillian F Cavell

Case study and questions

Day 1 Mrs MR, a 74-year-old lady, was admitted on a Friday night after being referred from her nursing home with a recent history of increasing confusion and urinary incontinence. A urinary tract infection was suspected. Her past medical history included atrial fibrillation, Type 2 diabetes mellitus and osteoporosis. The medication history documented on the GP referral letter included digoxin 0.625 mg daily, warfarin, furosemide 20 mg daily, gliclazide 80 mg twice daily, Tylex 2 four times a day for pain, alendronate and Adcal-D3. An allergy to penicillin was also noted by the GP.

On examination she was confused, appeared dehydrated and smelled of urine. Her blood pressure was 110/80 mmHg and her pulse was normal at 80 beats per minute. Her temperature was elevated at 38.5°C. She was noted to be confused and unable to answer questions put to her by the junior doctor. Her nursing home was contacted and they reported that she was normally quite well and her present condition was unusual for her.

Her serum biochemistry was as follows:

- Sodium 141 mmol/L (reference range 135–145)
- Potassium 3.6 mmol/L (3.5–5)
- Creatinine 128 mmol/L (60–120)
- Random blood glucose 16.5 mmol/L (3.5–10)
- Red blood cells (RBC) 5×10^9/L (4.5–6.5×10^9)
- White blood cells (WBC) 15×10^9/L (4–11×10^9)
- Haemoglobin 11.8 g/dL (13–18)
- International normalised ratio (INR) 2.3

A random sample of urine was sent off for microscopy, culture and sensitivity. In the meantime she was commenced on ciprofloxacin 250 mg orally twice daily to treat the urinary tract infection. An intravenous sliding-scale insulin regimen was commenced to reduce her blood glucose level. The furosemide was discontinued. Intravenous fluids were written up as follows: 40 mmol potassium in 1000 mL sodium chloride 0.9% infusion, followed by 1000 mL sodium chloride 0.9% infusion.

Q1   Comment on the medication history.
Q2   How should the medication history be confirmed?
Q3   Outline a pharmaceutical care plan for Mrs MR.
Q4   What hazards are associated with intravenous potassium replacement therapy?
Q5   Should concentrated potassium solutions be held in clinical areas?
Q6   What risks are associated with the use of infusion devices and how can they be managed?

Day 2   Mrs MR remained confused and was refusing to take anything orally. A nasogastric tube was passed to facilitate the administration of oral fluids and medicines.

Q7   What risks are associated with drug administration through enteral feeding lines and how can they be managed?

Day 3   The patient's drug chart was seen by the ward pharmacist on Monday morning. The pharmacist noted that the patient had received a dose of phytomenadione 1 mg, intravenously, on Sunday evening, in response to an INR of 8. Her warfarin therapy had been discontinued.

Q8   What was the most likely cause of Mrs Mr's elevated INR?
Q9   What action should be taken?

On the regular prescription Mrs MR was prescribed digoxin 0.625 mg daily, alendronate 70 mg at 8 a.m., Adcal-D3 2 at 8 a.m., Tylex 2 four times daily and lactulose 10 mL twice daily, in addition to ciprofloxacin 250 mg twice daily. She was also prescribed co-dydramol two tablets every six hours if required for pain relief. No allergy history had been documented on the drug chart.

Q10   Comment on the prescription. What changes would you recommend?
Q11   How might problems associated with misplaced decimal points be avoided?

The patient's prescription was corrected as recommended. Trimethoprim 200 mg twice daily was added to treat her urinary tract infection.

The alendronate prescription had been signed as given daily. The patient had been given three doses of 70 mg from a supply of alendronate 10 mg tablets dispensed for another patient.

Q12 What are the likely causes of this error?

Q13 Suggest ways in which this type of error might be avoided in future.

Her INR on Monday evening was 2.9 and warfarin was represcribed at her usual maintenance dose to commence on Tuesday.

Q14 What advice would you give the nurses to facilitate administration of the tablets through the nasogastric tube?

Day 5   Mrs MR was much improved. Her temperature had reduced to 37.2°C and she was much less confused and able to talk to her daughter who came to visit. Her INR had returned to within the target range for thromboprophylaxis in atrial fibrillation (2–3).

Q15 How should information about Mrs MR's medication be communicated to her GP?

Day 7   Mrs MR was discharged back to her nursing home.

Comment on the medication history.

A1 **The medication history is incomplete and appears to contain a dosing error.**

The digoxin dose is written on the GP referral letter as 0.625 mg, which is equivalent to 625 micrograms. This dose is unlikely to be correct. It is more likely to be a transcription error with a misplaced decimal point. Doses are missing for warfarin, alendronate and Adcal-D3.

How should the medication history be confirmed?

A2 **The medication history should be confirmed by contacting either Mrs MR's nursing home or her GP for a list of her current medication.**

A medication history can be confirmed in several ways: interview the patient; identify a list of prescribed drugs from the duplicate prescription the patient may have with them; identify a list of prescribed medication from a hand-written or printed *aide-mémoire* the patient may carry; identify the patient's current medication from the patient's own supply if it is available; contact the patient's GP to discuss the current medication regimen and doses with him, or contact the patient's nursing home and request a faxed copy of the medication administration record or a list of current medication.

As Mrs MR is confused and is cared for in a nursing home it would not be appropriate to obtain a medication history from her directly. Additionally, she is unlikely to be holding a copy of a repeat prescription or an *aide-mémoire* as she does not have responsibility for self-administration of her medicines. The most appropriate way of confirming the medication history for Mrs MR would be to try to obtain a faxed copy of her medicine administration record and, as she is on warfarin, the most recent entry in her yellow anticoagulant booklet. Any outstanding queries can be clarified by speaking directly to her GP.

Outline a pharmaceutical care plan for Mrs MR.

A3 **The pharmaceutical care plan for Mrs MR should include the following:**

(a) Ensure that the medication history for Mrs MR is accurate and complete.

(b)   Ensure all prescriptions are accurate, complete and unambiguous.

(c)   Ensure all medicines are prescribed according to the *British National Formulary* prescribing guidelines.

(d)   Ensure that allergy documentation is complete.

(e)   Monitor the prescription for drug interactions and therapeutic duplication.

(f)   Advise medical staff on the appropriate choice of antibiotic.

(g)   Provide advice to nursing staff on the safe administration of medicines.

(h)   Advise nursing staff of the availability of ready-made potassium-containing infusions.

(i)   Provide medication-related information appropriate to the needs of Mrs MR and/or her carers after discharge.

What hazards are associated with intravenous potassium replacement therapy?

A4   High concentrations of intravenous potassium administered rapidly can cause fatal cardiac arrhythmias. Such situations can arise as a result of accidental administration of concentrated potassium solutions or when concentrated potassium solutions are added to large infusions without adequate mixing during preparation.

Potassium chloride is one of the cocktail of drugs used to carry out the death sentence of convicted criminals in certain parts of the world. There have been reports in the literature of deaths associated with inadvertent use of potassium chloride in hospitals, where ampoules of concentrated potassium solutions have been mistaken for ampoules of sodium chloride 0.9%, Water for Injections or furosemide.

Should concentrated potassium solutions be held in clinical areas?

A5   Ideally, no. The storage of concentrated potassium solutions, including potassium chloride and potassium phosphate, should be restricted to critical care areas where infusions containing high concentrations of potassium are frequently administered to patients with close monitoring.

In order to reduce the risk of errors associated with concentrated potassium solutions in NHS hospitals the UK National Patient Safety Agency (NPSA) has made recommendations for the ordering, storage and use of concentrated potassium solutions in a Patient Safety Alert.

It is recommended that, wherever possible, intravenous potassium should be administered using commercially available, ready-mixed solutions. This reduces the need for ampoules of concentrated potassium solutions to be stored in clinical areas. Where it is necessary to store the ampoules in clinical areas their receipt and use must be documented in a register, and preparation and administration of infusions containing concentrated potassium must be double-checked.

Pharmacists should promote the prescription of intravenous potassium in amounts that correspond to concentrations in commercially available infusions.

Mrs MR was prescribed 40 mmol potassium in 1000 mL sodium chloride 0.9% which can be supplied by pharmacy as a commercially prepared infusion.

What risks are associated with the use of infusion devices and how can they be managed?

A6 **Because of the array of infusion devices available staff should be able to select the most appropriate device for the drug to be administered and be trained in the use of that device.**

Infusion devices are used widely in secondary care to administer potent drugs intravenously at a controlled rate. Mrs MR is receiving intravenous insulin at a variable rate to control her blood glucose. The rate of administration of the insulin needs to be carefully controlled to ensure that the dose administered is accurate and titrated to her current blood glucose measurement to avoid hypo- or hyperglycaemia.

Adverse incidents associated with the use of infusion devices can occur for a number of reasons, including failure of the device itself, user error, inadequate servicing and maintenance, inappropriate device selection and inadequate instructions for use. User error is the most frequent cause of infusion device-related adverse incidents. Errors may be a result of misloading the syringe, setting the wrong rate, not confirming the set rate, not confirming the pump type or syringe size and not stopping the pump correctly.

To reduce the risk of infusion-related errors staff need to be trained to operate any piece of equipment they are expected to use and be trained not to use equipment they are unfamiliar with. This may be difficult if a wide range of infusion devices is available in clinical areas. Some hospitals have introduced equipment libraries where infusion devices are procured, serviced and stored centrally. Such centralisation ensures that a range of appropriate, well-maintained devices is available for use, and support in the form of training and advice is available.

The UK Clinical Negligence Scheme for Trusts, Clinical Risk Management Standard 5, requires NHS Trusts to ensure the training and competence of all clinical staff in the use of equipment. For each piece of equipment, the users and their training needs are identified. Staff can then be trained and certified as competent in the use of equipment needed to carry out their clinical role.

What risks are associated with drug administration through enteral feeding lines and how can they be managed?

A7 In order to administer drugs safely through enteral feeding lines issues such as formulation, interactions with the feed and method of dose preparation need to be considered.

Not all formulations intended for oral administration are suitable for crushing for administration via enteral feeding lines. In addition, where patients also have intravenous access, there is a risk of inadvertent intravenous administration of oral medicines if an intravenous syringe is used to prepare the dose.

In order to administer oral medicines through a nasogastric tube they need to be either formulated as a liquid medicine or prepared by crushing and suspending oral solid dosage forms. Not all solid oral dose forms can be crushed without altering the pharmacokinetic profile. Modified- and controlled-release tablets and enteric-coated formulations should not be crushed for administration in this way. Where tablets are crushed they should be suspended in plenty of water and the tube flushed after administration to prevent it blocking. Some medicines interact with the feed, possibly reducing drug absorption. Depending on the drug being administered, the feed will need to be discontinued for a while before and after medicines administration.

In many hospitals intravenous syringes are used to administer doses of oral medicines to patients via enteral (nasogastric, gastrostomy or jejunostomy) lines and also to administer doses of liquid medicines which cannot easily be measured in a graduated measuring pot. When oral medicines are drawn up in intravenous syringes there is always the risk of wrong-route errors, e.g. inadvertent administration of an oral medicine via the intravenous route, especially if the patient has an intravenous access. There have been reports of fatalities as a result of the administration of oral medicines via the intravenous route. Part of the reason this risk exists is that the additive ports on the enteral giving-sets have Luer connectors which makes them *incompatible* with the tips of the oral syringes used to measure liquid medicines for children as out-patients, but *compatible* with intravenous syringes which have luer tips. If oral syringes are used to administer medicines via enteral feeding lines an adapter needs to be fitted to the tip to enable it to fit the luer connection.

Due to these risks, which have potentially disastrous consequences, the use of intravenous syringes for measuring oral medicines should be discouraged.

What was the most likely cause of Mrs MR's elevated INR?

A8   The elevated INR was most likely to have been caused by an interaction between ciprofloxacin and warfarin.
Ciprofloxacin enhances the effects of warfarin, leading to over-anticoagulation.

This event can be described as a clinically significant prescribing error. A prescribing error has been defined in the UK literature as follows: 'A clinically meaningful prescribing error occurs when, as a result of a prescribing decision or prescription writing process, there is an unintentional significant reduction in the probability of treatment being timely and effective or an increase in the risk of harm when compared with generally accepted practice'.

Prescribing errors often occur as a result of lack of knowledge about the drug or lack of knowledge about the patient. Errors can also occur where there is a lack of understanding of how the patient's clinical condition may alter the way the drug is handled by the body, e.g. renally excreted drugs in a patient with renal impairment. The majority of prescribing for hospital in-patients is done by junior doctors. Because of their relative inexperience, junior doctors are unlikely to have sufficient knowledge to prescribe in every situation without the support of senior medical and pharmacist colleagues.

In this instance, an incorrect prescribing decision has been made as a result of lack of knowledge of the interaction between warfarin and ciprofloxacin. The two drugs were then administered concurrently over the weekend when clinical pharmacy services were not available.

In the absence of computerised prescribing systems with effective decision support software there was no feedback to the junior doctor to alert him of the interaction and the risk of over-anticoagulation. Most hospitals only provide clinical pharmacy services to wards, including drug chart review, for all patients on a weekday basis. At weekends and on

Bank Holidays prescribing for hospital in-patients is not routinely reviewed for safety and appropriateness. Prescribing errors such as this are therefore unlikely to be identified before doses have been given and, in some instances, after patients have experienced an adverse event.

What action should be taken?

A9 **The prescriber should be contacted to advise him of the interaction.**

The pharmacist should discuss the interaction with the junior doctor and recommend a suitable alternative antibiotic according to local micro-biology guidelines. Ciprofloxacin should be discontinued to enable war-farin therapy to be restarted as soon as possible.

Comment on the prescription. What changes would you recommend?

A10 **The prescription contains a number of pharmaceutical care issues that need to be resolved.**

(a) Digoxin.

The digoxin dose has been erroneously transcribed from the GP letter as 0.625 mg. As has been previously discussed this is likely to be a 10-fold error caused by a 'slip' when the letter was being written, resulting in a misplaced decimal point. The correct dose needs to be established and the prescription amended accordingly.

(b) Alendronate.

The dose of alendronate was not specified on the GP referral letter. A dose of 70 mg has been prescribed to be administered at 8 a.m. This dose should however only be administered once a week. Alendronate should not be administered within 30 minutes of any other drug.

(c) Adcal-D3.

Adcal-D3, used as a calcium and vitamin D supplement, should not be administered at the same time of day as alendronate. Ideally, the calcium preparation should be administered in the evening.

(d) Tylex.

Tylex is a combination analgesic containing 30 mg codeine phosphate and 500 mg paracetamol (co-codamol 30/500). The indication for regular use of this analgesic is unclear and is likely to be contributing to constipation and confusion in Mrs MR.

(e)   Co-dydramol.

Mrs MR is receiving maximal daily doses of paracetamol as Tylex taken as a regular prescription. The concurrent prescription of an additional paracetamol-containing analgesic is inappropriate and may result in overdosage especially if the nurses are unaware that Tylex contains paracetamol.

(f)   Allergy history not documented on chart.

The patient was reported to have an allergy to penicillin in the referral letter; however, this information has not been transferred to the drug chart. If this information is not available at the point of prescribing, the allergy may be overlooked and the patient may be prescribed a contra-indicated drug with the potential for causing serious harm.

The following changes to the prescription should be recommended:

(a)   The digoxin dose should be changed to 62.5 micrograms daily.
(b)   The alendronate dosage frequency should be changed from daily to weekly.
(c)   The timing of the Adcal-D3 should be changed from 8 a.m. to 6 p.m.
(d)   The 'as required' co-dydramol should be discontinued and the need for the regular codeine-containing analgesic reviewed.
(e)   The ciprofloxacin should be changed to trimethoprim.
(f)   Mrs MR's allergy status should be documented.

How might problems associated with misplaced decimal points be avoided?

A11   Guidance on prescription writing is available in The *British National Formulary* which is published twice a year by the British Medical Association and the Royal Pharmaceutical Society of Great Britain.

As well as ensuring that prescriptions are legal and legible, the *British National Formulary* states 'The unnecessary use of decimal points should be avoided'. Because Mrs MR's dose of digoxin was less than 1 mg the prescription should have been written as micrograms, i.e. 62.5 micrograms. Had the GP and the junior doctor written the dose in micrograms the high dose of 625 micrograms would have been identified and corrected at the point of prescribing.

Mrs MR has received digoxin against the original prescription over the weekend. It will be necessary to try to establish exactly what dose has been administered by the nursing staff to determine whether there is a risk of toxicity.

Illegible, incomplete, ambiguous and incorrect prescriptions are an important source of medication error. The prescription writing standards in the *British National Formulary* provide pharmacists with a tool for auditing and improving the quality of prescription writing within their organisations.

Some electronic prescribing systems lead prescribers to select a correct dose or are programmed to only accept drug doses which lie within predefined limits. For example, if a doctor wants to prescribe digoxin he may be led to choose between the commonly prescribed doses of 62.5, 125 or 250 micrograms. The option of 0.625 mg or 625 micrograms does not exist. Alternatively if he is allowed to input 625 micrograms a warning may appear to advise him that a dose outside the recommended range has been prescribed.

An electronic prescribing system introduced into one hospital in the US reduced the incidence of medication errors by about 60%. The system eliminates the need for the transcription of orders and includes a dose selection menu, simple allergy and drug–drug interaction checking, and indicates routes and usual frequency of drug dosing. Error rates at all stages of the medication process, including prescribing, transcription, dispensing and administration, were reduced.

What are the likely causes of this error?

A12 **Daily and weekly doses have been confused, possibly as a result of lack of flexibility of the in-patient prescription chart and lack of knowledge of the different formulations of alendronate.**

There are a number of causes of this error. Typically hospital medication administration records do not facilitate the prescribing of intermittent doses. Even if a weekly prescription is intended, there is scope for daily administration of drugs unless the days on which doses are not due are crossed through on the drug chart to indicate that no dose is due. If the nursing staff are unfamiliar with the usual doses of the medicine or the availability of different formulations of a medicine, the risk of administration of daily high doses is compounded. Mrs MR's drug chart has not been reviewed by a pharmacist over the weekend and so no endorsement highlighting the need for a weekly dosing regimen has been made.

Mrs MR received the inappropriate dose of alendronate because the product was available in the medicine trolley having been dispensed for another patient. Medicines dispensed by hospital pharmacy departments and stored in medicine trolleys tend to be treated as 'stock' drugs and may be used for more than one patient. The increasing trend towards reuse of patients' own drugs in hospitals and bedside storage of medicines is likely to reduce this tendency to 'share' non-stock drugs between patients.

Fortunately, Mrs MR is unlikely to experience any permanent harm from the overdose, although her serum calcium and phosphate levels should be monitored due to the risk of hypocalaemia and hypophospha-taemia. However, the risks from similar errors with other medicines may be more significant. Confusion between daily and weekly doses of metho-trexate and vindesine have resulted in serious patient harm.

Suggest ways in which this type of error might be avoided in future.

A13 **Reporting and collating error reports in order to develop an understanding of how and why they occur is a way of reducing the incidence of errors. Where errors are known to occur, risks can be identified and solutions put into place.**

This is an example of an error which has resulted from multiple system failures rather than the action of any individual.

In the past, error reporting has tended to focus on the actions of individuals, and has been associated with blame and punishment. It is now recognised that errors occur as a result of *active failures* and *latent conditions*. Active failures are unsafe practices of people working with a system. Latent conditions are organisational issues, such as resource allocation, management, environment and processes which, either alone or in combination with an active failure, can result in error. Blaming individuals discourages error reporting, making it difficult for organisa-tions to identify trends in the types of errors that occur and understand their risks. By understanding the conditions that may predispose to error, safe systems of work can be developed to reduce future risks. In *An Organisation with a Memory*, the Department of Health highlights the need for the NHS to learn from its mistakes and set up the NPSA to collect, assimilate and analyse adverse incidents, and to propose solutions to prevent their recurrence.

Although this error is unlikely to result in permanent patient harm it is an example of an error which should be reported as an adverse incident through the Trust incident-reporting scheme to the NPSA.

The use of electronic prescribing systems could eliminate this type of error by preventing the daily prescription of a product which is designed to be prescribed and administered weekly. In the future, electronic prescribing combined with bar-code technology, in which the product to be administered is identified by scanning a bar coded prescription and the product bar code, may be a means of confirming that the product selected for administration is the correct one for the prescription.

What advice would you give the nurses to facilitate administration of the tablets through the nasogastric tube?

A14 **Wherever possible, liquid formulations or soluble tablets of the prescribed medicines should be administered, ideally by using a suitably sized oral syringe. For some drugs differences in the bioavailability between liquid and solid dosage forms will need to be considered.**

Digoxin and trimethoprim should be dispensed as liquids and the prescription endorsed to show that these formulations have been made available. Although digoxin elixir is more bioavailable than the tablets (80% for the liquid compared to 70% for the tablets) a dosage adjustment is unlikely to be needed unless the patient has significant renal impairment.

Adcal-D3 tablets may be crushed and suspended prior to administration.

Alendronate tablets cannot be crushed for administration in this way. Alendronate should be withheld until Mrs ME can swallow the tablets whole.

Depending on the outcome of the analgesic review a soluble paracetamol-containing analgesic could be supplied.

The feed should be discontinued before the medicines are administered and the line flushed with 20–30 mL of water using a large, ideally 50-mL, oral syringe. The medicines should be administered one at a time using an oral syringe, with flushing between each one. The line should be finally flushed through prior to restarting the feed.

How should information about Mrs MR's medication be communicated to her GP?

A15 **Accurate, complete and timely information about a patient's medication should be transferred to the patient's GP as soon as possible after her discharge. Ideally this should be done electronically.**

Medication errors can occur when patients move from one health care setting to another. Effective communications are especially important at these stages in the patient journey. On discharge, the patient's new drug regimen and treatment plan need to be communicated in a timely and reliable way to ensure safe and seamless transfer of care back to the Primary Care Team.

When patients move between health care settings communication is often slow and incomplete. Delays in communicating information about the discharge medication mean that the information may not be available to the GP when he next prescribes for that patient. The patient may then be inadvertently prescribed medicines that are no longer indicated, duplicate drugs, drugs that interact or even drugs that are contra-indicated. This can lead to readmission to hospital with a preventable, drug-related problem.

When Mrs MR is discharged from hospital it is important that changes in her medication are communicated with both the GP and the nursing home so that she does not continue to receive the medicines she was prescribed prior to her admission. There is also evidence that communicating with the community pharmacist helps to reduce the incidence of discrepancies between the discharge medication and medication subsequently prescribed by the GP. Ideally this information should be transferred electronically to reduce delays, reduce the risk of transcription errors and help to ensure seamless care at the interface.

Further reading

National Patient Safety Agency. *Patient Safety Alert (PSA01) 2002*. Available at: www.npsa.org.uk

Richardson N. A review of drug infusion incidents. *Br J Intensive Care* 1995; Suppl.

Phillips J, Beam S, Brinker A *et al*. Retrospective analysis of mortalities associated with medication errors. *Am J Health-Syst Pharm* 2001; **58**: 1835–1841.

Dean B, Barber N, Schachter M. What is a prescribing error? *Quality in Health Care* 2000; 9: 232–237.

Bates DW, Leape L, Cullen DJ *et al*. Effect of computerized physician order entry and a team intervention on prevention of serious medication errors. *J Am Med Assoc* 1998; **280**: 1311–1316.

Cambridgeshire Health Authority. *Methotrexate Toxicity. An Inquiry into the Death of a Cambridgeshire Patient in April 2000*. Cambridgeshire Health Authority, Cambridge, 2000.

Department of Health. *An Organisation with a Memory*. Department of Health, London 2000.

32

Medicines management

Kym Lowder

Case study and questions

Day 1 Mrs KW was visited in her own home by a Primary Care Visitor (PCV). A PCV is a qualified Health Care Assistant (HCA) who has been given additional training in how to assess clients at risk of falling, how to check need for social benefits, and how to carry out a general basic medical assessment. Basic training around commonly prescribed medicines and their problems, compliance issues, and key points to be aware of is provided to all PCVs by a Primary Care Trust (PCT) prescribing adviser. All visits are subject to the same format. The service is targeted at the over-75 population, who live alone and are not in regular contact with any medical or social care agencies.

The resulting medication report (see table on following page) and general health report (see below) was sent to the PCT prescribing adviser for comment.

- Date of birth: 4.12.27
- Resting BP 176/92 mm Hg
- Standing BP 180/92 mm Hg
- Lying BP 175/90 mm Hg

- Urine: nothing abnormal detected
- Falls in past 12 months: one
- Dizziness: occasional

Q1 Is Mrs KW's blood pressure a cause for concern?
Q2 Comment on the dose of aspirin.
Q3 Which medicines could be contributing to her dizziness?
Q4 Comment on the possible problems associated with purchasing ibuprofen over-the-counter.
Q5 What could explain the varying quantities of Mrs KW's medication?
Q6 What additional information might be provided through a pharmacist domiciliary visit?

Week 2 Based on the information received the prescribing adviser had decided that a domiciliary visit was indicated. Further details of Mrs KW's

Medication	Dose	Quantity in home
Glyceryl trinitrate (GTN) sublingual tablets	as required	2 × 50 plus 20
Aspirin dispersible	75 mg twice daily	30
Isosorbide mononitrate	20 mg twice daily	84 (takes a.m. and 6 p.m.)
Atenolol	100 mg daily	112
Fluoxetine	20 mg daily	65 (takes at night)
Co-codamol 30/500	two tablets four times daily as required	160
Lactulose	10 mL as required twice daily	400 mL
Senna tablets	two at night when required	98
Ferrous sulphate tablets	200 mg daily	30
Nitrazepam tablets	5 mg at night	44
Oxybutynin tablets	2.5 mg twice daily	140

PLUS: purchased ibuprofen tablets taken as required.

medical condition had been obtained from her medical notes at the surgery. They showed Mrs KW's main medical problems were stable angina and osteoarthritis of the hip (awaiting replacement). She was also being treated for moderate depression and nocturnal urinary frequency.

Q7 Outline the key elements of a pharmaceutical care plan for Mrs KW.
Q8 How would you recommend her medication regimen be rationalised?
Q9 Outline how you could change or withdraw Mrs KW's nitrazepam.
Q10 What additional drug therapy may be indicated for Mrs KW?

Over a cup of tea, during the pharmacist's visit, Mrs KW began to talk more openly about the way she managed her medication. She lived alone with occasional visits from her son who was particularly vocal about how she should take her pills. It became apparent that she was quite confused over why she was on *so* many tablets as they did not make her feel better; in fact, often worse. In a low voice she confessed that constipation particularly bothered her. She felt particularly sluggish and drowsy in the mornings, which in turn meant that she was often late taking her tablets, if she managed to remember at all. She was only taking her fluoxetine sporadically as she thought they were for when she was a little 'down in the dumps' and they didn't help her sleep anyway! However, her angina appeared to be well controlled as she rarely had to take the little white tablets that 'you have to put under your tongue'. The bottle of GTN looked somewhat aged and had no date of opening visible.

The pharmacist used the opportunity to explain the reasons for taking the medication she had been prescribed, and to discuss the possible significant side-effects. She suggested that Mrs KW take her fluoxetine in the morning, as it was then less likely to disturb her sleep. The need to take it regularly for it to work properly was emphasised. The pharmacist suggested that if she still felt 'down' after three to four weeks then she should see her GP again.

Q11 Why do you think Mrs KW is not taking her medication as directed?

Q12 What are the medicines management options to help Mrs KW remain independent and in her own home?

Q13 Which option would you recommend for Mrs KW?

Week 3   After discussions between the prescribing adviser and GP, Mrs KW's regular repeat medicines were amended in line with the advice from the prescribing adviser.

To give Mrs KW a fresh start with her medication all old medicines were removed from the house and a fresh prescription written so that all the medicines would finish at the same time, thus allowing rational ordering. The surgery would then also notice any subsequent abnormal ordering patterns. Although this might appear an expensive option in the form of wasted medication, the benefits in terms of keeping Mrs KW safely in her own home significantly outweigh this cost. Items that were no longer taken by Mrs KW were removed from the repeat slip to ensure that she could not order them in error.

The prescribing adviser visited the community pharmacist and discussed Mrs KW's problems and her identified pharmaceutical needs.

Q14 What role can the community pharmacist play in caring for patients like Mrs KW?

The prescribing adviser arranged a follow-up visit to Mrs KW to explain the changes to her therapy and answer any questions that had subsequently occurred to her.

Week 6   A follow-up appointment for Mrs KW showed that her blood pressure was well controlled at 148/85 mmHg. The results of her serum lipid test showed that a statin was indicated (greater than 30% risk over 10 years), but Mrs KW declined the therapy and 'informed dissent' was marked in her notes. Her osteoarthritis still troubled her at times, but she felt more in control of her pain and was much happier as she no longer relied on laxatives. She was still considering what to do about her nitrazepam as she had been on it for 15 years since her husband died. The ferrous sulphate therapy was discontinued as her haemoglobin level was 11.8 g/dL.

Her final list of medication was as follows:

- GTN spray sublingually when required for chest pain
- Aspirin 75 mg orally each morning after breakfast
- Monomax XL 60 mg orally each morning
- Atenolol 100 mg orally each morning
- Fluoxetine 20 mg orally each morning
- Paracetamol 1 g orally four times daily when required for pain
- Codeine phosphate 30 mg one orally when required for severe pain, up to four times daily
- Senna two orally at night when required for constipation
- Nitrazepam 5 mg orally at night when required to aid sleep
- Oxybutynin SR 5 mg orally each morning

Is Mrs KW's blood pressure a cause for concern?

A1 **Yes. Her blood pressure should be controlled to National Service Framework (NSF) standards for coronary heart disease (CHD).**

Mrs KW's blood pressure was taken whilst she was sitting, standing and lying. This was to exclude the possibility of postural hypotension, which can be a cause of dizziness in some patients.

Both her diastolic and systolic blood pressure is considerably higher than the British Hypertension Society and NSF guidelines. However, abnormal blood pressure readings should be repeated two or three times over a period of a few days to rule out the possibility of anxiety-induced raised pressure brought on by the PCV equivalent of 'white coat' syndrome. The target blood pressure for Mrs KW, who is not diabetic, but who suffers from ischaemic heart disease (IHD), should be 140–150/80–85 mmHg.

High systolic blood pressure is an independent risk factor for stroke, and hypertension in general is a major risk factor for worsening CHD and myocardial infarction. Mrs KW is already on a beta-blocker for her angina, so suitable choices for additional therapy would be a dihydro-pyridine calcium-channel blocker (CCB) or a thiazide diuretic. Angiotensin-converting enzyme inhibitors (ACEIs) are thought not to add significantly to the hypotensive effects of beta-blockers, and also are less effective in the older person due to less sensitive renin–angiotensin systems, so should not be considered as a first-line addition for Mrs KW. CCBs are well known for their adverse side-effect profile (e.g. headache and angioedema), which can lead to a 20% drop-out rate, so a trial of 2.5 mg bendroflumethiazide would probably be the best initial option. However, if Mrs KW's angina had been poorly controlled a CCB may have been a good option.

Comment on the dose of aspirin.

A2 **The dose of aspirin is higher than routinely recommended for CHD prophylaxis.**

Aspirin is one of the mainstays of cardiovascular event prophylaxis in patients with IHD. However, it comes with a risk of gastrointestinal side-effects that can be minor, in the form of dyspepsia, or fatal, in the form of a major gastrointestinal bleed, in susceptible individuals. The risk in the older person is significantly higher and IHD is also an independent risk factor for increased risk of bleeding. Aspirin-induced gastrointestinal bleeds are known to be dose-related and reducing Mrs KW's dose of aspirin to 75 mg will reduce her risk of bleeding by 40%. Various doses have been studied to try to establish the optimum level required to protect from a cardiovascular event. A meta-analysis of these studies has shown that 75 mg is an effective dose and therefore considering the risks involved it would be prudent to reduce her dose to 75 mg. The aspirin should be taken once daily, in water and after breakfast, to minimize gastrointestinal irritation and dyspepsia. The use of buffered or enteric-coated formulations has not been shown to be of any clinical benefit in reducing gastrointestinal adverse events.

Which medicines could be contributing to her dizziness?

A3   **Co-codamol 30/500, nitrazepam and oxybutynin.**

Dizziness can be caused by a variety of reasons, both physiological and pharmacological. As older people are already at increased risk of falling, due to muscle weakness and poor balance, it would be logical to ensure that all avoidable risks are either eliminated or minimised. Postural hypotension can be a problem but is not so in this case, according to the PCV's report. The cumulative effects of the following three drugs could, however, be contributing to Mrs KW's problems.

(a)   Co-codamol 30/500. The high dose of codeine prescribed that will accumulate in the older person's body due to failing liver function can cause significant daytime drowsiness, poor coordination and lethargy.

(b)   Nitrazepam. The role of long-acting benzodiazepines in causing falls and accidents is well documented. This effect is particularly pro-nounced in the older person due to an extended half-life and poor elimination. An alternative option would be to try to withdraw Mrs KW's hypnotic gradually or substitute a shorter-acting drug, like oxazepam, that may not cause the same 'hangover' effects.

(c)   Oxybutynin. This drug is known to cause cognitive impairment. There are several alternatives to oxybutynin and trospium is known not to cross the blood–brain barrier. However, switching would not generally be considered as a first-line option in Mrs KW's case, unless a direct link had been made between her fall and the initiation of therapy.

Comment on the possible problems associated with purchasing ibuprofen over-the-counter.

A4 **Self-medication is of concern in patients with other medical problems, especially when there may be no clinical input if purchasing occurs in outlets like supermarkets and garages.**

Medicines bought by patients over-the-counter will not generally appear on their medication records at the surgery or pharmacy unless it has been previously prescribed by the GP. This can lead to problems of over-medication, interactions, and side-effects that are not attributed to the over-the-counter product. Ibuprofen, although the non-steroidal anti-inflammatory drug (NSAID) with the lowest risk of causing gastrointestinal bleeds, could cause a fatal bleed in a susceptible patient particularly if taken regularly at high doses. In Mrs KW's case the prescribed aspirin and fluoxetine will also increase her risk of a gastrointestinal bleed. If Mrs KW's pain cannot be controlled with simple analgesia then NSAIDs may be the answer, but they should be prescribed under the supervision of her GP. A proton pump inhibitor would be required for gastric cover, or the prescription of a cyclooxygenase-2 selective inhibitor could be considered.

What could explain the varying quantities of Mrs KW's medication?

A5 **Erratic ordering, unmatched quantities and non-compliance.**

One common explanation is that Mrs KW is ordering unmatched quantities via her repeat prescription slip. Ticking all drugs for reorder, whether or not they are required, is a common occurrence. Patients will often have one, two or three months therapy as a standard ordering quantity on their repeat prescribing list. An immense amount of work is going on in many surgeries to rationalize repeat prescribing through improved processes and patient education. In some cases patients are asked to bring in all the medication they are currently taking and all tablets are counted. The repeat clerk will then get a repeat prescription issued for individual quantities to align all the medication, so that future ordering is rational. Compliance can also be monitored by the surgery repeat clerks. Repeat medication that has not been ordered for more than nine months is generally deleted from the repeat screen. Clinical issues are raised with the GP where appropriate.

Alternatively Mrs KW may be non-compliant, erratic or plain forgetful about her therapy.

What additional information might be provided through a pharmacist domiciliary visit?

A6   Insight into the patient's attitudes to medication, evidence of hoarding and social issues.

A domiciliary visit has the immediate advantage of assessing the patient in surroundings in which they should feel more comfortable and at ease. Time is not as limited as in the clinical setting and patients are generally more open about how they feel and cope with their medication. It is also an opportunity to ask to see where medicines are kept to check storage conditions and to review the quantities being held. Previously unmentioned over-the-counter medicines and herbal/vitamin supplements that may be of clinical significance can also come to light. Social problems may become apparent which can then be passed on to the appropriate agencies for further action.

Outline the key elements of a pharmaceutical care plan for Mrs KW.

A7   The pharmaceutical care plan should address each of Mrs KW's problems to ensure that positive, patient-centred outcomes are obtained for all of her medical conditions. Key issues include:

(a)   Optimise her medication regimen with respect to frequency of dosing, timing of dosing and continued therapeutic need for each medication.

(b)   Ensure that Mrs KW is fully informed about her medication, its basic mode of action, and the reason for its prescription.

(c)   Review medication that may be causing Mrs KW's problems due to side-effects.

(d)   Try to ascertain the cause of her fall and dizziness.

(e)   Ensure that medication, where applicable, is producing the desired effect, e.g. pain relief.

(f)   Monitor her therapy appropriately.

(g)   Question Mrs KW as to her own personal feelings and beliefs about her therapy and counsel accordingly, in order to help ensure she will be concordant with her therapy.

(h)   Identify ways in which she can be supported around her medication-taking so that she can remain independent.

How would you recommend her medication regimen be rationalised?

A8 **The aim will be to simplify the drug regimen to one that is best suited to Mrs KW.**

Clinically unnecessary medication should be stopped and dose frequencies that Mrs KW has trouble with remembering should be reviewed.

(a)   GTN tablets. This could be changed to a GTN spray. This will ensure that Mrs KW does not get muddled with more tablets. She will also always have an effective rescue therapy, which is not out of date, in the event of breakthrough chest pain.

(b)   Aspirin 75 mg. Reduce dose to 75 mg daily as discussed in Answer 2.

(c)   Isosorbide mononitrate 20 mg. An extended-release formulation of once-daily isosorbide mononitrate 60 mg may suit Mrs KW better and ensure that she has a nitrate-free period to avoid nitrate tolerance. Branded prescribing is now recommended in many Primary Care Organisations for sustained-release products and will ensure that Mrs KW will receive consistent therapy each month from the community pharmacy at an economic cost.

(d)   Atenolol 100 mg. This dose is correct for the treatment of angina.

(e)   Fluoxetine. This and other selective serotonin reuptake inhibitors (SSRIs) are known to cause sleep disturbance and therefore should not be taken at night. Mrs KW should be advised to take her medication regularly and in the morning.

(f)   Co-codamol 30/500. Paracetamol is the recommended treatment for pain relief due to osteoarthritis, so regular four times daily dosing is the best option. It is generally accepted that multiple dosing for pain relief is not a problem in the majority of patients as it enables them to manage their pain relief on an individual basis. Removal of regular, and high-dose, codeine from the regimen will significantly help Mrs KW's constipation and would also improve Mrs KW's daytime alertness and wellbeing. (See also Answer 3.)

(g)   Lactulose and senna. Lactulose is not a first-line treatment for constipation unless the condition is chronic. Adequate fluids, exercise and dietary fibre are the first approach to treating and preventing constipation, with senna used when required for acute episodes.

(h)   Ferrous sulphate. Iron salts are also known to cause constipation and at the dose prescribed is unlikely to be of therapeutic value. Withdrawal could be discussed with the GP.

(i)   Nitrazepam. The use of nitrazepam for Mrs KW's 'insomnia' is of particular concern. Its implication in falls has already been mentioned (see Answer 3). It also appears that Mrs KW is getting up in the night for the toilet, so the risk of falling is increased significantly.

(j)   Oxybutynin. The twice-daily dose could be changed to the once-daily sustained-release formulation.

Outline how you could switch or withdraw Mrs KW's nitrazepam.

A9   **Switching or withdrawal of hypnotics can be successfully achieved, but only with the close collaboration and commitment of the patient.**

Patient education is vital when trying to reduce benzodiazepine use. Mrs KW should be made aware of all the problems associated with benzodiazepine therapy and the benefits of therapy withdrawal. Benefits have been shown to include improved memory (which may improve compliance), better coping skills and increased dexterity. Mrs KW can be reassured that there is no evidence to show a relationship between decreased hypnotic usage and worsened sleep. Education regarding good sleep hygiene, which involves the use of relaxation strategies, hot baths, milky drinks, etc., can be provided.

There are two main options: either withdrawal of the nitrazepam in a managed way or by switching to a shorter-acting drug like oxazepam (equivalent doses are found in the BNF) and then withdrawal. As nitrazepam has such a long half-life, a managed gradual reduction in dose over a period of several weeks may be the most suitable option. Mrs KW would need to be fully committed to the reduction plan and regular support from a health care professional will be required. This service can be offered by GPs, nurses or community pharmacists and should, if possible, be backed up by counselling services.

What additional drug therapy may be indicated?

A10   **A cholesterol-lowering agent and the ACEI ramipril.**

Mrs KW's medical records should be checked for results of recent serum lipid tests. Current guidelines promote the use of lipid-lowering agents (generally statins) for secondary prevention in IHD if the total cholesterol is higher than 5 mmol/L. This option should be discussed with Mrs KW. Although Mrs KW is 75 years old, which was generally considered the cut-off age for statin prescribing, due to the evidence base, ageism is no longer acceptable in medicine. The decision to prescribe should be made based on a combination of the evidence base, patient wishes and the likely benefit the patient is likely to gain from the therapy (including biological age).

Ramipril, as a result of the HOPE trial, is licensed for the prevention of coronary events in patients over the age of 55 post-myocardial infarction or with IHD and one other risk factor (e.g. smoking, hypertension, diabetes). Again, Mrs KW should be fully informed as to the therapeutic options open to her.

If Mrs KW's blood pressure remained high over several readings then an additional antihypertensive, as previously discussed, would also be indicated.

Why do you think Mrs KW is not taking her medication as directed?

A11   **The reasons are probably multifactorial.**

Mrs KW appears to show key signs of lack of concordance/non-adherence. She would not be unusual in this as it is estimated that at least 50% of patients do not take their medication as the prescriber intended.

Lack of concordance is now regarded as a more accurate reflection of why patients do not take medication as the health care professional intends them to. Concordance demands that there is a negotiation between both the practitioner and the patient to achieve agreement about how their condition should be managed.

The following factors can affect concordance:

(a)   Satisfaction with the consultation.
(b)   Personality and credibility of the practitioner.
(c)   Severity of condition (perceived and actual).
(d)   Complexity of regimen.
(e)   Effectiveness.
(f)   Patients' expectations.
(g)   External influences (people).
(h)   'Who cares anyway?'

The first two points reflect the relationship the patient has with the practitioner, in this case her GP, and her previous experiences within the health service. A series of rushed and impersonal appointments at the surgery will not give the patient any confidence that she has been treated as an individual, or that her personal needs have been listened to and understood. These factors will undermine the importance Mrs KW places on her treatment and therefore the likelihood of her adhering to pre-scribed medication. The beliefs of the practitioner are equally important in that a GP who does not appear to believe in the course of action being prescribed will not engender any confidence in the patient that they are doing the right thing.

'Silent' illnesses like hypertension and hypercholesterolaemia gen-erally lead to lower levels of compliance because the treatments do not result in day-to-day observable benefit, whereas the pain brought on by the angina and osteoarthritis are regular reminders to patients like Mrs KW of the consequences of not taking their medication. In such cases a clear explanation to the patient about the nature of the problem and its possible long and short-term consequences is extremely important, as is quantifying any risks in terms that the patient can relate to real life. In addition, the effectiveness of the therapy should be regularly demon-strated to the patient through the sharing of results of tests and other clinical markers, so that the patient can 'see' progress being made. Results that are not as expected could indicate poor compliance; or ensure that therapy is regularly reviewed and adjusted by the doctor.

The patient should have realistic expectations about what their therapy is likely to achieve for them. In some cases this will be a total cure, in others a control of symptoms, and in some conditions the patient will not physically feel any different at all. A patient's personal health beliefs and previous successes or failures will also play a role in whether therapy will be adhered to or even accepted.

Influences from external sources, which can include friends, family, the media and the internet, should never be underestimated. Negative comments are much more likely to jeopardize the way a patient feels about their condition or therapy, than several positive or corroborative ones.

The patient's self-esteem and the place they hold in society will also affect concordance. A patient who feels that they are not valued, are a burden or nuisance will have no interest in ensuring their therapy is effective.

It has never been established that levels of compliance can be related to race, gender, intelligence, occupation, income, or cultural backgrounds. The relationship between age and compliance is also com-plex and, contrary to popular belief, some studies have shown that younger people are less compliant than their older counterparts.

The PCV's 'chat' with Mrs KW suggested that there had been little communication with her about her condition and treatment options, or if there had been, it had been forgotten or not understood.

What are the medicines management options to help Mrs KW remain independent and in her own home?

A12 Possible options include a domiciliary carer, help from neighbours/relatives, compliance aids and medication review.

Using her domiciliary situation to aid her memory should not be underestimated. Tick box charts on the fridge, tablets next to the kettle or by the toothbrush are all useful methods of aiding memory and therefore compliance. Help from other people such as neighbours or relatives, or someone supplied by a care agency or social services can support Mrs KW and also give her confidence to maintain her independence. Compliance aids (e.g. Nomad, Medidose) of various types and quality are available. Supplies of tablets or capsules are dispensed into cells for each specific dose period, or blister-packed into individual dose units. However, it should be remembered that some older people find these foil and blister packs very difficult to manage due to their reduced manual dexterity and finger strength. All of these systems can help those who get easily muddled with several different types of tablets but they will not solve problems due to failing memory, also known as poor (mental) capacity.

The value of medication review has already been discussed.

Which option would you recommend for Mrs KW?

A13 An easy 'domestic' memory aide that was individually suited to Mrs KW.

Following a discussion of the various options with Mrs KW, she considered that a tick box chart system on her fridge door would help her to remember her medication, plus, it would also ensure that she did not double-dose. Her son would check, weekly, that the system was working.

The idea of using a monitored-dose system (MDS) was ultimately rejected as Mrs KW, once her medication had been rationalised, felt that her own personal systems were less confusing and easy to use.

What role can the community pharmacist play in caring for patients like Mrs KW?

A14 The community pharmacist is ideally placed to advise and monitor Mrs KW about her prescribed medication and items she may wish to purchase over-the-counter.

As a result of the above initiatives Mrs KW had felt a lot more confident about managing her medication and said that, in future, she would not hesitate to ask her local pharmacist if she had any queries.

All of the information gained and the interventions carried out, require the intervening pharmacist, whether from primary or secondary care, to share the relevant information with Mrs KW's usual community pharmacist. Otherwise, there is a significant risk that the new care plans will not be continued as intended.

When the prescribing adviser talked to Mrs KW's local pharmacist she asked if it was possible for Mrs KW's medication to be dispensed into readily distinguishable packaging. For example, a mixture of large and small bottles, cartons, and bold writing for analgesics.

Other patients will of course require different solutions to their problems and the community pharmacist is ideally placed to make significant contributions. There are a number of local schemes already running that have been immensely successful in keeping older people in their own homes and out of costly Care Homes. One such scheme is the provision of MDSs to suitable clients paid for by the PCT. Access to this service is through referral from a variety of sources: secondary care, primary care, social services, and community pharmacists. The client is visited in their own home by a member of the PCT pharmacy team who assesses their pharmaceutical needs according to a standard form. Where appropriate, arrangements are made for an MDS to be supplied by the client's local pharmacy, which is then paid a fee for providing the service. In over 50% of cases referred it has been found that an MDS is either not necessary or unsuitable. Other problems that arise from this visit are dealt with by direct liaison with the GP or community pharmacist. It has been found that direct contact with the prescriber is essential to ensure appropriate action is taken.

PCTs are also using community pharmacists to refer medication issues back to surgeries in a variety of schemes that include: recommending aspirin for cardiovascular patients, reporting regimen problems, following-up patients on antidepressants by telephone and managing hypnotic withdrawal.

Further reading

Anon. Medicines management services – why are they so important? *MeReC Bull* 2002; **12**(6).

Department of Health. *National Service Framework for Coronary Heart Disease*. Department of Health, London, 2000.

Department of Health. *National Service Framework for Older People*. Department of Health, London, 2001.

Goldstein R, Rivers P, Close P. Assisting elderly people with medication – the role of home carers. *Health Trends* 1993; **25**: 135–139.

Lord SR, Anstey KJ, Williams P *et al*. Psychoactive medication use, sensori-motor function and falls in older women. *Br J Clin Pharmacol* 1995; **39**: 227–234.

Ogden J. *Health Psychology: A Textbook*. Open University Press, Buckingham, 1996.

National Pharmaceutical Association. *Medicines Management: Everybody's Problem*. NPA, St Albans, 1998.

National Pharmaceutical Association. *NSF for Older People: A Guide for Community Pharmacists*. NPA, St Albans, 2002.

Royal Pharmaceutical Society of Great Britain and Merck Sharp Dohme. *From Compliance to Concordance: Achieving Goals in Medicine Taking*. Royal Pharmaceutical Society of Great Britain, London, 1997.

Royal Pharmaceutical Society of Great Britain. *RPS ePIC References. Brown Bag and Medication Reviews*. Royal Pharmaceutical Society of Great Britain, London, 2002. Available at: http://www.rpsgb.org.uk.pdfs/brownbag medrev.pdf

Taylor K, Harding G. *Pharmacy Practice*. Taylor & Francis, London, 2001.

Index